HEALTH ECONOMICS

FUNDAMENTALS AND FLOW OF FUNDS

HEALTH ECONOMICS

FUNDAMENTALS AND FLOW OF FUNDS

Thomas E. Getzen

Temple University

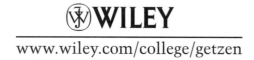

www.wiley.com/college/getzen

Acquisitions Editor   *Leslie Kraham*
Project Editor   *Cindy Rhoads*
Editorial Assistant   *Jessica Bartelt*
Marketing Manager   *Charity Robey*
Managing Editor   *Kevin Dodds*
Associate Production Manager   *Kelly Tavares*
Production Editor   *Sarah Wolfman-Robichaud*
Illustration Editor   *Benjamin Reece*
Cover Design   *Kris Pauls*
Cover Images   *© PhotoDisc, Inc/Getty Images; © Corbis*

This book was set in Minion by Leyh Publishing LLC and printed and bound by Hamilton Printing. The cover was printed by Lehigh Press.

This book is printed on acid-free paper. ∞

USA ISBN: 0-471-43203-2
WIE ISBN: 0-471-45176-2

Printed in the United States

10   9   8   7   6   5   4   3   2   1

To Bea, Bob, Karen, Matt, and Zoa.

CONTENTS

4 Insurance 67

7 **Medical Education, Organization, and Business Practices** 127

PREFACE

Health Economics: Fundamentals and Flow of Funds is a primer for the economic analysis of medical markets and the production of health. Its intended audiences are students of medicine, public health, and administration who wish to engage the central economic issues of their field without prolonged preparatory work; beginning students in economics who wish to study an applied area in detail without recourse to extensive mathematical manipulation; and more advanced students in economics who may be familiar with analytical techniques, but lack knowledge of the many institutional features which make the study of health and health care so unique and rewarding.* This book draws upon the work of many scholars, but in keeping with its design as a primer for introducing students to the principles and concepts of health economics rather than its literature and research methods, the use of attribution, footnotes and references is purposely limited. Suggestions for additional reading and more advanced source materials and databases are listed at the end of each chapter, and on the web site www.wiley.com/college/getzen.

The first twelve chapters use a "flow of funds" approach to describe the incentives and organizational structure of the health care system. Transactions between patients and physicians (and others) are examined to see how profits are made, costs covered, contracts written (or implied) and regulations formed. The long-term consequences of exchanging services for money in a particular way are revealed by exploring the historical development of those distinctive features which characterize the industrial organization of health care: licensure, third-party insurance, non-profit hospitals, and government regulation. The last seven chapters take a wider macroeconomic perspective in order to explore the dynamics of change within the health care system, and to explicitly consider determinants of national health spending and the role of governments in public and private health.

The introductory chapter lays out the overall flow of funds, schematically presents the complexity of medical care transactions, and introduces the basic principles that form the toolkit for economic analysis. Chapter 2 examines the economic concept of demand and compares it to the medical concept of need. Chapter 3 applies the basic principles of supply and demand, marginalism and equilibrium, using a cost-benefit approach in a clinical context. The more detailed investigation of medical care organization begins in Chapters 4 and 5 on insurance and third party reimbursement, which has become the dominant source of funds in medical care. Physicians, the patient's agent and a central player in all medical care transactions, are the subject of the next two chapters. Chapters 8 and 9 cover the reimbursement, regulation and cost structure of hospitals. HMOs and the other contractual networks used to manage care are discussed in Chapter 10, with particular attention to payment mechanisms and access to capital. The survey of providers is rounded out with

---

*The special features, which make medical care so interesting as a subject for economic analysis, also tend to make the application of simple models difficult or implausible. Those students who have the desire and opportunity to do so are well advised to get a firm grasp of basic principles using a text such as Heyne's *The Economic Way of Thinking* or Samuelson's *Economics* before attempting to grapple with the complexities and ambiguities of medical care.

chapters on long-term care and pharmaceuticals. Pharmaceuticals provide an exemplar of the modern "information economy" where the fixed costs of research and marketing outweigh the cost of production, and where competition relies on continuous innovation.

In order to understand the interactions between the parts, it is necessary to place health care in a macroeconomic context that includes redistribution, taxation, inflation, and growth. Chapter 14 explores the role of government, and Chapter 15 examines public goods as particular forms of market failure that requires intervention. The economic history of health is traced in Chapter 16, drawing on the contributions of demography and the cliometric work of Fogel and North. Chapter 17 provides international comparisons of health and medical care expenditures, using Kenya, Sudan, Mexico, Poland, Germany and Japan as illustrative examples. The dynamics of national health expenditure are presented in Chapter 18 as an application of the permanent income hypothesis. This model is then used to empirically assess the effectiveness of several attempts to control health care costs. A final chapter addresses the probable trends in health care spending, suggesting that the primary barrier to increased effectiveness and efficiency is poor allocation.

Health economics is fascinating to study, but is not easily summarized or readily captured in neat equations. In part, that is because the study of health economics is relatively new and still in the process of refinement, but primarily it is because the trades organized by doctors and hospitals are not simple, and cut to the heart of what it means to be human. What is the value of life? Who pays the price of pain, and what does it mean to trust a surgeon who profits because of a crisis? Since most medical care is funded through taxes and insurance, there is no direct linkage between the amount paid and the resources used in treatment. As a consequence, "prices" become more ambiguous and are often of less immediate relevance to the transaction than ongoing relationships of trust and professional behavior. It is important to understand how economic forces continue to operate when markets are indirect and inefficient, and how other organizing principles (professionalism, licensure, agency, regulation) act as substitutes for prices. While most of the special features of medical markets are there to make people better off, they have also been shaped by those groups who had the power to modify the rules in their own interest, subject to the controls of economic and political competition. Tracing the economic rationale and development of medical care organization, and making those forces more clearly visible and amenable to analysis, is the purpose of this book.

CHANGES FOR THE SECOND EDITION

The "flow of funds" approach that proved so successful in the first edition is still in use here. "Money" represents a point of structure on which all parties are forced to agree, and creates the budget constraint that determines hospital costs, physician incomes, pharmaceutical profits and insurance premiums. International examples have been expanded, with most now authored by experts discussing their own country, thus allowing for greater accuracy and authenticity. A number of illustrative "box" examples illustrating economic principles have been added (Substitutes: Another Diamonds-Water Paradox, RBRVS fee schedules, Physician Assistants and Comparative Advantage, Bankruptcy at Allegheny Health System, Claritin and DTC Advertising, Triple-tier Pharmacy Benefits). Most students need to obtain a set of skills, an economic toolkit, in order to work. This second edition includes more basic economic "principles" material (opportunity cost, scarcity, demand, marginal revenue, value, fundamental theory of exchange) in Chapters 1 and 2.

Additional materials on demand and supply curves, cost and production functions, market transactions and measurement of elasticity are downloadable from the Web site http://www.wiley.com/college/getzen/ as Appendices 1 and 2. For classes emphasizing economic evaluation, this more detailed quantitative and diagrammatic presentation can be quite useful. For general classes directed toward clinicians, administrators or policy makers, it can be a bit too long and dry, severely taxing their enthusiasm for health economics before they have fully worked through the mechanics of determining the marginal rate of technical substitution. I usually find time to review this material in most classes by adjusting the length of the presentation and the number of illustrative examples to the extent of familiarity within that particular class setting. Teaching notes and problem sets for these appendices, and for all other chapters, are found online.

WWW references are used throughout the text to provide access to constantly updated material. There are links to a variety of major sources of health economics data and commentary such as the WHO, OECD, CDC, CMS, GAO, and others. Some content created specifically to supplement the text has also been archived on the web. Additional problems, comments from students and professors, and breaking issues are linked to specific chapters and sections. Updates of critical legislation and statistics are also made available in this manner. Your comments and queries are welcome. For adopting professors, online help, answers to all problems, and chapter teaching guidelines are available through the text website, and also through email at getzen@temple.edu.

ACKNOWLEDGEMENTS

The writing of this book incurred intellectual and personal debts sufficient to preclude any complete listing of those who have contributed. My family and extended family (Rufus and Beverley Getzen, Sydney White, Bill W.) come first. My initial research on these topics began at the University of Washington, with the assistance of Yoram Barzel, Gardner Brown, Steve Shortell, Bill Richardson and Mike Morrisey, and while working under Gordon Bergey, who was an exemplar of the concerned physician and administrator. I am indebted to the efforts of Joe Newhouse, Mark Pauly, Tony Culyer, Morris Barer, Mike Drummond, Bill Swan and others who have done so much to build the field and create a rigorous body of literature in health economics, and thank them for their service to iHEA. Jeff Caswell at Ohio State created the instructor's manual. David Barton Smith, Patrick Bernet, Bill Aaronson, Chuck Hall, Jackie Zinn and other colleagues at Temple have shaped the health economics course as it was taught. Alan Maynard sheltered and inspired me during my sabbatical at York during which the first edition was begun, and Uwe Reinhardt keep me informed, amused and concerned at Princeton as the second edition was started. I also express my deep appreciation to the reviewers of the second edition who provided extensive comments that contributed to the quality of the book. The reviewers include Angela Dominelli, Albany College of Pharmacy; Howard Foreman, Yale University; Robert Rosenthal, Stonehill College; Antonio Trajillo, University of Central Florida; Joseph Lovett, University of California–San Bernadino; and John Goddeeris, Michigan State University. The usual and heartfelt disclaimer applies, all remaining errors are mine.

ABOUT THE AUTHOR

Thomas E. Getzen is Professor of Risk, Insurance and Health Management at Temple University and the founder and Executive Director of iHEA, the International Health Economics Association. After receiving an undergraduate degree from Yale University, he worked for the U.S.P.H.S. Centers for Disease Control Venereal Disease program in New York and Los Angeles, and then obtained an MHA degree in Medical Care Organization and Ph.D. in Economics from the University of Washington. Dr. Getzen's main research contributions have been in the areas of contracting, price indexes and forecasting of health care spending. His consulting work has included employee benefit negotiations, laboratory diagnostics, risk assessment, and capital financing for managed care. Dr. Getzen has been a visiting professor at the University of York (U.K.), the Wharton School of the University of Pennsylvania, and the Center for Health and Wellbeing of the Woodrow Wilson School at Princeton University. He has served on the boards of Covenant House, a local community health center in Northwest Philadelphia, MSI, a venture-capital financed managed behavioral health care corporation, CHE, a large provider system with over 60 hospitals and nursing homes. Dr. Getzen is a member of the editorial boards of *Health Economics* and the *Journal of Health Administration Education.*

FOREWORD

Public policy in almost any field depends on specific knowledge of the field, but it usually also depends (or should depend) on general principles of economics. For example, the building of a bridge requires knowledge of engineering, to know what is feasible; it requires knowledge of traffic patterns; and it requires knowledge of economic principles, to see if the traffic that will use the bridge and the value of the time saving to that traffic will justify the costs imposed by the engineering requirements. So, too, is there a need of economic analysis to help in the construction of a system of health care. First of all, indeed, we must know what medical care can do, and how much in the way of skilled professionals, other workers, machinery, and buildings it takes to achieve any given level of medical care. But second, we must analyze how the payment mechanisms to compensate for these supplies affect the delivery of medical care.

Medical care is indeed a more complex economic problem than bridge-building. Like some other professions but unlike many other goods and even services, it is difficult for the consumer (here the patient) to evaluate the quality of the services received. Much depends on the self-control and reliability of the individual practitioner, the supplying group, and the medical profession as a whole, in ways that the patient cannot readily check. Then, too, the service provided is needed only at unpredictable intervals, but it frequently is very important when it is needed. Further, the costs, a reflection of the resources used, are very uncertain and can be very high. All these reasons lead to the use of some form of insurance, a natural economic institution for improving everyone's welfare. But insurance reduces the incentive of an individual patient or physician to seek the most economical means of treatment. As a result, new institutions and regulations develop to overcome this "moral hazard," as it has been termed—institutions such as health maintenance organizations, managed care by insurance companies, and regulations such as those that govern Medicare expenditures. The standard paradigms of economics have been enriched to discuss problems such as this.

The difficulties of quality evaluation and moral hazard are special cases of a more general phenomenon, differences in information between the two sides of a transaction. These differences, though not confined to medical practice, are especially important there, and have further consequences beyond those already noted, as in the need for licensing physicians or the specially important role of nonprofit institutions.

The economic problems of allocating resources to medical care have long been a major part of government economic policy, more in other countries than in the United States. The steady rise in the expenditures on medical care, outstripping the rise in national income by a considerable margin, has brought these issues to the fore of public attention. Equally important has been the increase of explicit consideration of costs within the medical profession; the historically unwelcome trade-off between costs and treatment has come forcibly to the fore. The need for good education and good texts has become acute, and Professor Getzen's book is a welcome attempt to meet this strongly felt need.

Kenneth J. Arrow

CHAPTER 1

TERMS OF TRADE: THE FLOW OF FUNDS THROUGH THE HEALTH CARE SYSTEM

QUESTIONS

1. Who is made better off, the surgeon or the patient?
2. Who pays when you skip a workout to watch television?
3. Why does health care cost so much?
4. Is health scarce?
5. Who pays for it?
6. Does everyone get the same amount of care?
7. Is there trading in health futures?
8. Why is health care bought and sold differently from other goods and services?

Who gets a heart transplant? Why does surgery cost so much? Will insurance pay for AIDS treatment? How many children get immunized? Is Senator Smith's health plan worth voting for? These questions are dealt with every day in hospitals, in doctor's offices, and in people's homes. They are the subject of health economics, along with the more mundane decisions that cumulatively have an even greater impact on your personal health: how much exercise to get, the value of reducing cholesterol in your diet, whether to study until 3 a.m. or get a good night's sleep, and so on.

Conveying information and using it to make decisions is the stock in trade of both doctors and economists. By the end of this book, we will have discussed hospitals, nurses, ambulances, drugs, sex, extortion, kickbacks, government, family ties, love, international trade, sports injuries, and the next generation—the makings of several box office hits. The discussion will take the perspective of an economist, seeing things in terms of opportunity cost, budget constraints, monopoly, marginal productivity, and other analytical concepts. Some people claim that this takes all the fun out of drugs, sex, and business intrigue. Not so. Economic principles provide the motivations that shape this story, giving it character development and structure rather than just one scene after another as in some forgettable action movie. As a sophisticated student of human society, you seek full disclosure of the ambitions that lie behind the actions, the deviousness of self-interest cloaked in proclamations of public benefit, the pragmatism of those who use strategy and tactics to make the best of a bad situation, the tragedy of noble aspirations that fail because of human limits, the labyrinthine connections of one of the world's largest businesses, and the growing awareness that behind it all we will find money at the root of much that is evil, and even more that is good, in the search for health. This wealth of behind-the-scenes drama is what makes the economic perspective on health so compelling.

Looking carefully at how people make deals with physicians, with hospitals, and with each other to improve their health is the fundamental approach to health economics taken here. Simplified assumptions and abstractions are used to clarify the forces that lead to economic change. Tracing the flow of funds through the health care system will make it possible to apply the principles of price theory to situations involving life and death, non-profit organizations, professional licensure, addiction, and other issues. The powerful generalizations and concepts of microeconomics, macroeconomics, and industrial organization will allow us to see how medical transactions are like, and yet unlike, most of the rest of the economy. As a practical matter, it will be helpful if you already have a basic grasp of economics theory and applications. Reviewing a textbook, such as Paul Samuelson's *Economics*, Paul Heyne's *The Economic Way of Thinking*, or Campbell McConnell and Stanley Brue's *Microeconomics,* may prove useful. A student guide, instructor's manual, introduction to elasticity, cost and production functions, lecture slides, and current Internet resources are available at www.wiley.com/college/getzen, and you are urged to check out this site for current links, updates, and other material.

When someone says "economics" or "economic behavior," the sorts of things that probably come to mind—interest rates, unemployment, stock markets—seem far removed from the hospital emergency room. If I asked about your most recent contribution to the health sector of the economy, you might not even think of the little line on your paycheck stub labeled "HI" or "FICA:M" or "Medicare." Yes, that's 1.45 percent of your gross income that is taken out for Medicare, which you might not have realized you were paying. No, it's not your health insurance, because you don't become eligible for Medicare until you reach age 65 or become permanently disabled. Health care doesn't always conform well to the standard models economists use to analyze buying and selling wheat, or renting property, or the price of gold. However, money drives the health care system just as it does many other activities in a modern industrial society. Furthermore, economic development is by far the greatest cause of improvements in health, and the General Agreement on Tariffs and Trade has probably saved more lives than penicillin.

1.1 WHAT IS ECONOMICS?

The essence of economics is trade, or "making a buck." Its focal point is the market, the point where buyers and sellers exchange dollars for goods and services. Without buyers and sellers there would be no economy—no rich surgeons, no insurance companies, no hospital billing departments (or textbook royalties for health economists). To say that there would be no rich surgeons is not a statement of envy but one of fact. Without an advanced economy, a person could not spend 15 years studying and practicing eye surgery, and hence could not provide a highly specialized form of labor that is so valuable; therefore, patients could not reap the benefits of so much knowledge and training.

For a surgeon to be a seller, the patient must be a buyer. They both must agree on a price so that an exchange can occur. The surgeon would probably prefer that the price be higher and the patient would probably prefer that it be lower, but both must be satisfied in order for a trade to take place. As economists, we can observe that since a transaction took place, there must have been mutual agreement that made both the buyer and the seller better off. If the surgeon would rather have watched television than perform another operation, she would have turned down the case. If the patient would rather have saved the money, or gone to a different surgeon, he could have done so. The insight that both parties must be benefiting if they freely agreed to make a trade is central to an economic vision of the world, and is known as the Fundamental Theorem of Exchange.

Terms of Trade

The "terms of trade" specify what the buyer is to give to the seller, and what the seller is to give to the buyer in return. When you buy a common item in a store, such as aspirin, a simple price of $1.29 per bottle of 50 may tell you everything you need to know about the transaction. For services, and for medical care in particular, the transaction is apt to be much more complex. For example, consider the transaction for an operation to implant an artificial intra-ocular lens (IOL) in a patient's eye to replace the natural lens that has become clouded by cataracts. The patient is to pay a $200 deposit up front and $800 more within 30 days after the surgery is completed and all sutures are removed. Reduced to its most simple element, the terms of trade in this exchange can be expressed as a monetary price of $1,000 for the IOL implant. Yet much more than the $1,000 is being agreed to in this transaction. The physician agrees to provide not just any artificial lens, but to choose the correct one, continuously monitor the quality of the operation, and control adverse reactions to post-operative medications. The patient agrees to make payment in two parts, with a time limit, and may assume the operation will be redone without further charges if the first attempt is not satisfactory. Many of the agreed-upon conditions (that the physician is licensed, will use only qualified assistants, will not try to boost the bill needlessly to increase her fees, and will keep the patient informed of any possible adverse consequences, and that the patient will wear bandages as long as necessary and not go skydiving) will never be specified explicitly unless some disagreement and subsequent legal action force the doctor and patient into court.

In the simplified neoclassical model of perfectly competitive behavior with which most textbooks begin, price is the only term that matters in a transaction and both the buyer and seller are "price takers." That is, there are so many buyers that whether one person buys or not has little influence on the price in the market; therefore, buyers must "take" the price as given. Similarly, there are so many firms selling the same product that no single firm can affect prices; hence, all firms must take the price as given. This uncomplicated model of perfectly competitive behavior is not too distant from reality when you buy a

---

FUNDAMENTAL THEOREM OF EXCHANGE

The foundation of market economics is that trade makes both parties better off. People make a deal because they expect it will provide more satisfaction than not making the deal. The surgeon and the patient expect to gain from trade—the surgeon by receiving money and gratitude, and the patient by being healed. It may turn out that the patient dies, and the surgeon gets sued for malpractice, but both made the transaction with the expectation that they would become better off. Trade does not take advantage of people so that one party is made better off at the expense of the other (that is stealing). Trade takes advantage of differences in skills, endowments and tastes so that people can make exchanges that are mutually advantageous.

bottle of aspirin. The model works reasonably well for most of the purchases made by consumers, and thus can be used to frame the analysis of the economy as a whole. Yet buying a bottle of aspirin is not representative of most medical decisions, and an elementary model does not capture many of the essentials when life and death decisions are being made in the operating room. While the same principles used to analyze monetary prices can be applied to other stipulations in the terms of trade, a more detailed and explicit consideration of how transactions are made, and what is being exchanged and by whom and on whose behalf, is required. Although the analysis is made more difficult, it becomes more exciting. Economic organizations adapt creatively to the special demands of health care. Studying such adaptations reveals the potential of economics as a discipline in a way that the analysis of more standard markets cannot.

Value

Why does health care cost so much? Because health is so precious that its value exceeds that of the things we possess. What benefit do I get from spending my money on books or art or cars or clothes if I am dead? Sick and in pain, confronted with the possibility of death, people would be willing to spend almost any amount of money to get their health back. Health care costs so much because people are willing to pay so much for it. The many years a surgeon spends in training, the billions of dollars government spends on public health, and the comprehensive health insurance plans provided by employers are consequences of the value we as a society place on health care. They are effects, rather than causes. We are willing to spend so much on physician training, public health, and health insurance because what they produce is valuable to us. If we stopped caring about (or paying for) health, no new magnetic resonance imaging (MRI) scanners would be built, surgeons would stop spending years in training, and our taxes would go toward highways or national parks instead of AIDS and cancer research. Cows can get just as many diseases as humans do and we could put all those resources to work saving cows, but we don't. Cows, I am sure, would set priorities rather differently, but they are not paying the bills.

1.2   THE FLOW OF FUNDS

Goods and services are provided in a market economy only if the people who want them are willing to pay for them and if suppliers are willing to accept those payments in return. Exchange is based on voluntary agreement, so that trade between a buyer and seller occurs only when both parties believe that they will be made better off by trading (Fundamental Theorem of Exchange). In the simplest form of trade, consumers buy from businesses, exchanging money for goods and services in a two-party transaction.

Consumers make up the demand side of this simple service market, while firms make up the supply side. In legal terms, firms are contractual entities that can own, buy, and sell property and pay taxes just as real people do. To get the labor, land, and other inputs needed for production, the firm (the seller) in Figure 1.1 must also be a buyer, as shown in Figure 1.2. These secondary two-party transactions are characteristic of derived demand, purchases made as an intermediate step in production, rather than for final consumption. Firms are owned by individuals (or other firms) that provide the capital, labor, and organizational effort necessary to get them started and keep them running. Thus, every dollar that a consumer gives to a firm, whether used for wages, profits, or purchase of input from another firm, ultimately ends up in the hands of someone who wants to spend it. When workers or owners spend money, they become consumers, and therefore complete the circular flow of funds through the economy, as shown in Figure 1.3.

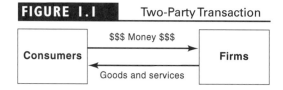

FIGURE 1.1   Two-Party Transaction

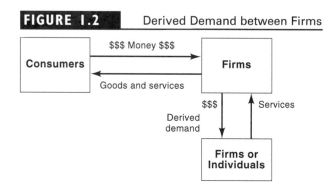

FIGURE 1.2   Derived Demand between Firms

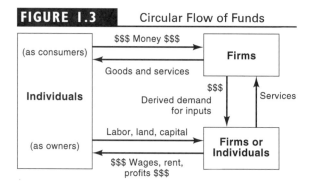

FIGURE 1.3   Circular Flow of Funds

Health Care Spending in the United States

Medical care in the United States is a trillion-dollar business, with an estimated average of $5,427 spent per person in 2002.[1] The 285 million citizens of the United States received services from more than 4,000 hospitals, 30,000 nursing homes, 750,000 physicians, 2.2 million registered nurses, and 8 million other health care workers. The major sources and uses of health care funding in 2002 are indicated in Table 1.1. Individuals paid $227 billion, or 15 percent of total funding; private (mostly employer-based) health insurance paid 35 percent; and government, the largest payer, paid 45 percent (17 percent Medicare, 16 percent Medicaid, 12 percent other government programs). The remaining 5 percent of total health care funding came from a variety of other private sources (philanthropy, industrial clinics, interest and rental income of providers). The largest use of funds was the $476 billion spent on hospital care, 31 percent of the total.

Figure 1.4 presents this information, highlighting a simple yet important fact: the "sources" and "uses" bars are of equal height because the total amount spent on health care must be identical to the total amount collected by providers. Every dollar spent by a patient, insurance company, or government is recorded as a cost, but is also recorded as income to a physician, hospital, agency, administrator, or other health employee. The flow

TABLE 1.1			U.S. Healthcare Spending, 2002		
Uses of Funds	**Percentage of Total**	**Amount Per Person***	**Sources of Funds**	**Percentage of Total**	**Amount Per Person***
Hospital	36%	$1,509	Medicare	19%	$ 813
Physician	20%	852	paycheck deductions		528
Dental	4%	175	Medicaid	14%	593
Drugs & supplies	8%	353	VA & DOD	3%	119
Nursing home	8%	340	Workers comp.	2%	93
Home health	3%	123	Other government	7%	297
Eye & equipment	1%	55	*Total government*	*45%*	*1,914*
Other	9%	375			
Admin. & ins.	5%	215			
Public health	3%	113	Employer ins.	34%	1,416
Research	2%	62	Self paid	17%	734
Construction	1%	54	Charity, etc.	4%	162

*Based on a projected U.S. population of 285 million.

Source: U.S. Office of the Actuary, National Health Projections, http://cms.gov/statistics/nhe/.

of money is circular. Money itself is only a way of keeping track of all the obligations within the economy. Every dollar spent by one person is, of necessity, a dollar of income for someone else. Tracing the flow of funds through this complex system provides some sense of the forces that shape the economy.

Sources of Funds

Health care spending has grown enormously. In 2002, it was 15 percent of the Gross Domestic Product (GDP) and accounted for 1 of every 12 employees in the labor force. That growth has been facilitated by the shift from individual payments to third-party financing. In 1929, 81 percent of medical expenditures came directly from individual "out-of-pocket" payments and only 19 percent from government and other third-party organizations (Table 1.2).

FIGURE 1.4	U.S. Sources and Uses of Health Care Funds, 2002

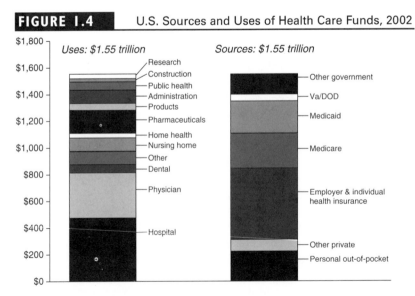

Source: Office of the Actuary, www.cms.gov.

TABLE 1.2	Sources of Payment, 1929, 1965, 2002		
	1929	**1965**	**2002**
Total health spending (millions)	$ 3,656	$ 41,012	$1,545,900
Adjusted for inflation (2002 $$)	32,400	192,300	1,545,900
Per capita (adjusted)	305	962	5,427
As a % of GDP	3.5%	5.7%	14.7%
% Paid by			
Self (out-of-pocket)	81%	44%	15%
Third parties	19%	56%	85%
Government	13%	25%	45%
Private insurance	< 1%	25%	35%
Philanthropy, other	6%	6%	5%

By 2002, this ratio had been reversed, with individuals paying only 15 percent directly and the remaining 85 percent of funds flowing through third-party transactions involving government, nonprofit organizations, and insurance.

All of the elements that characterized health care in 2002 were present in some form one hundred years ago, but their relative importance to the flow of funds has changed so much that the transactions look entirely different today.[2] Physicians, who in 1900 were tradespeople sometimes making do with partial payment in eggs or flour, have become highly paid and technologically sophisticated professionals who rarely talk to their patients about paying the bills. Hospitals, once minor supports for a few disabled and disadvantaged, are now technological palaces of intensive treatment and the largest users of U.S. health care funds. Whereas in 1900 hospitals were financed by a few donors and some patient fees, they are now financed almost entirely by third parties: either by government insurance such as Medicare and Medicaid or by private insurance provided through employment or purchased directly by consumers (Figures 1.5 and 1.6). For every $100 spent in the hospital, less than 2 percent comes from charitable donations. Even the 3 percent paid for by patients out-of-pocket does not really flow through a two-party transaction, because much of that 3 percent consists of co-payments, deductibles, and other fees related to third-party insurance payments.

There are many reasons health care spending has grown rapidly. An increasingly wealthy population is willing to spend more on all goods and services. Extra spending on health care has a greater appeal after basic necessities such as food and housing are taken care of. Technological advances make modern medicine more desirable. An aging population favors health care over other goods. Insurance now covers more of the cost. Shifting

FIGURE 1.5   Health Care Flow of Funds, circa 1900

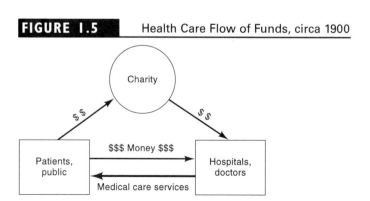

| **FIGURE 1.6** | Health Care Flow of Funds, circa 2002 |

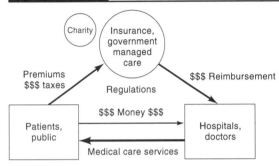

the financial burden from individuals to third parties through insurance not only changed the way funds flowed, but made more funds available, so that the health care system could grow rapidly and absorb an ever-larger share of total economic output.

Such "cost-shifting" has made the payment system complex and opaque—almost no one knows who is paying for what.[3] Billed charges bear little resemblance to what is paid, or what the provider receives, and provider revenues are usually identified not as "income," but as "reimbursement." Third-party payments are made with:

- Taxes paid to government agencies (Chapters 14 and 15)
- Employer and employee payments to commercial insurance companies (Chapters 4 and 5); for-profit and nonprofit managed care firms, including health maintenance organizations (HMOs), preferred provider organizations (PPOs), and other organizations (Chapter 10)
- Philanthropic contributions to charities (Chapters 4 and 14)

Each of these major categories of third-party payments exists in endless variations. The details differ widely, but from a flow-of-funds perspective, they all have a similar purpose: pooling funds from many people to pay the bills of the few patients who need care.

Who gets care and what kind of care are decisions made according to the rules of the group and the opinions of the professionals who run the health care system. In each case, indirect third-party payment weakens the monetary linkage between buyer and seller that characterizes the direct two-party transactions typical in most other sectors of the economy. For most medical transactions, there is no exchange of money between the recipient of services and the provider. The patients (or their families) pay insurance premiums and taxes, and the doctors and hospitals are paid by the government and insurance companies. In the absence of a direct link between the amount paid and the resources used in treatment, "prices" become more ambiguous and less important to the transaction than ongoing relationships of trust and professional behavior. One of the purposes of this textbook is to explain how economic forces continue to operate when prices do not function in a normal way and how other organizing principles (professionalism, licensure, regulation) serve as replacements.

Health Care Providers: The Uses of Funds

Payments by patients, government, and insurance companies have increased 200-fold over the past sixty years; thus, payments received by doctors, hospitals, and other care providers have increased by the same amount. In general, both the public, as users of the system, and providers, as suppliers of care, have been happy with this large increase in spending. The public has gotten a health care system that is technologically advanced and responsive to their needs. Providers have gained glory in the fight against disease and substantial gains in income, making them eager to continue the struggle.

Part of the increase in health care spending from almost $4 billion in 1929 to $1,546 billion in 2002 is just an accounting fiction due to inflation, because $1 in 1929 is roughly the same as $9 in 2002. Also, some of the increase reflects a rise in the number of people who must be cared for. Yet even after adjusting for changes in population and inflation, real per capita spending has increased more than ten-fold since 1929. Some of this real increase in spending is due to a real increase in wages. As per capita incomes rise, workers expect more real goods and services per hour of work. Therefore, expenditures on labor-intensive services tend to rise more rapidly than expenditures on goods and capital-intensive commodities. Furthermore, the wages of health care workers have risen more rapidly than for other types of labor.[4] This probably reflects both the increased education of health professionals today and the increased demand for their services. Increases in the quantity of services provided account for some of the growth in total expenditures, but the medical services most commonly counted, number of days spent in the hospital and number of visits to physicians, have actually declined since 1965 (see Table 1.3).[5] However, nursing home days and number of prescriptions per person have increased substantially.

After taking all these factors into account—inflation, higher health care wages, and use of services—there still has been a tremendous increase in expenditures over the last thirty years, more than 250 percent. How can spending increase so much more rapidly than the increase in the number of services, or in the wages of those who provide them? By increasing the **intensity and quality of services.** More tests are done for a patient in a modern intensive care unit during a single day than were done for a patient over the course of a month in his or her wooden bed in 1929. Many of those tests (MRIs, blood glucose, heart monitoring) were not available back then. The physician who drove to the patient's house and worked alone out of a black bag has been replaced by a team of therapists, technicians, and support staff assisting a group of physicians, many of whom are specialists

TABLE 1.3   Changes in the Use of Health Care

Funds over Seventy Years			
	1929	1965	2002
Spending per person (in 2002 dollars)	$305	$962	$5,427
Percentage			
Hospital	18%	34%	31%
Physician	36	21	22
Dental	12	7	4
Drugs	18	9	10
Other	1	6	6
Nursing home	na	4	7
Home health	na	na	3
Products	3	3	4
Admin. & insurance costs	3	5	7
Public health	3	2	4
Research	1	4	2
Construction	5	5	1
Total	100%	100%	100%
Hospital days (per 100 persons)	9.4	10.3	5.6
Hospital employees (per patient)	< 0.5	2.5	7.4
Physician visits (per person)	2.6	4.3	3.8

using an array of medical equipment. Another factor that explains some of the growth in spending is that, as some common, acute (short-term) diseases have become curable or preventable, medical care is increasingly applied in cases of chronic diseases that were once considered hopeless. The shift from simple caring to technologically sophisticated curing is reflected by shifts in the categories of expenditure; more is going to institutional care in hospitals and nursing homes, while the share devoted to personal services by doctors has declined. The fraction of the health care dollar spent for manufactured goods such as drugs has also fallen, while the cost of labor-intensive services has risen.

1.3   QUALITY

Medicine often involves life-and-death decisions. In these situations, quality is crucial and quantity is irrelevant. It doesn't help if a mediocre surgeon offers to give you a second operation at half price. A patient usually consumes one and only one "unit" of care—an operation in this case—for each illness. The only trade-off made is in the quality, not the quantity, of the procedure. Having budget decisions made over quality rather than quantity tends to complicate economic analysis. While it is reasonable to assume for most other goods that price per unit remains constant as the quantity increases or decreases, any change in quality must change the price. Quality cannot simply be added up or multiplied to arrive at a total spending limit the way quantity can.

The quality of medical care has increased over the last thirty years. But has it increased as much as, or more than, the cost? While measures such as the consumer price index (CPI) attempt to deal with these issues, there is no consensus on how accurate they are, or even on what these measures should be. Can quality be measured by number of lives saved, number of lives saved per dollar spent, number of tests or services provided, level of physician knowledge (should this count if the patient dies), or patient satisfaction? Historically, most emphasis on quality was at the level of the individual: a procedure, a patient, or a physician. Was the surgery done properly? Did the patient heal well and was he satisfied with the care he received? Was the doctor adequately trained for the procedure with a certified supporting staff? Recently, a more comprehensive statistical perspective has come to the fore. What percentage of patients suffer infections as a result of surgery? What percentage of patients requires a second operation? How do these rates compare with surgeons and hospitals in other states or countries? The development of information technology has provided a major impetus for the development of such **population health** measures, which shift the focus from individual errors and competence to assessment of system performance.

Even though quality of care can mean the difference between life and death, it is important to remember that medical care cannot permanently save a life since we will all die eventually. What medical care can do is prolong a life and make it more productive. (See discussion of quality adjusted life years [QALYs] in Chapter 3.) The extension of life is not, however, unambiguously good. Increasingly, we are asked to make decisions about end-of-life care, release from suffering, and quality of life not in terms of morbidity and mortality, but in terms of relationships, social connections, and spiritual concerns.

1.4   PUBLIC OR PRIVATE CHOICES

For some goods there is only one unit, which we consume collectively. The atmosphere is an example. Quantity is not economically meaningful for the atmosphere. Having "more" by breathing deeply, turning on a fan, or opening a window does not add value if the problem is pollution. Quality is the only relevant dimension. Air quality, the legal system, national defense, cancer research, transportation, and other goods that are similarly universal in consumption are known as "public goods." Being universal does not exempt them from scarcity. Scarcity of air quality (i.e., pollution) can be addressed through various improvements, each of which has a cost. Public funds, although much greater than those of any individual, are still subject to budget constraints. The price of better air must be paid by giving up some other public goods, or by all of us giving up some of our private goods by paying higher taxes.

Smoking has been banned on airplanes, trains, buses, and in office buildings of many firms, universities, and hospitals. Air quality has been improved without paying for pollution control equipment or raising taxes. Does this mean that these improvements in air quality came without a price tag or that no trade-offs had to be made? Of course not. Listen to the smokers gripe or to the complaints of non-smoking libertarians who worry that the next distasteful behavior to be banned will be drinking, or sex, or gun ownership. While it does not appear that anything has been bought or sold, a transaction has in fact taken place. The opportunity cost of a smoke-free workplace was a discernible, but small, loss of personal liberty. This is the "price" of the gain in air quality. People have made it clear that this is a price they are willing to pay—and just as clear that some measures advocated by health advisors are too costly to be implemented. Even though such collective relationships are inherently complex, involving millions of people, the fundamentals of opportunity cost, budget constraints, and trade-offs still apply. Price theory can be used to analyze what will happen.

"Private" and "public" are polar concepts. Few goods are so purely private that they are entirely unregulated regarding safety, ingredients, and disposal, and few goods are so public that there are no differences among individuals regarding use or quality.[6] The economic organization of medical care clusters more services toward the public end than is immediately apparent. Even though each of us goes individually to the hospital emergency room, in a small city we must all go to the same emergency room and, therefore, get pretty much the same quality of care. The mayor may get better service than a homeless person who is brought in off the street, but the mayor will be operated on by the same surgeon, will be cared for by the same nursing staff, and might end up in the same room as the homeless person. In a large city with many hospitals, there is somewhat more variation, but patients are rarely able to choose their surgeon, nursing staff, or room. Contrast that with the purchase of a coat, a birthday cake, or even a wheelchair, in which there are many more choices and much more individual control over quality.

Payment systems also tend to make medical care a public good. All employees in a firm often have the same insurance plan. Therefore, the mail clerk and the executive vice president are equally valued customers of the hospital. In Chapters 4 and 5 we will examine how the pooling of funds into insurance for payment of medical expenses can distort choices and obscure the nature of the budget constraint.

1.5 RESEARCH

Technology has been the driving force in the health care system—saving babies, lengthening lives, creating hospitals, linking medical records worldwide, and raising the American public's willingness to spend more than $1 trillion a year. One can easily imagine that spending would be doubled again without complaint if the research laboratories could come up with a vaccine for AIDS, a cure for cancer, and a reversal of Alzheimer's disease. Medical discoveries often have been fortuitous outgrowths of other activities (Pasteur's discovery of bacteria grew out of an investigation into the causes of spoiled wine and beer) or the refinement of insights from patient care. Historically, what little direct funding there was for research came mostly from philanthropists. Today, taxpayers are the largest source of pure research funding through support of the National Institutes of Health and similar programs. However, a much larger portion of research funding is hidden in the cost of patient care, as the work of physicians to develop and refine new technologies is covered through reimbursement. The most prestigious hospitals and clinics are deemed superior because cutting-edge research and innovative therapies are first applied there. Being on the cutting edge is expensive, and charges for patient care at the top academic medical centers are as much as three times higher than those at local community hospitals (see Chapters 8 and 9). This source of indirect funding may be under pressure as the growth of managed care increases price competition in the hospital services market (see Chapters 10 and 12).

Most of the cost of developing new types of surgery and diagnostic tools does not show up as research in the national health accounts because it is covered as part of patient care reimbursement. Similarly, most of the research and development (R&D) at pharmaceutical companies is buried as an overhead cost in the production of drugs. Even more hidden is the cost of administrative innovation. Developing new forms of contracting, such as HMOs, or new methods of delivering care, such as home health companies and life care communities, is very costly, largely because it is a trial-and-error process requiring many expensive failures before a better system can be found. Yet such organizational development is not usually even recognized as being research and its cost is almost never tallied alongside the cost of laboratories and biomedical scientists.

The cost of continually innovating and changing medical treatments and delivery systems is staggeringly high, yet the forgone opportunity cost of not innovating is much greater. What athlete injured today would wish to forgo arthroscopic knee surgery and accept a hot mustard plaster? Senior citizens may say they want to turn back the clock to the good old days, but any politician who threatens to take away Medicare, or even to cut benefits slightly, gets defeated at the polls. The American public demands a modern, constantly updated health care system. Research into new therapies and new forms of organization is the force that has made it worth spending $1,546 billion today versus $4 billion dollars one hundred years ago. Yet the flow of funds into research is hard to trace, the connection between spending and benefits is difficult to make, and the dynamics of technological and organizational change are among the most challenging of economic questions.

1.6   TIME

Time is more limited than money. You have just 24 hours each day. To use your money as a consumer you must have time. Given time, you can get money. Or, you can spend your time meditating, hunting for berries in the woods, or writing poems in the sand. At least you are alive. If you have money, but no time left, the money is worthless. Death is the ultimate budget constraint. Once the sum total of all your hours is gone, there are no second chances, no credit advances—and no more decisions to make. While all economists acknowledge that scarcity is fundamentally defined by the consumer's lifetime, this awareness is more acute among health economists because the business of medical care centers on life-and-death decisions.

It is difficult to improve your health once it has deteriorated. Spending money on medicine once you are seriously ill is a little like spending money on your car after the engine has begun to burn oil; regular maintenance is a lot cheaper. How healthy you are when you get old depends not so much on the medical care you get then, but on what you have done to and for your body over the years. Taking some of your time each week to exercise and giving up some tasty junk food (donuts, french fries, ice cream sundaes) can help you live longer and feel better in the future. Some people would call such behavior health consciousness, or following a healthy lifestyle. As economists, we call it savings and investment. What I am doing is reducing consumption now (less ice cream) so that I can consume more (have greater enjoyment) in future years. I invest in my body by exercising, just as a firm invests in a manufacturing plant by doing maintenance and construction. Most readers of this textbook are studying now for a future reward: knowledge, grades, a degree, career advancement. You are investing, giving up time (money) now to obtain more value in the future.

Medical school is a form of investment, usually a very good one (see Chapter 7). Similarly, the research done by pharmaceutical companies is an investment: forgo current profits to discover a new drug that will begin to sell fifteen years from now. In a society, the money used for medical schools and research, the loss of life due to trials of experimental drugs, and the difficult learning curve of surgeons in training (somebody has to be the first patient) are investments in the future of medical care. Current losses are real, and staggeringly large, but the rewards are greater. Imagine how many of your parents, or your classmates, would be dead if we decided as a society to stop the losses and practiced the best nineteenth century medicine for the next one hundred years.

1.7   THE STRUCTURE OF THE ECONOMY: CONTRACTS

A contract is an agreement to trade. In a two-party transaction, as depicted in Figure 1.1, the contract is often so simple that it is never written down and is specified in only a few words (e.g., "Will you take $5 for that lamp?"). Buying a new car is more complicated. There is almost always a sales agreement, the terms of which must be agreed to by a manager, and the real seller is not the salesperson but a corporation. Taxes must be paid. The buyer has a warranty against defects and malfunction, and in some states has a legal right to return the car without penalty within the next three days. Buying a house entails an even more intricate set of contracts, with obligations involving many firms and the government. The shape and responsiveness of an economy—its information structure or "neural network"—is determined by the contracts that link parties. It is made up of all the contractual entities: people, partnerships, corporations, government agencies, courts, constitutional conventions, legislatures, and even the police and military forces (since contracts engender disputes and force is the ultimate means of dispute resolution).

Medical care is part of, and contractually connected to, the larger economy as a whole.[7] Physicians earn money so they can buy cars and houses and CDs. The cost of care to patients is in forgoing cars and houses and CDs. While all parts of the economy exchange money and share certain features, many parts have special features and specialized contractual forms (movie studios, the National Football League, stockbrokers). Medicine is more special than most other types of economic activity because of extreme information requirements and risks entailed in treating disease. No one needs a prescription to rent a DVD. You don't have to have insurance or sign a consent form to have your car's fuel pump worked on, and almost anyone can cut your hair without a license. The degree of trust in a surgeon, and the reliance on professionals to enforce standards and maintain quality within the operating room, is quite special. The use of more extensive contractual structures (professional licensure, hospital staff bylaws, regulatory review) to meet such special needs is a standard and helpful response of a modern economy.

1.8 ECONOMIC PRINCIPLES AS CONCEPTUAL TOOLS

Questioning whether the effects of another course of chemotherapy are worth the possibility of surviving until your daughter graduates is highly personal, yet the principles involved are common to most economic problems: balancing costs and values within a set of constraints imposed by the situation. Structurally, it can be analyzed like other decisions: whether to apply to medical school, how many risks to take while skydiving, the choice between buying health insurance and taking a vacation. A list of seven principles useful as "conceptual tools" for analyzing decisions is provided here. Most of these will be evident to you based on your own experience or previous study. If not, you might wish to review some of the suggested introductory economics resources.

Trade

People engage in trade, exchanging things, time, favors, money, and information, because it makes them better off. Both sides must benefit, or they would not agree to trade. This is the Fundamental Theorem of Exchange and perhaps the most basic principle of economic reasoning.

Choice: Are Benefits Greater Than Costs?

Every decision involves a trade-off, giving something up in order to get something else, choosing the one that means more to you. This is obvious when you engage in trade with someone else. It is true whenever you make a choice, even though you "trade" only with yourself (e.g., giving up a workout at the gym in order to study, passing up a new CD in order to buy dinner at a restaurant, giving up some of your savings in order to take a trip to Cancun). Economists assume that people tend to make choices that make them better off in a way they value (not necessarily financially). This is known as the "benefit-cost principle."

Opportunity Cost

The best measure of what something costs is what you have to give up to get it. The trip to Cancun might cost you $750 in savings; an extra weekend date might cost you an A as your grade falls to a B+ because you gave up study time. Conversely, you might say that the decision to be a grind and get an A cost you a date. It is the decision you make, not the price tag or money, that really determines the cost of something. The primary cost of attending this class is the time it takes (the fun you could have had and/or the money you could have earned), not the amount spent on tuition and books.

Scarcity (Budget Constraints)

Why does a decision always involve giving something up? Because reality imposes limits, or constraints, on what you can do. The most basic limit is time. You have only 24 hours per day and once your days are gone (due to death) you have no more life to use in production or consumption. Your income and your bank balance, the place you live, the things and friends you have, and even your credit rating all put limits on what you can do to make yourself better off. Economists call them "budget constraints." This term applies not only to money, but also to time, things, relationships, and any other kind of constraint.

Maximization/Marginalism

Productive effort and exchange (trade) are ways people make themselves better off. What principle determines when to stop? When the benefits from the next step are outweighed by the costs. Each decision increment (read one more page, eat one more slice of pizza, play one more game) adds a little value (marginal benefit). Each step also takes a little more time or money (marginal cost). The real issue is not whether something (grades, food, playing time) is good, but whether you would be better off with more or less of it.

As more and more is done a point at which the benefits of each additional step become smaller and smaller (diminishing marginal returns) is usually reached, and the costs of an additional unit become greater. Maximum net benefits are obtained by pushing to the point at which rising marginal costs equal falling marginal benefits.

Money Flows in a Circle

When someone buys something, the money spent must be received by someone else. The seller wants those dollars for what he or she, in turn, can buy. The dollar is almighty because it flows—because it can be changed into anything else—not because there is any inherent value in a wrinkled piece of paper.

Contracts and Organization

The seller must have faith that the money obtained in trade will have value. The buyer must have faith that the goods received are what they are supposed to be. Both buyer and seller must be able to trust each other. The more complex the transaction, the more a buyer and seller have to trust each other and to rely on external guarantees. Buying on credit or for future delivery (mail order, new custom home, knee surgery) creates potential problems and requires an extended contractual framework. Uncertainties in value (a used car "as is," a share of stock in a start-up company, an experimental drug to treat your rash, trip insurance for your Cancun vacation) also force greater reliance on trust and contract specifications. Having to include a third party that handles the money (purchasing agent, insurance company) makes transactions even more complex and vulnerable to fraud. Two of the parties may collude to take advantage of the third party. Often, tracing the flow of funds helps reveal the underlying economic forces at work, even if the contracts are confusing or people lie.

Organizations evolve to build trust and increase the efficiency of exchange. Laws, rules, political parties, mandatory labels, certified measures, corporate financial statements, clubs, professions, and nonprofit organizations are in a sense market responses to market failure, as difficulties in making simple price transactions are resolved by more comprehensive contracts. Government is the most comprehensive of such social structures. Exchange and economic potential remain limited until a solid base of personal trust, laws, contractual organization (markets, firms, credit, regulations), and social structure evolves. The growth and output of an economy have more to do with the efficiency of organization than the endowment of natural resources, numbers of people, financial aid, or any other factor.

1.9   HEALTH PRINCIPLES

Medicine is not all, or even mostly, about money. Science, caring, professionalism, and even religious concerns regarding birth and death can be more important than dollars.

Economics gives one important and clear perspective, but it is a limited view—analogous to the kind of limited view that an X-ray provides of a person, or that radiology provides for all of medicine. Just as radiology has been expanded to include sonograms, computed tomography (CT), positron-emission tomography (PET), MRI scans, and other forms of diagnostic imaging, economics has expanded to examine social relationships, politics, and the financing of technological advances. Yet, no matter how powerful economics is for analyzing decisions, it still remains just one piece of a larger picture. Most of medicine and health lies outside the scope of this textbook, but a few simplified health principles within the expanding realm of economics are noted here.

Health Is Priceless

In a crisis, people will pay almost anything for medical care. The opportunity cost is too great to bargain over "how much" when your daughter's life is at stake. People do not want to make difficult decisions trading off dollars for health. This is why virtually every modern economy offers medical care on demand and extensive programs of health insurance. Much of the struggle in health economics is to face up to the inevitable trade-offs by stepping out of crisis mode and looking at the larger picture regarding costs and benefits.

And Yet, Money Still Determines Health

Everywhere we look, the rich are healthier than the poor. In unsophisticated rural villages and modern cosmopolitan cities, with health insurance or without, the rich tend to do better in terms of both mortality (death rates) and morbidity (illness rates). A particular rich person may be in worse health than a poor person, but in general, money has a strong positive impact on physical condition. Other demographic factors (age, sex, race) are often even more important.

Health Risks Are More Public Than Private

Just as your income depends more on the level of development of the economy into which you were born than on your individual skills and effort, so does the state of your health. Compared with starting your life in Switzerland, being born in a rural village in the Sudan severely curtails both your earning power and your life expectancy.

Individual Choices: Lifestyle Is More Than Medicine

To the extent that individual choices influence health, lifestyle matters more than medical purchases. It is not that medicine isn't important, but that most people will almost always pay for the important types of care. The remaining marginal choices, Branch Creek Hospital versus University Hospital, generic *naproxen sodium* versus *ALEVE*, doctor at the local health department clinic versus specialist in private practice, will not have a major impact on death rates, although they may have a lot to do with personal satisfaction and the quality of the experience. Flying first class on a major carrier is more comfortable than flying cut rate in economy class, but safety (the likelihood of dying in a crash) is about the same. Similarly in medicine, the available choices in a generally high-quality and highly regulated system mean that "better" care usually does not have a measurable impact on mortality.

Measurable Differences in Quality Over Time, or Regions, Are Greater Than Most Differences in Choices Faced by Patients

Heart surgery in 2002 was so much better than the kind practiced in 1962 that no one would choose the latter. Rich patients may fly from Guatemala to the United States for superior medical care, but few U.S. tourists would decide to have knee replacement surgery done in Guatemala while on vacation to save a few dollars. Individual market choices for quality are important and persistent for goods such as clothing and housing, but medical care is more like the market for computers and video equipment, in which most people pay for what is newest.

1.10 HEALTH AND THE ECONOMY

Spending money on medical care is only one of many ways that the economy affects people's health. Economic prosperity enables people to have a better diet, to avoid hazardous jobs, and to clean up the environment, as well as to purchase more medical care.[8] A major benefit of higher incomes is education, which changes values and production possibilities in ways that are favorable to health. Chapters 16 and 17 provide more detailed examination of the complex relationships between economic growth, income distribution, medical care, and health, but some basic facts provide a useful background for study of the health care system. Table 1.4 presents the results of a study of 320,000 middle-aged men enrolled in a trial of cardiac risk reduction.[9] Income for this study is based not on individual wages, but on the community in which the person lived (average per capita income of the ZIP code of residence). Reading down the columns, it becomes evident that men in poorer communities face a much higher risk of death each year, a finding that holds even as the groups are adjusted for age, unemployment, use of medical care, and other factors. Indeed, those living in areas with average incomes below $10,000 per year were twice as likely to die as those in areas with average incomes above $30,000 per year. Blacks were more likely to die than whites, largely because of living in lower income areas. Yet even after controlling for differences in income, black mortality is still significantly greater each year. Similar differences in morbidity and mortality rates by socioeconomic and ethnic grouping are observed among women, the elderly, and children.

Although insurance and government assistance has done much to equalize access to medical care, large disparities in actual health and life expectancy endure. Inequalities in health are found throughout the world. Countries such as Sweden and the United

TABLE 1.4	Annual Mortality Rate Among Middle-Aged Men	
	Mortality Rate	
Income Category	**White**	**Black**
< $ 9,999	0.918%	1.234%
$10,000 – $14,999	0.840%	1.123%
$15,000 – $19,999	0.706%	0.899%
$20,000 – $24,999	0.660%	0.867%
$25,000 – $29,999	0.591%	0.603%
$30,000 +	0.542%	****

Source: G. D. Smith et al, *American J. Public Health* 86: 486–504, 1996.

Kingdom, which have universal national health systems, also show substantial differences in mortality between groups, as do poorer countries such as Bangladesh and Ghana, where a national health infrastructure is almost nonexistent. Health economists are still working to understand the persistence of excess mortality among disadvantaged groups despite tremendous increases and redistribution in health care spending.

The effects of medical care on the economy are as profound as the effect of economics on health. Not only has medicine led to better health, greater longevity, and increased productivity, it has become one of the largest businesses in the world. Investments are made in hospital bonds and biotech stocks to make people better off monetarily, not just in terms of health. To those who directly or indirectly earn their living from medicine (physicians, nurses, hospital administrators, equipment vendors, and even health economists), the business aspects—the contracts that are used to allocate health services—are the most salient. The invisible hand plays a role in creating a demand for health economics that is just as powerful, and more direct, than the desire to improve the standard of living and care for the sick.

SUGGESTIONS FOR FURTHER READING

Health United States, 2002. U.S. Department of Health and Human Services (annual publication), (www.cdc.gov/nchs/hus.htm).

National Health Expenditures 1980-2001 and National Health Expenditure Projections 2001-2011, U.S.D.H.H.S., Centers for Medicare and Medicaid, National Health Accounts, (www.cms.gov/statistics/nhe).

Kaiser Family Foundation Health Policy Studies (www.kff.org).

Victor Fuchs, "Economics, Values and Health Care Reform," *American Economic Review* 86, no.1 (1996):1–24.

Paul Starr, *The Social Transformation of American Medicine* (New York: Basic Books, 1982).

SUMMARY

1. For people to get what they want from the system, exchanges between patients and providers must be made. **Trade** is the means, not the goal. **Health economics** is the study of how those transactions are made and of the bottom line results.

2. The **terms of trade** are the specifics of a transaction. Only in a very simple exchange are all of the terms of trade captured in the money price. The **Fundamental Theorem of Exchange** states that for a trade to take place, both the buyer and the seller must believe that it makes them better off.

3. **Value** is not inherent in a good, but in the trading relationship. **Health care costs so much because people are willing to pay for it.** As a wealthy country, the United States was willing to spend more than 1.5 trillion dollars in 2002, $5,427 per person, supporting a dynamic and technologically sophisticated health care system.

4. Health care costs have consistently **risen 3 to 5 percent more rapidly than incomes** and now account for **15 percent of GDP. Government** is the largest provider of health care funds (45 percent), and hospitals are the largest users (36 percent). **Physicians** account for about 0.5 percent of the U.S. labor force, about the same percentage as in 1880. However, the number of nurses and other health workers per physician has risen from 0.2 to sixteen.

5. Two major complexities in the economics of health are that most choices are made regarding **quality,** rather than price or quantity, and that there is **uncertainty** regarding the effects of medical care upon health.

6. **Costs are unevenly distributed.** Seventy percent of total health care dollars are spent on the 10 percent of people who become most ill during a year. Due to the uncertain and uneven distribution of medical costs, most health care payments flow through **third-party insurance** intermediaries, which pool and transfer funds. This system replaces the direct exchange of money for services between two parties (consumers and providers), which is common to most markets.

7. Some choices can be made only by society as a whole. Such things as airline safety, cancer research, and malpractice laws are **public goods.** Pooled financing through insurance can make medical care into a form of public good even though services are provided and consumed in private transactions between doctors and patients.

8. **Research** into new drugs and therapeutic techniques is very expensive, but the forgone opportunity cost of not innovating would be much greater.

9. Improvement in **health and longevity** has come mostly from **economic growth, social factors,** and inexpensive **public health** activities rather than the application of expensive medical technology. Insurance and government programs have greatly reduced disparities in the use of medical care between income groups, but **socioeconomic differentials in health status have persisted.** Residents of poor neighborhoods are twice as likely to die as are people of the same age and sex who live in wealthy neighborhoods.

PROBLEMS

1. {*economic principles*} What is the opportunity cost of going to a doctor to be examined for skin cancer?

2. {*economic principles*} What is the primary budget constraint facing an 84-year-old billionaire?

3. {*planning resources per capita*} Using the data in this chapter, calculate the number of physicians, nurses, hospitals, and nursing homes there would be in an average small town with 10,000 people (total U.S. population was approximately 285 million in 2002).

4. {*local estimates*} Using the telephone book for your city, try to determine whether the number of physicians, nurses, hospitals, and nursing homes is greater than or less than the number you calculated for Problem 3. Why is it more difficult to estimate the number of physicians than the number of hospitals? Why is it so difficult to estimate the number of nurses?

5. {*distribution of health expenditures*} Ranking everyone by the amount spent on medical care, 30 percent of the total (all expenditures for all people) is accounted for by the top 1 percent of patients. Take the overall average per capita personal health expenditure and determine how much on average is spent on each of these high-cost patients. The top half of the population accounts for 90 percent of total spending. What is the average amount spent on the remaining people in the bottom half of the distribution? Is the median (i.e., amount spent on the person who is at the middle of distribution, with half of all people spending more, and half of all people spending less) higher or lower than the mean?

6. {*philanthropy, $ versus %*} Has the dollar amount of charitable giving for health increased or decreased since 1900? Has the percentage of health expenditures paid for by charity increased or decreased?

7. {*manpower*} Which has increased more rapidly since 1900, the number of physicians or the number of ancillary health workers? As medicine becomes more technologically advanced, which will grow faster, the number of more-skilled workers or the number of less-skilled workers?

8. {*utilization*} Did people go to the doctor more often or less often in 2002 than in 1965? In 1929? Did they spend more or fewer days in the hospital? Why?

9. {*causality*} Have health expenditures increased because the number of people employed has increased, or has health employment increased because total health expenditures have increased?

10. {*causality*} Would eliminating research reduce or increase the cost of U.S. health care?

11. {*normative and positive judgments*} Are public choices better or worse than private choices?

12. {*Fieldwork*} Contact three people and find out how much they spent on health care last year. Try to estimate how much they spent out of their own pockets and how much was spent by their employers, insurance companies, or the government. Did the people with more serious health problems always end up spending more of their own money on health care? Did they personally end up paying a larger or smaller percentage of their total health bills out of pocket?

ENDNOTES

1. National Health Care Expenditures Projections 2001-2011. U.S.D.H.H.S., Centers for Medicare and Medicaid, National Health Accounts (www.cms.gov/statistics/nhe), accessed November 22, 2002. The CMS Office of the Actuary is the source for all expenditure estimates in this and subsequent chapters, unless noted otherwise.

2. Committee on the Costs of Medical Care, *Medical Care for the American People* (Chicago: University of Chicago Press, 1932); Odin W. Anderson, *Health Services as a Growth Enterprise in the United States since 1875* (Ann Arbor, Mich.: Health Administration Press, 1990).

3. The distribution of costs across individuals can be measured only for personal health care costs that are billed to individuals, not for overhead items such as public health, construction, and insurance administration. Such overhead items make up about 14 percent of national health expenditures. Hence, the "personal health expenditures" account for only 86 percent of national health expenditures in Table 1.1 and elsewhere. In truth, even when charges are billed to an individual, many costs have overhead components and are difficult to unambiguously assign to a single person, although they are clearly concentrated on the most ill and not evenly distributed. Many economists would argue that costs are more concentrated than statistics indicate (Figure 4.1 and Table 4.2) since hospitals and physicians typically overcharge the least complex patients to subsidize the most difficult and complex cases (see the discussion of "cost shifting" in Section 8.4).

4. Bureau of Labor Statistics, U.S. Department of Labor, *Employment and Earnings* (www.bls.gov). Bureau of Labor Statistics, U.S. Department of Labor, *Employment Cost Indexes and Levels, 1975–90*, Bulletin 2372, 1990.

5. U.S. Department of Health and Human Services, *Health United States 1975*, and *Health United States 2002* (www.cdc.gov/nchs/hus.htm).

6. Joseph E. Stiglitz, *The Economics of the Public Sector* (New York: W.W. Norton, 1986).

7. Paul Starr, *The Social Transformation of American Medicine* (New York: Basic Books, 1982).

8. Thomas McKeown, *The Modern Rise of Population* (London: Edwin Arnold, 1976); Massimo Livi-Bacci, *A Concise History of World Population*, trans. Carl Ipsen (Cambridge, Mass.: Blackwell, 1992). James P. Smith, "Healthy Bodies and Thick Wallets: the Dual Relationship Between Health and Economic Status," *Journal of Economic Perspectives* 13, no.2 (Spring 1999): 145–166.

9. G. D. Smith, J. D. Neaton, D. Wentworth, R. Stamler, and J. Stamler, "Socioeconomic Differentials in Mortality Risk Among Men Screened for the Multiple Risk Factor Intervention Trial," *American Journal of Public Health* 86 (1986): 486–504.

CHAPTER **2**

DEMAND

QUESTIONS

1. What is the difference between Mr. Axel's **demand** for physical therapy, and his **need** for physical therapy?
2. Why would a life-saving cardiac drug cost less than one providing only temporary symptomatic relief?
3. Do buyers and sellers face the same demand curve?
4. Is price the only thing that matters?
5. Can better quality actually decrease demand?
6. Which is more sensitive to price change—one person, one firm, or the whole market?
7. Do politicians face demand curves?
8. Is medical care a necessity or a luxury on which the rich spend more?

Health economists use the concept of demand to ask how the quantity of services used varies as price changes. Demand implicitly holds constant and largely ignores differences in illness and social conditions. The concept of a demand curve yields two fundamental insights: (1) providing more medical treatment means giving up something else (opportunity cost), and (2) as more and more care is provided, the benefit of each additional unit becomes smaller and smaller (downward-sloping demand). Health economists focus on trade-offs, choices that must be made, scarcity of resources, and allocating resources among competing needs, not on defining one specific need.

2.1 NEED VERSUS DEMAND

Decisions regarding who gets what medical services, and when, are made mostly by doctors.[1] Doctors tend to consider medical decisions in terms of **need**. This perspective frames each decision as a response to a technical question regarding the level of service required to adequately treat the illness of a particular patient. Such a need-based medical perspective focuses on differences in health status and ignores the role of prices and incomes in allocating scarce resources. To concentrate on patient needs, physicians try not to think about who pays (employer, patient, taxpayer) and who gets paid (themselves, hospitals) so as not to be distracted by economic concerns. Their task is to operate within a given system to allocate resources and to advocate for patients. Because physicians are supposed to act in a patient's best interest, they try to behave as though prices are set anonymously by somebody else, as if the bills get paid to some agency unrelated to their personal incomes and as if insurance payments are really paid by some insurance company rather than taken out of wages.

For decisions regarding individual patients, a need-based medical perspective is suitable. Within the health care system, most physicians strive to do the best for their patients, not to change the system or help people they have never met. We do not ask doctors to determine what is best for taxpayers or employers or insurance companies, yet someone must address this question. Economists are required to think about differences among systems: how choosing one set of insurance regulations means more children will get immunized, but fewer elderly will receive home care, while another plan might protect accident victims, reduce taxes, or provide more incentives to work. The trade-offs between medical care and other goods, among different groups of patients and different types of care, are the issues that health economics is designed to address.

Although *demand for medical care* is a concept that is awkward when applied to a specific individual who either is or is not sick, it is a tool that works well regarding groups of people or society as a whole. In large groups there is always a range of illnesses and a range of treatments available; therefore, the necessity for choices and balancing at the margin is obvious. Need and demand are different, yet complementary, perspectives on the complex set of human, financial, and scientific exchanges that constitute medicine. With care, the two perspectives can be combined to provide a fuller understanding of how the system works on different levels: the individual, the hospital, the company, the community, and society as a whole.

There is often an unnecessary and acrimonious division between economists and doctors in addressing medical care because the two are trying to answer different questions. For doctors, the question is: "If money is no problem, what should I do for *this patient?*" Economists, even health economists, have no particular skill at addressing such a question. They focus on a different issue: "Given that there is not enough for everyone to have all that they need, who should get treated? How should resources used for medical care vary across groups?" It could be said that, to some extent, doctors ignore economics, while economists ignore medicine. Bringing the science of medicine together with the structure of economic models is the interdisciplinary task of health economics.

2.2 THE DEMAND CURVE

Demand is the relationship between price and quantity. When an economist says "demand," the word "curve" is implicitly attached. A specific number is just one point on the curve and hence is known as the "quantity demanded." If a *Wall Street Journal* article stated that the "demand" for computed tomography (CT) scanners had risen to 50,000 machines, the punctilious economist would jump up to correct the assertion, noting that the "quantity demanded" had reached 50,000. The **demand curve** is drawn sloping downward to express the economist's insistence that the quantity demanded will always fall as prices rise (assuming all other conditions remain constant), a generalization known as the **Law of Demand.** For example, consider the development of an artificial heart. If each heart costs $1 million, they would only be used in matters of life and death. If further development reduced the cost of artificial hearts to $100,000 each, more people would get them (Figure 2.1). The artificial hearts would still be used only for people with serious illnesses, but they might be implanted long before a person's natural heart gave out. If the cost of making an artificial heart dropped to $100, one would be readily available to anyone who needed it. Consider

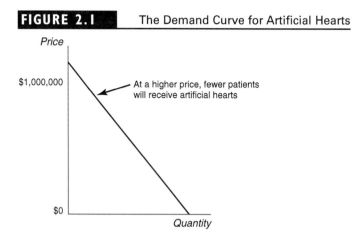

FIGURE 2.1   The Demand Curve for Artificial Hearts

what would happen if the cost of artificial hearts dropped to $10 and could be easily implanted during a 15-minute visit to the doctor. Some people who had never been ill but were just worried, or who thought that they were weak and wanted a supercharger to help them run faster, might have new hearts implanted.

The demand curve is a marginal benefit curve. At a price of $1 million, the artificial heart would be implanted only in people who believed they would receive more than $1 million in benefits. At a price of $100,000, the artificial heart would be implanted in people whose perceived benefit ranges from $1 million to $100,000. At $50,000, the artificial heart would be implanted in a few more people, whose marginal benefit falls between $100,000 and $50,000, who would be willing to pay for the operation, and so on. Note what the demand curve implies: there is no such thing as "the value" of an artificial heart. Its value depends on its scarcity and on how many are already in use. If only a few hearts were sold, their value would be fantastically high, costing millions and millions of dollars each. Once many artificial hearts were sold, their marginal value would be quite low.

The Diamonds-Water Paradox: An Example of Marginal Analysis

All ordinary economic goods show the same functional relationship between marginal benefit and quantity. They are extremely valuable when only a few units are available, of moderate value to a larger number of people, of less value as more and more people receive them, and almost worthless or even harmful if overused. The founder of modern economics, Adam Smith, was intrigued by the following problem: If water, which is necessary for life itself, is so valuable, why does it cost so little, and why do diamonds, which are simply ornamental, cost so much? Although Smith was a brilliant economist, he was never able to explain this phenomenon. With the benefit of price theory, the situation is easily explained by making the distinction between marginal benefits and total benefits. The value of the first ounce of water is very high because it can save the life of a dehydrated person. The second ounce is worth less and the third still less. In many areas, water is so plentiful that there are literally millions of gallons available, and few people have to pay more than a few cents for a glass of water. The total benefit, the value indicated by the area under the entire demand curve, is very large. The marginal benefit, the value of one more glass of water at this point (price) on the demand curve, is very small.

For diamonds, the situation is quite different. The area under the demand curve (total benefit) is not large (I can live very well with no diamonds at all). However, diamonds are scarce enough that the incremental benefit from obtaining one more is still substantial. This is shown in Figure 2.2. The decision to purchase is a decision made at the margin, whether the purchase is a bottle of water or a diamond or surgery. How much is it worth to pay for one more?

It is useful to keep the diamonds-water paradox in mind when analyzing health policy. Treatments that are highly beneficial to a few selected patients get supplied to so many people that the system is moved further and further down the marginal benefit curve, and eventually the bulk of the work is being done on patients for whom doctors can do little good. Efficiency in medical care is not just a matter of technical excellence and minimizing the cost of production. More often, efficiency depends on how much is produced and which patients get treated. Some of the nation's problems with the high cost of medical care come from using diamonds when a bandage around the finger would do just as well.

Angioplasty and Aspirin   "Diamonds-water" pricing can be found in medical care as well. Angioplasty, the procedure wherein a catheter is inserted through the major vein in the leg and up into the heart, can be used to diagnose and treat heart disease. The procedure is difficult and expensive, costing $5,000 to $25,000. Yet angioplasty works well only some of the time, provides only a temporary cure, and must often be repeated or followed up with major surgery. Research has shown that a low-dose aspirin tablet, taken daily, prevents many heart attacks, yet the price is minimal. Since firms can produce tons of aspirin for less than 1¢ per tablet, it remains by far the cheapest way to reduce cardiac mortality.

Perceptions: A Water-Water Paradox   Even water is not always priced the same. It may be available free from the tap or drinking fountains yet sell for a dollar or more in a store or restaurant. It is what buyers believe they are getting—not what they actually get—that counts here. Even though many people claim that bottled water is healthier, most biological analyses show little difference between it and tap water. (Much bottled water comes from the same source as tap water.) Yet they are not the same if we perceive them differently. If you think that Evian water is more purified and you value purity, you will pay extra for it.

FIGURE 2.2   The Diamonds-Water Paradox

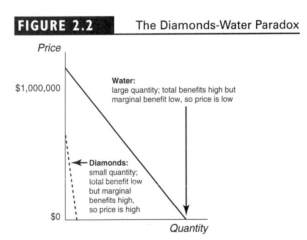

The dominance of perception is evident when examining treatment for breast cancer. For many years, even small lesions were removed using a radical mastectomy, in which all breast tissue, underlying muscle, and surrounding lymph nodes were removed. Subsequent research showed that much less invasive surgery (a lumpectomy) was usually just as effective, and often a patient could wait to see whether any surgery at all was necessary. The fact that millions of women had painful, disfiguring, and expensive radical mastectomies does not mean that they or their doctors were irrational, but rather that, at the moment they had to choose, they believed they were choosing the right treatment.[2]

Having to deal with uncertainty, as is usually the case in medicine, makes it clear that, at the moment of decision, expectations are more important than results. People buy lottery tickets, go on dates, book vacations, buy stock, major in computer science, or make appointments for surgery based on what they expect to get, even though many times they will be disappointed. Similarly, the outcomes from chemotherapy, infertility treatment, and heart transplants are never certain. When the purchase decision is being made, it is the expected value, not realized value, that counts (see Chapters 3 and 4).

Ceteris Paribus

Expectation is just one of the factors that can affect demand. Income, population growth, taste (i.e., personal preferences), health status, the availability of other goods, thunderstorms, war, and a host of other factors can influence the quantity demanded even when price is held constant. Such factors, usually known as **demand shifters,** are, in turn, the subject of economic analysis. At this stage, it is necessary to limit our discussion so that the effects of price and price alone can be examined. We will make use of the notion of *ceteris paribus,* a Latin phrase that means "all other things the same." This assumption—that all other factors besides the one under discussion are assumed to hold constant—is standard and usually unstated.

Derived Demand

You get medical care only if you need it, if you think that doing so will improve your health. No one buys heart surgery, chemotherapy, or X-rays just because these are fun things to have, or because the hospital is having a sale. As economists, you would say that the demand for medical care is **derived demand,** and depends on the usefulness of the treatment in providing health. This is the case with most goods. A cast-iron skillet is bought not for the metal, but as a utensil for cooking food. Skis are bought for skiing, not to take up space in the closet. The business of health, the actual transactions observed— doctor visits, surgery, prescriptions—are in the derived realm of medical care, they are not direct trades for health itself. If we could simply buy health—adding to life expectancy the way one picks up a three-year guarantee on a new computer—then much of what makes health economics special would simply fade away.

The flow-of-funds approach taken here starts with the **business of health**—that is, medical care. The more general biological consideration of how health itself is produced falls mostly outside the scope of this book. When medical care is viewed as derived demand, other health-determining factors—genetics, nutrition, lifestyle, environment—are seen as substitutes for that care. That is, instead of going to the doctor we could try to eat right, exercise, and start life with better parents. The cumulative impact of these other factors is much greater than any differences in the amount or quality of care received in the current U.S. health care system. Why then is so much money spent and attention focused on medical care, an input that makes such a relatively limited contribution to health?

At the moment of need, medical care is perhaps the only thing we can buy to make us better. The other factors that determine health (genetics, lifestyle, accumulated exposure to pollutants, luck, nutritional history) cannot be purchased on demand. None of us can buy new parents. In the United States, however, most of us can buy the surgical care needed to mend and straighten a broken nose.

Intermediate microeconomic theory courses build from an abstract base that begins with the ultimate source of demand, the utility function. Indifference curves, budget lines, and production functions are used to explore the mechanics of optimization. Such an approach is necessary for extending theory. It is possible to approach health economics in this way, but to do so is to risk losing track of all the structural features and organizational details that make medicine worthy of special study. In much the same way that music can be approached in terms of decibels and frequencies, and that French cuisine can be discussed in terms of vitamins and calories, health economics can be approached mechanically in terms of optima and tangency points, but doing so tends to miss the harmony and flavor that makes concentrated study worth doing. In this textbook we will often build from a particular illness or event to observe generalized economic principles at work. These principles can then be applied in new situations. In a sense, we will act as "economic naturalists," looking for patterns in human behavior and trade.[3]

Individual, Firm, and Market Demand Curves

So far, we have been rather casual about the distinction between the demand of an individual and the demand of a group. Let's be more precise. The definition of "demand" depends on the decision being made. To determine how many times Alice Anderson will visit the doctor, we look only at Alice's behavior. To estimate the use of ambulance services in Lockport, Maine, we look only at people in the town and the surrounding area, not the entire state. To project how a change in the hospital deductible for Medicare will affect spending, it is necessary to look at the entire elderly population, some 35 million seniors. The **market demand** is the sum of all individuals in that market (see extended discussion and diagrams in Technical Appendix 2). It is the decision being analyzed that defines the market. It may correspond to a geographic area, a group of friends, or all the people who visit a particular Web site.

If there were only one pharmacy in Lockport, it would be a **monopolist** (sole seller) and the demand of the market as a whole would be the same as the demand for the firm. Suppose instead that there are four pharmacies in Lockport. What demand curve is relevant to them? The pharmacies are concerned with more than individual demand, since each of them has many customers. Yet none of them fills all the prescriptions in Lockport; therefore, a pharmacy's own business is not the same as market demand. Rather, each pharmacy can sell a greater or lesser fraction of all the drugs sold in town by changing prices. Economists say that the pharmacy "faces a **firm demand** curve" of potential customers (which is some fraction of the entire market). If one pharmacy's prices are much cheaper than the others, it will get the bulk of business. Conversely, even a pharmacy charging high prices will get some business from customers who live nearby, or if it is the only one open in the middle of the night.

2.3 MARGINAL REVENUE

A firm's profits depend not on how many units are sold, but on the amount of money they bring in (revenue). In deciding whether to sell more, not only does price matter, but how much prices must be lowered to increase sales. If a pharmacy sells two bandages at $10 each, its total revenue is 2 × $10 = $20. To sell three bandages under the same circumstances, the pharmacy would have to lower the price to $8. At the lower price, the pharmacy's total revenue will rise to 3 × $8 = $24. The gain in total sales is just $24 − $20, or $4. This is the **marginal revenue** of the third unit of sale. One way of looking at marginal revenue is that to increase sales, the $8 received from the additional unit sold is partially offset by the $2 price reduction (from $10 to $8) of the other two units, so that the net gain is just $4.

Suppose your cousin Bob is a star plastic surgeon, doing rhinoplasties (nose reconstructions) for $10,000 each. He has bragged to you that each operation takes him only 2 hours, and that if he lost money in the stock market, he could make it up by doing more noses. Knowing how little he needs the money, you suggest he help out Cousin Jane, who has been struggling to save enough to pay for a nose job. "Give Cousin Jane a deal," you say, "Do her nose for $4,000." Bob explains the realities of business to you. "I really want to help Cousin Jane, I really do. But I can't do her nose for $4,000. That will make me look like I'm cheating all my other patients. And you know Cousin Jane—she'll have to tell everyone what a deal she got. Every other patient is going to come after me for a cut-rate price. Pretty soon, I'm just a run of the mill guy who gets $5,000 per nose job. Given my expenses, I'd be lucky to be able to keep the yacht, much less the beach house." The threat to Bob's income is not the loss on one operation. It is the way that a change in price affects all units sold. Without ever having taken an economics course, Bob is focused on the information relevant to his decision—marginal revenue. It is not how much Cousin Jane pays that matters, but rather how changing the price for her affects the revenues from all other patients.

It is total revenue and total cost, not the apparent "costs" and "charges" that appear on bills and accounting statements, that count. The way to maximize profits (*Total Revenues − Total Costs*) is to sell additional units as long as the marginal revenue is greater than the marginal cost. Once marginal revenue is less than marginal cost, the sale is a loser, even if the price is still above cost.

The concept of marginal revenue takes a while to grasp, but is essential for understanding business decisions. The relevant decision is about a bit more or a bit less, and how total revenue will change as a result: a decision *at the margin*. For students who need to review the concept, or who have not had a chance to learn it in depth, additional examples are provided on the Web in the Appendix materials for this book at www.wiley.com/college/getzen.

Price Sensitivity

The distinctive feature of the economic approach to demand is the emphasis on *change* rather than the amount. A measure is needed that focuses on movement and differences, on the sensitivity of the buying decision to an increase or decrease in price. Economists have borrowed a calculation from engineering, **elasticity,** to measure price sensitivity. A demand curve indicating that the quantity demanded will change a lot for any small change in price is said to be "price **elastic.**" If the quantity demanded barely budges when the price rises, demand is said to be **inelastic.** More precisely, price elasticity is measured by the percentage change in quantity demanded for each 1 percent change in price.

$$\text{Price Elasticity} = \frac{\%\text{ change in Q}}{\%\text{ change in P}}$$

The elasticity measure of price sensitivity can be used to investigate the similarities and differences in demand. If Alice's demand for Claritin is likely to decline by 25 percent if the price increases by 10 percent, then her elasticity is −2.5. If Alice's response is pretty much average, then even though we may be talking about thousands of prescriptions, the effect on the market as a whole will still be a 25 percent decline for a 10 percent price increase. That is, market price elasticity and average individual demand elasticity are the same, even though the total quantities are much different. This demonstrates one of the advantages of the elasticity measure—it is dimensionless. We could have measured quantity in terms of the number of pills or the number of bottles containing 50 doses for one person or for 10,000, and the percentage changes would still be the same.

What about the firm demand for Eastside Pharmacy in Lockport? Chances are, it will be more price sensitive than the individual or market demands. If Eastside Pharmacy raised prices, many customers would start buying from Central Pharmacy instead. Only if all four pharmacies in Lockport raised prices by 10 percent would it be likely that all four would experience a 25 percent decline in demand. Why is firm demand so much more price sensitive? Because the other firms in the market are good substitutes. The more substitutes available, the more price sensitive demand is.

To see how substitution affects price sensitivity, consider what would happen if there were 10 percent increases not just in the price of Claritin, but also in the prices of all allergy medications. Alice would not be so quick to cut her purchases of Claritin since all of her alternatives had also increased in price. Considering the range of substitution provides more insight into why so much medical care is price inelastic. If I think that a particular medication is best for me, or that my doctor is the only one who can understand my headaches—that there are no good substitutes for the care she provides—I am not likely to be very sensitive to price. On the other hand, if I consider all doctors and allergy medications to be pretty much the same, I will be quite happy to switch to save a few dollars.

The change in demand due to a change in price also depends on the amount of time available to find a substitute. Acute need (heart attack, stroke) makes it impossible to shop around for the best price in medical care. However, you might have a long time to look for a surgeon to operate on your sore knee, or to find a nursing home for your grandfather. With an extended time horizon, demand is more sensitive to price.

Price Elasticity and Marginal Revenue

If the percentage change in price is equal to the percentage change in quantity, demand is said to be "unit elastic."[4] Such demand has a special property. If the price of drugs went up by 2 percent, causing the quantity of prescriptions filled to decline by 2 percent, the total amount spent would remain unchanged (see Figure 2.3).

Most medical care is relatively insensitive to price. Pain, critical needs, fear of uncertainty, and the prevalence of insurance tend to attenuate the role of price in patient decision making. Note what happens to a firm selling more of an inelastic good. Since increasing the quantity sold by 2 percent requires a large decline in price, perhaps

---

SUBSTITUTES—ANOTHER WATER PARADOX

Why are there so few drinking fountains at sports arenas? By reducing the number of substitutes, soda vendors can increase demand and decrease the price sensitivity of consumers. Such attempts to shift demand are common in most commercial activity. At games, fans expect to pay more to eat and drink and park, and understand that such overcharges are part of the price they pay to see their team in action. Are there analogues in the medical arena? What does this behavior, limiting substitutes for soda, suggest about the enthusiasm of surgeons to provide information about massage, chiropractic treatment, or drugs as alternatives to an operation?

FIGURE 2.3   Effect of Raising Price on Total Revenue: Elastic, Unitary, and Inelastic Demand

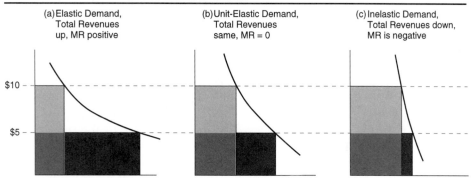

(a) Elastic Demand,
Total Revenues
up, MR positive

(b) Unit-Elastic Demand,
Total Revenues
same, MR = 0

(c) Inelastic Demand,
Total Revenues down,
MR is negative

The dotted area shows total revenue (Price × Quantity) at price of $10, the shaded area shows total revenues at price of $5.

10 percent, the firm will actually lose money. For example, a firm that lowers price from $99 to $90 will see a 2 percent increase in units sold from 300 to 306, but will find that total revenue declined from $29,700 to $27,540. If demand had been unit elastic so that quantity rose by 10 percent to 330, total revenue would have remained unchanged at $29,700. If demand were elastic, so that the 10 percent price reduction led to a 50 percent increase in quantity (from 300 to 450), then total revenue would rise from $29,700 to $40,500. Conversely, the firm facing inelastic demand that sells fewer units will be able to raise price by a larger percentage and will actually take in more, not less, total revenue for a smaller quantity sold. For example, if raising price from $10 to $11 reduced sales only slightly, from 50 units to 48, the marginal revenue from raising prices and selling fewer units would be 48 × $11 − 50 × $10 = +$28. To summarize, raising prices (and reducing quantity) increases total revenue if demand is inelastic, and decreases total revenue if demand is elastic. Since most hospitals face very inelastic demand, especially for emergency services, it follows that they are charging less than profit-maximizing prices. Why don't they charge more if it would increase profits? The reasons are many, ranging from desire to help the poor to administrative controls over allowable changes. Also, the sensitivity to price change today is significantly less than the ultimate response to a price change in the long run (after people organize protests, build another hospital, or shift their business across town).

Some medical goods—especially those for which consumers have several choices and good information in advance of purchase, such as allergy medications—are price elastic. For these goods, firms would reduce total revenues if they raised prices. Thus, it is more likely that a medical provider facing elastic demand is behaving more like a standard profit-maximizing firm. However, price controls, informal norms about overcharging, and other deviations from perfect competition may still be significant even in the more price-sensitive medical markets.

Firms facing inelastic demand find that total revenue goes down when they sell more units. Firms facing elastic demand find that revenues increase when prices are reduced to sell more units. Firms facing unit elasticity find that total revenues remain unchanged. It follows that there is a generalizable relationship between price elasticity and marginal revenue. This is expressed in the following formula (remembering that price elasticity is always a negative number):

$$\text{Marginal Revenue} = \text{Price} \ (1 + 1/\text{elasticity})$$

Price Discrimination

A firm does not necessarily face the same price elasticity in each market in which it operates. Where should it try to raise prices? In the market that is least price sensitive. Consider a young radiologist, Dr. Almon, who is starting a practice in Los Angeles. He works at a posh Beverly Hills clinic on Tuesday and Thursday, seeing a few patients, and on Monday, Wednesday, and Friday in a crowded clinic in East L.A., seeing a multitude of patients. Initially, he charges $25 to read a routine X-ray in both places. He finds that raising prices to $35 makes little difference in Beverly Hills, but he loses half his clients in East L.A. He can increase the profits of his overall practice by raising prices in Beverly Hills to $45 and lowering prices to $20 in East L.A. He is just as busy as he was before, but he is making more money.

Charging different prices in different markets is a standard strategy used by both business and nonprofit organizations to increase revenues. The practice is known as "price discrimination." Hot dogs cost more in baseball parks, clothes cost less if you work in the store (being there gives you great information and increases price sensitivity, you may get an employee discount), and scholarships reduce the price of a college education for students who have the most choices (athletes and scholars). Price discrimination is socially accepted and pervasive in medicine. The most common form, charging patients with higher incomes and/or better insurance more, has the advantage of appearing socially beneficial and fair. Even the federal government practices price discrimination, making higher income states pay a higher proportion of Medicaid expenditures. It seems right to charge less to those who can afford less, but is it? Milk and bread are not sold at a discount to people with less money, so why should radiology or physical therapy be? One major reason is that any attempt to sell bread and milk cheaper would be undercut by **arbitrage** (see glossary for definition): rich people would drive to East L.A. for low-priced groceries.

Why is there no arbitrage between Beverly Hills and East L.A. for Dr. Almon's services? Some patients will switch clinics to obtain a lower price, but only a few. Service markets are much easier to separate for purposes of price discrimination than goods markets because the patient actually has to show up at the office to receive services. First, they must find out that the price differential exists and then be willing to incur the extra travel costs.

The profit-maximizing price for a monopolist to charge in a market depends on the price elasticity. Dr. Almon can charge more in Beverly Hills because his patients are less price sensitive there, not because they have higher incomes, or can afford more, or deserve to pay more (even though these reasons may count for something as well). He will choose to set prices in each market relative to the price elasticity demand among consumers there. Looking at Figure 2.3, he would raise prices in (c) where demand is inelastic, and reduce prices in (a) where demand is elastic. It would be a mistake to assume that rich people are always less price sensitive than poor people. For example, inner city patients often lack transportation, which makes it difficult to shop around for the best prices. Many pharmaceuticals are priced higher in low-mobility city neighborhoods than they are in suburbs, where patients can easily drive to several stores and price competition is intense.

Just as markets can be separated by distance, they can also be separated by time. All that is needed for price discrimination is that consumers not be able to arbitrage by easily transferring goods from a low-price period to a high-price period. Movies are cheaper in the afternoon because customers are more price sensitive then—and they cannot transfer the picture to view it later in the evening.[5] Dining out is often less expensive during the week than on Saturday night for the same reason. Computer makers routinely roll out the newest machines at a high price to pick up the dollars of customers who must have a new machine now, then gradually reduce prices. Many CD and videocassette manufacturers practice price discrimination over time in the same way. One interesting question is why some forms of temporal price discrimination are discouraged. For instance, it would be considered highly unethical for a doctor to charge a patient more during an emergency than for similar services on a routine visit, even though it is clear that patients are very price inelastic during a medical emergency.

The frequency with which price discrimination is practiced in medicine was one of the factors that first convinced economists that physicians had a substantial monopoly power even though there are many physicians competing for patients in every city. The evidence that physicians use monopoly power to increase their incomes is well established, but tells only a small part of the story since there is even more persuasive evidence that physicians do not behave as profit-maximizing monopolists. Charging lower prices in poor neighborhoods may help increase total revenues, but providing care for free (which many physicians routinely do) is altruistic behavior inconsistent with profit maximization. As noted above, physicians also tend not to exploit patients' willingness to pay more during medical emergencies. Even more interesting to many economists is the evidence that for much of the medical care provided in hospitals and doctors' offices every day, demand is inelastic, but prices do not rise. As demonstrated earlier, a profit-maximizing firm would keep raising prices in the face of inelastic demand until it reached an elastic portion higher up the demand curve. It is evident that, while demand and supply analysis can give us some insight into the economics of medicine, it does not account for many of the features that make medicine a notable profession with a special place in human society rather than just another way to make money.

2.4 IS PRICE THE ONLY THING THAT MATTERS?

What does it mean to pay for something? To a politician, it may mean losing some votes or giving up a pet project. To a student going out partying on Sunday night, it may mean a headache and a lower grade on Monday's exam. To someone who wants a driver's license, it may mean hours of anxiety. In each case, something has to be given up to get something else. Economists often use the term "price" to refer to all of the things one has to give up to get some desirable good in trade. For medical care, it is common to talk about time, pain, and risk of death as part of the price of treatment. The concept of a **time price** was developed in recognition that the time spent traveling to and from the hospital, in treatment, and confined to bed in recovery has an opportunity cost. At the margin, the cost of time is roughly equivalent to the time price, and so a net price of time + money can be calculated. Pain is far more difficult to value since there is no objective measure for it. A monk and a businessman can go through identical operations, and one have much more pain than the other. Furthermore, even if the pain were in some technical sense the same, the two patients might value it differently. Some people can function well with a level of pain that would make others miserable. For hazardous therapies such as thoracic surgery and chemotherapy, it may not be pain but the risk of death due to the procedure that is the most important cost associated with treatment.

Services can be allocated to patients through time, pain, and risk just as they can through money. In Canada, where patients do not pay directly for most doctors' services, waiting times have increased. By discouraging those who are not willing to spend time waiting for care, the number of patients treated is limited just as effectively as it is when price is used to discourage those who are not willing to pay money for care. An example of allocation by pain is provided by pain clinics that insist on screening patients with an uncomfortable diagnostic procedure known as an electromyelogram (EMG). Patients who are not willing to undergo an EMG cannot obtain clinic services.

A fundamental difference between a money price and a time price or a "pain price" is that the money price is paid to the other party in the transaction. If an arm brace costs $10, the store receives $10. In contrast, if a patient has to wait six extra hours in the waiting room, no one receives those six hours. If an EMG is painful, a patient's willingness to undergo it may convince the therapist that the patient needs services, but the pain does not yield pleasure to the therapist. The patient's time and pain is a personal cost that does not directly benefit the provider. Economists tend to favor money prices as a rationing mechanism because they entail fewer such "deadweight" costs.

2.5 PROFIT-MAXIMIZING FIRMS, SUPPLY, AND MARKETS

Competitive **markets** use prices *to allocate* goods and services to consumers who want them the most (in monetary terms) and *to pay* suppliers for producing those goods and services. As noted above, most real markets, and virtually all medical markets, depart to some degree from the model of perfect competition. Nevertheless, it is a useful starting point for analyzing the underlying economic forces that shape human transactions even when time, pain, uncertainty, and tradition cause substantial deviations from the simple model.

The demand curve has been discussed at length. But what about supply? Again, it is vital to note that the economic concept of supply is always a **supply curve.** This curve emphasizes change, allowing us to focus on a range of responses indicating how firms will vary the amount supplied as the price increases or decreases. The supply curve also relies on the *ceteris paribus* assumption, implicitly holding many factors constant that are not being talked about. Just as the demand curve is a marginal benefit curve, showing how people in the market are willing to pay for one more unit of a good, under perfect competition *the supply curve is a marginal cost curve,* showing how much must be paid to induce firms in the market to supply one more unit.[6]

In most competitive markets with which you are familiar, supply and demand are quite distinct, and the process of organization and maximization is straightforward. The firms set whatever price they choose, and consumers decide how much to buy. Firms experiment with different prices to maximize profits; just as consumers experiment with different patterns of consumption to maximize the benefits they can obtain within their budgets. Price is the point at which all the stresses are met and balanced. The decision rule for a profit-maximizing firm is quite simple. Sell more (lower your price) if the marginal revenue (MR) obtained is greater than the marginal cost (MC) of providing the goods. The firm will continue to lower price until the gains from additional sales are offset by the costs, that is, where MR = MC.

In medical care, hospitals and doctors are often not allowed to set their own prices, but must accept prices that are set administratively by government or insurance companies. Patients buy what is needed (i.e., what sellers think patients should buy) and do not pay any price directly, but rather pay some amount indirectly through taxes and premiums. The transactions are highly regulated, and some of the funding comes from grants and philanthropy rather than sales. This is so different from the model of perfect competition that legislators and actuaries want information that spells out what would happen if medical transactions were "normal." Chapter 3, Economic Evaluation, provides cost-benefit and cost-effectiveness estimates that are used to derive the values that would be obtained ("shadow prices") and the decisions that would be made under regular economic principles (opportunity cost, marginalism, and so on). As practiced by health economists, economic evaluation for the most part replicates on paper what a market would do if it existed, but with some of the rules changed: acting as if rich and poor had the same purchasing power, assuming that decisions are made in advance rather than at a time of crisis, and assuming decisions are rationally based on medical evidence rather than on patient expectations and fears.

2.6 EFFICIENCY

Every economy must address certain basic questions: What should it produce? How? For whom? These are never purely technical questions, but at this stage, it is useful to concentrate on only partial answers—looking at the efficiency of production. However, even if we assume away all conflict over values, distribution, and culture, the question of production efficiency can become very complicated. For the sake of clarity, the following discussion simplifies a complex interdependent process into a set of discrete steps (see Table 2.1).

The first step, often forgotten, is *management*. Labor, capital, and other inputs do not produce anything unless effort is put into making them do so. If the machines or the workers are idle, if supplies are being pilfered, or if directions are not being followed, output falls. The second step concerns process—what *technology and techniques* to use. This decision depends not only on the state of knowledge at the time, but also on the price of labor, capital, and other inputs, as well as on external conditions. A "just-in-time" inventory system is not very efficient for a field hospital operating in the Cambodian jungle. Given adequate management and a choice of technology, the third step is the choice of the optimal combination of inputs to produce a specified level of output at the lowest cost. In many textbooks, the first two steps are called the **production function** and, in combination with input choice, are defined as **cost minimization.** Yet the production of output is not an end in itself. (A detailed exposition of production and cost functions is provided as a technical appendix at www.wiley.com/college/getzen).

What should that specified level of output be? The task of management is to provide benefits to customers and to satisfy salaried workers, unions, government, other interested parties, and vendors who supply inputs. Both demand- and supply-side considerations must enter into deciding how much to produce and how to distribute goods to consumers and income to producers. Jointly maximizing the total value of output is necessary to achieve *allocative efficiency*. In the abstract world of perfect competition, the optimum is identical to the profit-maximizing solution, in which marginal revenue equals marginal cost for all goods and services. In the real world, this is not always possible (see Chapter 14). We often care more about who gets care than about how much care is produced, or about making it possible for the incomes of surgeons or pharmaceutical companies to rise.

Minimizing the cost of production and distributing output is not sufficient to guarantee efficiency. In health care, insurance, finance, and other complex systems, the costs of transacting and exchange are especially high, and far exceed the direct costs of production.

TABLE 2.1	Efficiency: Steps in the Decision Process
How do we get the most out of these inputs?	*Supervisory efficiency*
What processes should be used?	*Technique efficiency*
What combination of inputs should be used?	*Cost minimization*
How much should be produced?	*Allocative efficiency (Profit maximization)*
How should contracts be formed with customers and suppliers?	*Transactions efficiency*
How should production change over time?	*Dynamic efficiency*
What is best overall (externalities)?	*Social efficiency*

Salespeople, insurance agents, lawyers, clerks, computer programmers, and accountants are all components of *transactions costs.* Many of the chapters in this book address how an organization may be structured—through property rights, professional associations, and regulations—to economize on transactions costs and promote efficiency. Understanding *dynamic efficiency* (i.e., how to create technological and organizational change to improve economic efficiency in the future) is even more challenging. In his *History of Economic Analysis,* Joseph Schumpeter attributes growth in a mature market economy to a process of "creative destruction," yet little is known about how entrepreneurial renewal occurs, except that some current efficiency must be sacrificed.[7] A purely cost-minimizing organization is not likely to be the most creative. In order to make new discoveries, scientists need time to tinker undisturbed, while managers need free time to come up with ideas for new products and service delivery systems. Finally, the effects of economic decisions on everything else that matters must be factored in. The externalities and social costs of cloning, antibiotic use (and overuse), the creation of bacteria that excrete gold (yes, it is possible), muscle and brain enhancements, and the extension of life beyond 200 years, cannot be taken lightly.

How can an organization lower costs? Why would it want to? Do not assume that more competition and greater efficiency is always good and desired by everyone. Competition is beneficial for the system as a whole, but for any given individual, more competition means more anxiety, more work, and a higher chance of failure. Greater efficiency comes at a cost to the individuals involved. First of all, change itself is difficult and often painful. Some workers will not be able to make the transition. Those who do must be willing to try harder, spend time learning new techniques, and make mistake after mistake in order to improve the process. All of the effort required to increase efficiency is clearly beneficial to the firm and to the economy, but it is worthwhile to the worker only to the extent that he or she shares in the benefits (e.g., through higher wages, greater job security, or more time off). If workers are paid by the hour regardless of the organization's output, why should they innovate or exert themselves? Capturing the benefits of increased productivity requires managers who know what gains are possible, an awareness of the costs to all of the people in the organization, and a willingness to share some of the gains with them.

SUGGESTIONS FOR FURTHER READING

Paul Heyne, *The Economic Way of Thinking* (Upper Saddle River, NJ: Prentice Hall, 2002).
Joseph Newhouse, *Pricing the Priceless* (Cambridge, Mass.: MIT Press, 2002).
Thomas Rice, *The Economics of Health Reconsidered* (Chicago: Health Administration Press, 1998).

SUMMARY

1. The **law of demand** states that a rise in prices will, *ceteris paribus* (all other things being constant), cause the quantity purchased to fall. It is a reflection of the most fundamental trade-off a buyer must make, recognizing that having more of one good means having less of something else.

2. The concept of **need,** a professional assessment of the quantity of services required regardless of price or other trade-offs, is appropriate for individual decision making when price, cost, budget constraint, and other monetary factors have already been decided—for example, within a fully insured system. The concept of **demand,** a functional relationship (curve) showing how quantity changes as price changes, is

more useful for decisions balancing the need for medical care with other goods, or allocating care among groups of people.

3. **Value** in trade is determined by supply and demand, not the inherent worth or usefulness of a medical treatment (the diamonds-water paradox).

4. The demand curve is a **marginal benefit** curve, tracing how much each additional unit of service is worth. Much of the total value of health care may lie in only a few units of service targeted to those most in need, with many subsequent services provided to a large number of people for little additional benefit. Some things that are essential to health (nutrition, exercise, preventive care) are plentiful and trade at a very low price in the market, while some services that make only a marginal contribution but are scarce (neurosurgery for someone who is already seriously ill) command a high price.

5. **Prices** arise from **transactions,** the actual exchange of money for service. Since most health care is funded by government or third-party insurance, there is no real price and therefore careful attention must be paid to the use of demand curve analysis, which depends on well-defined goods exchanged in markets that depend only on price.

6. The major demand shifters for most goods are income, prices of substitutes and complementary goods and services, population growth, and the catch-all term for everything else, "taste." In medical care, **quality** and **illness status,** personal characteristics that would usually be lumped in with taste and not analyzed separately, are of greatest importance. In making a decision about value, **expectations** or perceptions, not actual results (which cannot be known in advance, or maybe ever) are what matter.

7. **Elasticities** measure the percentage change in one variable (quantity) with respect to the percentage change in another (price). Elasticities have the advantage of being dimensionless; they do not depend on units of measurement or the size of the market. Elasticity is virtually always larger the longer the **time allowed for adjustment.** The price elasticity facing a single firm, which has many other firms competing for the same customers, is much greater than the price elasticity of the market as a whole, or of any individual consumer. A monopolist may use **price discrimination,** charging higher prices for the same good to consumers in the market with less price sensitivity (New York City versus Mexico City, insured versus uninsured, midnight versus daytime) to increase total revenues.

8. Empirical estimates of the demand for **medical care usually** show that it **is quite inelastic,** in the range of 0 to 0.5. However, elasticity is greater for items that are viewed as discretionary (dentistry, counseling) and less fully covered by insurance, and may well exceed 1.0 over the long period of time required to change health habits and beliefs.

9. **Marginal revenue,** the additional revenue that can be obtained by selling one more unit, is always less than average revenue (price), since a firm must reduce the price of goods to sell more. How much the price must be reduced depends on the elasticity of demand, so that marginal revenue can be calculated from the formula **MR = Price (1 + 1/elasticity).** A firm facing elastic demand that raises prices will see total revenues fall because the quantity demanded will fall by a larger percentage than the increase in price. A firm facing inelastic demand can raise prices and increase revenues because there will be only a small decrease in quantity sold.

10. **Management** is necessary to make labor and capital productive and requires **converting economic principles into rules of behavior** that can be clearly communicated to employees, bosses, clients, and other partners. Management is not simple, because it is people, not things, that have to be managed, and because **decisions** must be made under **uncertainty,** based on **expectations,** without ever really knowing all the facts one would like to have.

11. **Efficiency** of the health care system depends not only on how effectively it is producing medical services and reducing costs, but also on its **dynamic** ability to generate new medical technology and on the performance of the system in meeting broader **social welfare** goals.

12. For manufactured goods, supply and demand are clearly separated, with interaction occurring only through market forces. For health care, several factors make such a separation untenable: a strong physician-patient relationship of trust, the difficulty of making choices and obtaining information about life and death matters, and pervasive uncertainty. The tools of supply and demand analysis must be used with care and sometimes must be modified to conform to the realities of the health care market.

PROBLEMS

1. What is the difference between Mr. Axel's demand for physical therapy, and his need for physical therapy?

2. What determines the value of a knee brace? How can an economist maintain that I am better off if I paid $7,000 for an operation that made my twisted knee worse rather than better?

3. Which are more elastic, dental visits or visits for the treatment of diabetes? Physician visits or hospital days? Psychiatry or orthopedics? Why?

4. If the price of office visits increases from $20 to $22, and the number of visits per family per year declines from 12 to 10, what is the price elasticity of demand?

5. If most college students are poor, why do they spend so much on discretionary goods, such as CDs? Are the ones who go on to medical school richer or poorer than the ones who take jobs upon graduation?

6. In the year 2005, in Anytown, suppose that one person is willing to pay $1,000 for relief from hay fever; another two are willing to pay $350; about five more are willing to pay $50; one is willing to pay $40; one is willing to pay $35; one each is willing to pay $34, $32, $30, and $28; about a dozen are willing to pay $10; four are willing to pay $5; and half of the rest of the town (another 75 people) are willing to pay $1.

   a. Draw the demand curve for hay fever relief in Anytown.

   b. What is the potential total benefit from relief of hay fever if it is provided to everyone who asks? To everyone willing to pay $35 or more?

   c. If the price of hay fever medication is $20, what is the quantity demanded? What is the quantity demanded if the price is $50? $5?

7. Suppose Betty's demand for physician visits is Quantity = 10 − (0.2 × Price).

   a. Draw Betty's demand curve.

   b. What is the quantity demanded at a price of $10 per visit? $25?

c.   At what price will she buy four visits? Eight visits?

d.   If the government agrees to pay half of her health care bills, what would her quantity demanded be at a price of $10 per visit? $25? Draw the new, subsidized demand curve.

e.   What is the elasticity between a price of $5 and $6 per visit? Around a price of $30? Around a quantity demanded of eight visits?

f.   Calculate the elasticity of the new, half-subsidized demand at a price of $30 per visit and compare it with the elasticity you obtained from the original demand curve. What is the new elasticity around eight visits?

8.   Is chemotherapy a substitute for or a complement to cancer surgery?

9.   Provide your own example of a diamonds-water paradox in medicine, in which the clearly more valuable service is provided at a much lower price.

10.   In what units is Prozac purchased? What are the units in which psychotherapy is purchased?

11.   If the price of a post-operative follow-up visit is reduced from $40 to $30, the number of patients returning for follow up increases from 18 to 25.

a.   What is the marginal revenue (MR)?

b.   What is the price elasticity?

c.   What would your estimate of MR and price elasticity be if the quantity demanded moved from 18 to 20 (instead of 25)?

12.   Dr. Old requires that all services be paid for at time of treatment, in cash. If he decides to allow patients to pay with credit cards, will this increase or decrease demand? Will it increase or decrease price elasticity?

13.   Which is more price elastic, the demand for Cesarean sections or the demand for vaginal deliveries? Why?

14.   Ask four people what they have paid for (a) a drug, (b) minor care (office visit, physical therapy session), and (c) major care (hospitalization, surgical procedure). Find out how price sensitive they think they were for each. Do they think that everyone else receiving similar care paid the same amount as they did?

15.   Our Lady of Dollars Hospital needs to increase total revenue to build a new chapel. The hospital wants to keep the total number of patients in each service area (emergency room, obstetrics ward, operating room, laboratory, cardiac ward) the same. How can the hospital use price discrimination to achieve this objective?

16.   Give an example that shows how the health care system is willing to give up some current efficiency in the production of medical services to (a) increase dynamic efficiency by providing money for research and (b) increase social welfare.

17.   Explain how current proposals to increase insurance for mental health services would affect the market for psychiatrists. Discuss short-term and long-term effects, equilibrium, and disequilibrium. Illustrate with supply and demand graphs.

18.   If people are healthier, will their demand for medical care increase or decrease? (Careful, this is a tricky question. Consider some analogues: If people become more coordinated, will their demand for athletic equipment rise or fall? If they become more knowledgeable, what happens to their demand for books?)

ENDNOTES

1. John Eisenberg, *Doctor's Decisions and the Cost of Medical Care* (Ann Arbor, Mich.: Health Administration Press, 1986).
2. Barron H. Lerner, *Breast Cancer Wars* (New York: Oxford University Press, 2001).
3. Robert Frank, "The Economic Naturalist: Teaching Introductory Students How to Speak Economics," *American Economic Review Papers and Proceedings* 92, no.2 (May 2002): 459–462.
4. Although, of course, opposite in sign due to the law of downward sloping demand—as price goes up, quantity goes down.
5. Video rentals cost the same whether you get them in the morning (when demand is low) or in the evening, because the customer can hold on to the disc and play it when they want to. However, video stores can still practice a form of "time price discrimination." My local store allows you to return a video "late" (until noon the next day) without penalty, since almost no one wants to watch videos in the early hours.
6. This perfect correspondence holds only under many simplifying assumptions. Supply curves may deviate from marginal costs, may be flat or upward sloping as well as downward sloping, and so on. These are complexities that must be faced, but are beyond the scope of this textbook. Too much attention to technical details relying on unreal assumptions (constant technology, perfect information, no charity) tends to obfuscate rather than clarify the workings of medical markets for most readers. A useful overview of some of the issues is provided in *The Economics of Health Reconsidered* by Thomas Rice, which is listed among the suggestions for further reading.
7. Joseph Schumpeter, *History of Economic Analysis* (New York: Oxford University Press, 1954).

CHAPTER **3**

COST-BENEFIT AND COST-EFFECTIVENESS ANALYSIS

QUESTIONS

1. What is the value of life? Is one life worth more than another?
2. Is the effort expended to save one more life a total or a marginal cost?
3. Can the statistical probability of death among teenagers be compared to mortality among the retired elderly?
4. Is there necessarily a trade-off between health and money?
5. Is it more beneficial to screen high-risk or low-risk people for disease?
6. Do decisions based on the average benefit from treatment lead to excessive use of medical care?
7. Why do economists insist on discussing every choice as if it could be converted into dollars?
8. Which are better measures of the value of care: patient choices or professional judgments?

Every choice involves a trade-off, giving up something to get something else (see Chapter 1, Section 1.8, Economic Principles as Conceptual Tools). **Cost-benefit analysis (CBA)** replicates on paper the balancing of pros and cons, of advantages and disadvantages, that occurs implicitly in the marketplace. CBA is also used for public decision making to protect the interests of children, homeless people, people with mental illness, people with substance abuse problems, and other disenfranchised individuals, as well as people of future generations who are not adequately represented in the marketplace. Moreover, many health care decisions are sufficiently complicated and threatening that the individual, even though otherwise competent, may have to depend on the judgment of physicians and other professionals to identify alternative treatments and determine the relative value of medical outcomes, rather than depending on his or her own informed choices. When decisions must be made involving third-party financing or multiparty public issues, an explicit decision-making process such as CBA replaces the independent market decisions of consumers. **Cost-effectiveness analysis (CEA)** is a truncated form of CBA, fully analyzing the cost side but not translating the benefits (lives saved, illnesses prevented, a patient's additional days of activity, extent of a patient's sight restored) into dollars. CEA is used in decision making to determine which alternatives are cheaper. A study evaluating whether hypertension screening, nutrition counseling, medication, or cardiac bypass surgery would provide the most additional years of life expectancy for each dollar spent is a cost-effectiveness study. A study evaluating whether cardiac bypass surgery adds a sufficient number of years to life expectancy to justify the cost is a cost-benefit study.

3.1   COST-BENEFIT ANALYSIS IS ABOUT MAKING CHOICES

"It is best to think of the cost-benefit approach as a way of organizing thought rather than as a substitute for it."

— *Michael Drummond*[1]

Every decision—whether in the market, the public sector, or the family—involves a form of CBA. Usually the consideration of costs and benefits is informal and internal; therefore, we are not conscious of it. Only the behavior that results from this internal weighing of costs and benefits can be observed. A recent study by Orley Ashenfelter and Michael Greenstone addressed the increase in traffic fatalities caused by the decision to raise speed limits on major interstate highways from 55 mph to 65 mph.[2] Raising speed limits allows cars to go faster and can reasonably be expected to cause more traffic fatalities. This study showed that higher speed limits led to slightly faster travel, about +2 mph (many people routinely exceed posted speed limits), saving approximately 45 million hours of travel time each year. However, faster travel led to more deaths, approximately 360 additional fatalities per year. Doing some simple calculations translates these findings into a cost of 125,000 hours per life. Valuing time at a wage rate $12.80 per hour yields an estimate of the value of time gained per life lost of $1.6 million. Differences in assumptions or in the estimation procedure can lead to a higher or lower value (the range here was $940,000 to $10 million). The point of the study is that the lives lost were not the result of a mistake or bad luck—they were a choice. We, the public, decided that it is worthwhile to have more people die on the road to save travel time for the rest. While economic analysis reveals the implied dollar value of this legislative choice, it is people's behavior, not economic analysis, that puts a value on human life.

An Everyday Example: Knee Injury

Life, and the health care system in particular, confronts us with difficult choices every day. Is it worth taking three hours, and possibly paying $80, to go to the emergency room (ER) so that a doctor can examine the throbbing knee you injured playing soccer? Since pain makes it difficult to think, it can be helpful to make a list of the pros and cons (see Table 3.1).

If you believe that the benefits of going to the ER outweigh the costs, you will go to the ER. Even if you do not write down the pros and cons, a similar sort of balancing takes place inside your head. CBA is the explicit and formal presentation of that mental balance sheet. Economics does not provide answers or make it easier to take bitter medicine, but it does clarify *how to ask the questions* to make decisions more rational and more consistent. First, you must *enumerate* the benefits and costs. Then, you must *quantify* each benefit and cost as accurately as possible, given what is known about the situation. For example, it is impossible to tell exactly how much time it will take in the ER, but you think a range of

TABLE 3.1	Cost-Benefit Analysis (CBA) of Knee Injury (first step)
PROS (go to ER)	**CONS (don't go to ER)**
It might stop the pain.	It will cost $50, $100, or more.
It could prevent long-term injury.	It will take at least two, maybe four, hours.
I will feel stupid if something was wrong and I did not go.	Even if the injury is serious, surgery could make it worse.
I can't get any work done anyway while I sit here worrying.	My friends on the team will think I am not tough.

two to four hours is likely. You must then place a value on each benefit and cost. A balance sheet can be added up only if every line is expressed in the same terms, usually dollars. It does not make much sense to compare a benefit of $50 with a cost of ¥910 (yen), and there is no rule for determining how many hours of pain are worth avoiding a permanent limp; however, it is very clear that a cost of $500 is less than a benefit of $1,000.

This hypothetical knee injury can be used to illustrate CBA. The direct dollar cost of the ER visit is expected to be about $80 and you expect to wait for three hours. Since you could have been at a job where you were making $7 per hour, we can add $21 for the *opportunity cost* of the waiting time. (We will later consider the fact that surgery could make you worse instead of better.) Feeling that you are not as tough as other members of the team seems silly, but it is worth something. How much? Suppose that you were willing to pay $40 for crutches you really did not need, just to keep your friends from making fun of you. This $40 reveals your dollar value of avoiding a "wimp" label. Adding all the items, your estimated comprehensive total cost for going to the ER is $80 (charges) + $21 (time) + $40 (fear of being called "wimp") = $141 (see Table 3.2).

It is reasonable to assume that if your knee does not get better, you will eventually seek treatment, even if you don't go to the ER immediately. Let's suppose that before you injured your knee, you already had an appointment to go to the sports medicine clinic a week from Thursday. Therefore, the relevant costs and benefits are for treatment today versus treatment ten days from now, rather than for treatment versus no treatment. *Only count items that change as a result of your decision—the marginal benefits and costs.* The potential that an ER visit will stop the pain is counted on the list of pros and cons as a benefit. The labeling of pros and cons is somewhat arbitrary, and it is equally correct to say that the potential for continued pain is a cost of not going to the ER. A reduction in cost is the same as a benefit, since both are expressed in dollar terms. It is this equivalence that makes it possible to create a balance sheet for decision making. If benefits and costs are not expressed in the same terms (dollars) with opposite signs (+ or −), one cannot say which is greater.

What is it worth to stop the pain? Suppose that instead of going to the ER, you call the clinic and ask that someone phone in a prescription to the pharmacy. How much would you be **willing to pay (WTP)** to get the prescription rather than endure the pain? It is difficult to study, and may be impossible to work, when you are in pain. It is also difficult to sleep, or even enjoy watching television. You might be willing to pay as much as $150 for relief from pain for the next ten days. This WTP is the correct measure of the value of benefit received. WTP is the mirror image of opportunity cost, the "highest-valued opportunity forgone." Different people put different values on what it is worth to endure pain. Furthermore, your estimate of its worth to you will be imprecise, because you don't frequently make deals trading money for pain. However, let's assume that if the pills cost $200, you would not buy them. That refusal would demonstrate that the value of pain relief is less than $200 for you. The value is somewhere between the lower ($0) and upper ($200) bounds. Is pain relief worth $40, $50, or $150? There is no way to tell unless we observe your entire demand curve.

TABLE 3.2	Knee Injury as an Example of Cost-Benefit Analysis

Scenario: I injured my knee playing soccer this afternoon. I called and got an appointment to go to orthopedics/sports medicine clinic in ten days, next Thursday. However, it has now begun to hurt a lot and I wonder if I should go to the emergency room (ER) right away.

CONS (don't go)

Visit to ER will cost $50, $100, or more. (direct personal cost, ignores cost to insurance)	average	=	$80
I will have to wait for at least 2, maybe 4 hours. (opportunity cost)	3 hours × $7	=	$21
My buddies on the team will think I am a wimp. (willing to pay $40 for crutches just to look good)	willingness to pay	=	$40
Even if the injury is serious, surgery could make it worse. (The issue is treatment today v. Thursday, rather than treatment v. no treatment, so only incremental costs count.)	sunk cost	=	$0
	Total Cost		**$141**

PROS (go to ER now)

Might stop the pain. (pills stop pain with certainty, going to ER just a 1-in-3 chance)	$150 × 1/3	=	$50
Could prevent long-term injury. (WTP knee surgery $50,000, 1/200 chance, discount 7 years @ 5%)	$50,000 × 1/200 × .71	=	$178
Will feel stupid if something was wrong and I did not go. ("worried well" WTP for regular office visit)	willingness to pay	=	$20
I can't get any work done anyway while I sit here worrying about it. (time has same $ value for benefits and costs)	6 hours × $7	=	$42
	Total Benefits		**$290**

Observed behavior just gives us a lower bound that benefits exceed costs (>$141). Another observation, that I did not go when the wait was 5 hours and ER charges were $250, could provide an upper bound as well (<$325).

There is an overstatement of benefits here, since the pills are virtually certain to relieve pain, whereas the visit to the ER may not. Clearly a chance of reduced pain is worth less than the certainty of reduced pain, but how much less? An approximate **adjustment for risk** can be made by calculating the **expected value.** Assume that we have made enough observations to know that the average person would be willing to pay $150 for relief of knee pain. If we think there is a one-in-three chance that going to the ER now will stop the pain, the expected benefit of this one-third chance of pain reduction is one-third of the $150 I would be willing to pay for certain pain reduction (i.e., $50).

The most important benefit of prompt treatment is probably a reduction in the risk of permanent injury. People are willing to pay thousands of dollars and undergo multiple operations to try to fix their knees. Although your personal valuation is the only one that is truly relevant, the values established by other people may provide a useful guide since you have not had hundreds of opportunities to figure out how much an injury is worth. Let's say your estimate of the loss imposed by a bad knee is $50,000. This is a lot of money, but the possibility that going to the doctor this week rather than next week will make a difference is slight, maybe 0.5 percent (1 in 200). Thus, the expected value of prompt versus delayed treatment is one two-hundredths of $50,000, or $250. Furthermore, it is likely that if the knee does cause you a problem, it will be some years in the future. While that is still bad, it is not as bad as being harmed today. To take into account the fact that the problem will not occur for a while, we should **time discount** the $250, using the methods provided in section 3.6. This reduces the expected marginal benefit of prompt treatment to $178.

The fear of looking stupid for failing to seek treatment for a problem that could have been cured if treated promptly is common. Indeed, some studies have estimated that more than 70 percent of all initial visits to the doctor are made by the "worried well," people who have some vague symptom and just need evaluation and reassurance rather than treatment.[3] A modest lower bound for the value of worry reduction might be the price of a brief diagnostic office visit, or $20. What about the loss of work time due to pain and worry? These hours should be valued the same as the waiting time in the ER, or $7 an hour (the assumed hourly wage). If you think that a prompt visit will help you avoid six hours of wasted time between now and the appointment next Thursday, the prompt visit is worth $6 × $7, or $42. The sum total of all the benefits is $50 (pain) + $178 (prevention) + $20 (worry) + $42 (time) = $290.

You go to the ER. You may not realize it, but you have done a CBA—even if you never thought about the injury in these quantitative terms. Your action (going to the ER) reveals that your subjective estimate of total benefits ($290) outweighs your subjective estimate of total costs ($141). You don't find yourself being wheeled into the ER saying "I'm happy because I've got a projected consumer surplus of $149 ($290 – $141) from coming here." You just do it, or you don't. An economist considers your choice the true indicator of your personal and largely unconscious CBA. Your preferences would be revealed in more detail if we could observe you in another situation in which you chose not to go to the ER. Suppose you arrived at the ER and found that the wait would be five hours instead of three, so you decided not to stay (in dollar terms used above, the time cost to you would have been $250 instead of $80). This would provide an analyst of your behavior with a second set of costs, which in this case exceeded benefits and set an upper bound on estimated total benefits.

Opportunity Cost: Looking at Alternatives

"Growing old is a pretty lousy thing to have happen to you, until you consider the alternative."
—*George Burns* (and lots of others who were not comedians)

Costs and benefits are not intrinsic or absolute values; they are comparative values. Once a patient is diagnosed with pancreatic cancer or human immunodeficiency virus (HIV) infection, all the alternatives are pretty bad, but four years of life might be a lot better than two years of life, and the ability to play tennis a lot better than continuous nausea. On the other hand, all the alternatives facing a student graduating with a master's degree in medical information systems may look good, yet living in San Francisco might be more appealing than living in San Antonio, and the possibility of moving up into corporate systems management within a national health care chain might be more appealing than remaining the director of records in a small community hospital. To make a decision, the relevant question is not how good or how bad the situation is, but rather: What are the options? The appropriate measure of economic cost is **opportunity cost,** determined by the highest-valued alternative forgone when a decision is made. Thus, in choosing a $45,000 job in San Francisco, the graduating student who gives up a $50,000 job in San Antonio is "paying" an opportunity cost of $5,000. The cost of not taking an experimental drug is the forgone chance of living an extra two years or feeling better.

Although it might seem obvious that opportunity cost is the correct measure of costs, many discussions that purport to be logical distort, rather than clarify, decision making. A common tactic is for a supporter of a program to compare it with an alternative that is obviously bad, which makes it possible to overstate costs and benefits (e.g., "Do you want to go to the dentist today, or would you rather have all your teeth fall out?" or, "The proposed health insurance program can save the country from socialized medicine.") Most of us are able to detect such bias in the presentation of arguments, but we may miss more subtle distortions. Often a decision is presented as all or nothing, when the real alternatives are between different levels of action. The choices are not limited to flossing your teeth every day or never, they include flossing occasionally, every other day, or after each meal.

Expected Value

The general principle is to make a decision in which benefits (B) are greater than costs (C), or B > C. But suppose benefits or costs are uncertain. Five hundred grams of Xloxidine might cure you or leave you in the same condition. Surgery may cause you to miss one or five weeks of work. A choice must be made, based on the best possible information or the best guess, long before the outcome of treatment is revealed. The estimate of what is likely to happen is called the **expected value**, a core concept of risk analysis. If the analysis concerns many people, in which case the law of large numbers applies, the expected value is just the average.[4] For a single person facing an event that either will or will not happen, the expected value is the value of that event (benefit or cost) multiplied by the fraction of the time that the event will occur:

Expected Value of Z = (Probability Z will occur) × (Value of Z)

A patient receiving chemotherapy with a 70 percent chance of death may live, while a patient receiving surgery with a 20 percent chance of death may not. Yet the decision must be made in advance and should maximize expected welfare in the face of this uncertainty. Of course, after the fact, the patient's family may wish that they had done something differently. To say that the optimal choice sometimes turns out worse is simply to recognize that life is full of risks. CBA is based on the best available estimate of probability. It may be a guess or, preferably, an extrapolation from well-designed studies reported in scientific journals to which the analyst refers. "I don't know," or "I need more information," are not valid responses, since a decision is going to be made regardless of how much is known. The job of the analyst is to get the best estimate and indicate the sources of information and the range of variability. A clear discussion of the alternatives in specific terms is required. Under this useful shorthand formula, an option is chosen if

(Probability of Gain) × (Benefit) > (Probability of Loss) × (Cost).

In this formula, attention is focused separately on the uncertainty and the relative values that interact in the decision-making process. Judgmental advice, such as "it is better to get the operation and risk dying than not get the operation and remain impaired" jumbles probabilities and values together, hiding information and making communication more difficult. Such commingled statements do not make the patient think about how much it is worth to live impaired compared with dying, or to consider specifically the percentage probability of partial recovery or death. An explicit recognition of benefits, costs, and risks provides a better ground for shared decision making between physician and patient.

For situations involving many people and events with more than one outcome, the expected value is a weighted average of all possibilities. The calculation must be summed (Σ) across all categories of people and all possible outcomes to arrive at the expected value for the group as a whole:

$$\text{Expected Value} = \frac{\Sigma[(\text{probability that } \mathbf{Z} \text{ will occur for person } i) \times (\text{Value of } \mathbf{Z}_i)]}{\text{number of persons}}$$

Maximization: Finding the Optimum

More medical care usually makes people healthier. Physicians, rightly, concentrate on benefits as opposed to costs and often try to do as much as possible. However, people who use more resources to obtain medical care have fewer resources available for food, enter-tainment, housing, and other goods they want. Economics is concerned with trade-offs. What is the appropriate balance between medical care and other goods? How many doc-tors, nurses, and hospitals should there be? Economists insist that both costs and benefits be considered in making a decision. Economists also approach the decision differently from most physicians, asking not what is right or wrong, but whether a little more or a little less would make things better or worse. An economist will use marginal analysis to **optimize,** moving toward a maximum net benefit in small steps. To apply principles of maximization and use mathematics to estimate values, economists must abstract from other elements, ignoring some of the complexity of medical conditions and framing the issues in terms of dollars. Prices, costs, taxes, bids, contracts, and so on are the language used by economists to communicate human desires and limitations. The task of CBA is to make that language clear and applicable to the situation at hand, and to present the essential facts and trade-offs in a way that is easily understood by physicians, the public, and politicians.

Defining Marginal: What Is the Decision?   The term "marginal," much favored by economists, means "the change in *xxxx*." The decision being made defines the margin. Sometimes, the margin is how many patients should be admitted for treatment. For the example in section 3.2, screening for colon cancer, it is assumed that everyone will get screened; therefore, the margin is the number of times the test is repeated to increase accu-racy. Economists use a powerful analytical rule to simplify decision making: **the decision between alternatives depends only on factors that change.** Therefore, it is not necessary to examine the full range of possibilities, but only to look at doing a little more or a little less (i.e., to consider changes at the margin) to determine whether a decision is optimal. If the marginal benefits of a therapy are greater than the marginal costs, more should be done. If marginal costs are greater than marginal benefits, less should be done.

Declining Marginal Benefits   The marginal benefit is the value to consumers of one more unit of service. Willingness to pay for additional care declines as more and more is pro-vided; therefore, the curve slopes downward. It looks like the demand curve; in fact, the mar-ginal benefit curve and the demand curve are the same. To see why, remember that the demand curve is a schedule showing what quantity a consumer will buy at different prices. As long as marginal benefit exceeds the price, consumers will continue to buy. The quantity at which they have had enough and stop buying is the quantity at which the marginal benefit has fallen to the point where it is just equal to price. The quantity bought at price $P is the same as the quantity at which marginal benefit is $P; the marginal benefit (stated in dollars) of one more unit for a consumer who already has quantity Q is the same as the price they are will-ing to pay for one more unit.

Even though society benefits from having more medical care, the additional incre-ment of benefit from each additional hospital day or doctor visit tends to become smaller and smaller as more services are provided. There are two reasons for declining marginal benefits. As more treatments are provided, they are given to less and less severely ill peo-ple, who are less likely to benefit. In ERs and Army field hospitals, the process of giving treatment first to those who are most likely to be helped is known as triage, and although it does not use all the mathematics or geometry or technical terminology, triage operates on the same principles as economic maximization. Second, for any single person, the ben-efit from having one more medical service tends to decline as more and more services are used, just as benefit from consuming additional pizzas or sodas or pretzels per day tends to decline as the second, third, and fourth are consumed. In Figure 3.1a, the fact that more medical care will improve health is shown by the rise in the total benefit curve. The fact

FIGURE 3.1 Total, Net and Marginal Benefits and Costs

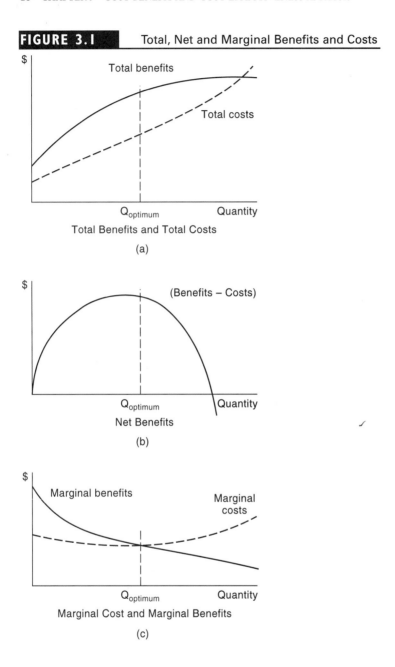

Total Benefits and Total Costs

(a)

Net Benefits

(b)

Marginal Cost and Marginal Benefits

(c)

that marginal benefits become smaller as more and more services are used shows up as a lower rate of increase, reducing the slope to make it flatter.

Optimization: Maximum Net Benefits Costs are the other side of the decision. Every additional unit of treatment adds to total costs. After start-up, the marginal cost of producing another unit of medical treatment is usually constant or rising as the total number of treatments increases. Each additional hospital bed tends to cost as much or more than the last one, and each additional nurse who is hired expects to get paid as much or more as the last one hired. At some point, the additional costs of extra treatments will outweigh the additional benefits. An optimum is where the net gain (benefits – costs) is largest. This can be found diagrammatically by plotting both benefits and costs on the horizontal axis and choosing the point where the distance between them is greatest (Figure 3.1a), or equivalently by plotting net gains on the horizontal axis and choosing the quantity of care where it peaks (Figure 3.1b), or finally by plotting the marginal benefit and marginal cost curves and choosing the point where they cross (Figure 3.1c).

A geometric property in Figure 3.1 is frequently used by economists to determine the point at which a maximum is reached: at the peak of the net gains curve it is flat (horizontal); therefore, its slope is 0 (Figure 3.1b). The total benefit and total cost curves (Figure 3.1.a) have a corresponding property: at the point where net gains are maximized, their slopes are equal; therefore, the difference in the slopes is 0. More generally, since "net gains" are defined as (benefits – costs), $slope_{net\ gains} = slope_{benefits} - slope_{costs}$, and at the maximum, $slope_{net\ gains} = 0$. These principles of maximization common to geometry and calculus can be stated in everyday terms. As any curve or function approaches a peak, the incremental increases become smaller and smaller. The maximum occurs at the turning point, where the curve goes from rising (positive) to falling (negative). To the left, marginal gains are positive, and to the right, marginal gains are negative. Here, as the optimum is reached, the marginal gains from adding a bit more or a bit less are 0. To determine the maximum distance between two curves, the focus is on the incremental or marginal change of one curve relative to another. If the additional (marginal) benefit from providing one more treatment is larger than the additional (marginal) cost, providing more treatments will make society better off (Figure 3.1.c). If the additional benefit from providing one more treatment is smaller than the additional cost, providing more treatments will make society worse off. At the optimum, the additional benefit will just offset the marginal cost; therefore, there is no change in net gains (marginal gain = 0).

Maximum net gains at: Marginal Benefit = Marginal Cost *so that* MB – MC = 0

Average, Total, and Marginal Costs

Although we can use geometry or calculus to determine the average cost and average benefit (the slopes of a line from the origin to the total benefit curve or total cost curve, respectively), these common accounting measures are not especially useful for determining optimization. The largest average gain usually occurs at a point to the right of where marginal costs have long exceeded marginal benefits. **A society that uses average benefits and average costs to make medical decisions usually ends up providing far too much medical care.** To see why, consider the following example. Suppose that a new operating suite for cardiac surgery is built. The first operation will be performed on the patient who needs it the most, one who gets a major reduction in mortality (risk of dying from cardiac disease), perhaps 50 percent. The next patient selected will not need the operation as much and will obtain a significant, although smaller, reduction in mortality, perhaps 40 percent. The third and fourth patients will obtain mortality reductions of 30 percent and 20 percent, respectively. At this point, the operating suite is full. How much benefit would be obtained by increasing capacity so that a fifth patient could be treated? If expansion allowed a fifth patient, whose mortality will be reduced by 10 percent, to be treated, the marginal benefit is 10 percent. However, the **average** mortality reduction is much greater, 50% + 40% + 30% + 20% + 10% ÷ 5 = 30%, making the expansion appear much more worthwhile than it really is. Whether that extra patient is scheduled to come in first or last does not matter. The relevant issue is that the more limited operating room space would be given to the patients who need the operation most; therefore, the marginal benefit of adding one more patient

(10 percent gain) is less than the average benefit (30 percent gain). In other words, the over-all average gain per patient treated is a poor indicator of the marginal benefit to be gained by treating one more patient.

3.2 AN EXAMPLE OF MARGINAL ANALYSIS: COSTS AND BENEFITS OF A SIXTH STOOL GUAIAC

Colon cancer is a serious illness. In the United States, 109,000 new cases are diagnosed each year, of which 64,000 are fatal, accounting for about 10 percent of all cancer deaths. One way to reduce deaths is early detection of asymptomatic cases through screening. A "stool guaiac" is a commonly used screening test. A positive test result means that occult blood is present in the feces, possibly indicating cancer (i.e., the cancer is causing minuscule amounts of internal bleeding that shows up in the feces). However, a "false positive" result may occur due to bleed-ing from ulcers, diet, or random errors. Therefore, each positive test is followed up with a more specific test, such as a barium enema, which can detect early and precancerous growths and rule out other causes of a positive test result. Since a single test may fail to pick up these early signs of cancer, it is common to test repeatedly even if the patient's results are negative the first time. In 1974, the American Cancer Society endorsed a protocol recommending that all people receive six stool guaiac tests in a row to screen for colon cancer. If any one of the six tests came back positive, the person screened would be referred for further cancer evaluation. However, two researchers, Duncan Neuhauser and Ann Lewicki, decided to examine the incremental gains and costs of using five, four, or fewer tests, rather than the recommended six.[5] Their study illustrates the substantial difference between marginal and average costs.

The expected incidence of asymptomatic colon cancer among a group of 100,000 people is about 720 cases. It is assumed that the initial stool guaiac, costing about $4, would detect 90 percent of the undiagnosed colon cancer, or 648 cases ($.90 \times 720$, see Table 3.3).[6] However, this test would also give false positive results for about 20 percent of the people screened; therefore, the total number of positive tests among the 100,000 people screened would be 20,648. Each positive test result, whether true or false, would require a confirmatory barium-enema test costing $100. Following up on false positive results would account for 80 percent of the $2.5 million total program costs. The cost of cancer detection using a single test on each patient is $2,464,800 ÷ 648 cases = $3,804 per case found. While hardly trivial, this does not seem like an outrageous amount to spend for early detection of an often life-threatening cancer.

The second test would cost $1 and pick up 90 percent of the remaining undiagnosed colon cancers, or 64.8 cases. The incremental cost for the second test, $1.7 million, is less than the initial test, but the number of additional cases detected is far lower; therefore, the average cost per case detected with two tests is higher, $5,852. More important, the mar-ginal cost of cancer detection with the second test is much higher, $26,335 per additional case found ($1.7 million in additional costs divided by 64.8 additional cases).

Each of the third, fourth, fifth, and sixth tests would cost $1 and pick up 90 percent of the colon cancers not yet diagnosed. These additional tests are finding very few cases of cancer, but are still generating a substantial number of false positive results. Since five tests will have uncovered almost all (719.9928 out of 720) the cancers, the additional cases of cancer detected by the sixth test is a negligible, at .0065. However, the sixth stool guaiac will still account for 100,000 tests and another 6,554 false positives; therefore, the marginal cost per case detected for the sixth stool guaiac is $755,400 ÷ .0065, an astronomical $116,574,074 per additional case found.

To complete a CBA, the dollar value of early cancer detection must be estimated. The discussion of valuation methodology is deferred to section 3.5, but to illustrate the

TABLE 3.3 Calculating the Costs of Using Stool Guaiac Tests to Detect New Cases of Colon Cancer

Number of Tests	Cases		New Cases Found	# Tests Positive	Costs of Screening Program				Cost Per Case Detected	
	Detected	Not			Testing	Confirmation	Total	Marginal	Average	Marginal
0	0	720	0	0	$0	$0	$0	$0	$0	$0
1	648	72	648	20,648	$400,000	$2,064,800	$2,464,800	$2,464,800	$3,804	$3,804
2	712.8	7.2	64.8	36,713	$500,000	$3,671,300	$4,171,300	$1,706,500	$5,852	$26,335
3	719.28	0.72	6.48	49,519	$600,000	$4,951,900	$5,551,900	$1,380,600	$7,719	$213,056
4	719.928	0.072	0.648	59,760	$700,000	$5,976,000	$6,676,000	$1,124,100	$9,273	$1,734,722
5	719.9928	0.0072	0.0648	67,952	$800,000	$6,795,200	$7,595,200	$919,200	$10,549	$14,185,185
6	719.99928	0.00072	0.00648	74,506	$900,000	$7,450,600	$8,350,600	$755,400	$11,598	$116,574,074

Source: Adapted from "What do we gain from the Sixth Stool Guaiac?" by Duncan Neuhauser and Ann Lewicki, *New England Journal of Medicine,* Volume 293, pp. 226–228 (1975). The table assumes that 100,000 people are to be screened, and that if perfect, the test would detect 720 cases of colon cancer. Each additional test will find 90% of the undetected cases, so that the first test will find .90 × 720 = 648 cases, the next test will find an additional .90 × 72 = 64.8 cases, and so on. However, the test will be falsely positive for 20% of the people who do not have cancer. Thus with one test, about 20,000 people with no cancer as well as the 648 with cancer will test positive. With two tests, about 36,000 false positives will occur (i.e., 20,000 from the first test, plus 20% of the 80,000 cancer-free people who were negative on the first test). It is assumed that the cost of stool guaiacs is $4 for the first test, and $1 for each additional test, and that each person who tests positive will be given a barium-enema test costing $100 to confirm whether or not cancer is really present.

process, an arbitrary benefit per case of cancer detected of $100,000 is assumed, with comparisons to a range of other values (from $1,000 to $10 million) to see how significantly different measures of benefits would change the results. Total benefits can be determined by multiplying value per case by the number of cases detected. Using one test will detect 648 cases, which, at $100,000 each, implies total benefits of $64,800,000. With two tests, 712.8 cases are detected, for total benefits of $71,280,000. With six tests, 720 cases are detected, for total benefits of $72,000,000. Total benefits and total costs for the range of decisions (zero to six tests) are illustrated in Figure 3.2a. The total benefit

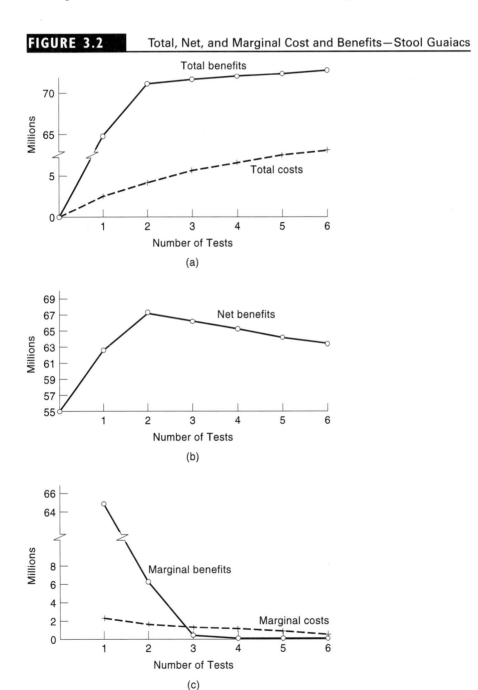

FIGURE 3.2 Total, Net, and Marginal Cost and Benefits—Stool Guaiacs

curve is above the total cost curve throughout, indicating that any amount of stool guaiac screening from one to six tests generates positive net gains over the no-screening alternative. The maximum net gains (benefits minus costs) are obtained using a screening program that uses two tests, as shown in Figure 3.2b, or using the marginal curves (Figure 3.2c). The marginal cost of the third test is $1,380,600, while it detects only 6.48 additional cases of cancer, for marginal benefits of $648,000. The first test yields very large gains and is clearly worthwhile. The second test has a marginal cost of $1,706,500 and detects 64.8 cases, generating marginal benefits of $6,480,000 and thus is also seen as providing net gains. Marginal analysis shows that the optimal level of screening is obtained by using just two tests. The conclusion that two tests are "better" than three tests depends on the value the analysis places on detecting a case of cancer (here assumed to be $100,000). Three tests will find 6.48 more cases, and potentially allow treatment to extend someone's life, but the additional health benefits are deemed to be worth less than the cost: $648,000 versus $1,380,600. The original program with six tests is better than doing nothing, as indicated by the fact that the average cost per case of $11,598 is less than the $100,000 average benefit, but the fact that the marginal cost of $116,574,074 is much higher indicates that a screening program using fewer tests will provide greater net gains (see Table 3.4).

The cost per case of cancer detected in this example depends on several factors. If the prevalence of colon cancer in the group being screened is greater than 720 cases per 100,000 population, more cancer would be detected and the cost per case (both marginal and average) would be lower. Conversely, a population with lower colon cancer prevalence would have a higher cost per case, and a larger percentage of those who tested positive would, in fact, turn out to be false positives. A better test would be more specific to colon cancer, with a lower false positive rate. If the stool guaiac did not indicate cancer so frequently when no cancer is present, the cost per case detected would be much smaller. The appropriate level of testing also depends on the estimated benefits of detection. Most of the cases, and most of the benefits, are found with the first test. If the value per case is $10,000, just one test per person would be optimal. If the value per case is $1 million, three tests would be optimal. Trying out different assumptions regarding costs, benefits, therapeutic effectiveness, and disease prevalence to determine how much they affect the results of CBA is called "sensitivity analysis." Here, a hundred-fold variation in estimated benefit (from $10,000 to $1 million) only changes the recommendations slightly, from one test to three tests. A little algebra and examination of Table 3.4 shows that any level of estimated benefit per case between $27,000 and $210,000 would lead to a recommendation of two tests per person. While the exact value of early cancer detection is difficult to estimate, it is unlikely that it falls much outside the range that would support one to three tests, and it is

TABLE 3.4   Calculating Benefits and Optimal Level of Stool Guaiac Testing

Number of Tests	Cases Detected	Total Benefits	Total Costs	Net Benefits	Marginal Benefits	Marginal Costs
0	0	$0	$0	$0	$0	$0
1	648	$64,800,000	$2,464,800	$62,335,200	$64,800,000	$2,464,800
2	712.8	$71,280,000	$4,171,300	$67,108,700	$6,480,000	$1,706,500
3	719.28	$71,928,000	$5,551,900	$66,376,100	$648,000	$1,380,600
4	719.928	$71,992,800	$6,676,000	$65,316,800	$64,800	$1,124,100
5	719.9928	$71,999,280	$7,595,200	$64,404,080	$6,480	$919,200
6	719.99928	$71,999,928	$8,350,600	$63,649,328	$648	$755,400

Source: See Table 3.3. Table 3.4 assumes value of each case detected is $100,000. For alternate assumptions, see text.

certainly less than the $100 million needed to justify doing all six tests, as originally proposed. The Neuhauser and Lewicki study and subsequent cost-benefit studies were influential in convincing the American Cancer Society to revise its recommendations in 1980, and again in 1992, to take a more conservative stance. Now, routine stool guaiac screening is recommended only for individuals over age 50 or whose family history places them at high risk for colon cancer.[7]

This study illustrates several important elements of CBA. First, the marginal cost is often considerably different from the average cost. Second, the direct cost (screening) may be much less than the indirect costs of dealing with unintended side effects (e.g., from the barium-enema test to rule out cancer among those with false positive results). Together, these observations suggest the following *rule for making medicine cost-effective:* **target diagnosis and treatment of persons at highest risk.** However, this basic principle is routinely violated. Our desire to do as much as possible for as many people as possible means that effective screening programs are extended to everyone—including healthy young people with almost no risk of disease—making the marginal cost per case very high. At least some of the rapid increase in medical care costs can be attributed to this general failure to distinguish average costs from marginal costs, when marginal costs are most relevant to the question of how much medical care should be provided. Thousands of lives are saved by modern medicine each year, and more than 90 percent of those lives could still be saved even if half the medical care system were eliminated, as long as we continued to screen and treat those at highest risk.

3.3 MEASURING BENEFITS

For most medical programs, the three major types of benefits are as follows:

- Health
- Productivity
- Reductions in future medical costs

Health

Better health is the most direct and important gain from medical care. Yet it is often difficult to determine how much change in health status actually results from medical care, and how much results from waiting for things to heal, random variation, nutrition, and other factors. If a cancer patient lives eight months, is that six months longer than the patient would have had without treatment, or four months fewer, since chemotherapy is so toxic?[8] Such obstacles to valid measurement of the effects of treatment usually limit CBA to studies of large groups of patients where statistics can be used to estimate average effects. After the effect of therapy is measured, the problem of placing a dollar value on the improvement in health must be faced. If faster treatment can give the average heart-attack victim four more months of life, is that worth $1,000? $100,000? $1,000,000? Or perhaps $19.95? Most people would agree than gaining an extra year of life is worth more than $1,000 and less than $1,000,000. Deciding exactly where, within that range, the appropriation valuation lies is crucial in determining whether it is worth spending $50 million to upgrade the 911 emergency telephone system in order to treat people quicker. Some innovative techniques for measuring the value of life are explored in section 3.5, but it is important to recognize now how difficult and ambiguous the measurement process is. Most health care provides more subtle gains (e.g., physical therapy improves mobility, medication lessens the pain from a headache), which are even harder to measure in dollar terms.

A significant fraction of all visits to the doctor, perhaps as many as half, do not make a difference in health status. Either the symptoms that led people to seek care were not caused by anything serious, or the condition was such that medical care could not change the course of the disease. These visits provide care, reassurance, and social support, but not cure. The benefits of caring are often left uncounted because they are small relative to the gains from a dramatic cure. Also, much the same benefit can often be obtained regardless of the type or scientific validity of the treatment (e.g., a naturopath may provide sympathy as well as or better than a trained neurologist). When one considers how many more people obtain the benefits of caring from medical professionals than obtain large health gains from cures, the cumulative importance of subjective personal assessments look quite large.

Productivity

The earliest economists were not so much interested in the value of health itself, as in how much a healthier workforce could contribute to the economy. In 1667, Sir William Petty proposed a plan to improve the treatment of the plague in England and wrote an analysis showing that the additional costs would be more than covered by the additional taxes obtained from having more people at work.[9] When modern economists turned their attention to evaluating health programs in the 1950s and 1960s, the difficulty of directly measuring and valuing health improvements led them to consider increases in earnings due to greater life expectancy and reduced sick days as proxy measures. Such gains can be measured with precision, are objectively verifiable, and are easy to obtain from existing labor statistics. These advantages made earnings the primary measure of benefits in CBA for the next twenty years, but now they are considered inadequate. Are women's lives worth less than men's because women's earnings are lower on average? Are elderly people worthless once they stop working? Contributions to society through the labor market are a clear benefit of health care, but by themselves form an incomplete and biased measure.

Reductions in Future Medical Costs

Many diseases are less costly to treat if care is given early and if treatment is done correctly the first time. Vaccination now can prevent hospitalization in the future. Better infection control allows patients to be discharged from the hospital sooner. Yet good medical care is not always, or even usually, cheaper. The least expensive way to treat heart attacks is never to attempt resuscitation. A transplant may mean ten more years of life, but it will certainly mean hundreds of thousands of dollars in additional care. Reductions in cost, while not insignificant, can hardly constitute the primary justification for medical care.

3.4 MEASURING COSTS

Following are the primary types of medical costs:

- Medical care and administration
- Follow-up and treatment
- Time and pain of patient and family
- Provider time and inconvenience

Medical Care and Administration: Charges Versus Costs

Unlike prices for other goods, most medical prices are overstated to cover related expenses for education, research, community outreach, and care for patients who cannot pay. Health economists use three methods to determine the direct costs of medical care: adjusted charges, cost accounting, and extrapolation from comparable services.[10] **Adjusted charges** for U.S. hospital care are usually estimated by multiplying billed charges by the Medicare cost-to-charge ratio (see chapter 8, section 2). The actual cost of hospital services is, on average, only about 60 percent of billed charges. The cost of some services, such as laboratory work and drugs, may be as little as 15 percent of charges, while for ER and obstetric services, actual costs may be as much as 125 percent of billed charges. Per-unit costs are always estimates and are subject to interpretation, since they depend on numerous assumptions regarding overhead allocation, counting, and the averaging of quality and quantity. **Cost accounting** for CBA uses the same principles as job costing in other industries. Resources (e.g., nursing hours, technician time, space, supplies) are estimated from direct observation, and their costs are estimated using prevailing wages, prices, and so on. An overhead charge is then applied for administration, utilities, and other central services. Specialized job costing studies for the most expensive elements of care are often combined with the more readily available adjusted charges for other services. **Extrapolation from comparable services** is used when charges are not available and cost accounting is too time-consuming. For example, the cost of keeping patients in the hospital when they need only custodial care could be extrapolated from the cost of a day in a nursing home. Likewise, the cost of services provided by salaried physicians in a public health clinic may be extrapolated from adjusted charges for similar services in nearby communities.

Follow-up and Treatment

While direct costs are almost always counted, most medical care creates **secondary treatment costs,** which are not always counted. In the colon cancer example, the largest cost is not the screening test itself, but the additional laboratory work done on those who never had the disease but whose initial test results were false positive. Similarly, the surgical cost of a knee operation for a seventy-year old widower may be much less than the cost of post-operative admission to a nursing home for weeks of recovery because he cannot climb the stairs of his apartment. With surgery, it is usually necessary to include as a cost the possibility of serious complications and death, which are worse than the condition being treated. The point is that most medical care (and other human attempts to do good) involves many secondary or unintended effects that must be included to ensure that the cost accounting is comprehensive.

Time and Pain of Patient and Family

The time patients lose and the pain they suffer often outweigh direct medical costs. It is common to value patient time at the average wage rate for all employed workers, as was done for the traffic fatality (55 mph versus 65 mph) study discussed in section 3.1.[11] Using different rates for men and women, children, elderly people, and minorities usually contributes little to the analysis and may incorporate institutionalized discrimination. However, such differentials may explain many individual differences in behavior because they are very real to the person choosing whether to obtain care. Pain, suffering, anxiety, and death are most appropriately valued according to a person's willingness to pay. An analyst may not consider a particular patient's point of view and his or her specific pain and time costs, which could explain why many beneficial treatments are not sought.

Provider Time and Inconvenience

The supply-side reason for not undertaking many medical activities is that providers are not compensated for their time and inconvenience. For example, while there is a tremendous need for organ donations, the physicians who must obtain the families' consent are the ER doctors, neurosurgeons, and internists present at death who find it burdensome to speak with the families and try to get them to agree to donate their loved ones' organs. Taking time to explain the issues, dealing with emotional distress, and facing frequent refusals are costs for which they obtain no direct benefits. Such "hassle costs" are a disincentive that greatly reduces the number of organs made available for transplant. Similarly, the requirements that every hospital admission or referral to a specialist be documented imposes a hassle cost on the primary physician, and leads predictably to a lower number of hospital days and specialist referrals. This reduction in services may make it look as if managed care plans ration the number of services to reduce costs and make profits. However, it is important to remember that the services forgone are those which the patient's physician was unwilling to write a letter or make a phone call to support and, therefore, are unlikely to have been considered critically important.

3.5 THE VALUE OF LIFE

> "A man who knows the price of everything and the value of nothing."
> — *Oscar Wilde's definition of a cynic*

Isn't health priceless? Some patients and physicians protest that it is impossible to measure the priceless benefits of medical care with the crude yardstick of money. Regardless of whether people think it is right or proper, their actions place a dollar value on human life when they make a decision to provide or deny treatment. If an 87-year-old patient in heart failure is transferred from a nursing home to a cardiac care unit for ten days, the physician affirms through his or her actions that living another six months in a nursing home is worth more than $15,000. Immediately discharging this patient with instructions to take four aspirin every six hours affirms the physician's belief that it is not. Our actions place a dollar value on life even if we do not choose to recognize this fact. We live in a world of scarce resources and must make decisions within these limitations. We place a value on (and a limit on the value of) health whether we wish to or not, with money as a generalized expression of this value.* Perhaps the most important role of economists in the CBA of health care is pointing out this reality.

Valuing human life places special but unavoidable demands on economists. For activities that are traded in the market, such as medical care, work time, drugs, and transportation, valuation may be complicated by risk and discounting, or blurred by overhead allocation and wage differentials. Nevertheless, the process of connecting resources and

---

*A decision maker's preferences are said to be "lexicographic" when everything depends on one factor, with other factors allowed to affect choice only when they are equal to the primary factor. For example, a parent might say to a physician, "Do whatever you can to minimize my child's chance of dying. Given that, if one treatment is less painful, or costs less, you can do that one." This decision is lexicographic since one factor, the probability of the child's survival, dominates all others. In such a case, there are no trade-offs and hence no necessity to make an economic analysis such as a CBA. Computers sort alphabetical lists lexicographically: by the first letter, then by the second, and so on. People often claim that one thing is important above all others (survival, honor, religious purity) even though most behavior indicates that trade-offs are made. Even saints respond to pain, and parents are not acting nobly if they do everything to try to save one child and in the process harm their other children and their own lives. Arguing that medical decisions should only be based on costs when there is no chance that doing so will affect quality or risk lives is the same as saying that money does not matter in the real world.

program effects to specific dollar amounts is understandable and familiar. Considerations of life and death or pain and suffering are not so clear. Since there is no explicit market for post-operative pain and mortality, a way must be found to reflect the value that people place on these events. By choosing to buy a car that is cheaper but less safe, a person is making an implicit trade between money and the risk of dying. That trade is also made in buying smoke detectors, choosing to accept a more dangerous job assignment for higher pay, refusing to fill a prescription because it costs too much, and flying to the Mayo Clinic to get the best possible treatment for a rare disease. People buy and sell health all the time, but they do not do so in an organized market like the New York Stock Exchange. **Economists do not put a value on life or illness; they measure the value that consumers put on life and illness as shown by their behavior.**

One attempt to provide an explicit dollar value for life is described by Michael Jones-Lee.[12] It was observed that people would run across a highway (at a small but noticeable risk of dying) rather than spend the time going around to a pedestrian overpass. Through observations and questionnaires, it was established that people were willing to accept a risk of .000002 of death to save seven minutes (0.117 hours) of walking. Valuing their time by an average wage rate of $20, the value of life as can be extrapolated as follows:

Value of Life: Jones-Lee Approach

$$\text{Value of Life} = \frac{(\text{Value of Time}) \times (\text{Hours used})}{(\text{Risk of death per hour saved})} = \frac{\$20 \times .117}{.000002} = \$1,170,000$$

A more sophisticated approach is to consider the value of life as the additional wages required to get someone to take a more dangerous job. A statistical regression[13] of the association between wages and risk showed that for each .0001 increase in risk of death, there was an additional $240 in annual salary; therefore, the estimated value of life measured by the method used in this study was $240 ÷ .0001 = $2.4 million. Other studies using similar methods have estimated values of life from $800,000 to $6 million.[14] One problem with occupational risk estimates is selection bias: the people who are less risk-averse or mistakenly underestimate the true risk are the ones most likely to apply for the more dangerous jobs. A study that captures the behavior of the more safety-conscious individuals was conducted by Rachel Dardis.[15] The author measured the number of people purchasing smoke detectors as a function of price to construct a demand curve (Figure 3.3). In 1974, the price of a smoke detector was $52, and only 1.8 million were sold (adjusted for inflation, $52 in 1974 is worth $177 in 2002, and Dardis estimated an annualized operating cost per household of $24 in 2002 dollars). By 1979, the price had declined to $12, and 10 million were sold (which is $28, inflation-adjusted, and yields an annualized cost of $3 a year). Each smoke detector was estimated to result in a .000036 reduction in the risk of death and a .000023 reduction in the risk of injury. Using these probabilities, Dardis estimated that those who purchased smoke detectors when they first came on the market at $177 made decisions consistent with a value of life of $2 million; those who waited until prices dropped to below $30 implied a lower value of life, less than $400,000. The Dardis smoke detector study brings home the relevance of the first law of demand: even for life itself, people will buy less as the price increases.

We must all die sometime; therefore, no medical treatment can truly save a life. A problem with efforts to estimate the value of life is that the rhetoric itself reinforces denial, making it seem as if the purpose of medical care is to save lives. The real task of medicine is to reduce suffering and anxiety while extending the expected length of life by a few years. Glorified language can thwart clear thought and practical action. It may provide a convenient way to avoid admitting in public that the life of an eight-year-old child is valued more

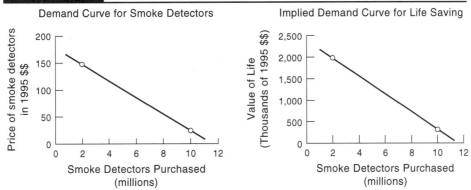

FIGURE 3.3 Value of Life: Smoke Detector Study

Changes in the number of smoke detectors purchased as prices fell from $150 in 1974 to $24 in 1979 are interpreted as a derived demand for life saving, implying a "value of like" demand that exceeds $2,000,000 for early purchasers, and $305,000 for late purchasers.

Source: Rachel Dardis, *American Economic Review,* 70: 1077–1082, 1980.

than the life of an eighty-year-old grandparent. Such avoidance does not make the difference in valuation any less true. Economists use the decisions made by state legislatures, families, and patients to show that they value the length and quality of life, which can be changed by medical care, rather than the fact of mortality, which cannot.

3.6 QUALITY-ADJUSTED LIFE YEARS (QALYs)

The average dollar cost of providing one additional year of life expectancy has become a standard method for evaluating many health programs. Yet a year spent sick and in pain is worth less than a year lived in perfect health, free of symptoms. A significant risk of surgical mortality may be worth accepting to treat a disease and alleviate pain. But how much risk? Researchers use econometrics, surveys, and professional judgments to estimate the value of a year spent in different states of disability.[16] Such **quality-adjusted life years (QALYs)** rate quality of life between 0.0 (death) and good health (1.00). In the survey results presented in Table 3.5, respondents indicated that living for three months confined to a hospital for tuberculosis treatment was worth only 1.8 months (.60 × 3 months) of regular time spent at home in good health.[17] The value of living in the hospital declines further when it is not temporary, but permanent. Living ten more years confined in a hospital being treated for a contagious disease was considered to be worth only 1.6 years of normal life. Although such conditions were not included in this survey, people consider some illnesses to be worse than death; therefore, each additional year lived in such misery has a negative value.

Discounting Over Time

The value of an additional year of life fifteen years from now is worth less than increasing the probability of living today. The *present value* of an additional year of life obtained fifteen years from now is calculated by discounting over time, the same as the present value of an additional dollar obtained fifteen years from now. If the rate of discount (interest rate) is 5 percent, the present value of receiving a dollar next year is $1 \div (1.05) = \$0.952$,

TABLE 3.5	Quality of Life Adjustment Factors	
Duration	**Health State**	**Adjustment**
	Reference State: Perfect Health	**1.00**
3 months	Home confinement, tuberculosis	0.68
3 months	Home confinement, contagious disease	0.65
3 months	Hospital dialysis	0.62
3 months	Hospital confinement, tuberculosis	0.60
3 months	Hospital confinement, contagious disease	0.56
3 months	Depression	0.44
3 months	Home dialysis	0.65
8 years	Mastectomy for injury	0.63
8 years	Kidney transplant	0.58
8 years	Hospital dialysis	0.56
8 years	Mastectomy for breast cancer	0.48
8 years	Hospital confinement, contagious disease	0.33
life	Home dialysis	0.40
life	Hospital dialysis	0.32
life	Hospital confinement, contagious disease	0.16
	Reference State: Dead	**0.00**

Source: Sackett, D. L., and G. W. Torrance, (1978). "The Utility of Different Health States as Perceived by the General Public." *Journal of Chronic Diseases* 31 (11): 697–704.

and the present value of receiving a dollar in fifteen years is $1 \div (1.05)^{15} = \$0.479$. Analogously, the 5 percent discounted value of an additional year of life fifteen years from now is about half the current value.

QALY League Tables

The costs of medical care can be compared with benefits by calculating the cost per adjusted year of life gained. On the benefit side, each additional life year is discounted for risk (expected value), time, and quality of life. On the cost side, adjustments are made for any differences between charges and actual costs, expected reductions in days lost from work, and reductions in the cost of medical care for related conditions. Consider the hypothetical example in Table 3.6. The patient can expect to live three years with medications alone, but will live five years, with a better quality of life, if the surgery is successful. However, the surgery is effective only 40 percent of the time, it costs $30,000, and there is a 3 percent chance of immediate death due to surgical mortality. The estimated cost per QALY gained is $44,000. Similar estimates have been made for a number of medical interventions so that relative costs can be calculated and presented in QALY league tables, such as Table 3.7.[18] From these results, it can be seen that it costs more than seven times as much ($15,000 versus $2,000) to increase QALYs by one year with a heart transplant as it does with a pacemaker implant. Trying to extend and improve life by using coronary artery bypass grafting to treat minor two-vessel disease with mild angina is still more expensive, $42,000 per QALY gained. QALY rankings can be used to assess which medical treatments should be expanded and which should be cut back to optimize system efficiency. When the state of Oregon decided in 1993 to enroll more poor residents in its Medicaid program, funding those extra people by eliminating coverage of medical services deemed to be of lowest benefit, legislators used a decision-making process analogous to the construction of a QALY league table.

| TABLE 3.6 | Hypothetical QALY Calculation Example |

	Year 1	Year 2	Year 3	Year 4	Year 5	Total
Time discounting factor	1.00	0.95	0.91	0.86	0.82	
Baseline						
Quality of life	0.60	0.50	0.40	*(dead)*	*(dead)*	
Discounted value	0.60	0.48	0.36	0.00	0.00	1.44
Quality adjusted life expectancy without surgery, 1.44 years						
Successful surgery						
Quality of life	0.90	0.80	0.70	0.60	0.50	
Discounted value	0.90	0.76	0.63	0.52	0.41	3.23
Quality adjusted life expectancy without surgery, 3.23 years						
Net gain in QALYs			1.79	*(3.23–1.44 discounted years)*		
Probability			40%			
Expected value			0.72			
Less surgical mortality			−0.04	*(3% of baseline 1.44 years)*		
Expected net QALY gain			0.68			
Cost of surgery			$30,000			
Cost per QALY gained			$44,000	*($30,000 ÷ 0.68)*		

| TABLE 3.7 | QALY "League Table" |

Treatment	Present Value of Extra Cost Per QALY
Physician advice for smoking cessation	$450
Pacemaker implantation for heart block	$1,900
Hip replacement	$2,000
CABG for severe angina LMD	$2,800
Control of total serum cholesterol	$4,600
CABG for severe angina 2VD	$6,200
Kidney transplant	$8,200
Breast cancer screening	$9,500
Heart transplant	$14,000
CABG for mild angina 2VD	$35,000
Hospital hemodialysis	$38,000

CABG: "coronary artery bypass graft."
LMD: "left main disease."
2VD: "two vessel disease."
Source: A. Williams, "Economics of Coronary Artery Bypass Grafting,"
British Medical Journal, 291: 326–329 (1995).

3.7 PERSPECTIVES: PATIENT, PAYER, GOVERNMENT, PROVIDER, SOCIETY

How much has to be paid for treatment, and how much the treatment is worth, depends on whose perspective the cost-benefit analyst is taking. From the individual's point of view, treatment that makes an infectious disease less communicable is of no direct benefit, and medical costs may be relatively unimportant because he or she has insurance.

From a group perspective, reducing communicability to neighbors is a major benefit of treatment, and hospital charges are important because total insurance premiums for the group as a whole will rise. The broadest perspective is that of society as a whole, including future generations.

Many of the conflicts over health policy arise from the difference in perspectives of different groups. For gay men in San Francisco, many of whom are infected with HIV, research and prevention of AIDS is the most important health issue of our time, while finding drugs to assist in stroke rehabilitation is not.[19] For residents of the Christian Acres Retirement Community in a small Midwestern town, these priorities may be reversed. An economist hired by Medicare to do a CBA on whether a new type of surgery should be covered must ask, "Am I to consider primarily the effects on the Medicare budget, or should I also include benefits to hospitals, doctors, and state legislatures?" The treatment of taxes and transfers is crucial in this regard. If new Medicare regulations cost Medicare $100, but reduce state Medicaid expenditures by $40, is that reduction to be counted? From the state's perspective, it is a windfall gain of $40. From the perspective of the U.S. budget and the Medicare administrator, it is a cost of $100. From a social perspective, the shifting of costs from state to federal budgets is irrelevant, and the cost is the net amount, $60. Consider also the effect of taxes. If a 10 percent tax on health care raises the price of a visit to the doctor from $20 to $22, the extra $2 is a relevant cost to the patient or the insurance plan, but not to society. If there were no "health taxes," that $2 would have to be obtained elsewhere by raising other taxes or by reducing government spending, perhaps on roads or defense.

Distribution: Whose Costs and Whose Benefits?

In the real world, people may think that they should consider benefits to society as a whole, but they act according to a more immediate calculus of benefits and costs to themselves as individuals and to the groups (teenagers, steelworkers, residents of Lancaster, Hispanics, senior citizens) to which they belong. A major barrier to actually implementing a project is raised by the following question: What about the losers? Laser surgery for cancer may help thousands of people who would not have survived with the chemotherapy previously used, but it will kill some people who would have lived. Development of a new home health system means that the hospital down the street will find even more of its beds empty and will have to lay off some employees. It is almost impossible to make a major change that hurts no one. Unfortunately, it is also almost impossible for a politician to vote for a project that clearly hurts some identifiable person. Programs are more likely to pass when the costs are diffused over a large number of people and thus are difficult to identify. For example, a requirement for more extensive testing of drugs or better disposal of toxic waste leads to a general rise in the cost of medicine. Even though in total it amounts to millions of dollars, it takes only a few pennies per prescription and thus is ignored. Conversely, imposing a loss of a few thousand dollars on a single individual or firm is sufficient to get them to file a lawsuit to stop the program. The relative power of the group that must bear most of the costs often determines the political feasibility of any change.

CBA Is a Limited Perspective

While CBA is a powerful tool for policy analysis, it can be quite limited. It is impossible to do an economic analysis unless the medical facts are well known. How many people have the disease, what is the cure rate from therapy, and what levels of disability are likely to result? These clinical questions must be answered before any assessment of costs and benefits is attempted. The strength of CBA as a tool lies in its ability to interpret medical issues as choices in a market. Yet to do so, it must force health and human caring into such a rigid economic model that it tends to overemphasize efficiency and may entirely fail to recognize the most important ethical and social values that underlie medical practice. Medicine as a profession rests on the dignity and sanctity of life, a philosophy and practice that resists overt commercialization.

CBA and Public Policy Decision Making

Cost benefit analysis is a way of looking at past behavior, at decisions actually made, so that future decisions can become more clear, rational, and consistent. A decision being made by a single person was used in the knee injury example. In practice, CBAs are almost never done for a single case since it takes too long, costs too much, and depends on statistical assumptions that are more valid for large groups. When a single person is involved, that person knows his or her personal costs and willingness to pay better than any analyst. Formal analyses are apt to be most useful under the following circumstances:

- Large amounts of resources (millions or billions of dollars) are involved.
- Responsibility for decisions is fragmented (government agencies, large corporations).
- The goals and objectives of different groups are at odds or unclear.
- Alternative courses of action are radically different.
- The technology and risks underlying each alternative are well understood.
- A long time frame is involved (e.g., strategy versus management).

Econometrics, balance sheets, surveys, decision trees, and other tools of the economics trade are usually applied to large projects and long-standing problems. For example, is screening blood donors for HIV and hepatitis worthwhile? How often should they be screened, and with what tests? Is inpatient alcohol treatment better than outpatient and, if so, is it enough to justify the increase in costs? The treatment of millions of people costing billions of dollars over many years is involved in these issues, each of which has been given full formal CBA. The test of what is important ultimately lies in the judgment of those who are most affected by the decision. Health CBA almost always counts two things, death and money, because they are routinely recorded. A good analysis is able to capture other factors that are significant and yet keep the presentation simple enough that the costs and benefits of alternative courses of action are clearly seen.

SUGGESTIONS FOR FURTHER READING

David M. Cutler and Mark McClellan, "Is Technological Change in Medicine Worth It?" *Health Affairs* 20, no.5 (September 2001): 11–29.

A.S. Detsky, "A Clinician's Guide to Cost-Effectiveness Analysis," *Annals of Internal Medicine* 113, no. 2 (July 15, 1990): 147–154.

Michael F. Drummond, Greg L. Stoddart, and George W. Torrance, *Methods for the Economic Evaluation of Health Programmes* (Oxford: Oxford University Press, 1997).

J.M. Eisenberg, "Clinical Economics: A Guide to the Economic Analysis of Clinical Practices," *Journal of the American Medical Association* 262 (1989): 2879–2886.

M.R. Gold, J.E. Siegal, L.B. Russel, M.C. Weinstein, eds., *Cost–Effectiveness in Health and Medicine* (New York: Oxford University Press, 1996).

B.J. O'Brien, D. Helyland, W.S. Richardson, M. Levine, and M.F. Drummond, "Users Guides to the Medical Literature XIII: How to Use an Article on Economic Analysis of Clinical Practice (B)—What Are the Results and Will They Help Me in Caring for My Patients," *Journal of the American Medical Association* 227 (1997): 1802–1806.

Martin I. Meltzer, "Introduction to Health Economics for Physicians," *The Lancet* 358 (September 22, 2001): 993–998. Available free from www.theLancet.com.

T.O. Tengs, M.E. Adams, J.S. Pliskin, et al., "Five Hundred Life Saving Interventions and Their Cost-Effectiveness," *Risk Analysis* 15 (1995): 369–90.

M.A. Testa and D.C. Simonson, "Assessment of Quality of Life Outcomes," *New England Journal of Medicine* 334 (1996): 835–840.

Mark S. Thompson, "Willingness to Pay and Accept Risks to Cure Chronic Disease," *American Journal of Public Health* 76, no.4 (1988): 392–396.

SUMMARY

1. **Every act is a judgment about value.** When people act, they show by that act that they think the gains are worth more than the costs. Economists look at decisions patients and physicians have made in the past to estimate the value they place on health outcomes.

2. **Cost-benefit analysis (CBA)** does not make decisions. It is a **framework** that can be used to make the decision-making process more rational, more consistent, and more clearly communicated. The cost-benefit analyst organizes the facts provided by clinicians and the public's values to present data in a way that is useful for making policy decisions. Although some form of cost-benefit trade-off occurs in virtually all decisions made by consumers, a formal CBA is used only for large-scale government or corporate projects with a long time frame and many parties involved in the decision-making process.

3. **Cost-effectiveness analysis (CEA)** compares the cost of two different methods of reaching the same goal (immunizing 100 children, preventing 10 cases of flu, adding one extra year of life) but does not attempt to measure the benefits in dollars.

4. The appropriate measure of costs is the **opportunity cost** (i.e., what is given up). The appropriate measure of benefits is **willingness to pay (WTP),** what the patient or society is willing to give up to attain an improvement in health.

5. In choosing between alternatives, it is the change in benefits (**marginal benefits**) and the change in costs (**marginal costs**) that matter, not the average or per person value.

6. **Marginalism** is the process of trying out small adjustments and moving always in the direction of adjustments that make things better, until no further improvements are possible. With marginalism, we do not need to know whether a decision is good or bad, only whether it makes things better or worse. If a manager keeps choosing in a way that makes things better, eventually the organization will reach the best possible decision (i.e., its **optimum**). Economists have found that to evaluate an organization they need not look at everything, but rather need only to examine the organization's **behavior at the margin** to determine whether it can do better.

7. The primary **benefits** to be accounted for in health care projects are as follows:
    a. Health (extend life or reduce morbidity and pain)
    b. Productivity (decrease time lost from work)
    c. Reductions in future medical costs

8. Following are the major categories of **costs** to be accounted for:
    a. Medical care and administration
    b. Follow-up and treatment damages (side effects)
    c. Time and pain of patient and family
    d. Provider time and inconvenience

9. Since marginal benefits are usually declining and lower than the average benefits as health programs increase in size, it is important to **target treatment toward those individuals most in need.** Many useful medical technologies become wasteful when they are expanded to include low-risk individuals.

10. Benefits are rarely certain. The **expected value** of a medical treatment is the product of the likelihood of success multiplied by the magnitude of the health gain that will occur if treatment is successful. A useful shorthand for dealing with risk is to examine whether:

    (Probability of Gain) × (Benefit) > (Probability of Loss) × (Cost)

11. Years of life must be discounted if the quality of life is reduced. Questionnaires are used to estimate how many years of life a person with a disability would be willing to give up to gain one additional year of life without the disability, or to reduce the risk of death. In this way, **comparisons can be made between treatment alternatives in terms of quality-adjusted life years** or **QALYs.** Since an additional year of life expectancy in the distant future is worth less than an increase in health now, it is also necessary to use an interest rate to discount benefits over time.

12. Comparing medical therapies in standardized units, such as cost per QALY gained, can help decision makers determine which programs should be expanded and which should be cut back, and thus lead to better public policy.

PROBLEMS

1. {*expected value*} **a.** Successful rehabilitation of a shoulder injury obviates the need for reconstructive surgery costing $6,000. However, rehabilitation is successful only 70 percent of the time. What is the expected value of rehabilitation?

   b. Treatment for endocarditis is risky. The patient will either (a) die in the hospital, (b) partially recover, or (c) fully recover. With full recovery, the patient can expect to live for another 20 years, but only 25 percent of patients fully recover. With partial recovery, the patient can expect to live 10 more years. However, 20 percent of patients die in the hospital. Assuming patients usually live just one year without treatment, what is the expected value of the treatment expressed as additional years of life?

2. {*marginal cost*} **a.** A course of chemotherapy costs $8,000. If give to patient A, it will increase life expectancy by two months; for patient B, by six months; for patient C, by one month; for patient D, by five months; and for patient E, by four months. If all five patients are treated, what is the average cost per year of life gained? If only one patient can be treated, which one should it be? If only two patients are treated, which ones should they be? What is the marginal cost per additional year of life for the patient most likely to benefit? What is the marginal cost per additional year of life for the patient least likely to benefit? Draw the total and marginal benefit curves (label the Y axis "Years of life gained" and the X axis "Number of patients treated"). If all five patients are treated, what is the average cost per year of life gained? The marginal cost? If patients are treated in alphabetical order, which one determines the marginal cost per year of life gained, patient A, patient E, or some other patient?

   {*demand curve*} **b.** Assuming that each additional year of life is worth $60,000, draw the demand curve for chemotherapy. Draw the supply curve. What is the relationship between the demand curve and the total and marginal benefit curves you drew in part A of this question?

3.   {*downward-sloping demand*} Government programs that send doctors to reduce infant mortality direct most of the doctors to poorer neighborhoods. Pediatricians setting up new practices are more likely to locate in wealthier neighborhoods. Explain why both doctors can be said to be obeying the "law of downward-sloping demand," even though they move toward opposite ends of the income distribution.

4.   {*direct versus indirect costs*} A school district determines that less than 70 percent of first-grade students have completed all recommended immunizations. A task force suggests two ways to reach the goal of 95 percent immunization: (1) hire 20 visiting nurses to do outreach in the community or (2) pass a law mandating that children will not be allowed to attend school unless they bring documentation showing evidence of complete immunization. Which plan is more cost-effective? How is the distribution of costs and benefits different under the two plans?

5.   {*need versus demand, opportunity cost*} Many experts recommend that people get at least 30 minutes of vigorous exercise three to five times a week; however, actual participation in exercise is less than the amount (a) needed or (b) demanded? Why do most college students get more exercise in summer than in winter? Does need, demand, or a difference in the opportunity cost of time account for the fact that most actors get more exercise than most accountants?

6.   The World Health Organization (WHO) is considering sending in a team of experts to deal with an outbreak of schistosomiasis in a distant country. Sending a larger team will allow WHO to prevent more fatalities, and they estimate the following effectiveness:

# of team members	# of deaths
0 (i.e., no action)	1,200
5	500
10	200
15	100
20	60
25	40
30	30
35	25
40	22
45	20
50	20

a. It costs $5,000 for each team member sent. Calculate the *total, average,* and *marginal* cost of life saving through this effort and display it on a graph. If saving a life is valued at $100,000, what is the optimal number of people WHO should send to combat the epidemic? If saving a life is valued at $10,000, what is the optimal number? What team size gives the most "bang for the buck" (i.e., the largest number of lives saved per dollar spent)?

b. Each person sent must be taken away from a disease-fighting team at work elsewhere in the world. What is the appropriate opportunity cost measure of sending people to fight the new epidemic: the transportation cost of $5,000 or the reduction of life-saving efforts from the job they are pulled away from?

7.   {*willingness to pay*} What determines the value of a cure for acne? For ALS (amyloid lateral sclerosis, or Lou Gehrig's disease)? For Alzheimer's disease? Which discovery is worth more to a pharmaceutical firm that is able to patent a cure?

8. {*QALYs*} Patient BN is a 36-year-old female with a type of organ failure that reduces her quality of life to half of what it would be in good health. Without treatment she can expect to live only two years. With a successful transplant, BN can expect to live four years and have a quality of life that is near (80 percent) of what she would enjoy in good health. However, the transplant costs $100,000, plus $10,000 each year for drugs and follow-up care, and carries a 15 percent risk of rejection resulting in immediate death. What is the cost per additional year of life gained (without discounting for time or quality of life)? What is the cost per discounted QALY gained (assuming a 5 percent time discount rate)?

9. {*interest rates and future value*} As a health economist for the U.S. Centers for Disease Control and Prevention, you have been asked to analyze a number of programs targeting different diseases and recommend which should receive priority, given that budgets are limited. As part of your analysis, you will have to determine what interest rate is appropriate for discounting future costs and benefits. You are going to be visited by an economist from AARP, formerly the American Association of Retired Persons, and another economist from the Children's Defense Fund. Which group will lobby harder for a lower discount rate? Why?

ENDNOTES

1. Michael Drummond, *Principles of Economic Appraisal in Health Care* (Cambridge: Oxford University Press, 1981), 17. Several sources and texts are listed at the end of this chapter as suggestions for further reading. Good current examples of cost-benefit analyses and reviews of the literature can be found in journals such as *Health Economics, American Journal of Public Health, Medical Decision Making, New England Journal of Medicine,* and *Journal of the American Medical Association.*

2. Orley Ashenfelter and Michael Greenstone, "Using Mandated Speed Limits to Measure the Value of a Statistical Life," *National Bureau of Economic Research Working Paper w9094,* August 2002 (http://www.nber.org/papers/w9094).

3. S. R. Garfield, et al., "Evaluation of an Ambulatory Medical Care Delivery System," *New England Journal of Medicine* 294, no. 8 (1976): 426–431; P. J. Wagner and J. E. Hendrich, "Physician Views on Frequent Medical Use: Patient Beliefs and Demographic and Diagnostic Correlates," *Journal of Family Practice* 36, no. 4 (1993): 417–422.

4. The "law of large numbers" says that the observed average will be close to the "true" mean if the number of observations is large enough.

5. Duncan Neuhauser and Ann Lewicki, "What Do We Gain from the Sixth Stool Guaiac?" *New England Journal of Medicine* 293 (1975): 226–228.

6. Some of the assumptions used by Neuhauser and Lewicki have been modified slightly to facilitate exposition. For a more current assessment of the sensitivity and specificity of stool guaiac screening tests, see J. E. Allison et al., "A Comparison of Fecal Occult-Blood Tests for Colorectal-Cancer Screening," *New England Journal of Medicine* 334 (1996): 155–159, and for a critical assessment of the assumptions presented there, see the editorial by D. F. Ransohoff and C. A. Lang in the same issue, pp. 189–190.

7. American Cancer Society, "Guidelines for the Cancer-Related Checkup: Recommendations and Rationale," *CA—A Cancer Journal for Clinicians,* 30 (1980): 230; Bernard Levin and Gerald Murphy, "Revision in American Cancer Society Recommendations for the Early Detection of Colorectal Cancer," *CA—A Cancer Journal for Clinicians,* 42, no. 5 (1992): 296–299.

8. Michael Ibrahim, "Rules of Evidence," in *Epidemiology and Health Policy* (Rockville, Md.: Aspen Press, 1985), 39–49.

9. Sir William Petty, *The Economic Writings of Sir William Petty,* ed. Charles Henry Hull, [1662-1687] reprint (New York: AM Kelley, 1963), 108. This anthology includes *A Treatise of Taxes and Contributions* (1662), *Political Arithmetik* (1676), and other writings. Petty's plan primarily involved the forced closure of houses where the plague appeared, with resettlement of the families at government expense at farms forty miles outside of London for three months. Arguably the first real economist, Petty was no stranger to self-interest or pride. He asked that two percent of the net increase in tax revenues from his plague treatment plan be given to him as a reward from the King for his brilliant idea. He did not fully specify how those gains would be figured. Had he done so, health economists today might be much more effective, competing for millions of dollars in health benefits royalties.

10. Thomas E. Getzen, "Medical Care Price Indexes: Theory, Construction and Empirical Analysis of the U.S. Series 1927-1990," *Advances in Health Economics* 13 (Greenwich, Conn.: JAI Press, 1992): 83–128.

11. See the discussion in the "Suggested Readings" by Drummond et al. and others.

12. Michael W. Jones-Lee, *The Economics of Safety and Physical Risk* (Oxford: Blackwell, 1989), 67, based on data and extrapolations from S. J. Melinek, "A Method of Evaluating Life for Economic Purposes," *Accident Analysis and Prevention* 6 (1974): 103–114.

13. *Regression Analysis* is covered in virtually all standard statistics textbooks. There is also a short description provided in S. Folland, A. Goodman, and M. Stano, *The Economics of Health and Health Care* (Upper Saddle River, N.J.: Prentice Hall, 2001), 59–67.

14. M. Moore and W. Kip Viscusi, "Quality Adjusted Value of Life," *Economic Inquiry* 26 (1988): 369–388.

15. Rachel Dardis, "The Value of a Life: New Evidence from the Marketplace," *American Economic Review* 70 (December 1980):1077–1082.

16. M.E.Backhouse, R.J. Backhouse, and S.A. Edley, "Economic Evaluation Bibliography," *Health Economics* 1(Supplement) (1992): 1–236. John Hutton and Alan Maynard, "A NICE Challenge for Health Economics," *Health Economics* 9, no.2 (2000): 89– 94.

17. D. L. Sackett and D. W. Torrance, "The Utility of Different Health States as Perceived by the General Public," *Journal of Chronic Diseases* 31, no.11 (1978): 697– 704.

18. Alan Williams, "Economics of Coronary Artery Bypass Grafting," *British Medical Journal,* 291 (1985): 326–329; Julia Fox-Rushby, Anne Mills, and Damian Walker, "Setting Health Priorities: The Development of Cost-effectiveness League Tables," *Bulletin of the World Health Organization* 79, no. 7 (July 2001): 679–680; Tammy O Tengs et al., "Five Hundred Life-saving Interventions and Their Cost-effectiveness," *Risk Analysis* 15, no. 3 (1995): 369–390.

19. T. R. Fanning et al., "The Epidemiology of AIDS in the New York and California Medicaid Programs," *Journal of Acquired Immune Deficiency Syndromes* 4 (1991): 1025–1035.

CHAPTER **4**

INSURANCE

QUESTIONS

1. Who takes care of people when they need medical care they cannot afford?
2. Who pays for losses: insurance companies or the people who buy insurance?
3. How does pooling of funds reduce exposure to risks?
4. Is a favor from a friend similar to a loan from a bank?
5. Do insurance companies take risks, or do they just put a price on risks?
6. What is an "actuarially fair" premium?
7. Are people who think they will become sick more likely to obtain insurance?
8. Are people with insurance more likely to sustain a financial loss?
9. Does insurance increase or decrease the demand for medical care?

Breaking an arm, catching pneumonia, having a heart attack—there are a dizzying array of risks that could disrupt your life. We hope none of these bad things will happen, but if they do, most of us can rely on insurance to cover some of our financial losses. From an individual perspective, insurance generates net benefits by allowing trade between two possible states of the world: a little money in the usual state (when a person is healthy) is given up to get a lot of money in the unusual and more difficult state (when a person is sick). From society's point of view, insurance is a method of pooling risk so that one person's loss is shared across many people rather than being borne by that person alone. If all people contribute, the pool of collected funds will be sufficient to compensate the unlucky few. All participants gain peace of mind, knowing that they can obtain necessary medical care with limited financial risk. The next two chapters examine the operations, history, and theory of health insurance. To grasp how insurance works , it is necessary to understand that it is a means for both individual maximization of utility and for social promotion of group values such as respect for life, care of people with disabilities, equal opportunity, and political unity.

4.1 METHODS FOR COVERING RISKS

What would you do if you broke your arm? Who would take care of you? How would you eat and pay your rent while you were out of work? Who would pay for the doctor and hospital care? There are several ways this loss could be covered.

Savings

The first economic consequence of a loss is to use savings to pay for current expenses. *Savings* can be thought of as a trade between time periods. People do not save to pile up money. They save so that they can consume more in the future, either because they plan to do so (e.g., for retirement or a vacation) or to protect themselves against the unexpected (e.g., accident, illness). Savings provide a buffer against random losses, smoothing out consumption over time so that you can still eat if you are not working, still pay the rent if you incur a $600 doctor bill immediately after your vacation, and still pay tuition bills if you need expensive prescription drugs to get you through your final exams. The ability to smooth out the amount of consumption over time improves utility. The difference between a planned variation (a vacation trip) and a risk (a broken leg) is the element of uncertainty. Saving is limited as a risk management tool because it allows individuals only to trade with themselves at different time periods; it does not spread a catastrophic loss over a large group of people so that it can be borne more easily. Although people can plan a vacation or retirement within their budgets, they may face an extraordinary loss (e.g., spinal injury, cranial fracture) that is far too expensive to be handled by their own resources.

Family and Friends

Young people who have not had a chance to accumulate their own savings must depend on their families' financial resources to carry them during an illness. Although family assistance may be freely and generously given, it creates an obligation to pay your family back when you are well, to be grateful, and to help other family members in the future when they need it. Thus, the family engages in a form of exchange among people as well as among time periods.[1] Your current loss is covered by someone else's current savings, which gives you an obligation to cover someone else's loss in the future. Whereas individual savings allow one person to trade among his or her own time periods to optimize consumption, families trade over time and people; therefore, they can absorb the shock of a loss without a disastrous decline in living standards more effectively than an individual alone.

Favors that friends do for each other occur so frequently and unconsciously that it seems strange to look at them as trades. When I carry books for someone whose leg is in a cast or take notes for a classmate who has the flu, I am simply being nice and not looking to receive anything in return. Yet ultimately, families and friendship are based on a sense of mutual obligation and reciprocity.[2] If someone consistently fails to help me, eventually I will stop being helpful to him or her. Furthermore, I might let others know how inconsiderate and selfish that person is so that they won't waste their time assisting him or her. It is by such means that the informal rules of exchange among friends and families are enforced. Helping out might not be legally binding, but it is socially binding.

Charity

The obligation to help extends beyond friends and family to people we have never, and may never, meet and who can do nothing for us in return. We still care about people even if we don't know them. Mutual caring makes people a society rather than just a random collection of individuals.[3] The first hospitals were caring institutions, substitute homes for people who did not have a home, and for people who were ill or had a disability but whose families were too poor to take care of them.[4] Charity as a means of social exchange predates formal insurance contracts by thousands of years and has been far more important as a way to pay medical bills for most of that time. Yet charity is limited in scope and the extent to which most people feel responsible for someone else's misfortune has declined as formal market institutions have arisen to provide coverage for risks.

Private Market Insurance Contracts

Bad things happen. We cannot always do anything about them. When we can do something, it often costs a great deal of money. Suppose that I am one of one hundred middle-aged executives sent by XXumma Corp. to Eastern Europe for a year. We can assume that several of us will get sick during the year. Suppose we knew that one of us was going to have a heart attack. An operation could help, a coronary artery bypass graft (usually known by its initials CABG and pronounced like "cabbage"), but this operation, with all its attendant aftercare, costs about $50,000. The person who has the heart attack will suffer financially as well as physically. A way of making a bad situation a little better is for us to form a club. Each person puts in $500 and the unlucky one who has a heart attack gets the operation paid for. This is known as "risk pooling," which is an essential feature of all insurance.

Although no one can predict who will be the unlucky one, for large numbers of people, the **risk**—the expected value of all losses averaged over all people—is quite predictable. From the individual perspective, insurance is a trade between two possible states of the universe: one in which the person has a heart attack and one in which he or she does not. Money is shifted from the state in which individuals have more (when they are healthy) to the state in which they have less (when they are sick), similar to the way saving shifts money from good periods to pay for the bad periods. From a societal point of view, insurance is a collection of trades between people. Money is shifted from people who have plenty of money (those who are healthy) to people who suffer losses (those who are sick).

Insurance pools losses; it does not get rid of the losses or even reduce them. The group members must pay for all losses (plus some administrative fees) with the **premiums** they pay. Insurance companies do not like to take risks. They like to sell insurance to large groups of people with predictable (average) losses. This way the insurer's revenues and expenses, and therefore its profits, are very stable and predictable from year to year. Insurance companies specialize in pricing risks, not in taking risks. They try to predict exactly how large premiums need to be to cover all the predicted losses. This specialty, known as actuarial science, uses information on previous losses to make accurate predictions of the amount of money required to pay for future benefits. For this example, the probability (one in one hundred) and size ($50,000) of the loss is well known, so it is simple to determine the **actuarially fair premium,** $1/100 \times \$50,000 = \$500$. An actuarially fair premium is the same as the *expected value of a loss* discussed in Chapter 3 with regard to cost-benefit analysis.

Insurance must be priced above the actuarially fair premium to cover the expenses of administering the insurance plan and to provide profit to the owners who put up their expertise and capital. The difference between the actual premium and the actuarially fair premium is known as the ***loading factor.*** It may be as small as 5 percent or 10 percent for group policies covering large businesses and may exceed 100 percent for individual policies.

Traditional insurance plans simply paid for all (or a defined part) of the medical bills a person incurred. Such **indemnity** plans have become rare. People want insurance companies to bargain for lower prices with hospitals and physicians, to evaluate whether new variations on an old drug are really worth twice as much, and to process all paperwork. **Managed care** plans provide a package of services at a cost lower than people could obtain if they tried to do it all on their own (see Chapters 5 and 10).

Social Insurance

Market contracts are mutually beneficial to people who purchase insurance and to the companies that act as financial intermediaries. However, they do nothing for people who cannot afford to buy insurance or for people excluded from purchasing insurance (e.g., people with disabilities). Market contracts do not pay for medical research or education programs to promote healthy lifestyles, nor do they provide outreach to teenage mothers or people with mental illness. In short, they do nothing to strengthen the social contract that binds the people of a nation together in support of each other. The informal obligations of citizens to society expressed in charitable giving are extended and formalized in social insurance programs such as Medicare and Social Security in the United States, the National Health Service in the United Kingdom and Canada, and the health care systems of most countries.[5] Contributions to social insurance are not voluntary, but mandatory through the tax system. Who will pay and who will receive are determined by concerns common to all and the political process rather than through individual choices made in the marketplace.

As explained in Chapter 1, the U.S. health care system is a blend of private and public financing. Medicare, a social insurance program that covers medical bills for most elderly people in the United States, is larger than the many private for-profit companies combined. Even when insurance is privately paid and managed by profit-making firms, government regulations mandate who is covered, what services are offered, and how prices are set. Therefore, even private insurance is forced into some conformity with social insurance principles.

Strengths and Weaknesses of Different Forms of Risk Spreading

Individual savings are quite limited as a form of risk management since the resources of only one person are used. There is no way that a person born with a genetic defect can save money to cover that risk. Most young people cannot save the $20,000 or so required to treat a broken leg, and a serious illness would exceed the financial capabilities of all but the wealthiest individuals. Trades involving more than one person are needed for coverage. Taking money from family and friends spreads the risk more widely, but this larger group may have difficulty telling whether you really need assistance. In addition, if family and friends do contribute toward your medical bills, they may also want to give you lots of unwelcome advice and intrude in your personal affairs. Charity brings in an even broader group, but the sick individual has less incentive to minimize waste, since he or she is spending other people's money. Charity also tends to be unreliable and even more meddlesome.

WHY DO POLICE OFFICERS AND FIREFIGHTERS HAVE SUCH COMPREHENSIVE INSURANCE?

Medical coverage for those who put their lives on the line for the good of the community remains comprehensive even though many employers and government agencies are cutting back on benefits. There is a symbolic importance to this insurance that goes beyond financial considerations. If the community is not willing to do everything possible to protect the health of these public servants, why should these servants continue to risk it all to save lives? Similar considerations lie behind the willingness of an Army troop to go to great lengths to recover a wounded or dead comrade when such efforts don't seem to be worthwhile from a cost-benefit perspective and have led to the creation of a $20 billion system to care for disabled veterans.

The extent of resources available is limited by how much people care, and charity alone could never fund a modern medical system.

Markets create impersonal contracts to pay for services. They can draw on financial resources from around the world. Your insurance may be handled by a company in the Netherlands that neither knows nor cares about you as a person, but fully meets your needs as long as the doctor bills get paid on time. Yet markets are driven by profits, not love, and each participant must pay his or her own way. Nothing will be done for a child with a genetic defect unless a parent has a policy that includes dependents. A lawyer's interpretation of a contract replaces family concerns as the factor determining which kind of medical care will be provided. The movement from individual to group to market financing reveals a trade-off: the individual is most sensitive to his or her own needs, but has the smallest span for risk pooling (savings, trade over time periods). The market is global in reach, but impersonal and willing to help only when there is a profit to be made (see Table 4.1).

Social insurance combines the humanitarian thrust of charity with the financial strengths of the market, but it provides only a compromise, not a reconciliation. Social insurance can be comprehensive only if contributions are made compulsory through taxes. As the base of funding is broadened to include more people, social insurance grows ever more divorced from personal empathy and becomes just one more government service provided through the political process. As taxpayers, we are willing to provide some medical care for everyone, but not necessarily the best quality in the best rooms of the most modern hospitals. In addition, some taxpayers may be downright hostile about spending millions of dollars on patients who, for example, spent their money on entertainment rather than medical care or who have worsened their own illnesses through substance abuse or unhealthy lifestyles. Social insurance requires that society reach a consensus on who deserves what and how medical care should be delivered. Such a consensus currently exists in the United States only for the elderly under Medicare, and even that can fall apart, as it did in 1989 when revisions to cover pharmaceuticals and catastrophic expenses were passed, implemented, and then repealed by Congress after a revolt by older taxpayers.[6]

4.2 WHY THIRD-PARTY PAYMENT?

As medical care became more expensive, the potential cost of illness went from burdensome to overwhelming. In 1929, $200 was an unusually large medical bill. In today's high-tech intensive care units (ICUs), hospital costs of $100,000 or more are common, with extra payments needed to cover surgery, anesthesia, laboratory tests, and drugs. Few individuals can afford to pay the high cost of advanced modern treatment for serious illness, but few are willing to forgo treatment if they become seriously ill. Insurance makes it possible for most people to obtain care when they need it without going bankrupt. Regular

TABLE 4.1	Types of Risk Protection	
Method	**Reduces Effects of Loss By:**	**Depends On:**
Savings	Shifting consumption between periods	How much I personally have now
Family, Friends, Charity	Sharing between people	How much people care about me
Insurance Contract	Trading between possible states of the world through financial markets	Ability to price risk

withholding of premiums and taxes spreads the financial risk across many people and makes catastrophic expenses bearable.

Insurance would not be necessary if everyone's medical expenses were near the average of $5,427 per person per year. Instead, there is a great deal of variation—much more than that for food, housing, clothing, transportation, and other major expenses. Most people are healthy during any given year, with 15 percent having minimal costs (less than $500) for medical care (see Table 4.2 and Figure 4.1).[7] However, each individual from the 9 percent of the population that needed hospitalization in 2002 averaged more than $20,000 in medical expenses. Only 1 percent of patients had expenses that exceeded $100,000, but this 1 percent accounted for 30 percent of total health care dollars spent. Indeed, it took just 10 percent of all patients to account for 70 percent of the costs.[8] For this group of 28 million people, average medical expenditure exceeded $35,000 for the year.

Although each of us would prefer to pay nothing, most of us can afford to pay for at least some of the cost of the care we expect to receive if we get sick. Even if we are healthy, it is reasonable to be asked to contribute something toward the expenses of those who are not. But how much? A $150,000 bill could be staggeringly difficult to pay. We might not even think that we can afford $5,427, the average annual cost of medical care per person. But whether we wish to pay that much or not, an average of $5,427 per person must be extracted through taxes, bills paid by individuals, insurance premiums paid by employers (who must therefore reduce wages), or some other means, such as charitable giving, to keep the system running. These funds are needed to keep hospitals open; pay doctors, nurses, custodians, and clerks; keep research laboratories investigating new cures; and so forth.

Most of us are not aware of the financial burden we bear for health care provided to ourselves and others. For most workers, employers pay about $2 an hour (11 percent of compensation) for health benefits, reducing the amount that can be paid out as wages.[9] Even if an employer does not provide health insurance, something is deducted each week as taxes, which is often labeled "H.I." or "FICA:M." This is hospital insurance, not for the employee, but for the elderly and people with disabilities on Medicare. Every time we buy a candy bar or a gallon of gasoline, we pay state taxes that fund Medicaid for indigent people. On the other hand, senior citizens might complain bitterly about the cost of drugs and hospitals and nursing homes, with little awareness of how much subsidy they are receiving. Even if senior citizens pay thousands of dollars out of pocket, more than 90 percent of hospital bills, half of nursing home bills, and almost one-third of the costs of their drugs are being borne by other people, mostly younger working people.

Variability

The chance that an insured group will have extraordinarily high or low losses declines sharply as the number of people in the group increases. Figure 4.2 shows how risk declines with the size of the risk-bearing pool. It assumes that each person in the group has a one in one hundred chance of sustaining a $50,000 loss. The expected loss ($500 per person) is the same regardless of the number of people insured. With just 10 people insured, it is

TABLE 4.2	The Concentration of Personal Health Expenditures				
		Top		Middle	Bottom
	All	**1%**	**Next 9%**	**75%**	**15%**
Persons (000s)	285,000	2,850	24,650	213,750	42,750
Health $ (millions)	$1,545,900	$436,400	$646,000	$455,770	$7,730
Per person	$ 5,427	$153,126	$ 26,210	$ 2,135	$ 184

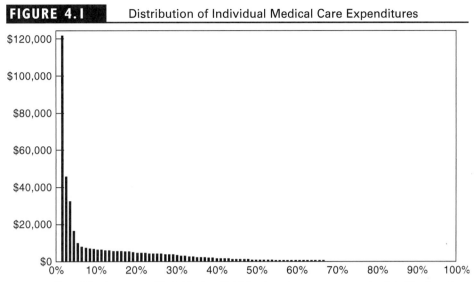

FIGURE 4.1 — Distribution of Individual Medical Care Expenditures

Note: The 1 percent of individuals with highest cost consume approximately 30 percent of total services, and the top 5 percent consume about 50 percent.

impossible for the loss to be equal to the expected loss of $500. With 100 people in the risk pool, it is possible (37 percent of the time) that one of them will get sick, thereby making the loss equal to the expected value of $500. Just as often (37% of the time), however, no one will get sick and losses will be 0. About 18 percent of the time two people in the group will get sick, making the average loss $1,000, and 8 percent of the time three or more people in the group will become ill. With 1,000 people in the group, it is unlikely (0.005 percent) that no one will have an illness. Most (99 percent) of the time the average loss will be between $1,000 and $100 per person. These are known as 99 percent confidence intervals, which are represented in Figure 4.2 by the dotted lines that start far from the mean and gradually move closer as the number of people in the group increases. With 10,000 people in the risk-pooling group, the chances of no one getting sick are vanishingly small, as are the chances that the average loss will exceed $1,000. The group will experience losses between $370 and $630 per person 99 percent of the time. An insurance company is quite confident doing business with a group this large. On the other hand, a company with fewer than twenty-five insureds has a sizable chance of losses that are more than double the expected value (about 22 percent of the time).

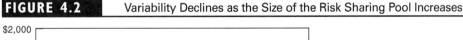

FIGURE 4.2 — Variability Declines as the Size of the Risk Sharing Pool Increases

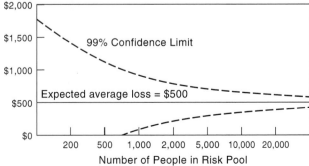

4.3 RISK AVERSION

Would people be willing to pay even a 10 percent load (mark-up) just to get their premium money back as benefit payments? To the extent that people can easily fund routine losses through personal savings, they won't be willing to pay the mark-up, which is why most routine losses are not insured. Only large and potentially catastrophic losses are worth paying extra to insure against.

Suppose the premiums required in the earlier heart attack example were not the actuarially fair $500, but $750, or $1,000, or even $1,500? This is still better than having to sell your house, being in debt for twenty years, or—perhaps worse—not being able to have an operation that could save your life if catastrophe strikes. To an economist, the fact that people are willing to pay more than the expected value of the loss for insurance is evidence that they think they are better off with insurance than without it. The desire to replace an uncertain loss with a steady and certain premium payment is known as **risk aversion.** Some people feel very strongly about risk and will go to great lengths to avoid it. Most people choose not to take financial chances unless they have to or are well paid for doing so (e.g., risky investments provide a higher rate of interest than safe government bonds). Others are willing to take some chances. To some extent this is a matter of taste, similar to how spicy you like your food. Your aversion to risk also depends to some extent on how much income you have—going from $2 million a year to $50,000 is not nearly as scary as going from $200,000 to $5,000, which would provide you with less than $100 a week to spend on food, rent (forget it—you're living at your parent's place again or homeless), and travel (mostly by bus).

With insurance, people can obtain medical care they otherwise could not afford. What if a $350,000 liver transplant could extend your life expectancy by 10 years? If you value your life at $100,000 per year (see Chapter 3, section 5), the benefit-to-cost ratio of treatment is 3 to1 and clearly worthwhile. Yet you, like most people, do not have $350,000 in cash to spend and cannot get a bank loan for that amount, without collateral, just to possibly extend life. Insurance expands the choice set of patients facing serious illness and gives us all peace of mind. Economist John Nyman estimates that this **access to treatment** (affordability) gain is more valuable than pure risk sharing in ordinary financial insurance by an order of magnitude.[10] When it comes to life and death, being able to get help is extremely important.

Given that most people are risk averse, why aren't all risks insured? Life is full of risk. I buy an airplane ticket for a spring vacation even though I could die before I ever get to use it. My bicycle might be stolen. Some people study for a profession, such as accounting or computer science, only to find that job market conditions have changed by the time they graduate. As you take the exam for this course, at least some of the result (I hope not all) will be random (e.g., which questions were asked during class, when television commercial breaks occurred during your study time). Only a few risks in life are insured. Why? For one reason, it is costly to write up and specify insurance contracts, pay claims, and so on. Most small losses will, on average, balance out over time and thus can be handled by savings. In addition, several structural incentive problems occur with insurance (e.g., moral hazard and adverse selection, which are discussed later in this chapter) that reduce its value.

ARE YOU RISK AVERSE?

Here's an easy test. Imagine your boss offering to flip a coin to determine whether to double your monthly paycheck or take it away. If the prospect of losing your paycheck is much more unpleasant than the chance of doubling it, you, like most people, are risk averse and a good candidate for insurance.

In most property and casualty insurance, the losses that are insured are large, infrequent, and random (unpredictable). Many medical expenses meet these criteria, but not all do. For example, most doctor visits for colds and the flu are small, frequent, and fairly predictable. Although the magnitude of the financial losses incurred might explain why some medical expenses are insured, it does not explain why insurance coverage is so extensive in health care, covering many minor and routine services as well as catastrophic events. Three special factors must be recognized in considering the market for health insurance. One is the belief that everyone has a right to medical care. Another is the effectiveness of medical providers in promoting insurance because it provides benefits to them, not the least of which is removing the doctor-patient relationship from the world of commercial trade and haggling over price. Third, and perhaps most important, is the near impossibility of patients acting as informed consumers and smart shoppers. Trying to determine what medical care to get, whether treatment A is really worth $1,500 more than treatment B, or whether having an operation now will save money in the long run, is too difficult. We turn to intermediaries, to doctors and insurance plans, to make many of these decisions for us.

The fact that we are not insured against all risks raises an interesting question: If people are so risk averse, why do they gamble (by playing the lottery or at casinos)? It is clear why people may gamble on an investment in stock or land. They are compensated by getting (on average) higher returns than they can obtain with less risky investments. But in the casino form of gambling, you don't get paid for taking risks; you have to pay for the privilege of taking on risk. The truth is, people gamble this way mostly for fun. It is something exciting to do, like going to a sports event. Sometimes people gamble because they do not understand that the odds are against them—that if they keep playing long enough they are bound to lose. And then there are a few people who gamble because it is their job, and like casinos, they almost always win when we put our money on the table. Don't envy the professional gambler too much, though. For this person, gambling is work rather than a diversion, and the hardest thing is finding willing customers—which is also the case for insurance salespeople.

4.4 ADVERSE SELECTION

Risk pooling works well because everyone in the group is at risk and therefore has an interest in making sure that solid insurance benefits are provided. Consider the heart attack example again, and suppose that instead of the risk being purely random, you knew that you were the one who would end up in the hospital. In this case, you would make sure that you got insurance and might even be willing to pay an astronomical premium to get it. However, if you were certain that you were not going to be the one ending up in the hospital, you would not try very hard to be part of the insurance group and might not be willing to pay $500, or even $50.

If higher risks result from something the insurance company can observe in advance and that both the insured and the company acknowledge, adjusting premiums up or down to account for varying risk categories causes no difficulties. For example, pricing by age is common, such as charging $300 per month for people 35 and younger, $500 for people 35 to 50, $650 for people 51 to 60, and $850 for people 61 and older. Adverse selection creates difficulties when some risk factors are known to the insured, but not to the insurance company (e.g., my chest hurts every time I go walking, I enjoy fried foods and recreational drugs, my brother and sister recently died from heart attacks). Difficulties arise even when the risks are well known but it is considered "unfair" to charge for them (e.g., female employees paying less than males, doubling the premiums for people age 61 and older, charging unmarried men more because of the perceived higher risk of HIV/AIDS). If an employer subsidizes an optional health plan for its workers, the ones most likely to buy insurance are those at high risk. This is called **adverse selection** and means that the average losses in the insured group will be larger than the expected value for the employees as a whole. If young, healthy workers do not participate, premiums have to increase. At the extreme, the plan may be left with only those who were ill to begin with and who knew that they would collect benefits, which is not considered insurance at all because there is no risk pooling. For this reason, insurance companies require that all or at least a majority of the employees in an organization be insured.

A more subtle form of adverse selection occurs when a company offers two kinds of plans, a basic plan and a more comprehensive option for which employees pay extra. Who will choose the comprehensive plan? Some people will choose it because they are very risk averse and therefore willing to pay extra for the more comprehensive benefits. This causes no difficulty for the insurance plan since the actuarial risk (expected loss) of such people is about average. The difficulty arises because there will also be a disproportionate number of high-risk individuals (e.g., those who are older or overweight) who buy the comprehensive plan. As more and more high-risk people sign up for the comprehensive plan, their medical expenses will exceed the expected value and even the "high" premium will not be sufficient

---

ADVERSE SELECTION AT HARVARD: GETTING PUSHED OUT OF THE PPO

In 1994, Harvard University faced a substantial deficit in the employee benefits budgets. For years, Harvard had offered both HMO and PPO health insurance plans, with the more expensive PPO plans being more generously subsidized by the university. In order to reduce cost, Harvard in 1995 implemented a new program in which they contributed the same dollar amount regardless of which plan the employee chose (although the amount contributed is larger for low-income employees). While employee contributions went up for all plans, they went up more for the relatively generous PPO Flex plan (see Table 4.3). In response, enrollment in this high-option plan began to fall. David Cutler and Sarah Reber examined the characteristics of those employees who switched out of the high priced plan.[11] As theory predicts, those who switched were more likely to be healthy, they were younger on average and had spent less on medical care in prior years than those who elected to pay more and stay in the high-option plan. Hence it is not surprising that the high-option PPO Flex lost money in 1995. To compensate, PPO premiums were raised an additional 16 percent for 1996, which pushed even more young healthy employees into the HMO plans, and the PPO lost even more money. In 1997, the pattern was clear and the high-option plan was discontinued, completing an adverse selection death spiral in only three years.

TABLE 4.3		Changes in Employee Premiums and Enrollment at Harvard					
		Employee Pays		**Enrollment**			
	Premium	**Old**	**New**	**1994**	**1995**	**1996**	**1997**
Individual							
PPO Flex	$2,773	$ 555	$1,152	16%	13%	8%	discontinued
HMO	$1,980	$ 277	$ 421	84%	87%	92%	100%
Family							
PPO Flex	$6,238	$1,248	$2,208	22%	18%	11%	discontinued
HMO	$5,395	$ 776	$1,191	78%	82%	89%	100%

Source: Cutler and Rebler (1998).

to pay the bills. Thus, the extra premium for comprehensive insurance must be raised still higher. As the premium goes up, fewer and fewer low-risk people are willing to pay for the better coverage. Eventually, only the chronically ill who are certain to sustain a big loss will sign up for the comprehensive plan. As the difference in premiums between the basic and high-option plan becomes greater, fewer and fewer people at low risk are left in the high-option pool. The principle of risk sharing is defeated by the progressive separation of risks between the groups. This death spiral ends with the termination of the high option plan.

The more differences there are in expected costs of illnesses and the more inside information people have about their own health, the greater the potential for adverse selection. The elderly are particularly problematic because many of their medical expenses are for chronic illnesses that are well known to them, and not random. Insurers' major method for reducing adverse selection, insisting that all employees in a company be included in a group plan, is not available for the elderly since most of them are retired. The ultimate solution for adverse selection is to include everyone in a social insurance system, similar to what the United States did for the elderly by creating Medicare.

4.5 MORAL HAZARD

A person with medical insurance is more likely to go to the doctor because of a sore throat than someone who is not insured. If sent to the hospital, an insured person is more likely to pick a nicer and more expensive facility than an uninsured person. These changes in behavior cause the expenditures of people with insurance to be greater than what an actuary would have predicted from observing the records of people without insurance, and this increase in loss is known as **moral hazard.** One form of these behavioral changes can be illustrated using ordinary demand curve analysis (see Figure 4.3). The demand for physician visits by people without insurance is shown in line D. With insurance picking up 80 percent of the costs, the net "price" (P_i) that a patient has to pay personally is just 20 percent of the actual price; therefore, consumption will increase to Q_i. This increase in visits resulting from being insured is attributable to moral hazard.

Is it likely that people will consume medical care with little health benefit just because it is free? For heart surgery, no. Pain and the loss of time are sufficient to keep most people from undertaking surgery just for the fun of it. But what about routine office visits? Many of them are for minor symptoms that will go away without treatment. Insurance makes people much

---

DO PEOPLE CHOOSE TO DIE?

Actuaries have found that people who buy life insurance are more likely than average to die prematurely.[12] The reasons have less to do with the drama depicted in Arthur Miller's *Death of a Salesman* (since suicide invalidates most policies) than with mundane adverse selection. For example, people who know that their parents died young or that their heart palpitates, or who worry about their lack of physical activity since they turned fifty, are more apt to buy life insurance when it is offered. Conversely, those who buy annuities (policies that pay insureds a certain amount per year as long as they live) show positive selection and are less likely than average to die prematurely. Questionnaire respondents who reply "yes" when asked, "Do you expect to live a long time?" do, in fact, enjoy longer lives than those who respond "no," even after adjusting for the effects of age, blood pressure, cigarette smoking, and all other measurable health risks. This indicates that individuals do have private knowledge that they can use to select coverage that is most favorable to them, but costly to the insurer.

FIGURE 4.3 Moral Hazard

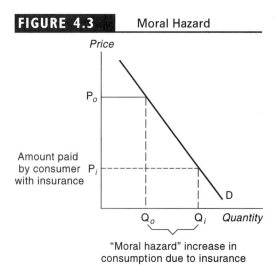

"Moral hazard" increase in
consumption due to insurance

more likely to seek treatment for minor symptoms and thus to increase the overall cost of insurance. Even some surgical procedures are of limited value and are likely to be undertaken only if insurance pays. Suppose seventy-six-year-old uncle Al has a liver infection. It is probable that he will die from the infection no matter what we do, but there is a chance that he could live several more months or even years with a liver transplant—at a cost of $100,000 for the surgery and $5,000 per month after that for drugs and after care. If Uncle Al or the family had to pay directly out of their own pockets, they would probably decide that it was not worth paying so much for such an expensive operation that is unlikely to be successful. However, if insurance is picking up the tab, or if Medicare is passing the cost on to all other taxpayers, Uncle Al and the family might go ahead and try for an improbable cure.

Figure 4.4 shows that the extent of expenditure increase due to moral hazard increases with the price elasticity of the demand curve. For services that are not very price sensitive (D_1), the fact that people are insured will not cause them to purchase many more services; therefore, there will not be much of a distortion in consumer behavior due to insurance. On the other hand, for services that are very price elastic (D_2), the fact that people are insured can cause a very large increase in the quantity they consume (which insurance will pay for), thereby making moral hazard a large problem. This theoretical result provides us with a hypothesis about which services will be covered by insurance. Since moral hazard reduces gains from risk pooling, types of medical care for which there is considerable moral hazard (services with high price elasticity) will be less likely to be covered by insurance than services for which there is very little moral hazard (those with low price elasticity). A number of studies have shown that this is the case.[13] Services such as hospital care and surgery with lower price elasticity of demand are more likely to be insured than services such as nursing home care, physical therapy, mental health care, dentistry, and drugs, which have a higher price elasticity of demand. Exchange must make all parties better off, and when problems such as moral hazard reduce the value of transacting, there will be less pooling of risks through the insurance market.

Welfare Losses Due to Moral Hazard

The extra services people consume just because they are covered by insurance result in some economic waste. If it costs $20 to produce an X-ray, but the X-ray is only worth $5

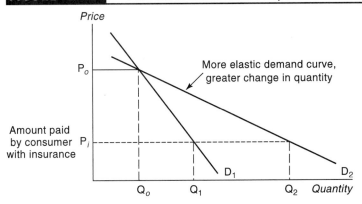

FIGURE 4.4 Amount of Moral Hazard Depends on Price Elasticity of Demand

to the patient, there is a net loss of value of $15. This loss of value is often called the **wel-fare triangle** because the area of the triangle between the price that the insurance company must pay and the demand curve yields a good measure of the size of the loss (see Figure 4.5). If insurance pays 80 percent of the bill, the number of X-rays consumed rises from five to nine. The cost of each X-ray stays the same, $20. The sixth X-ray is worth only $16, for a loss of $4; the seventh is worth $12, for a loss of $8; the eighth is worth $8, for a loss of $12; and the ninth is worth $4, for a loss of $16. The total amount paid for the four extra X-rays is $80, and the welfare loss is about half that, $40.[14]

Who loses? All members of the insured group lose because their premiums must be higher to cover this excess use of services. In fact, even the person getting the extra service probably would prefer a tighter contract that provided only worthwhile services at a lower premium. This is why so much work is done using contract exclusions, fee limits, second opinions, and so on to make sure that reimbursement is provided only for necessary serv-ices. There is a demand for the "hassle" of making patients and physicians justify their use of services because it reduces premiums. Evidence of this demand is that consumers choose policies that include restrictive contractual language rather than policies that pay for everything without question but cost more. This does not mean that it is pleasant when you are sick to go through all sorts of bureaucratic hoops to get a claim paid; it does mean

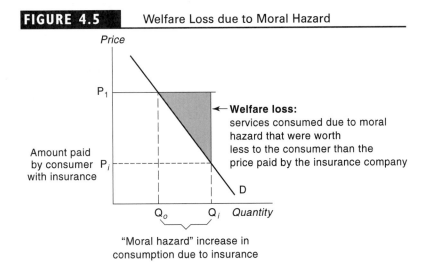

FIGURE 4.5 Welfare Loss due to Moral Hazard

that the effort is justified in terms of reduced premiums—or else you would choose a different plan. Insurance companies will give customers whatever they want, including aggravation, to make a profit.

Welfare losses due to moral hazard are to some extent unavoidable. They are part of the cost of insurance, the way that an unwanted orange peel is part of the cost of an orange. On net, people are better off with the insurance (including moral hazard) than without it. If people are buying insurance, the gains from trade due to risk pooling must be exceeding the welfare losses from moral hazard. If the losses were larger than the gains, people would not buy. However, when the purchase of insurance is subsidized by the government, this may no longer be the case. The extra insurance bought due to tax subsidization creates additional excess utilization of services that are not highly valued by consumers.[15]

There is a systemwide welfare loss caused by insurance that is more difficult to see. Insurance tends to increase demand and make patients less price sensitive, which increases prices overall. Whether or not one person becomes insured will have little effect on the price of X-rays. Yet if everyone who now has insurance had it taken away, demand would fall and the price of X-rays would surely decline. People who are uninsured are worse off because other people are insured, because those other people's insurance raises the price that uninsured people have to pay in order to obtain care.[16] It is even possible that we all would be better off if we were all uninsured, even though each one of us individually is better off with insurance. This paradoxical (and quite unlikely) result would only occur if the gains from risk pooling are smaller than the increase in prices resulting from universal insurance. However, the systematic distortion of prices resulting from insurance raising overall demand probably does create a larger welfare loss than the moral hazard welfare triangle attributable to tax subsidy. Such systemwide effects are difficult to gauge because looking at individual behavior may not tell us what is happening to the system as a whole. One way to measure systemwide effects is to compare different health care systems in different countries that use different types of insurance to see how well each one works and what they cost, but this ambitious effort is left for later (see Chapter 17, International Comparisons).

4.6 OPEN OR CLOSED FUNDING?

Funding for health care can be open ended, dependent on the individual decisions of many people and firms and expanding if demand increases, or closed, with a fixed total budget, usually set by the government (Table 4.4). In open-ended systems, if there are excess demands, either the insurance pool runs a deficit or individuals must reduce other consumption to pay medical bills. If excess demands are placed on closed systems with a fixed budget, no more money is spent, but troubles arise due to poor service, long waiting lists, and other frictional costs that lead to patient dissatisfaction. The National Health Service (NHS) in the United Kingdom is a notable example of closed or "global" budgeting.[17]

Parts of the U.S. health care system have had closed-end budgets (e.g., immunization programs, city health clinics, Department of Veterans Affairs hospitals, state mental hospitals). Yet traditionally, the United States relied on open-ended health insurance provided by employers, Medicare, and Medicaid. Patients were entitled to a specified set of services for which the payer had to cover all costs, regardless of the amount and types of services used. Insurance companies did not care about the size of the bill, since they were merely third-party intermediaries, raising premiums to match the rise in the cost of services. Patients had little incentive to moderate utilization, since services were being paid for with "other people's money" (i.e., taxes, insurance, employers' reserves).

TABLE 4.4		Comparison of Open-Ended and Closed-End Health Care Financing		
Open-Ended Entitlement Funding				
Patients	**Providers**	**Insurance**	**Short-Run Problems**	**Long-Run Problems**
Demand care	Produce services	Pays bills *(all risks are here and purely financial)*	Variability in costs	Costs escalate uncontrollably
Closed-End Budget Funding				
Government	**Providers**	**Patients**	**Short-Run Problems**	**Long-Run Problems**
Allocates budget *(no financial risk—political unrest)*	Produce services *(consumer complaints)*	Receive care *(quality/quantity risk)*	Government blamed for everything	Stagnant, unresponsive system since customers carry no $$

Hospitals, physicians and other providers had even less incentive to hold the line on costs, since larger total insurance reimbursements implied larger total payments to providers. The end result was that costs soared out of control. Eventually employers, Medicare, and Medicaid were all forced to make changes to reduce expenditures. In Medicare and Medicaid, the freedom of doctors and hospitals to charge what they wanted was replaced by controlled administrative prices under the prospective payment "Resource Based Relative Value System" (RBRVS) (see Chapter 6) and "Diagnostically Related Group" (DRG) system (see Chapter 8). Corporate health insurance started to control costs by using managed care contracts (Chapter 10). All these contractual innovations can be viewed as attempts to combine open and closed funding to simultaneously control costs and maintain patient satisfaction.

SUGGESTIONS FOR FURTHER READING

Health Insurance Association of America, *Source Book of Health Insurance Data*, 1999 (www.hiaa.org).

Employee Benefit Research Institute (www.ebri.org).

Institute of Medicine, *Employment and Health Benefits: A Connection at Risk.* (Washington, D.C: National Academy Press, 1993).

David M. Cutler and Sarah J. Reber, "Paying for Health Insurance: The Trade-Off Between Competition and Adverse Selection," *Quarterly Journal of Economics* 113 (May 1998): 433–466.

Paul Gertler and Jonathan Gruber, "Insuring Consumption Against Illness," NBER working paper w6035, May 1997, available at www.nber.org/papers/w6035.

John Nyman, *Health Insurance* (Stanford University Press, Palo Alto, Calif., 2002).

Mark V. Pauly, "Taxation, Health Insurance, and Market Failure in the Medical Economy," *Journal of Economic Literature* 24, no.2 (June 1986): 629–675.

SUMMARY

1. From an individual perspective, **insurance is a form of trade** between time periods or between different possible states (healthy or sick) in the future. From a societal perspective, insurance is a method of **pooling risks** so that the burden of financial loss is distributed over many people. An individual's **savings** can spread the cost of illness over time. **Family, friends, and charity** voluntary spreads risk across people. **Private insurance contracts** spread risk through organized markets. **Social insurance** uses taxation to spread risk over all citizens.

2. Due to the uncertain and **uneven distribution of medical care costs,** with 70 percent of total dollars being spent on behalf of the 10 percent of people who become most ill during a year, most health care payments flow through **third-party insurance** intermediaries that pool and transfer funds, which differs from the direct exchange of money for services between two parties (consumers and providers) common to most markets.

3. An **actuarially fair premium** is equal to the **expected value** of a loss, the dollar amount multiplied by the probability of occurrence. The "law of large numbers" means that higher losses for some will be offset by lower losses for others; therefore, for a large group the overall loss usually will be close to the expected value. If each person contributes an average amount, the pooled funds will be enough to pay for all the individual losses.

4. **Insurance companies do not pay for losses,** people do. The entire cost of medical care, including the costs of administration and use of financial capital, is paid through premiums, taxes, or patient coinsurance (e.g., deductibles, co-payments) collected for each service rendered. Therefore, only large, random, infrequent losses are worth insuring. Insurance covering small, regular losses raises costs while providing few benefits from risk reduction.

5. People prefer having an income that is certain rather than the same average income subject to random fluctuations. Because of risk aversion, consumers are willing to pay more than the expected value of a loss to obtain insurance coverage. From the supply side, the excess of premiums received over benefits paid is called the load or **underwriting gains** of the insurance company.

6. People who know that they are likely to sustain a loss are more likely to purchase insurance, resulting in **adverse selection,** a change in the composition of the insured group. This difficulty in the grouping of people for insurance is to be distinguished from an increase in the average loss due to a change in the behavior of individuals.

7. **Moral hazard** occurs whenever having insurance leads individuals to increase the amount spent, or to increase the risk of loss. In health economics, moral hazard most commonly refers to the increase in utilization of medical services that results from being insured. The **welfare loss due to insurance** occurs because people who do not have to pay the bills tend to consume some care that is worth less to them than what it costs to provide. The gains from risk reduction must be worth more than these welfare losses or people would choose to go without insurance. However, the subsidy provided by exempting employer-provided health insurance benefits from taxes encourages extra insurance coverage. There also may be a general rise in the price of medical care because insurance increases the demand for services. This clearly causes a loss of welfare to those who are uninsured and, by increasing overall costs, creates a systemwide distortion that reduces economic efficiency.

8. The **escalation in costs** due to **open-ended entitlement financing** through indemnity insurance that paid bills without imposing restrictions on use has been the primary force driving the development of more extensive contractual solutions through managed care.

PROBLEMS

1. {*cost sharing*} Find four people who have been treated for illness in the past three years. Ask them the following questions.

a. How much did you pay for insurance?

b. How much did the insurance really cost (i.e., what you paid plus what the employer or government paid)?

c. How much did you pay in medical bills?

d. How much did the medical care really cost (i.e., what you paid plus what the insurance company or government paid)?

2. {*actuarially fair premium*} A company with 617 employees had the following experience this year:

	Cost (each)
14 hospitalizations	$5,600
37 physical therapy sessions	$340
9 births	$1,800
4.1 physician visits per employee	$55
2.4 prescriptions filled per employee	$21

Assuming that the cost of medical care rises 7 percent over the next year, what would the actuarially fair premium per employee be for the next year?

3. {*size of risk pool*} Use the information in Figure 4.2 pertaining to a loss of $50,000 that occurs randomly with a probability of one in one hundred. If the insurance company charges $750 per person per year, what is the load above the actuarially fair premium? If one hundred people are in the group, will the insurance company show an underwriting profit? Will the insurance company ever break even? How likely is it that the plan will show a loss next year? With 50 people in the group, is it more or less likely that the plan will show a loss? What about with 500 people? How large does the group have to be before the insurance company can be 99 percent sure that it will show an underwriting gain for the year?

4. {*savings, social insurance*} Explain which mechanism (savings, charity & contributions from friends, private insurance, or social insurance) you believe would cover losses resulting from each of the following conditions:

a. seasonal hay fever

b. congenital birth defects

c. schizophrenia

d. Alzheimer's disease

e. preventive dental cleaning

f. post-traumatic jaw reconstruction

g. cigarette-induced chronic pulmonary obstruction

5. {*adverse selection*} In each of the following pairs, which situation would pose the largest problems regarding adverse selection?

a. A policy covering accidents for all children attending YMCA camps or **b.** A policy covering accidents for college students traveling abroad

c. Inclusion of HIV/AIDS treatment in the standard benefit package offered to teachers or **d.** An optional rider providing HIV/AIDS coverage for an additional premium

e. Basic medical services insurance package offered to students entering college or **f.** Basic medical services package offered to professors seeking early retirement

g. Optional mental health coverage offered to employees of ABC Inc. or **h.** Optional mental health coverage offered to children of ABC Inc. employees

6. {*moral hazard*} Explain which of the following types of insurance coverage would most likely cause the biggest problems resulting from moral hazard.

   a. Indemnity payments of $10,000 for each eye or limb lost or **b.** Indemnity payments of $50 for each day spent in a nursing home

   c. Treatment in an emergency room or **d.** Treatment in an intensive care unit

   e. Arthroscopic surgery for knee injuries or **f.** Amputation for foot injuries

   g. Family counseling or **h.** Electroconvulsive therapy

   i. Decongestants or **j.** Antibiotics

7. {*moral hazard*} The following table gives the demand curve for doctor visits for Ralph, who doesn't have health insurance. Assume that Ralph responds only to the amount he must pay out of pocket when deciding how much care to use. By filling in the blank lines, calculate Ralph's new demand curve if he obtained insurance coverage that paid 80 percent of the bill. If the charges are $100 (i.e., Ralph pays $20 out of pocket), how many of the additional services Ralph uses are worth less (to him) than what they cost? Worth less to him than what he pays?

Price per visit	Number of visits	Out-of-pocket cost with insurance	Number of visits with insurance
$0	20	—	—
$20	18	—	—
$50	15	—	—
$100	10	—	—
$150	5	—	—

8. {*welfare loss*} Bill's new insurance policy contains a prescription plan that provides all drugs through a local pharmacy with a $2 co-payment. Under the old insurance, Bill had to pay for his own medication and purchased 9 inhalers at $17 apiece to help control his asthma. With the new plan, Bill purchased 15 inhalers, keeping some as spares in his glove compartment and desk, since he only had to pay a $2 co-payment for each one. How much are the six additional inhalers worth to Bill? How much do they cost him? How much do they cost the insurance company? Is Bill better or worse off under the new plan?

9. {*incidence*} When medical care is reimbursed through employer-provided insurance, whose welfare is ultimately affected when the cost of medical care rises: the owners of the firm that pays the premiums (employer), the government whose revenues are reduced because insurance benefits are not taxable as wages, or the public in their roles as workers, consumers, and taxpayers? Is there any difference between short-term and long-term effects?

ENDNOTES

1. Gary Becker, *A Treatise on the Family* (Cambridge, Mass.: Harvard University Press, 1981).
2. Robert H. Frank, *Passions Within Reason: The Strategic Role of the Emotions* (New York: Norton, 1988).
3. Edward O. Wilson, *On Human Nature* (Cambridge, Mass.: Harvard University Press, 1976); Jerome H. Barkow, Leda Cosmides, John Tooby, eds., *The Adapted Mind: Evolutionary Psychology and the Generation of Culture* (New York: Oxford University Press, 1992).

4. Rosemary Stevens, *In Sickness and In Wealth: American Hospitals in the Twentieth Century* (New York: Basic Books, 1989); John D. Thompson, *The Hospital: A Social and Architectural History* (New Haven, Conn.: Yale University Press, 1975).

5. William A. Glaser, *Health Insurance in Practice: International Variations in Financing, Benefits, and Problems* (San Francisco: Jossey-Bass, 1991).

6. William Aaronson, Jacqueline Zinn, and Michael Rosko, "Medicare Catastrophic Health Insurance," *Journal of Health Politics, Policy and Law* (1993).

7. *Health Care Financing Review, Medicare and Medicaid Statistical Supplement, 1995,* p. 35; Marc L. Berk and Alan Monheit, "The Concentration of Health Expenditures, Revisited" *Health Affairs*, 20, no.2 (March 2001): 9–18.

8. The distribution of costs across individuals can be measured only for personal health care costs that are billed to individuals, not overhead items such as public health, construction, insurance administration, etc. Such overhead items make up about 10 percent of national health expenditures, and hence the "all persons" average in Table 4.2 is only 90 percent as large as the per capita average for all national health expenditures reported elsewhere. In truth, many costs have overhead components and are difficult to unambiguously assign to a single person, although they are clearly concentrated on the most ill and not evenly distributed. Many economists would argue that costs are even more concentrated than Table 4.2 indicates because hospitals and physicians typically overcharge the least complex patients to subsidize the most difficult and complex cases (see the discussion of "cost shifting" in Chapter 8).

9. Bureau of Labor Statistics, U.S. Dept. of Labor, *Employment Cost Indexes and Levels, 1975-90,* Bulletin 2372, 1990.

10. John A. Nyman, "The value of health insurance: the access motive," *Journal of Health Economics* 18 (1999): 141–152.

11. David M. Cutler and Sarah J. Reber, "Paying for Health Insurance: The Trade-Off Between Competition and Adverse Selection," *Quarterly Journal of Economics* 113 (May 1998): 433–466.

12. Lewis C. Workman, "Life Annuities," in *Mathematical Foundations of Life Insurance* (Atlanta, Ga.: Life Office Management Association, 1982), 155-195.

13. Kevin F. O'Grady, Willard G. Manning, Joseph P. Newhouse and Robert H. Brook, "The Impact of Cost Sharing on Emergency Department Use," *New England Journal of Medicine* 313 (1985): 484–490; Mark V. Pauly, "Taxation, Health Insurance and Market Failure in the Medical Economy," *Journal of Economic Literature* 24, no. 2 (June 1986): 629– 675.

14. The size of the welfare triangle is $(P_{original} - P_{insured}) \times (Q_{insured} - Q_{original}) \div 2$, which for this example would be $(\$20 - \$4) \times (9 - 5) \div 2 = \$32$. This is slightly less than in the numerical example because with discrete units (i.e., one, two, . . . eight, nine X-rays, with no fractions) the demand curve is not a continuous straight line, but a step function, and so the area between the original \$20 line and the demand curve is somewhat larger. In most cases, economists use the continuous formula, since with many consumers buying many units of service, the individual bumps are less important and the demand curve approximates a continuous line.

15. Martin S. Feldstein, "The Welfare Loss of Excess Health Insurance," *Journal of Political Economy* 81, no. 2 (1973): 251– 280.

16. Gina Kolata, "Medical fees are often higher for patients without insurance," *New York Times*, April 1, 2001(http://www.nytimes.com). However, it is *sometimes* the case that the profits that hospitals make from insured patients are used to provide charity services to the uninsured (see discussion of cost-shifting in Chapter 8). Whether or not an uninsured person is made better or worse off depends upon whether or not they receive services for free, or with sufficient subsidy that the price to them is less than the market price would be without insurance.

17. Alan Maynard and Karen Bloor, "Introducing a Market to the United Kingdom's National Health Service," *New England Journal of Medicine*, 334, no.9 (1996): 604–608.

CHAPTER 5

INSURANCE CONTRACTS AND MANAGED CARE

QUESTIONS

1. Who benefits from insurance: patients, physicians, or insurance companies?
2. Who is the third party? Who controls the flow of funds?
3. Who is the largest health insurer?
4. Do taxes on wages make employees prefer receiving insurance benefits instead of wage increases?
5. How is a state mandate to cover alcoholism treatment similar to a tax?
6. Why are so many Americans uninsured?
7. Who really pays when the cost of medical care rises: employers, employees, government, or insurance companies?

Insurance modifies the nature of economic exchange by redirecting the flow of money. It changes who negotiates prices, who bears responsibility for mistakes, and who has the right to profit from directing business to one hospital instead of another. The standard market model with one group (consumers) determining demand and a different group (firms) determining supply is left behind when we enter the medical world with patients (who receive care but do not directly pay for it), insurance companies (who neither supply nor consume, but pool risk and profit from handling funds), and providers (who are reimbursed by a *third party,* insurance, on behalf of a group of patients, rather than being paid directly). See Figure 5.1.

5.1 THIRD-PARTY TRANSACTIONS

What does each of the three parties in an insurance contracting network gain? *Patients* gain by pooling risks to eliminate financial uncertainty and make expensive treatments affordable (see Chapter 4). *Insurance companies* benefit from profits. Even when the underwriting gains (the difference between premiums paid in and benefits paid out plus administrative costs) are negative, an apparent loss, companies may still make money because they will hold the premiums for six to twenty-four months before paying out benefits. At 8 percent, the interest on $1 million dollars in premiums for two years is $(1.08) \times (1.08) \times (\$1,000,000) - (\$1,000,000) = \$166,400$, which is not a bad profit for a firm that some

FIGURE 5.1   Third Party Contracting

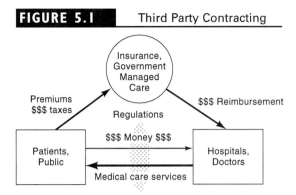

reports might claim made no money because benefit payouts exceeded premium revenues. In addition, insurance companies usually get higher returns on investments than individuals because insurers are so large, with better opportunities and specialized investment staffs. Insurance companies are regulated and taxed as large financial investment institutions, with underwriting gains and losses treated as secondary. This does not mean that underwriting and risk selection are not important, only that expected investment returns are already built into the price of the premium.

Providers gain from an increase in demand and regularity of payment. When patients are covered by insurance, they are more apt to come in for care and less likely to argue about price. Traditionally, patients have expected doctors and hospitals to be more lenient than landlords and bankers about late payment, and many medical bills went unpaid or were paid only in part. Falling demand and irregular payment during the Great Depression in the 1930s forced many hospitals to close due to bankruptcy and led to the start-up of the largest private insurance plan in the world (Blue Cross) as a method of insuring patients so that provider revenues could continue.[1] Like all great ideas, insurance had to benefit all parties so that all parties would enthusiastically cooperate.

Benefits from Exchange		
Patients	**Insurers**	**Providers**
risk pooling	profits	increased demand

Tax Benefits

There is a less visible and more diffuse fourth party in most insurance transactions—the government. Many governments take on the social obligation to provide medical care directly, as is done by the National Health Service in the U.K. and by the Swedish health system. Some countries have chosen to build on employee health insurance plans to create universal coverage for all citizens, such as the German Krankenkassen or the Japanese employment societies. The United States is somewhat unique in that insurance is encouraged but not universally required. The U.S. government, through Medicare, directly provides insurance for all people 65 and older and through Medicaid for many people who are classified as being indigent or disabled. The U.S. government also provides tax incentives for many others to be insured through the private sector. The primary tax incentive is that health benefits are nontaxable compensation for employees but still allowed as deductible expenses for the employer. The following example shows how this tax incentive works.

Employee Pays for Medical Care		Employer Pays for Insurance
$1,000	company labor cost	$1,000
none	insurance premium	($200)
$1,000	gross paycheck	$800
($350)	taxes (at 35%)	($280)
$650	net paycheck	$520
($200)	medical bills	none
$450	**available for spending**	**$520**

The employer spends the same for labor either way and does not care whether insurance premiums are taken out of a paycheck or paid later from the employee's bank account. With insurance taken out, the employees' gross income is less and therefore the amount of taxes paid is less. The employee with the larger paycheck, after paying for medical care with after-tax dollars, has less money left for spending than the employee whose health insurance premiums paid for the same amount of medical care on a pre-tax basis. As long as the administrative load is less than the tax rate, it is cheaper to buy medical care pre-tax using employer-paid insurance than for the employee to pay the bills directly. This tax break for employer-paid health insurance is a substantial and important part of the voluntary system of health care that Americans have come to depend on. Without the tax incentive, most working people would not have health insurance as an employee benefit.

Who Pays? How Much?

There is a popular misconception that when insurance pays for something, it is free. Unfortunately, while we may not realize who pays because third-party transactions are indirect, every dollar spent on medical care is paid by you, or by me, or by someone just like us. Insurance companies and the government never really "pay" for anything. For the most part, individuals pay for medical care by paying higher taxes and/or taking home lower wages. Even the tax advantage for employee benefits does not mean that we are able to get something for nothing. (There are no free lunches!) The government still has to pay its bills. If fewer dollars are collected through wage taxes, more dollars must be collected through gasoline taxes, property taxes, income taxes, Social Security taxes, or other taxes to make up the difference. When a hospital provides "free" care to someone as charity, it must raise charges to those who are insured (and the few who cover their bills out of their own pockets) to pay for it. Insurance does not reduce the cost of medical care, rather it redistributes costs so that different people end up paying.

Under third-party payment systems, the connection between what the first party (the patient) pays and what the second party (the provider) receives is indirect at best. The "charges billed" for a visit to the emergency room often bear little resemblance to what you have to pay or what the hospital receives. In health economics, one must give up the familiar realm of simple two-party transactions in which "bought" and "sold" happen at the same price. This chapter discusses how much the patient (or his or her family) pays, not how much the doctor or hospital actually receives, which is usually quite different (see Chapters 6 and 8). As pointed out in Chapter 1 (Table 1.1 and Figure 1.4), the total of all money paid by patients and families (as out-of-pocket charges, premiums, and taxes combined) will automatically match the total money received by all providers (e.g., hospitals, physicians, drug companies, nursing homes). However, for any particular subgroup or set of transactions, this equivalence is unlikely. Insurance breaks the linkage between what the patient pays and the amount the provider is paid.

People pay premiums to be insured, but then do not pay directly for the medical care they use. Health insurance is similar to having a credit card that allows you to buy whatever you need, but for which payment is set at $100 per month regardless of the number of purchases you make. As you might expect, since one does not have to pay any extra for more purchases, the amount spent tends to rise uncontrollably (see Figure 9.6 for one illustration). That is why most **indemnity insurance plans** providing unlimited reimbursements in return for a fixed premium have disappeared from the market. Most people are now covered by **managed care plans,** in which they allow the insurer to exercise some control over the number and type of services covered in return for more affordable premiums. Managed care plans use their control over purchasing to negotiate lower prices from hospitals, doctors, and drug companies. In a sense, managed care represents the evolution of the insurer from a passive financial intermediary to an active purchasing agent.

5.2 MANAGED CARE PLANS

The fundamental difference between traditional indemnity insurance and managed care is that a manager intervenes to monitor and control the transaction between doctor and patient (Figure 5.2). The management company acts as the patient's agent, trying to get better care and lower prices. An outside party, such as the plan medical director, a trained utilization review nurse, or a software program, identifies episodes of care that could be at variance with accepted clinical practice. This may be done through a statistical profile of each physician's practice, assessment of laboratory testing, or review of individual cases. The manager examines the process of care and controls the flow of funds, facilitating payments in some circumstances and holding back in others. Since the **managed care organization** (**MCO**) takes financial responsibility for medical care, it has an incentive to provide care efficiently. To remain viable, the MCO must compete on the basis of both quality and cost. A delicate balance must be maintained among expenditure control, administrative process, and medical uncertainty.

The most loosely organized MCOs are referred to as **preferred provider organizations** (**PPOs**) or **point-of-service plans** (**POSs**). The insuring MCO negotiates contracts with a set of doctors and hospitals (the network) to obtain care at a discount. Patients receiving care within the network pay only a small co-payment. Patients may obtain care outside the network, but may have to pay substantially more or receive a referral from their regular doctor stating that such specialty care is medically necessary. In a **health maintenance organization** (**HMO**), referrals are necessary for most specialty care, the insurance only pays for care

FIGURE 5.2   Flow of Funds with Managed Care

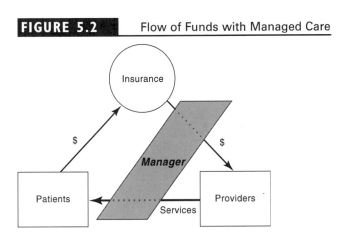

within the network, and the networks are usually more limited than under POS or PPO plans. A **closed-panel HMO** is an organization that provides all care in-house using its own doctors and hospitals. The largest closed panel HMO is Kaiser Permanente, which has more than 7 million members, mostly in the western United States (see Chapter 10).

5.3   HOW ARE BENEFITS DETERMINED?

Insurance is a legal contract that is specific regarding how much will be paid, to which providers, and under what conditions; the evidence of loss required; and who will arbitrate disputes. Health insurance isn't based on sickness at all, but rather on incurring an expense for medical treatment. Most people will never see the complete contract drawn up by their employer and the insurance company; they will only see informational pamphlets, hear descriptions during new employee orientation, and so on. All such benefit descriptions, even in an advertisement or brochure written in Spanish or another language, are legally binding contracts. If a policy states that it covers eye examinations, it covers eye examinations. If a policy states that it will pay $16 for filling a tooth cavity, it will pay $16. In some sense, every set of documents constitutes a slightly different insurance plan. The insurance plan must pay any amount that a court decides a reasonable person reading such descriptions would expect the insurance plan to pay. Furthermore, any benefits routinely paid in previous years and not explicitly revoked, become a precedent, even if those benefits are not mentioned in the contract. The use of fine print to leave the insured burdened with thousands of dollars of unexpected bills is simply not allowed and, in fact, would be self-defeating for an insurance company. Over time, premiums will be adjusted upward to cover whatever medical costs are incurred.

5.4   TYPES OF INSURANCE PLANS

Of the 285 million people in the United States, most have some form of private health insurance, usually through an employer. Government programs, mostly Medicare and Medicaid, cover 24 percent of the population, and about 25 million people, 9 percent of the population, purchase private insurance individually. That leaves about 44 million people, or 15 percent of the population, uninsured (see Table 5.1).[2]

Employer-Based Group Health Insurance

Three factors explain why more than half of the U.S. population is covered by employer group health insurance:

- Covering a large group under a single contract reduces transaction costs.
- Group coverage mitigates adverse selection.
- Employer payment yields a tax benefit.

An employee usually obtains insurance by choosing one of the options offered, deciding whether to include children and other dependents, and contributing a small amount toward the total premium (see Table 5.2). Almost all large employers provide health insurance benefits, but less than one-third of small employers (fewer than 10 employees) do so and often make the employee pay a large part of the premium, so that fewer people choose to participate (see Figure 5.3).[3] The largest employee groups are usually self-insured (i.e., the employer bears the risk although it may use an insurance company to administer benefits).

TABLE 5.1	Health Insurance Coverage of the U.S. Population

	Non-Elderly	Elderly
Total people	250 million	35 million
With insurance	74.2%	99.3%
Employment	34.9	34.1
Employment (dependent)	33.5	***
Other private insurance	5.7	27.9
Military	2.8	4.3
Medicare	2.2	96.9
Medicaid	10.4	10.1
Uninsured	15.5	0.7

Note: Percentages add to more than 100% because many people have multiple coverage.

Source: Robert J. Mills, Health Insurance Coverage: 2000, Current Population Reports, www. census.gov.

TABLE 5.2	Annual Premiums for Employee Health Insurance Coverage, 2002

	HMO	PPO	POS	Indemnity	Average
Single					
Total premium	$2,764	$3,119	$3,175	$3,582	$3,060
Employee pays	$ 455	$ 432	$ 527	$ 426	$ 454
Family					
Total premium	$7,541	$8,037	$8,173	$8,479	$7,954
Employee pays	$1,960	$2,152	$2,186	$1,630	$2,084
% of all insured employees	26%	51%	18%	5%	100%

Source: Kaiser/HRET *Employer Health Benefits Survey,* www.kff.org.

FIGURE 5.3	Percentage of Workers Insured

Size of Employer

Self-Paid Private Insurance

Nine percent of the population, mostly people who are self-employed or who work for small companies that do not provide employee benefits, purchase private health insurance individually. Individuals acting on their own behalf lack group purchasing power and often pay significantly higher premiums even for reduced levels of coverage.

Medicare

Since many elderly people do not belong to employer groups and would be subject to severe adverse selection if purchasing insurance individually, the U.S. government created **Medicare,** which covers the 12 percent of the population over age 65 and some people with disabilities. A substantial portion of the money for Medicare comes from a tax of 2.9 percent on all wages, half paid by the employer and half paid by the employee, with the remainder coming from general tax revenues and premiums.

Medicare is split into two parts, Part A (hospital) and Part B (physician and outpatient services). While the specifics of coverage can be complex, clear and detailed descriptions of benefits are readily available at www.medicare.gov. Part A coverage is provided on application to people age 65 or older and to those entitled to specified programs, such as Social Security and programs for people with end-stage renal disease. To obtain Part B coverage, beneficiaries must pay a premium ($54 a month in 2002), which is supposed to cover a quarter of the actuarial cost but usually falls short because of the reluctance of politicians to offend groups that lobby for the elderly. Since Part B coverage is so heavily subsidized and Part A beneficiaries are usually enrolled unless they explicitly choose to opt out, almost all Medicare insureds (98 percent) have both Parts A and B. In addition, 88 percent of those with Medicare have supplemental "Medigap" insurance or HMOs[4] that cover co-payments, deductibles, drugs, and some other expenses (Table 5.3).

Medicaid

People who are poor cannot pay for insurance and many of them (10 percent of the population) are covered under the government **Medicaid** program, which also provides supplemental coverage for a substantial number of elderly people, including a majority of those living in nursing homes.

Medicaid is funded jointly by the states and the federal government. The federal government may pay as much as 80 percent of the total program cost for low income states, but only half for wealthier states. Program design (which differs from state to state), beneficiary enrollment, and other factors, as well as per capita income, can affect both the total cost and the financing split. Although Medicaid was designed to cover mothers with low incomes and their children, it has become the dominant funding mechanism for nursing homes. This has occurred primarily because Medicare has very limited nursing home coverage; therefore, as the elderly incur expenses during long nursing home stays, they become poor enough to qualify for Medicaid and switch to government funding.

Other Government Programs and Charity

Charity paid for about $58 billion in health care in 2002. Workers' compensation, automobile accident insurance, and similar programs paid more than $25 billion. The Department of Veterans Affairs received $22 billion in funding, with a somewhat smaller amount being paid for dependents through the Department of Defense. Programs sponsored by the

TABLE 5.3   The Ten Standard Medicare Supplement Plans

Medigap policies (including Medicare SELECT) can only be sold in 10 standardized plans. This chart gives you a quick look at all the Medigap plans and their benefits. Read down to find out what benefits are in each plan. If you need more information, call your State Insurance Department.

Basic Benefits must be included in all plans, and cover Part A coinsurance plus hospitalization for 365 days after Medicare benefits end; Part B coinsurance (generally 20% of Medicare-approved expenses) and copayments, and the first 3 pints of blood each year. Note that many people choose to purchase a comprehensive HMO benefit under the MEDICARE + CHOICE plan rather than Medigap insurance—you do not need both.

A	B	C	D	E	F*	G	H	I	J*
Basic benefits	Basic benefits	Basic benefits	Basic benefits	Basic benefits	Basic benefits	Basic benefits	Basic benefits	Basic benefits	Basic benefits
		Skilled nursing coinsurance	Skilled nursing coinsurance	Skilled nursing coinsurance	Skilled nursing coinsurance	Skilled nursing coinsurance	Skilled nursing coinsurance	Skilled nursing coinsurance	Skilled nursing coinsurance
	Medicare Part A deductible	Medicare Part A deductible	Medicare Part A deductible	Medicare Part A deductible	Medicare Part A deductible	Medicare Part A deductible	Medicare Part A deductible	Medicare Part A deductible	Medicare Part A deductible
		Medicare Part B deductible			Medicare Part B deductible				Medicare Part B deductible
					Medicare Part B excess charge (100%)	Medicare Part B excess charge (80%)		Medicare Part B excess charge (100%)	Medicare Part B excess charge (100%)
		Foreign travel emergency	Foreign travel emergency	Foreign travel emergency	Foreign travel emergency	Foreign travel emergency	Foreign travel emergency	Foreign travel emergency	Foreign travel emergency
			At-home recovery			At-home recovery		At-home recovery	At-home recovery
							Basic drug benefit ($1,250 Limit)	Basic drug benefit ($1,250 Limit)	Extended drug benefit ($3,000 Limit)
				Preventive care					Preventive care

*Plans F and J also have a high deductible option.

Source: 2002 Guide to Health Insurance for People with Medicare, CMS Publication No. 02110, www.medicare.gov.

WHAT DO PEOPLE BUY WHEN THEY DON'T BUY HEALTH INSURANCE?

Most of the time, being uninsured is a matter of choice. It may not be a sensible choice or may be the result of a choice no one would want to face (buy the children food or buy health insurance), but it is a choice nonetheless. Knowing what people buy when they do not buy health insurance provides insight into their choice.

A study by Helen Levy and Thomas DeLeire from the University of Chicago indicates that what people buy with the money they save from not purchasing health insurance depends significantly on whether they are poor or relatively well-off.[8] According to the study, for people in the bottom quartile of the income distribution, the money they did not spend on health insurance went mostly toward food, rent, and other necessities. For people in the upper income quartile, the spending pattern was quite different—the largest type spending increase was for transportation, specifically, for expensive used cars (Jaguar or Ferrari anyone?). The study indicates that programs trying to help people who are truly needy may inadvertently subsidize people who are uninsured simply because they want to spend on other things.

Maternal and Child Health Bureau, Substance Abuse and Mental Health Services Administration, Bureau of Indian Affairs, and a variety of other programs accounted for about another $28 billion in health care.[5]

The Uninsured

Despite the wide variety of health insurance plans, 40 million Americans, about 15 percent of the population, have no health insurance.[6] Uninsured individuals needing care must try to pay with their own limited resources, find a special government program, depend on charity, or simply present themselves at a hospital or clinic and ask to be treated free of charge. The percentage of the population without coverage depends significantly on the efforts of local and state governments. States choosing expansive Medicaid programs and broad outreach to the working poor can reduce the number of uninsured individuals substantially. Iowa, Rhode Island, Minnesota, and Massachusetts insure all but 8 percent of their citizens, while Texas leaves 24 percent of its population without insurance.

While some uninsured individuals pay large sums out-of-pocket when they get sick, a much greater number stay healthy and pocket the cash or, having no resources, depend on charity when they are ill. That is why the problem of so many uninsured individuals is so intractable. For many of the uninsured, not having insurance is a rational economic decision. Three-fourths of the uninsured are under age 35, and people this young tend to be healthy, to be enrolled in college, or to earn low wages. For them, paying $300 a month or even $100 a month for health insurance does not make sense.[7] People over age 35 who are working in low-paying jobs often need the money to eat and pay rent more than they need it to provide protection from uncertain medical bills that may never materialize. There is also a small number of people who are chronically ill and would not pass even a cursory medical exam, and hence can be insured only if they take a job in a large firm that provides group coverage.

It would be easy to insure everyone by mandating universal coverage, yet this is unlikely to happen in the United States because it is politically unpopular. Most of the suggested reforms intended to bring about a voluntary increase in coverage would affect only a few people at the margin and would not have a major impact, since those currently without insurance are often uninsured because of rational economic choices made by themselves or by insurance companies.

State Children's Health Insurance Program

The State Children's Health Insurance Program (SCHIP) was enacted by Congress in 1997 as Title XXI of the Social Security Act to provide $40 billion to increase coverage for the 10 million children under the age of 18 who were uninsured. However, the program works through state governments and some have used available funding for other purposes, leading to great unevenness in implementation. Almost 5 million children eligible for SCHIP or Medicaid have not been enrolled. Less than 5 percent of children in Rhode Island, Connecticut, and Pennsylvania are uninsured, while almost 20% of children in Texas and New Mexico are left uninsured.[9] The fact that so many children are still uninsured reflects the choices made by the public and their elected representatives. In this regard, it is probably worth mentioning that children do not vote, and that the parents of poor children are much less likely to vote than the senior citizens who qualify for Medicare.

Medical Savings Accounts (MSAs) and Defined Contribution "Voucher" Plans

Insurance provides protection against the cost of medical care. Inevitably, this protection makes people less sensitive to costs; that is, they are more willing to use extra services and less concerned about finding the best price for the services they use.

Medical savings accounts (MSAs) and defined contribution plans are attempts to make patients more aware of costs and force them to act as smart shoppers.[10] In an MSA, a person deposits a set amount of money each year in a tax-advantaged account, which can then be used to purchase medical services. Any money left in the MSA at the end of the year can be rolled over to the next year or eventually used to fund retirement. With an MSA, the patient bears the marginal costs of medical care in full. The MSA pays until the account is depleted and every additional dollar of medical care after that takes $1 out of the patient's pocket. This is a high-powered incentive to motivate people to pay attention to costs, shop for the lowest prices, and avoid unnecessary services. To provide protection against really big losses, the MSA is usually packaged together with a high-deductible major medical plan (e.g., insurance that pays a specified percentage, such as 90 percent, of all expenses above a limit, perhaps $5,000). Some economists have been vocal in advocating for the "market incentives" provided by MSAs, and some corporations view them as a good way to set a limit on the total amount they must pay for health benefits, an advantage that is particularly appealing in a time of rapidly rising medical costs.

Using MSAs to increase patients' incentives to save money may solve some problems, but could create others. Since risks are not being pooled in a group, the individual is largely at risk for mid-range expenditures (between $1,000 and $5,000). This makes MSAs attractive to relatively young and healthy employees who expect to be able to keep total medical spending below the annual MSA contribution amount in most years, but not to older employees or those with dependents suffering from chronic illnesses. Such adverse selection means that the premiums for employees who do not choose the MSA are almost certain to rise (see Chapter 4, Section 4.3). Also, the bulk of medical costs are not in the low or middle range, but

---

SAMPLE DEFINED CONTRIBUTION MSA PLAN

Employer: Contributes $100 (pre-tax) per month and provides catastrophic major medical insurance that pays 90 percent of all expenses above $5,000 in a calendar year

Employee: Pays all bills, first using money in his or her MSA, and when that is gone, uses own money for the rest up to $5,000 and 10 percent of all bills in excess of $5,000

attributable to those few unfortunate patients who get really sick and have costs at the high end, where the major medical coverage kicks in and reduces the incentive to save money.

A conundrum of the insurance market is that you tend to get what you pay for—if you only insure catastrophes, you'll get a lot of catastrophes. If the catastrophic plan provides full coverage above a limit, then patients (and hospitals) have no incentives to control costs. Conversely, trying to get patients to pay more to make them cost-sensitive in this range might seem cruel and not work well in practice—the employee with a disability trying to come up with 20 percent of a $450,000 liver transplant bill is not going to be happy and will find many newspaper reporters sympathetic to his complaints that this kind of insurance is not fair.

Ultimately, it is up to the market to decide which kinds of incentives are appropriate for health insurance. So far the market has not been kind to the defined contribution MSA approach. After a decade of trying, the market share of these plans is still less than 1 percent. So far, employees have been reluctant to try something new that they find difficult to understand, which provides benefits mostly to the employers (a cap on total health benefit contributions) and to the market (aggressive shopping to hold prices down), but does not do very much to increase the protection they receive personally to ward off the risk of high medical costs.

5.5 A RANGE OF RISK BEARING: FIXED PREMIUMS, ADMINISTERED SERVICES ONLY, AND SELF-INSURANCE

An employer can purchase insurance at a fixed price and bear no risk, or it can pool its own funds, handle all claims, and self-insure while bearing all risks. In between these two options there are a range of contracts that split the risk and claims-processing burden: experience rated, retention ratio, minimum premium, and administered services only (ASO) plans (Table 5.4). Negotiating price is a major problem in contracting for insurance. **Experience rating,** by allowing the price to rise or fall to match the dollar amount of claims submitted by employees during the previous year (experience), avoids costly and contentious haggling. A **retention ratio** agreement makes a similar adjustment, but in the current year. The employer and insurer estimate losses, and if claims turn out to be smaller than expected, the insurer returns most of the difference, retaining only a percentage (the retention ratio) for administrative expenses and profit.

Two things make it difficult for an employer to act as its own insurance company: catastrophic losses and claims processing. To some extent these difficulties can be ameliorated through contractual arrangements. Economies of scale in risk-bearing can be obtained contractually through **reinsurance,** which is a type of major medical coverage for employers, a policy for the group as a whole that covers 90 percent of the cost of any individual above a specified amount (perhaps $50,000) or an aggregate loss of the group as a whole that is above the expected value (perhaps above $5 million). Of course, reinsurance is quite costly; therefore,

TABLE 5.4	Range of Insurance Contracts			
Insurer Bears Risk, Processes Claims ←				→ **Employer Bears Risk, Processes Own Claims**
Fixed Premiums	**Experience Related**	**Retention Ratio**	**ASO**	**Self-Insurance**
Pay pre-set amount for coverage	Premiums changed each year to reflect last year's actual claims	If losses are less than expected, insurer gives back part of premium	Administrative services only, insurance company pays claims using the firm's own funds	Firm pays claims, acts as their own insurance company

coverage is usually purchased for extraordinary losses only. Claims processing is apt to create administrative difficulties, because a company is usually better at its own line of business than at the business of managing and paying insurance benefits. Economies of scale in claims processing can be obtained contractually through **administered services only (ASO)** contracts in which an insurance company processes the bills, pays the claims, and settles disputes for a set fee per year or per claim, but all funds for paying benefits come directly from the employer.

Under "normal" circumstances the costs of experience rated, retention ratio, ASO, and self-insurance contracts should converge toward the same amount; however, circumstances are rarely normal. When a firm accepts bids for an experience rated plan, it is not uncommon for an insurance company to try to "buy the business" by setting the premiums very low in the first year. Then it will use the bad experience during that year to force a high premium in the following year. The employer who got such a good deal is now stuck and must accept a substantial premium increase or incur the costs of going out to bid again, often finding that with such a record of underwriting losses, few insurers want to bid. Also, a group with higher-than-expected losses may find that their insurer starts to give poor service and gets very nasty about paying claims (and thus is able to hold onto premium dollars longer). On the other hand, employee groups often try to take advantage of insurance companies by dropping them after a bad year (thus allowing no time to make up the extraordinary losses through experience rating) or repeatedly going into the market to search for low bids. The more flexible retention ratio agreement is like a partnership. The insurance company and the employee group get together in a long-term arrangement in which initial pricing is not so important. Year-to-year conflicts are avoided. However, the downside of this more integrated contract is that if things do go wrong, it is much worse for both parties.

The Underwriting Cycle

In the long run, the increases in premiums match the increases in underlying health care costs. Yet in any given year, the rate of increase could be higher or lower. Economists have observed that most insurance markets (e.g., property and casualty, malpractice, health) tend to have a cycle of overcharging and undercharging that lasts about 7 to 10 years.[11] At the peak of the cycle, premiums are high relative to costs, profits are fat, and competitors are attracted to start the cycle. As more insurance companies enter the market, premiums are driven downward. In the trough of the cycle, rates are low as insurance companies compete vigorously to gain market share. The lack of profitability eventually takes a toll, some insurance companies exit the market, and rates increase. Eventually, rising prices and good profits start the cycle over again. Figure 5.4 shows how premiums and costs have risen and fallen over the last decade. In the early 1990s, hefty double-digit premium increases built profitability. The rise of managed care and the overhanging threat of government intervention kept medical costs very low in the middle of the decade—but insurers trying to get a larger piece of the market drove premiums down below costs. The combination of low premiums and rising costs crushed profits, pushing several HMOs and insurance companies to the edge of insolvency. The years 2001 and 2002 were catch-up time, with insurers once again trying to build reserves. It is expected that premiums will increase even more in 2003, perhaps by as much as 15 percent. While some of this increase will be given up to hospitals and doctors (and, therefore, allow for some increases in underlying costs), eventually the protests of benefits managers and hard-pressed employees will lead to moderation that should cause the cycle to turn down again by the middle of the decade.

5.6 ERISA, TAXES, AND MANDATED BENEFITS

The employee benefits offered by a company are determined largely by competitive conditions in the labor market as the company tries to hire new workers or directly through

| FIGURE 5.4 | The Underwriting Cycle of Health Insurance, 1988–2002 |

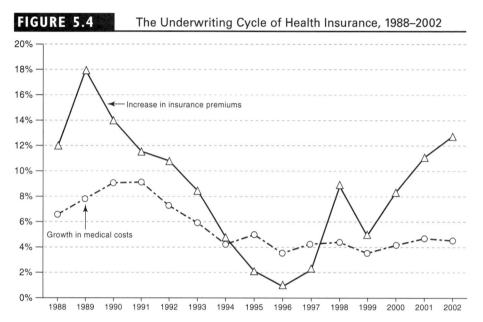

Source: Kaiser/HRET *Employer Health Benefits Survey* and U.S. National Health Accounts.

negotiations with the unions that represent the workers. Companies view benefits as a way to retain workers, and workers view benefits as a way to protect themselves against losses. The interests of both companies and workers are represented in the final outcome.

Sometimes a broader public interest is imposed in the form of **mandated benefits,** regulations promulgated by the government stating that specific benefits (e.g., substance abuse treatment, AZT treatment for HIV infection) must be provided. If such benefits are a good thing, why don't they arise naturally in the course of competitive contracting? Consider the case of substance abuse benefits. Without such benefits, insurance will pay for treatment of liver damage, but not for the excessive drinking that caused it. From a social perspective, it is much more efficient to treat the underlying cause (alcoholism) than to treat just the symptom (liver damage). However, a company is not interested in the productivity of society as a whole, but in the productivity of its work force. A quite reasonable profit-maximizing response to alcoholism is to fire the employee and push him or her out onto the streets, where the burden is borne by the rest of society. Adverse selection can also play a role. A company with especially generous benefits for HIV/AIDS treatment will find its premiums going higher and higher as more chronically ill people try to get jobs there. Eventually, if adverse selection is severe enough, only people with a very high risk of HIV/AIDS would be willing to accept the low wages paid by this company in order to get the benefits.

Mental illness poses similar problems of adverse selection because the benefits are highly concentrated, with most of the dollars spent on just a few people, who, with their families, are much more aware of the risks than the insurance company. In a competitive market, insurance contracts reflect the interests of companies and most employees, but not society as a whole. If such benefits are not mandatory, only a few companies will offer them.

Insurance is primarily regulated by the states. Some states, such as Arizona, impose very few mandates, while Massachusetts has more than thirty. Employers operating in multiple states need uniform national laws because it is difficult to maintain many different sets of benefit plans and give more or less to an employee depending on place of residence. Under the Employee Retirement and Income Security Act of 1974 (ERISA) and later amendments, self-insured firms are regulated under national **ERISA** rules and thus are exempt from state mandates. Because only large firms are able to self-insure, the attempt to increase coverage through mandates may have the paradoxical effect of reducing the number of people insured, as small firms opt to provide no health insurance at all.

State taxes provide another incentive to self-insure. Most states impose a premium tax of 1 percent to 2 percent that can be avoided through self-insurance or ASO contracts. Minimum premium plans in which the employer pays the first $X million (usually about 90 percent of estimated losses) and the insurer pays the rest exist primarily to avoid state taxes, since they are no different from fixed-premium full insurance with regard to risk or claims processing. Several innovative state health care financing plans have been challenged under ERISA. For example, New Jersey funded a special program for the uninsured through a 30 percent surcharge on all hospital bills. After large companies won ERISA exemption, only small employers and individuals were left paying the surcharge; therefore, the state was forced to dismantle its program.[12]

If mandated benefits are a good idea, why don't the states just pay for them? The answer is that they would have to raise taxes to do so. A mandated benefit, although it operates like a tax on firms, is counted as a regular cost of business to the firm. It does not appear on the government's budget and thus is not recognized by many voters. Although the public ultimately will lose more in forgone wages than in taxes avoided, this fact is not obvious to voters when they go to the polls. For this reason, any national insurance plan enacted in the United States is almost certain to be based on employer contributions. People who would never vote to increase taxes to fund national health insurance will calmly vote to have government insist that every employer provide benefits—and so our government will rationally follow the path of least resistance.

Insurance, by channeling funds through different organizations and contractual arrangements, has a tendency to obscure the actual costs of medical care. Pretending that a mandated insurance benefit will somehow make these services cost less than if they were funded through a tax increase has misled some people, while companies have misled the public by claiming to have paid a "fair share" for their own workers, but never dealing with the issue of how health care for people who are homeless, have a mental illness, or have HIV/AIDS will be paid for. A health care system that helps only the healthy is cost-effective in one sense and worthless in another. Perhaps the worst aspect of the complex system of health insurance that has arisen in the United States is this obfuscation of reality that allows interested parties to avoid responsibility and never face up to the hard decisions on how to pay for health care. It is, therefore, worthwhile to examine how this complex system came to be and why some organizations and contracts have dominated in the United States while different forms of insurance developed in other countries.

5.7   HISTORY OF HEALTH INSURANCE

In some sense, risk pooling has always existed—people have always taken care of each other during times of need. Financial contracts for pooling risk did not become important until the Industrial Revolution, when economies moved from the medieval manor system, where most people worked the land, to a wage-based economy centered in cities and towns. Freemen who left the medieval estates and gathered in towns to practice skilled trades, such as printing and goldsmithing, often became quite wealthy, but were potentially subject to catastrophic losses if they become ill. While gaining freedom, they had given up the protection and security that went with being part of an estate. If they became sick, they might have become destitute. The guilds were organized to further their interests collectively and became natural vehicles for sharing risks. Initially this took the form of soliciting donations from all other guild members "passing the hat" when someone became ill or died. Then more formal institutions evolved that accumulated funds over time. A "subscription" would be regularly collected that could be used to pay benefits. In this early form of insurance, there was no distinction made between the loss of wages due to illness and the costs of medical care (or burial). Insurance was simply a way to provide money in time of need. The guild members knew each other well and therefore the definition of loss was made by a consensus of the leadership, not the existence of a doctor's bill.[13]

Early industrialists also recognized the need to provide wages and medical care for workers when they were sick. It is unlikely that funds were set aside for this purpose. Rather, sickness funds were drawn out of daily business receipts. Most such benefits were informal, provided at the discretion of the business owner, and not part of the official employment contract. In this sense, early industrial benefits were quite similar to the paternalistic obligations owed to the serfs by the manorial lords who owned the land they worked on, except that as factories and wages replaced farms and tenant shares, the benefits were money payments rather than direct care. By the nineteenth century, some industries that were particularly dangerous and in remote locations had developed contracts with a "company doctor" so that there was always regular medical care available. In other industries, it was the workers who organized to provide sickness benefits. As unions became an important means for furthering the interests of workers, they found that they needed some way to keep the membership involved (and paying dues) throughout the year and not just when a strike was threatened. Medical coverage became the preferred union benefit. It was always needed, made the workers and their families grateful, and attracted newcomers. In those days care could be provided at relatively low cost through clinics or "dispensaries" staffed by young doctors hired by the union to practice several nights a week. Company and union clinics, mutual benefit societies, and other forms of prepayment had become common by 1850, but still provided medical care financing to only a small fraction of the population, probably less than one-twentieth. As wages rose above the subsistence level and workers became more assertive, it became evident that insurance would have to be extended to cover more of the population.

The first national health insurance program was implemented in Germany in 1893. Bismarck, the chancellor who had unified the German Lander (provinces) into a nation, saw that his political successes were threatened by the popularity of socialist causes among workers. By putting together a social security system with medical insurance and retirement benefits for industrial workers, he pre-empted one of the main goals of the socialist movement and was able to maintain popular support.[14] National health plans were established in England in 1911, Sweden in 1914, and France in 1930. At first, only salaried workers in the major manufacturing plants were covered, usually with a lesser degree of coverage for dependents. Other workers, such as agricultural and retail workers, day laborers, shopkeepers, and the self-employed, had to take care of themselves. Over the next fifty years, coverage was successively broadened. By 1980, almost every developed country had health insurance coverage for all citizens, either through a national health service (United Kingdom) or a universal insurance plan (Canada) or by coordinating all employer-based plans and providing government insurance for the rest of the population (Germany, Japan).[15] Evolution of health insurance in the United States was much different, and a large segment of the population still lacks health insurance today.

The United States depended on voluntary private initiatives to develop health insurance, with much less reliance on government. There was a recognition that the population needed protection against losses due to illness, and in 1929 the independent Committee of the Costs of Medical Care began a fact-finding study, eventually producing a twenty-eight-volume report that was very influential in shaping the growth of voluntary insurance in the United States.[16] In this same year, Baylor hospital proposed to the local teachers' association that it would provide all the care needed to anyone who would pay a premium of $0.50 a month. The plan proved to be very popular, and similar plans were started by other hospitals nearby. One problem with a "hospital prepayment" plan was that a patient whose doctor worked in a different hospital, or who needed a special type of care elsewhere, got no benefits. The solution was to combine all the separate plans under the sponsorship of the state hospital association so that one plan covered all hospitals; thus, Blue Cross was born. It grew rapidly, from 3,000 members in 1930, to more than 10,000 in 1932, to more than 1,000,000 by 1936. In 2002, 84 million people were insured through Blue Cross/Blue Shield plans.[17]

The imposition of wage and price controls during World War II provided an indirect but powerful boost to voluntary insurance. Employers were not allowed to raise wages, but they could provide additional benefits.[18] With wartime production booming and many laborers drafted into the military, most companies desperately needed to attract more workers. In less than twenty years, health insurance went from being an occasional perk that covered just 5 percent of the population to a routine benefit that was expected to be part of any good job, and covered more than 50 percent of the population. Even with favorable tax treatments and active encouragement, however, voluntary insurance could not be extended to cover two of the groups who needed it most: the elderly and the poor. The poor were simply not able to afford health insurance. Furthermore, while policy makers and hospital administrators might think that paying premiums to prepare for future medical expenses was one of the most important things a family could do with its money, many of the poor did not. Since there was always some form of care available, usually in city clinics and hospitals, the poor often chose to spend what little discretionary money they had on better housing, better food, or some entertainment, rather than insurance premiums.

The difficulties of the elderly in obtaining insurance were largely attributable to adverse selection and the discounting of consumption over time.[19] While younger people were formed into risk pooling groups on the basis of employment, many older people were not attached to an employer. There was no natural grouping by which risks could be shared, and there were no tax advantages to insurance premiums paid out of savings or retirement benefits rather than wages. Furthermore, the differences in the expected costs of medical care between individuals are much greater for older people, making it more difficult to constitute risk-sharing pools. Whereas many of the illnesses that strike younger people are essentially random events of low probability, many medical expenses of the elderly are for chronic conditions. There is no reason for a healthy seventy-two-year-old to want to be in a group paying the same premium as someone with cancer or arthritis who is likely to have high medical expenses for many years. Elderly people often know much more about the potential cost of their health conditions than any insurance company can and thus create adverse selection problems when allowed to purchase insurance individually. These difficulties are exacerbated by the need to save early in one's career to pay for medical expenses that come after retirement. There must be a mechanism for transferring dollars from consumption at early ages toward old age. The Social Security Acts of 1965, which established the **Medicare** (Title XVI) program for the elderly and **Medicaid** (Title XVII) for the indigent, created fundamental changes in the U.S. health care system and made government a major partner in financing medical care.[20] Adverse selection was no longer a problem for the elderly, because everyone age 65 or older was insured. Poverty no longer excluded the indigent from health insurance, because the government made these benefits available at no cost.[21]

After a century of development, health care financing in the United States is still in flux, with a mixed public and private system in which government accounts for 45 percent of total funds (55 percent if tax subsidies are counted), private insurance accounts for 35 percent (including Blue Cross/Blue Shield, self-funded employer plans, commercial insurance companies, and HMOs), charitable contributions and various programs account for 5 percent, and the remaining 18 percent is paid directly by patients and family members out of pocket. A sizable fraction of those out-of-pocket costs are for deductibles and coinsurance and thus, in one sense, could be considered part of the third-party insurance payments.

Among this variety of health insurance organizations, government (Medicare in particular) is the dominant payer. During the 1950s Blue Cross set the tone and structure for insurance coverage and Medicare copied the Blue Cross reimbursement system. Since then, the balance of power has changed dramatically. Blue Cross has fragmented, reducing what was once a pervasive community voluntary organization to a set of franchisees linked by a trademark, with the largest (California, New York) transformed into independent, and essentially faceless, for-profit insurance companies with no specific ideology or geographic ties. Conversely, Medicare has become such a central player that no hospital and few doctors can afford to be without a Medicare contract. Every provider is thus compelled to use the complex and highly regulated Medicare cost and activity reporting scheme. Other insurers find it easier to adapt the Medicare payment system than to develop their own, making the influence of Medicare even greater than its percentage share of the market.

5.8 INCENTIVES—TO PATIENTS, TO PAYERS, AND TO PROVIDERS

Which type of insurance plan encourages patients to use a more expensive, higher-quality hospital? Which type of plan encourages longer stays? The insurance contract not only provides coverage for risks, it also structures the incentives. Being reimbursed a fixed number of dollars per hospital day gives patients an incentive to a) find a hospital that is priced near that amount but not below and b) to stay as long as they want since each additional day is covered. It may also make patients try to bargain with the hospital to accept the amount of reimbursement provided as payment in full. If the per day maximum applies only to hospital charges, both the hospital and the patient may have an incentive to get laboratory fees, drugs, physical therapy, and other care billed separately by an outside firm.

HMO and PPO contracts use reduced deductibles and co-payments to provide incentives for patients to use only hospitals for which the HMO or PPO has negotiated volume discounts—and it is the promise of additional volume that makes hospitals offer discounts. Most drug reimbursement is now of the "triple-tier" form: a low per prescription fee for generic drugs, a moderate per prescription fee or percentage for drugs on an approved list (formulary), and a higher per prescription fee or percentage for "off-list" drugs (see "triple-tier" pharmacy plans in Chapter 10). Indeed, often it requires a physician to write a letter (a significant disincentive) for the patient to get any reimbursement at all if the prescribed drug is not on the list. By structuring incentives this way, insurance contracts can reduce or increase the use of certain services, steer patients to approved providers, and affect the sort of price negotiations that take place.

Insurance, like many other business arrangements, tends to serve the interests of those who write the contracts. Thus, the original Blue Cross plans, developed by hospital associations, were beneficial to hospitals; the generous reimbursement with no patient charges and community rating kept hospital beds full and revenues flowing. The entry of commercial insurers depended on their ability to offer a lower-priced product using co-pays and deductibles to reduce premiums and reduce services (not something in the interest of hospitals, which wanted more business, not less). If these contractual stipulations caused some "positive selection"—discouraging sick people from purchasing commercial insurance and making them stick with Blue Cross—this was fine with the commercial insurers and the employers who purchased commercial coverage for workers. They had no desire to cover more "high-cost" people. Of course, the hospitals worried because they still had to care for the high-cost people and the uninsured.

In the long run, contracts must meet the needs of all parties, but it can take a long time to get there. Also, it is possible to structure contracts so that the interests of some parties are ignored. For example, a corporation may be willing to eliminate coverage for alcoholism since they could just fire an employee rather than rehabilitate them, or be willing to put an annual maximum on the number of days of hospital treatment to discourage people with HIV/AIDS from taking a job there. Universal national health insurance coverage would put everyone under the same contract so that no one could be excluded. However, with everyone insured under the same plan, no one has incentives to shop around for better prices, no ability to pick and choose which coverage is or is not worthwhile, and no chance to go somewhere else if the service provided by the insurer is unsatisfactory. Insurance contracts in the real world represent a balancing of incentives and interests, a balance that is changing all the time.

SUGGESTIONS FOR FURTHER READING

Employee Benefit Research Institute, *Employment Based Health Insurance Coverage, 2000* (serial publication) (www.ebri.org).

Health Insurance Institute of America. *Sourcebook of Health Insurance Data* (Washington, DC: HIAA, annual), (www.hiaa.org).

Kaiser Family Foundation and HRET Employer Health Benefits, 2002 Annual Survey, (www.kff.org).

SUMMARY

1. Paying medical bills with **insurance makes health care a third-party transaction.** All three parties, *i)* patients, *ii)* providers, and *iii)* insurers, must benefit from the transaction. However, **separating the flow of funds from the flow of services obscures the real cost** of medical care. Health care is paid for by people (as patients, taxpayers, or employees giving up some wages to get health benefits), not by corporations.

2. The **government is the single largest insurer,** paying for 45 percent of all medical care. Medicare, which pays for the medical care of the elderly, is the largest and most influential government program, although the state/federal Medicaid program dominates long-term care reimbursement. Tax advantages have fostered the growth of health insurance as an employee benefit. Private health insurance covers 62 percent of the population, but pays only 36 percent of the total bills. About 17 percent is paid for out-of-pocket by patients or their families.

3. About 40 million Americans, **15 percent of the population, are uninsured.** For many of them it is a rational decision to go without insurance based on their youth, good health, and/or low current earning power. For some, going without insurance is the result of a chronic disease, bad luck, or the size of the company they work for.

4. Insurance comes in a range of contractual forms, from pure insurance with fixed premiums, to various forms of risk sharing, to administered services only, to self-insurance plans in which the employer bears all the risk. Obtaining **tax benefits and exemption from state-mandated** coverage under ERISA has been a major reason for companies to self-insure.

5. Historically, the development of voluntary insurance plans in the United States was led by groups of hospitals and doctors who were interested in **assuring payment to providers** as well as protecting patients from losses.

6. Insurance **contracts create incentives** for patients, providers, and insurance companies to behave in ways that affect the market. Almost any contract will favor some interests and harm others.

1. {*gains from trade*} Who benefits from a three-party transaction?

2. {*accounting, incidence*} How can a patient benefit if the premiums paid are more than the cost of the medical care received? How can an insurance company benefit if the medical care it provides costs more than the premiums paid in?

3. {*marginal incentives*} Explain how one insurance contract can provide more or fewer incentives to do the following:

   a. Choose a higher-quality (more expensive) hospital
   b. Spend more days in the hospital
   c. Use more drugs
   d. Choose a higher-quality (more expensive) surgeon

4. {*uninsured*} The law now gives a worker who becomes unemployed the right to buy continuing health insurance coverage after leaving the company. Why might it be rational for a factory worker who loses his or her job to give up this legal right to purchase coverage and become uninsured, even knowing that he or she is at risk for high medical expenditures?

5. {*mandated benefits*} Prior to 1970, maternity was usually treated differently from other medical expenses, either excluded entirely from coverage or subject to a flat lump-sum cash (indemnity) benefit. Why? During the 1970s, 23 states mandated that treatment related to pregnancy be covered the same as any other type of treatment, and in 1978, such coverage became uniform throughout the United States. Would mandated maternity benefits make working in a salaried position more or less attractive to women? Would it make women of childbearing age more or less attractive as employees? Would it increase or decrease the number of births performed by Cesarean section? Who do you think bore the expense of implementing this mandate? (For a discussion of these issues see "The Incidence of Mandated Maternity Benefits," by Jonathan Gruber, *American Economic Review* 84, no.3 (April 1994): 622–641.

6. {*ownership*} Why was it more common for railroads and timber companies to provide health insurance in the early 1900s than for textile mills or accounting firms?

7. {*ownership*} Who controlled Blue Cross when it was formed? Did this form of insurance generate profits for its owners?

8. {*adverse selection*} Which government insurance program is more affected by adverse selection, Medicare or Medicaid?

1. C. Rufus Rorem, "Sickness Insurance in the United States," *Bulletin of the American Hospital Association* (June 1932). Odin W. Anderson, *Health Services as a Growth Enterprise in the United States since 1875*, 2nd ed. (Ann Arbor, Mich.: Health Administration Press, 1990).

2. Estimates of coverage are from William S. Custer and Pat Ketsche, *The Changing Sources of Health Insurance*, Health Insurance Association of America, 2000 (www.hiaa.org) and Employer Health Benefits, 2002 Annual Survey, Kaiser Family Foundation and HRET, 2002.

3. Employer Health Benefits, 2002 Annual Survey.

4. Laschober, Mary A. et al., "Trends in Medicare Supplemental Insurance and Prescription Drug Coverage, 1996-1999," *Health Affairs* 21, no. 2 (April 2002): 11.

5. U.S. National Health Accounts, Office of the Actuary, CMS (www.cms.gov/statistics/nhe/).

6. U.S. Census Bureau, Health Insurance Coverage: 2001 (www.census.gov/hhes/www/hlthin01.html). J.P. Vistnes and S.H. Zuvekas, *Health Insurance Status of the Civilian Noninstitutionalized Population, 1997* (Rockville, Md.: Agency for Health Care Policy and Research, July 1999). MEPS Research Findings #8, AHCPR Publication No.99-0030.

7. The 19–24 age group is more than twice as likely to be uninsured as other age groups (35 percent versus 15 percent, see Vistnes and Zuvekas, 1999). Helen Levy and Thomas DeLeire, "What Do People Buy When They Don't Buy Health Insurance?" Harris Graduate School of Public Policy Studies working paper, University of Chicago, June 26, 2002, (www.jcpr.org/wpfiles/levy_delire.pdf).

8. Helen Levy and Thomas DeLeire, "What Do People Buy When They Don't Buy Health Insurance?" Harris Graduate School of Public Policy Studies, University of Chicago, working paper June 26, 2002 (www.jcpr.org/wpfiles/levy_deleire.pdf).

9. Lisa Dubay, Ian Hill, and Genevieve Kenney, "Five Things Everyone Should Know About SCHIP," Series A, No.A-55, The Urban Institute, October 2002 (www.urban.org/url.cfm?ID=3105707); Elizabeth Thompson Beckley, "Missing the SCHIP," *Modern Physician* (September 2002):10; also see (www.insurekidsnow.gov).

10. Mark Pauly et. al., "What Would Happen If Large Firms Offered MSAs?" *Health Affairs* 19, no. 3 (May 2000): 165–172; Deborah Chollet, "Why the Pauly/Goodman Proposal Won't Work," *Health Affairs* 14, no. 2 (Summer 1995): 273–274; Jon B. Christianson et al., "Defined-Contribution Health Insurance Products: Development and Prospects," *Health Affairs* 21, no. 1: 49–64.

11. Bradley C. Struck, P.B. Ginsburg, and Jon R. Gabel, "Tracking Health Care Costs," *Health Affairs* (September 25, 2002 Web supplement),(www.healthaffairs.org/WebExclusives/Strunk_Web_Excl_092502.htm); P.J. Feldstein and T.M. Wickizer, "Analysis of Private Health Insurance Premium Growth Rates: 1985-1992," *Medical Care* 33, no. 10 (October 1995): 1035–1050.

12. Howard S. Berliner and Sonia Delgada, "From DRGs to Deregulation: New Jersey Takes the Road Less Traveled," *Journal of American Health Policy* 3 (July/August 1993): 4448.

13. R. Munts, *Bargaining for Health: Labor Unions, Health Insurance and Medical Care,* (Madison, Wisc.: University of Wisconsin Press, 1967). David T. Beito, *From Mutual Aid to the Welfare State: Fraternal Societies and Social Services 1890-1967* (Chapel Hill: UNC Press, 2000).

14. Peter A. Kohler and Hans F. Zacher, eds. *The Evolution of Social Insurance 1881-1991: Studies of Germany, France, Great Britain, Austria and Switzerland* (New York: St. Martin's Press, 1982).

15. William A. Glaser, *Health Insurance in Practice: International Variations in Financing, Benefits, and Problems* (San Francisco: Jossey-Bass, 1991).

16. Committee on the Costs of Medical Care, *Medical Care for the American People* (Chicago: University of Chicago Press, 1932).

17. Robert Cunningham III and Robert M. Cunningham Jr., *The Blues: A History of the Blue Cross and Blue Shield System* (DeKalb: Northern Illinois University Press, 1997). Laura B. Benko, "The Blues Rise Again," *Modern Healthcare* (September 9, 2002):14–15.

18. Institute of Medicine, *Employment and Health Benefits: A Connection at Risk* (Washington, D.C.: National Academy Press, 1993), 70. Melissa A. Thomasson, "The Importance of Group Coverage: How Tax Policy Shaped U.S. Health Insurance," NBER working paper (February 2000): 7543 (www.nber.org/papers/w7543).

19. Herman M. Somers and Anne R. Somers, *Medicare and the Hospitals: Issues and Prospects*(Washington, D.C.: The Brookings Institution, 1967).

20. W.J. Cohen, "Reflections on the Enactment of Medicare and Medicaid," HCFR(supplement): 3-16. Theodore Marmor, *The Politics of Medicare* (Chicago: Aldine, 1973).

21. Note, however, that may people you might consider "poor" are not eligible for Medicaid, a major reason that there are still 40 million uninsured. Typically the "working poor" have income above the poverty line, but lack employer-provided insurance. Single persons without children usually do not qualify, even if their incomes are very low (hence the acronym TANF —"Temporary Assistance to Needy *Families*").

CHAPTER **6**

PHYSICIANS

QUESTIONS

1. How are physicians paid?
2. Which types of physicians earn the highest incomes?
3. How much does it cost to practice medicine?
4. Is it doctors or patients who decide which hospital to use, which drugs to buy, and which specialist to see for a second opinion? In what sense is the doctor the patient's "agent"?
5. Are rising malpractice insurance premiums a major cause of higher doctor bills?
6. Is medical care "sold" like other goods and services?
7. Why are licensure restrictions more strongly enforced for some types of medical care than for others?
8. Is the American Medical Association (AMA) a professional society serving science, or a union serving the economic interests of its members? Is it both?
9. Which is more competitive: the market for health insurance or the market for medical care?

At the center of medical practice stands the physician. Physicians direct the flow of patients by controlling admissions, referrals, regulations, insurance reimbursements, and prescriptions. A very powerful and special bond exists between doctor and patient. This relationship is based on medical science—and ethics and emotions—as well as economics.[1] Even when a transaction does not directly involve a physician financially, the physician still plays a dominant role. In the preceding chapters we discussed health care from the perspective of the patient. Now we switch to the perspective of the provider—not the payer, but the payee. For the physician, medical expenditures are not *costs*; they are *revenues*.

6.1   PHYSICIAN PAYMENT: HOW FUNDS FLOW IN

While most of the labor force is employed and paid a salary by a large organization, most physicians are independent entrepreneurs or partners running what are, in effect, small businesses.[2] The income of physicians in solo or group private practices mostly comes from **fee-for-service** payments, a specified amount paid for each visit or procedure, although an increasing amount is coming from complex, negotiated third-party contracts.

In the 1930s, physicians were essentially free to charge whatever they decided was appropriate but often collected much less than what they charged. Today, 88 percent of physician revenues come from third-party payments[3] and most fees are subject to some form of external review or control (see Table 6.1).

It is important to distinguish between what the physician **charges** (i.e., the amount that appears on the bill) and the actual payments made by the insurance company, which may be considerably less. One of the initial steps in the evolution of physician payment in the United States was the development of usual, customary, and reasonable (UCR) fee schedules. The Blue Shield plans, which then provided the largest portion of physician insurance and operated with the support of local medical societies, collected information on what each physician charged for each service in a local area during the previous year. When a physician submitted a bill, it was checked to determine whether it was above his or her median charge for the same service the previous year (usual), above the 75th percentile of charges by all doctors in the area (customary), or justifiably higher because of a patient's complicating secondary illness or another acceptable reason (reasonable). When Medicare was implemented in 1966, it adopted the Blue Shield UCR method of paying physicians.

An effort to reduce payments, particularly for certain services, led insurers to promulgate **fee schedules.** A fee schedule is like a menu that specifies how much the insurance company will pay physicians for particular services. Fee schedules can be proposed by the sellers (physicians) to try to keep prices up or by the buyers (Medicare, insurance companies) to try to keep prices down. A major difficulty with fee schedules is the amazingly large number of services that must be priced. It is easy to come up with a reasonable price for a coronary bypass operation or services associated with a normal birth, but what about for oblique lateral pelvic X-rays, measurement of bilirubin or potassium levels, management of schizophrenia, and a host of other medical services?

To bring order to fee schedules, organizations have devised **relative value scales,** which give each service a point value. A common service (e.g., standard office visit, hernia repair surgery) is usually given a weight of 1 point and all other services are given point values relative to that standard unit of service (e.g., 5 points, 0.2 points). After the physician and insurance company agree on the value per point, payment for each service is determined (e.g., if value per point is $20, a physician providing a 3.5-point service is paid $3.5 \times \$20 = \$70$). In 1992, the Medicare resource-based relative value scale (**RBRVS**) was implemented. A team of health economists and health services researchers, led by William Hsiao of Harvard University, studied the resources used in providing physician care to estimate a point value for each service based on (1) physician time, (2) intensity of effort,

TABLE 6.1	Types of Physician Payment

Charges: The amount appearing on the bill, without insurance.

Fee-for service: A specified payment for each unit of service provided.

Fee Schedule: A set "menu" of prices for each service agreed upon in advance.

UCR: A method for denying bills that are out of line with the "usual, customary and reasonable charges made by this and other physicians for the same service last year."

RVS: A schedule based on objective standards showing relative value points for each service compared to a common unit (i.e., regular office visit). Deciding a dollar value per point converts it into a fee schedule.

RBRVS: The relative value schedule set by Medicare for physician fees.

Capitation: A set payment per person per month regardless of the number of services used.

Salary: A paycheck from an employer.

(3) practice costs, and (4) costs of advanced specialty training.[4] The Centers for Medicare and Medicaid Services (CMS) of the U.S. Department of Health and Human Services, which administers the Medicare program, set the dollars per point for 2003 at $34.59, with adjustments for geographic variation in practice costs and for malpractice insurance (see the RBRVS Fee Schedule box).

The Medicare physician reimbursement system provides a kind of "public good" (see Chapter 15) for other insurance programs; that is, a universally understood and practiced standard fee schedule they can adopt or easily modify by changing the dollar conversion factor or separating certain categories. Medicaid, Blue Cross, and commercial insurance contracts that cover the 87 percent of the population under age sixty-five often base their payments on a modified form of the Medicare RBRVS or use Medicare payment levels as a benchmark.

RBRVS FEE SCHEDULE

Medicare relies on a resource-based relative value scale (RBRVS) to determine the fees it will pay physicians to treat its beneficiaries. A fee is calculated by multiplying a service's relative value units (RVUs) by a conversion factor, adjusting for geographic cost variations. Medicare also uses the RBRVS to pay for certain services furnished by allied health professionals (e.g., physician assistants, nurse practitioners, certified registered nurse anesthetists, physical therapists).

Relative Value Scale

An RBRVS is a list of physician services with RVUs assigned to each service. The units indicate a service's cost relative to that of the typical physician service, which has a relative value of 1.0 units. A service with 1.559 units is therefore 55.9 percent more costly to provide than the typical service, while a service with 0.693 units is 30.7 percent less costly to provide than the typical service.

A service's total RVUs are spread over the following three major components:

- Physician Work (pw)—The time spent, effort exerted, and skills used by the physician to furnish the service. This component includes pre-service, intra-service, and post-service work related to the physician's encounter with the patient.

- Practice Expenses (pe)—The wages, salaries, and fringe benefits the physician provides office staff and money spent on other office expenses, such as rent and supplies. Many physician services have two practice expense RVUs—facility practice expense units and non-facility practice expense units, the latter almost always higher than the former. This site-of-service differential recognizes that the physician does not absorb the full cost of services provided in a facility setting. Part of the cost is paid by the facility and, therefore, is included in the amount the facility is reimbursed.

- Malpractice Insurance (mi)—Separated from other practice expenses, largely because it varies significantly among specialties and across states and fluctuates markedly with oscillations in malpractice awards. Recently, malpractice expense has significantly increased.

Physician work accounts for approximately 55 percent of total RVUs, followed by 42 percent for practice expenses, and 3 percent for malpractice insurance.

Level 1 of the CMS Common Procedure Coding System is used to identify the physician services a patient receives. Level 1—Current Procedural Terminology, fourth edition

(Continued)

RBRVS FEE SCHEDULE (CONTINUED)

(CPT-4)—is the most widely used coding system for office visits, consultations, surgery, imaging, and other physician services. Approximately 7,500 CPT codes are paid under the RBRVS fee schedule. Certain physician services may be performed by nurse practitioners, nurse midwives, or other mid-level or nonphysician practitioners. These practitioners may practice independently or under a physician's supervision, depending on state law. The same CPT code is used to document a service, regardless of who performs it.

Table 6.2 shows Medicare's RVUs for calendar year (CY) 2003 for selected physician services, which range from under 1.0 to nearly 29. The table shows the following:

- The RVUs for a new patient's office visit exceed those for an established patient's office visit; the units for both types of visits vary directly with the level of care.

- The RVUs for major surgical procedures (e.g., CPT 69501) include the cost of services and items that are bundled with the procedure, such as the surgeon's initial consultation, preoperative visits, treatment for complications after surgery, and postoperative visits to the surgeon for 10 to 90 days after surgery.

- Diagnostic and therapeutic radiology services have a professional and technical component. The professional component represents the portion of the service associated with the interpretation of the test. The technical component is the portion associated with the performance of the test. Often, a physician is paid for the professional component while the hospital where the service is furnished is paid for the technical component.

The RVUs are adjusted for geographic variations in wage rates and other prices that physicians pay for the resources used to produce patient care. The adjustment is based on geographic practice cost indexes (GPCIs) for physician work, practice expenses, and malpractice insurance. As of January 1, 2003, there were about 90 Medicare payment areas nationally, including statewide areas and metropolitan statistical areas. GPCIs vary noticeably across payment areas.

TABLE 6.2   Proposed Relative Value Units for Ten Physician Services, CY 2003

HCPCS/CPT Code	Description	Physician Work	Facility	Non-Facility	Malpractice Insurance	Facility	Non-Facility
99202	Office or other outpatient visit, new patient, level 2	0.88	0.32	0.77	0.05	1.25	1.70
99204	Office or other outpatient visit, new patient, level 4	2.00	0.72	1.49	0.10	2.82	3.59
99212	Office or other outpatient visit, established patient, level 2	0.45	0.16	0.52	0.02	0.63	0.99
99214	Office or other outpatient visit, established patient, level 4	1.10	0.40	1.03	0.04	1.54	2.17
99283	Emergency department services, level 3	1.24	0.32	na	0.08	1.64	na
30400	Reconstruction of nose	9.83	8.81	na	0.80	19.44	na
35501	Artery bypass graft	19.19	7.43	na	2.33	28.95	na
42800	Biopsy of throat	1.39	2.62	3.09	0.10	4.11	4.58
69501	Mastoidectomy	9.07	8.07	na	0.65	17.79	na
70336	Magnetic image, jaw joint	1.48	na	11.67	0.56	na	13.71
	Professional component	1.48	0.51	0.51	0.07	2.06	2.06
	Technical component	0.00	na	11.16	0.49	na	11.65

Note: na = not applicable.
   Non-Facility = outside of hospital.

Source: Federal Register, "Medicare Program," vol. 67 (December 31, 2002), Appendix B.

(Continued)

RBRVS FEE SCHEDULE (CONTINUED)

Conversion Factor

The dollar value of an RVU is called the conversion factor (CF). This factor ($34.59 for CY 2003 for all physician services except anesthesia) is multiplied by the RVUs to calculate the fee for a given service. At times, Medicare's conversion factor serves as a floor for private health plans and ceiling for state Medicaid programs. Given the following assumptions for CPT 99283, CF = $34.59, RVU_{pw} = 1.24 (RVUs for *physician work*), RVU_{pe} = 0.32 (RVUs for *practice expenses*), RVU_{mi} = 0.08 (RVUs for *malpractice insurance*), $GPCI_{pw}$ = 1.032 (GPCI for *physician work*), $GPCI_{pe}$ = 1.109 (GPCI for *practice expenses*), and $GPCI_{mi}$ = 1.215 (GPCI for *malpractice insurance*), the fee would be $59.90.

$$\text{Fee} = \text{CF} \times [(RVU_{pw} \times GPCI_{pw}) + (RVU_{pe} \times GPCI_{pe}) + (RVU_{mi} \times GPCI_{mi})]$$
$$\$59.90 = \$34.59 \times [(1.24 \times 1.032) + (0.32 \times 1.109) + (0.08 \times 1.215)]$$

If the annual Medicare Part B deductible has been met, Medicare would pay 80 percent of the lower of the calculated fee or the amount the physician actually charged for the service (see Chapter 5, Section 4). The patient would be responsible for paying the balance plus any extra amount that Medicare allows a non-participating physician to charge.

Fee Updates

In general, the conversion factor is updated annually for changes in the costs physicians incur to provide patient care. Medicare's update factor equals the compound rate of change in the following items:

- Medicare Economic Index—Measures the weighted rate of change in the cost of physician and non-physician labor, supplies, and other resources used to produce patient care. The calculation includes a downward adjustment for productivity growth.

- Performance Adjustment—Made when actual and allowed Medicare expenditures for physician services differ. The allowed amount is a target designed to slow spending growth. Spending above the target is deducted from future fee increases; spending below the target is added to future fee increases.

- Other Factors—May cause Medicare spending to increase or decrease. Examples include an expansion of the physician services that Medicare covers or new statutory or regulatory requirements that affect practice costs (e.g., the Health Insurance Portability and Accountability Act [HIPAA]).

Note: This box on RBRVS was prepared by health finance consultant and lecturer Paul L. Grimaldi, Ph.D © 2003. For additional discussion on this topic, see Paul L. Grimaldi, "Medicare Fees for Physician Services are Resource-Based," *Journal of Health Care Finance* (Spring 2002): 88–104.

Co-pays, Assignment, and Balance Billing

Medicare and other insurers' contracts not only state what they will pay the physician, but also often specify what the patient must pay. A **co-payment** of $5 or $10 per visit is often required, both to reduce premiums and, by forcing the patient to bear some costs, to reduce the number of services utilized. Some plans may also have a **deductible,** which requires the patient to pay the first $100 or $500 out of pocket per year or per illness. **Coinsurance,** with patients paying 10 percent or 20 percent of the bill, is a common part of major medical benefits. The contracts are so complex that it is often difficult for either the patient or the physician to know exactly who is responsible for which part of the bill. Two forms of payment can be distinguished: individual reimbursement and assignment. Under **individual reimbursement,** the patient pays all the charges, sends copies of the bills to the insurer, and is reimbursed for the medical expenses that are covered. Under **assignment,** the physician sends the bill to the insurer. The patient is charged for the co-payment and may be **balance billed** for the difference if the physician's charges exceed the maximum fee allowed by the insurance contract. Under the Medicare participation agreement, a physician who accepts assignment agrees not to balance bill for any charges over the Medicare payment. Patients like assignment because they do not have to handle paperwork and are not stuck with additional fees. Physicians like the fact that they are paid directly and more rapidly, but do not like being denied the right to charge as much as they believe their services are worth. Indeed, the prohibition of balance billing in Canada led to a national physician's strike when the rule was first imposed.

Under current U.S. Medicare rules, physicians are limited to an additional 15 percent above the Medicare fee for balance billing if they choose not to accept assignment and are penalized by receiving only 95 percent of the regular fee schedule for services. In effect, Medicare has ruled out balance billing by making it economically unattractive. Medicaid rules are often more stringent and have significantly lower payment rates, which is why many physicians choose not to participate in the Medicaid program. Some physicians choose not to participate in Medicare to avoid the payment limits imposed by the RBRVS system, but since 20 percent of all physician bills are paid for by Medicare, this is difficult to do unless their practice is mostly obstetrics, sports medicine, or another specialty in which they treat few elderly clients.

Physician Payment in Managed Care Plans

As insurance companies have tried to control their costs by exercising market power, the passive payment of bills has given way to a system of **negotiated fees.** For some common and easily specified services purchased in large volume (intra-ocular lens implants, psychiatric evaluations for drug abuse), the insurance company can often obtain a low fixed price set in advance in return for guaranteeing the physician a certain number of patients or procedures. When individual fees are not negotiated, it is common for managed care contracts to specify **discounted fees,** offering perhaps 75 percent of what the physician would ordinarily bill other patients. The complexities of per unit service pricing are bypassed completely under **capitation,** a fixed payment per person per month regardless of the number of services used (see Chapter 10). A **health maintenance organization** (HMO) using a capitation rate of $30 per month pays that amount to the physician for each of the HMO members enrolled with that physician whether the member visits the doctor's office once, twice, ten times, or not at all. **Independent practice association** (**IPA**) **HMOs** that contract with many physicians use capitation rates to pay physicians, but a staff HMO hires physicians to work exclusively in the HMO's facility and pays physicians a **salary,** with perhaps some bonus based on productivity or on the profitability of the HMO. With this arrangement, the physician, in effect, becomes an employee of a large medical care firm (even though legally the physician may still be considered an independent practitioner because of laws in many states prohibiting the corporate practice of medicine). Salaried physicians are also found in administrative posts and in research and teaching organizations. About 40 percent of physicians are now salaried employees, and the number continues to grow as health care organizations become larger and more complex. Chapter 10 presents a more extensive discussion of managed care contracting.

Incentives: Why Differences in the type of payment matter

How physicians are paid determines the incentives they face to work harder, raise prices, or admit patients to the hospital. Under fee-for-service insurance, a physician gets paid more for doing more. Under HMO capitation, the payment is the same regardless of the number of services provided; therefore, a physician may do less. Under a relative value scale, payment is based on the number of points; therefore, physicians may push to classify the service in a higher point category (the ensuing gradual rise in total points while the number of services provided remains constant is known as "code creep"). In an intriguing experiment, half the doctors in a pediatric clinic were randomly selected to be paid on a fee-for-service basis and half were selected to be paid a salary.[5] The fees were set so that the average doctor seeing the average number of patients would earn the same on either a fee-for-service or salary basis. In practice, the fee-for-service doctors saw more patients, recalled them for more visits, and generally exceeded the normal guidelines for the amount of services, while the doctors who were on salary saw fewer patients, had them return less frequently, and more often provided fewer services than indicated by standard guidelines. This randomized control trial demonstrates that economic predictions regarding the incentive effects of different types of payment are borne out in a practice setting.

Payment type may affect patients' access to physician care as well. The Medicaid program has come under severe budgetary constraints and thus tends to pay physicians less well than Blue Shield, HMOs, and commercial insurance. Although physicians are constrained by ethics and law to provide high-quality care to all who need it, economic theory predicts that government imposition of mandatory price controls leads to shortages. A group of experimenters called 300 physician offices and requested an appointment, identifying their type of insurance as Medicaid.[6] Almost half the physician offices said that they were not accepting new patients, and when the experimenters did get an appointment, the average wait was two weeks. The experimenters then called back, identifying themselves as having commercial insurance, and 78 percent of the doctors' offices gave them an appointment within two days. Physicians try hard to provide adequate care to the poor, but if the payment levels are consistently lower, the level of service will be lower.

A Progression: From Prices to Reimbursement Mechanisms

As the medical care system moved away from fee-for-service arrangements and closer to salaried arrangements, the linkage between the flow of funds from patients and the flow of funds to physicians was attenuated, and finally severed. Although there may be some "price" attached to each service under Medicare RBRVS, the price bears almost no resemblance to what that would mean in a normal market: the patient does not pay the price, nor does the price allow the supplier to match output to demand, because it is imposed externally by the government. In such an environment, equilibrating varied interests through individual decisions based on price is replaced by a collective political market. Who is paid and how much is determined in part by concerns about how the elderly will vote in the next presidential election, the effectiveness of insurance lobbies, or a need to find the least difficult way of balancing the budget. Tracking the flow of funds to and from physicians is further obscured by referring to all payments as *reimbursement*, even though insurance companies do not "reimburse" physician costs (physician time is the bulk of the expense) and payments are more accurately termed physician *fees* or *revenues* or *salary*.

6.2 PHYSICIAN INCOMES

Physicians are among the most highly trained and well-compensated workers in the United States. The median physician income was $160,000 in 1998, four times the average worker's salary. Physician earnings grew more rapidly than average workers' earnings for most of the twentieth century. During the period 1982 to 1998, when average workers' earnings were almost flat (up only 2 percent in fifteen years after adjustment for inflation), physician earnings rose about 2.2 percent each year, or 24 percent over the fifteen-year span. To a large extent, these high earnings were attributable to the quality of those who entered the profession (almost all were in the top quarter of their college graduating classes), the long years of post-college training required, the extra effort (most physicians worked about 50 percent more hours than the average salaried worker), and compensation for having to act as entrepreneurs and manage a medical business (self-employed physicians earned 50 percent more than those who chose to work on salary). However, even after adjusting for all these factors, there is still a premium obtained for becoming a physician. Perhaps even more important than higher incomes is the implied "floor"; physicians virtually never face unemployment and many are able to accept "low-paid" positions (i.e., those that pay less than $100,000 per year) to follow their own interests in helping the poor, working with children, traveling to exotic locations, or studying interesting diseases.

Even during training in residency programs, physicians earn about $35,000 a year, which is about the same as the average worker, although certainly less than the opportunity cost of their time (see discussion of the costs of time and returns in Chapter 7). As with most workers, physicians' earnings grow rapidly early in their careers, rise to a peak around age fifty, and decline thereafter (see Table 6.3).

There is a marked difference in earnings by specialty. Generalists and family practitioners are at the low end, with pediatricians and psychiatrists only slightly above. The high end is made up of the surgeons, radiologists, and anesthesiologists. While numerous factors are involved, much of the difference in incomes among specialties is attributable to the reimbursement system: physicians get paid more for doing something (e.g., reading an X-ray, performing an operation) than for caring or thinking (e.g., listening to a patient's history, deciding which path of treatment to follow, helping the family of a dying person). The reimbursement system is driven by the "billable event." Although a colleague or a manager might be able to assess all the work a physician does on behalf of patients, the financial system is not able to do so. A physician always finds it easier to get paid for a procedure, since it is observable and has a standard billing code, than for a personal interaction or conceptual effort.

A desire to rebalance incomes across specialties and provide more payment for thinking and caring is an important part of the design of the Medicare RBRVS system, but this system is only partially successful. Health insurance is designed to protect individuals against potentially large but infrequent losses while minimizing moral hazard from excess purchase of discretionary services. While correct from a risk management perspective, in practice this means that fees for some specialties are almost fully covered (e.g., surgery, anesthesia), leading to increased demand and higher incomes, while other specialties are subject to co-payments and deductibles that limit demand and incomes (e.g., pediatrics, psychiatry). The bottom line for the physician is that the income potential from choosing a particular specialty has more to do with how the services of that specialty are treated by insurance than with the work or training involved.

6.3 PHYSICIAN COSTS: HOW FUNDS FLOW OUT

Physician Practice Expenses

The expenses of maintaining a practice take up almost half of all the funds flowing into physician offices (see Table 6.4). Physicians must pay for other medical professionals and assistants who help them take care of patients, as well as taxes, rent, utilities, supplies,

TABLE 6.3   Physician Characteristics and Incomes

813,770	Total number of U.S. physicians
647,430	Active in patient care
95,725	Residents in training programs
207,678	International medical graduates

Median Income

$160,000	*All physicians*	*100%*
126,000	Pediatrics	9%
130,000	Psychiatry	6%
130,000	General/Family practice	13%
140,000	General internal medicine	19%
184,000	Emergency medicine	3%
184,000	Pathology	3%
200,000	Internal medicine/subspecialty	10%
200,000	Obstetrics/Gynecology	6%
210,000	Anesthesiology	5%
215,000	General surgery	5%
230,000	Radiology	5%
249,000	Surgical subspecialty	8%
141,000	Employee or contractor	41%
162,000	Self-employed solo	26%
221,000	Self-employed group	33%
199,000	2 physician partners	9%
222,000	3 physician group	6%
238,000	4–8 physician group	12%
213,000	9+ physician group	7%
122,000	Younger than 35 years	17%
167,000	35–44	28%
179,000	45–54	28%
161,000	55–64	15%
107,000	65 or older	12%

Source: AMA Physician Characteristics and Distribution in the U.S., 2002-2003 and AMA Physician Socioeconomic Statistics, 2000-2002 and earlier years.

malpractice insurance, and so on. In addition to all these ongoing expenses, it usually takes at least $100,000 in start-up capital to equip even the most basic office, and an elaborate suite housing an active practice in specialties such as plastic surgery could cost several million dollars. One reason for physicians to work together in group practices is to obtain economies of scale from sharing office space, equipment, and information systems. Only a large group can afford to have assistants who specialize in support functions, such as laboratory technicians, billing and appointment clerks, physical therapists, and so on. Yet closer examination of the data reveals an apparently anomalous finding: even though it seems that a large group practice would use ancillary help and equipment more efficiently, such expenses take a greater percentage of total revenues for groups than for solo physicians who practice alone. To understand why a more efficient practice uses more, rather than less, non-physician inputs, it is necessary to consider a basic result from the microeconomic analysis of firm production. To reduce per unit costs, firms must use more of the inputs whose output per dollar is higher and/or use less of the input whose output per dollar is lower.[7] At the optimum, the ratio of marginal productivity to input price is the same for all inputs.

TABLE 6.4		Physician's Office Practice Revenues and Expenses		
$375,000	100%	Gross revenues	*100%*	
			Private Insurance	*45%*
			Medicare	*28%*
			Medicaid	*13%*
			Patients paid	*14%*
$195,000	52%	Net income		
$ 61,500	16%	Non-physician employee wages (3.5 FTE per physician)		
$ 9,000	2%	Employee physicians		
$ 45,000	12%	Office rent & expenses		
$ 15,750	4%	Medical supplies		
$ 17,250	5%	Malpractice liability insurance		
$ 6,750	2%	Equipment		
$ 24,750	7%	Other expenses		

Worked an average of 57 hours per week, seeing 105 patients, and giving 4 hours of charity/uncompensated care. The average charge for a new patient visit was about $136 in 2002.

Source: AMA *Physician Socioeconomic Statistics, 2000-2002.*

$$\frac{\text{Marginal Productivity}_{\text{input A}}}{\text{Price}_{\text{input A}}} = \frac{\text{Marginal Productivity}_{\text{input B}}}{\text{Price}_{\text{input B}}} = \ldots$$

$$= \frac{\text{Marginal Productivity}_{\text{input Z}}}{\text{Price}_{\text{input Z}}}$$

Larger and more organized physician groups are able to make better use of non-physician inputs, raising their marginal productivity. Therefore, groups use more of these inputs relative to physician time. Efficiency is not defined as having the lowest amount of overhead, or even the highest number of patient visits per physician hour, but rather the lowest cost (physician and non-physician) per visit. This raises the following question: what "price" should be applied to physician time?

The Labor-Leisure Choice

A physician-entrepreneur has an "income" of revenues less expenses, a flow that would be called *profit* by the Internal Revenue Service (IRS). Most of the income is not economic profit but compensation for all the hours of work put in. How should this time be valued? What is its opportunity cost? For a young physician starting out with relatively few patients, it is common to take on a temporary part-time moonlighting job in a hospital emergency room or in a well-established senior practice with many patients for wages of $75 to $150 per hour. Since doctors give up those jobs as their practices become established, their time must be worth more than that, but what forgone opportunity defines this higher hourly rate? What a busy physician gives up is leisure: time to be with family, time to run and swim and watch television, and even time to sleep. The more lucrative each hour of practice and the more hours the physician puts in, the more each hour of forgone leisure is worth. Most doctors work very hard, averaging more than fifty hours per week. Furthermore, once they make $150,000 or $250,000 per year, a little time off may well be worth more to them than earning an extra $5,000 by working late. This is one reason the supply of physician time is not very elastic; even doubling or quadrupling physicians' income could not get them to double the number of hours worked. Indeed, it is even possible that for some physicians, supply is "backward bending"—higher income per hour may make them feel sufficiently rich that they work fewer rather than more hours.[8] If backward bending supply seems difficult to understand, think about how much you would work if I paid you $100 per hour, $1,000 per hour, or $100,000 per hour. Eventually you would decide to work less and enjoy leisure more because additional money simply would not mean that much to you. One difficulty physicians have in making the labor-leisure choice is that their income often depends on putting in many hours per week early in their careers, when the rate of pay is low or even zero. This is similar to the problem facing most college students: getting into the best business or law school and making partner depends on excess hours put in now to obtain future income. To fully analyze the trade-off between labor and leisure, it is necessary to recognize that some work is done more for its value as investment in future earnings than for current earnings.

The Doctor's Workshop and Unpaid Hospital Inputs

Almost every doctor needs to use a hospital to provide patient care. Some specialties (anesthesiology, thoracic surgery, pathology) are practiced almost entirely inside hospitals. Yet physicians do not pay the hospital for the privilege of working there and usually are not employees of the hospital. In terms of an influential model proposed by Mark Pauly and Michael Redisch, the hospital functions as the "doctor's workshop" and is a source of unpaid inputs in production.[9] Since the efforts of hospital nurses, laboratory technicians, and record keeping professionals do not "cost" the physician anything, physicians tend to overuse them to supplant the use of similar inputs in their offices. It is easy to see how they might favor a system of nonprofit hospitals supported by the community and government subsidy because the value added to their practices by these hospitals far exceeds the hours physicians are expected to "give" to hospital educational and administrative functions.

The hospital-based specialties of radiology and pathology are a special case, with high incomes that clearly depend on hospital practice. Since physicians in these specialties spend virtually all their professional time within the hospital, have a regular flow of work, and do not meet individually with patients, it appears that they might most readily be paid on salary. Yet historically, radiologists have strongly opposed salaried practice, favoring fee-for-service arrangements, contracts in which they operate the diagnostic facility for a percentage of gross, or paying rent to the hospital. Their opposition was sufficient to force Medicare to separate the professional fee for reviewing X-rays and specimens from the hospital charges for producing them. The primary issue is control—over professional activity and over money. If the pathologist runs the lab, he or she in effect "owns" the captive block of business constituted by the hospital's patients. However, if the hospital runs the lab, pathologists must compete on the basis of price (i.e., take a lower salary) and accept hospital direction over their working conditions. Consider the case of a sixty-year-old pathologist who has been head of the lab for twenty years and is friendly with most of the surgeons on staff. If it is his lab, he can bring in a junior pathologist to do the day-to-day work and go into semi-retirement to play golf with the hospital administrator and his surgeon friends. If it is the hospital's lab and he is on salary, the hospital can threaten to fire him and hire the junior pathologist to save money, unless the senior pathologist is willing to accept a pay cut and work harder. The issue of who "owns" the patient's business arises repeatedly in our examination of the organization of medicine and is central to the managed care revolution currently taking place in the medical marketplace (see Chapter 10).

Malpractice

One of the most contentious physician practice expenses is malpractice insurance. The rationale for allowing medical malpractice suits is that they improve incentives for safety by forcing doctors to behave more carefully when treating patients. Malpractice is not a good way of compensating patients for harm done to them, since it costs $1.20 in legal fees for every $1 a patient receives.[10] About one in twenty physicians will incur a malpractice claim in any given year, and two in five will be sued at least once during their careers. The premium for a physician's malpractice insurance averages about $20,000 (5 percent of gross revenues), but ranges from just $5,000 or less for family practitioners to $100,000 and more for orthopedic and neurosurgeons. While malpractice premiums have risen rapidly in some years, virtually all the additional costs are quickly passed on to patients and their insurance companies in the form of higher fees.

Malpractice is a real problem, but the current malpractice system may not be the best solution. Studies have shown that a negligent iatrogenic injury (i.e., caused by the physician) occurs approximately once in every 100 hospital admissions. Only a tenth of those injured will file a claim, and less than half will gain compensation through the courts. At the same time, there will be a larger number of suits filed when there was no negligence, and some of these patients will win despite the lack of any physician error. The randomness of the legal process, as well as the fact that most physicians are almost fully insured for losses due to malpractice, limits the effectiveness of the system to change behavior. However, being sued is costly in terms of lost time and increased anxiety, and most physicians exercise extraordinary care in treating patients. After all, they became physicians because they wanted to care for patients, not because they wanted a job that was easy. Although some physicians have claimed that the fear of being sued has raised medical costs by forcing them to practice "defensive medicine," studies have shown that higher levels of liability or a greater number of suits do not necessarily lead to higher numbers of tests per patient, more admissions, or more prescriptions.[11] Since most suits are filed for a procedure that a doctor has done, rather than for something not done or for a diagnosis that was missed, the lack of excessive testing or other medical treatment attributable to malpractice is not surprising.

Does the malpractice system deter negligence by physicians? Only to a limited extent, and at considerable cost. Yet while the ability of malpractice suits to compensate patients for damages or to force doctors to practice better medicine has been roundly criticized with good reason, it has not been easy to find a solution that is clearly more efficient or acceptable to both doctors and patients.

6.4 THE TRANSACTION BETWEEN DOCTOR AND PATIENT

The bond of trust between doctor and patient is one of the strongest professional relationships in society. When patients show up at a doctor's office, they are apt to ask two questions: "What is wrong with me?" and "What should I do about it?" If told that they have a disease, most patients trust the doctor to perform the right diagnostic and therapeutic procedures, with little idea of what those might be or what the charges will add up to.[12] If a surgeon is called in, he or she is likely to be a complete stranger who asks for thousands of dollars to make an evaluation and incision. Patients who agree to surgery can only hope that in the long run it will do some good, since postoperative pain and mortality will make them worse off in the short run. Unlike a person shopping for a car, a suit, or a haircut, patients do not know what they need, what it should cost, and even, once paid for, how much good the treatment actually did. Instead of a clear specification of what is to be expected from both parties, the patient must trust the doctor to do what is right and to bill fairly for the necessary care (which will mostly be paid for by insurance).

Asymmetric Information

It is the superior ability of the physician to answer those two questions that tends to make the doctor-patient relationship so much different from an ordinary commercial transaction.

While the physician's information is not perfect, it is much better than that of the patient, and the physician is able to seek additional information required for treating an illness at much lower cost. This disparity is known as **information asymmetry.** When it is necessary to decide which test to perform, which drug to prescribe, and whether to perform surgery, all these choices can be made better and at lower cost by a physician. An exchange relationship in which one party makes choices on behalf of the other is known as **agency.**[13] Just as a purchasing agent buys supplies for a company and an actor's agent represents the actor in negotiations, a physician is the patient's agent in deciding which treatment is appropriate and which medical services to buy. The reason that agents act on behalf of another is that the agent's information and transaction costs are lower. It is cheaper for a physician to make medical choices on behalf of a patient than for the patient to go to medical school to make a decision.

While many goods and services are transacted under conditions of less-than-perfect information, it is the magnitude of the disparity that sets medical care apart. For example, although I may not know what my mechanic is doing, I can readily observe whether my automobile is working better when it comes back from the shop. Poor quality parts can be repaired or replaced. At most, I might ask for my money back. Bad surgery not only is difficult to detect, it can be disabling or even fatal. Once you are dead, repairs, replacements, and even outrageously large malpractice settlements are irrelevant.

6.5 UNCERTAINTY

In what is perhaps the most well-known and often-cited paper on health economics, Nobel laureate Kenneth Arrow stated: "The special economic problems of medical care can be explained as adaptations to the existence of uncertainty in the incidence of disease and in the efficacy of treatment."[14]

As discussed in Chapter 4, uncertainty "in the incidence of disease" refers to the random occurrence of illness—one never knows when one will get sick or how bad the illness will be. The problem of randomly occurring losses can be offset to some extent by pooling risks through insurance. The losses still occur and must be paid for, but the financial uncertainty is removed.

Uncertainty "in the efficacy of treatment" refers to the inability to know whether the chosen treatment will work. In theory, it might be possible to "insure" against such losses, but in the real world there are no meaningful guarantees for medical care. A cardiologist treating you for a heart attack does not guarantee that you will be able to run marathons again, nor does an oncologist guarantee that she can cure your cancer. The most either will promise is to provide you with everything modern medicine has to offer. Why can't they give a guarantee? First of all, because it is so difficult to tell how ill you were in the first place, it is often impossible to tell whether treatment has improved your health. Second, unlike a car or a house, there is no way to replace your body. While almost any ordinary loss can be fixed with sufficient compensation, a monetary guarantee is an empty promise if you are dead.[15]

The distinction between the two types of uncertainty and the economic response to them is shown in Figure 6.1. Note that in each case, there is a transfer of responsibility away from the patient. Under insurance, the responsibility for payment is transferred to the insurance company, relieving all actual and potential patients of the uncertainty of financial losses due to illness. Under agency, the responsibility for making a decision on appropriate care is transferred from the patient to the physician. Agency creates gains because it substitutes professional control for costly patient monitoring of quality. It is much cheaper for an experienced and highly educated physician to determine which treatment is best than for a patient to try to do so.

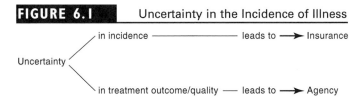

| FIGURE 6.1 | Uncertainty in the Incidence of Illness |

Uncertainty in the incidence of illness can be ameliorated by the use of insurance. Uncertainty in the outcome and quality of treatment can be ameliorated by exchange using an agency relationship; licensure and trust in physicians, nonprofit ownership, and government regulation.

6.6 LICENSURE: QUALITY OR PROFITS?

Licensure is a collective extension of the doctor-patient relationship of agency. Not only do individual patients trust their physicians to act as their personal agents, all of us together have collectively chosen to let the medical profession act as our public agent, deciding who is qualified to practice medicine. Through the institution of **licensure,** the medical profession serves as a sort of quasi-governmental body making decisions of behalf of all consumers.[16] Consumers do not examine each doctor's credentials and legal records, they turn that responsibility over to licensure boards. It is cheaper for knowledgeable professionals to do this once for all consumers rather than having each patient individually try to determine whether the person listed as a "doctor" in the phone book is qualified to practice medicine. The government does not make laws regarding the practice of medicine, but uses laws to enforce the decisions made by voluntary and independent professional boards.

It is often debated in the media and among economists whether licensure serves the interests of patients (by improving the quality of care) or of physicians (by raising prices and incomes).[17] Such a debate, framed in terms of one side or the other, misses the point: any public policy in a democracy is in fact a form of trade that must serve the interests of both parties if the policy is to be upheld. By the fundamental theorem of exchange, both physicians and patients must be made better off by licensure.

How Does Licensure Increase Physician Profits?

Licensure radically changes the market structure. A flexible supply curve is replaced by a fixed supply—diagrammatically a vertical line, since quantity does not change as prices rise or fall (see Figure 6.2). To the extent that the supply of doctor services is reduced under licensure, prices are higher so that all doctors enjoy higher incomes (of course, this means that some people who wished to become doctors are not allowed to do so). These profits are maximized if the profession acts as a monopoly in determining how many doctors are allowed to practice. Supply can also be reduced by work rules that control total productivity. For example, it is common for dental practice regulations to determine how many assistants each dentist can supervise (and therefore the number of total patients who can be seen). Extending the physician's training period also serves to reduce the effective doctor supply, since each graduate has fewer remaining years of productivity.

Thinking of the demand for physician services as derived demand suggests two further possibilities for raising income: 1) increasing the price of substitutes such as chiropractors and nurses and 2) increasing demand for output. The effective price of many physician substitutes can be made prohibitively large by prohibiting them from performing some acts (prescribing drugs, performing surgery, admitting a patient to the hospital). Less extreme, but also effective, are rules that limit health insurance to reimbursement for services performed by or under

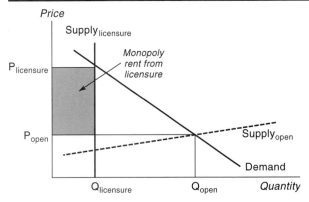

FIGURE 6.2   Demand and Supply with Licensure

the supervision of a physician. Even if a substitute provider is willing to provide services at a much lower price, it will still cost patients more because they will have to pay the entire bill out of pocket. Insurance has been the most important factor in increasing the overall demand for medical care. Physicians have played a major role in the spread of insurance and the creation of payment system rules (e.g., UCR fees, separate professional fees for radiologists and pathologists), which increase physicians' economic power. Hospital-based specialists such as radiologists and pathologists have fought the implementation of RBRVS and bulk-purchase managed care contracts that tend to give more control to payers and increase price competition among suppliers. Professional activities also directly increase demand both through new medical discoveries and by monitoring and controlling quality so that patients are more willing to visit any licensed practitioner.

Supply and Demand Response in Licensed Versus Unlicensed Professions

To illustrate the differences in market dynamics between licensed and unlicensed labor supply, physicians are compared with health administrators in Figure 6.3. Health administrators often earn a master of health administration (M.H.A.) degree early in their careers, but many rise through the ranks without attending graduate school and others obtain master of business administration (M.B.A.) or master of science (M.S.) degrees in schools of business, medicine, public health, public policy, or human services.[18] The crucial point is that there is no central control over the number of people who can enter the profession, no licensure or specific educational requirement, and no legal restriction on practice by outsiders. Administrators usually start at modest salaries ranging from $30,000 to $60,000, like most people with an M.B.A. degree, and work their way up the organizational ranks. While some administrators eventually earn large salaries, many tend to get stuck in the middle ranges and some are pushed out of the field entirely. Thus, administrator earnings are related to individual characteristics and experience and hence are rather variable. Physician earnings are in part monopoly "rents," increased profits shared by the profession as a whole, and thus are not only higher, but also more stable. While both physicians and administrators see their earnings increase as they gain more experience, for physicians, the growth is more regular and virtually never interrupted by unemployment.

The comparative effects of an increase in demand are shown in Figure 6.3. For physicians, who are licensed, virtually all the increase in demand goes into higher incomes because there is no flexibility for supply to increase. For unlicensed administrators, higher wages attract more and better entrants so that part of the increase in demand goes into an

FIGURE 6.3   Comparison Demand and Supply with and without Licensure

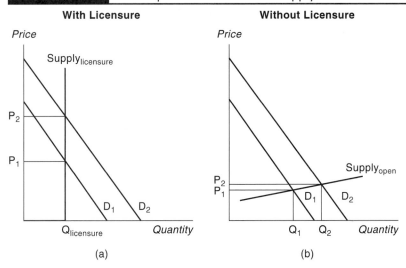

(a)   (b)

increase in the quantity of labor supplied and only partly into an increase in incomes. Although increased demand leads to more applicants to medical schools, no new medical schools will be built because these numbers are controlled by the AMA, American Association of Medical Colleges (AAMC), and affiliated professional bodies. In contrast, increasing demand for health administrators has caused graduate programs to spring up around the country as universities compete to attract students.

How Does Licensure Improve Quality?

It is possible to improve quality by revoking the licenses of physicians whose medical practices are shown to be inferior, but such removals are rare.[19] The quality of physicians in practice depends much more on the initial selection of who is allowed to enter the profession, the training they receive, and efforts by practicing physicians to monitor one another and impose informal sanctions (ostracism from professional groups, denial of hospital privileges, refusal to refer new patients or share business opportunities).[20] *The ability of sanctions and selection to improve quality would be greatly reduced if there were no monopoly profits.* Because licensure restrictions guarantee successful applicants a career with high income and prestige, many outstanding students seek admission to medical school. After becoming doctors, they work very hard not to lose that title. The money and power that come with being a physician, a form of monopoly profits, are too attractive to give up. If a doctor could earn more money and satisfaction working in a bank, an insurance company, or another career, why worry about losing a medical license? The opportunity cost of losing a license is so significant that the threat of losing a license is enough to make it rarely necessary for the profession to actually revoke a license and terminate a physician's right to practice.

The value of a license depends on the prestige of the medical profession as a whole; therefore, each doctor has an incentive to maintain the professional franchise by selecting only the best candidates to enter the profession and by continuing to make sure that all doctors are as good as they can be at caring for patients so that demand remains high.[21] Choosing only the best candidates for admission to medical school means that the graduates will be superior regardless of how much they learn during medical school. Prestige and income play a large part in attracting outstanding students. The incentive for a student to train long and hard is also related to the expectation of high income in the future. After graduation, the threat of losing these extraordinary returns provides an incentive to maintain competency and support licensing boards. The existence of monopoly profits serves as a monetary performance bond that can be lost, a kind of collective collateral put up by the profession to ensure good service on the part of all its members.

Observing that some specific restrictions on medical practice have no direct bearing on quality has led some economists to question whether licensure boards are committed to protecting the public interest or the private economic interests of their members. Application of the fundamental theorem of exchange indicates that there is no conflict between the two objectives and that they may reinforce each other. A particular restriction on medical practice may not directly improve quality, but removing it could cause quality to deteriorate by reducing the monopoly profits that provide incentives for the profession to police itself. A better test of whether licensure improves quality is to look at how the strength of licensure restrictions varies by type of medical practice—where and when the "licensure contract" is most apt to be approved by both patients and physicians.

A Test of the Quality Hypothesis: Strong Versus Weak Licensure

The timing of licensure legislation suggests that until the level of a doctor's training can significantly affect quality and the probable outcome of treatment, effective professional licensure is unlikely to occur or will be very weakly enforced. Before 1900, licensure was clearly desired by physicians to improve their economic status, as demonstrated by their vociferous support of such laws in state legislatures. Yet licensure laws could not get popular political support until medical science advanced to the point at which knowledge made a real difference.[22] The strength of licensure was related not only to the increased effectiveness of new treatments, but also to the increased danger posed by the use of surgery and powerful drugs.

Some types of medical care, such as cardiac surgery, are inherently dangerous and demand great skill. Bad heart surgeons may have a mortality rate five times higher than good heart surgeons.[23] Given the great impact of measurable physician quality indicators (training, medical practice records, opinions of peers), we would expect licensure to be very strong for heart surgery (see Table 6.5). That is the case. Although legally one need only be licensed as a physician in order to perform heart surgery, in practice doctors are virtually prohibited from doing so unless they have completed a residency, completed a fellowship in the specialty, and been given special hospital privileges after a review by peers who have observed them acting as assistants on a number of operations. These additional mandatory checks make it evident that heart surgery has strong licensure restrictions. Conversely, there are other types of medical care that are much less dangerous and demanding, such as surgery to remove corns from the foot. Although such surgery can be practiced with greater or lesser skill, it is not likely to cost a life. One does not need a residency or hospital medical staff review to remove corns, and indeed corns are often removed by podiatrists, who are not licensed doctors of medicine (M.D.s), although they are usually licensed doctors of podiatric medicine (D.P.M.s). The lack of special medical staff restrictions and the existence of alternative professional certification show that care of the foot has weak licensure. Refractions to prescribe eyeglasses are similarly performed by competing professions (M.D. opthamologists and O.D. optometrists) under weak licensure. Mental health is a specialty with a wide array of professionals—psychiatrists (M.D.'s), psychologists (Psy.D. doctors of psychology or Ph.D. doctors of philosophy), family therapists and counselors (C.A.C., M.S.W., AAMFT, and other designations), and even psychics (palm readers, speakers for past lives, aura visionaries)—and such weak licensure that virtually anyone can offer to help you with your problems. There are substantial risks to life in mental illness, and more people die from substance abuse and depression than from many other conditions, but the professional does not always have substantial advantage over the client in choosing therapies and therapists, because personality match is so important. It is

TABLE 6.5   Weak Versus Strong Licensure

Weak ← ——————— Licensure ——————— → **Strong**

Consumers can choose	Only trained professionals choose well
Low risk	High risk
Uncertainty small	Information asymmetry high
Examples: podiatry, eyeglasses	Examples: neurosurgery organ transplants

hard to gain insight from a psychologist you despise, or who despises you, but a cardiac surgeon can be totally lacking in human interpersonal skills and still perform a good operation.

As the extent and value of the information asymmetry between patients and professionals increases, licensure becomes stronger. In types of care in which the differential is small, licensure is weak. For heart surgery, technical quality is paramount and well evaluated by professional standards. Medical licensure is supplemented by hospital privilege reviews, insurance restrictions, and so on. For a broken heart, an M.D. psychiatrist may be no more effective than a sympathetic psychic whom the patient trusts and, for counseling, there are multiple forms of licensure, all rather weakly enforced.

SUGGESTIONS FOR FURTHER READING

American Medical Association, *Socioeconomic Characteristics of Medical Practice*, published annually (www.ama-assn.org).

Kenneth Arrow, "Uncertainty and the Welfare Economics of Medical Care," *American Economic Review* 53, no.3 (1963): 941–973.

Atul Gawande, *Complications: A Surgeon's Notes on an Imperfect Science* (New York: Holt & Co., 2002).

Paul L. Grimaldi, "Medicare's Physician Fees Are Resource Based," *Journal of Health Care Finance*, (Spring 2002): 88–104.

George D. Lundberg, *Severed Trust: Why American Medicine Hasn't Been Fixed* (NY: Basic Books, 2001).

Institute of Medicine, *To Err Is Human*, (National Academy Press, April 2000), (www.nap.edu/books/0309068371/html); and *Crossing the Quality Chasm* (July 2001), (www.nap.edu/books/0309072808html).

Michael Millenson, *Demanding Medical Excellence: Doctors and Accountability in the Information Age* (Chicago: University of Chicago Press, 2000).

SUMMARY

1. **The relationship between doctor and patient stands at the center of the medical care system.** Although payments to physicians constitute only 22 percent of total health care expenditures, the special characteristics of this exchange influence the organization and financing of all other parts of the system.

2. Over time, physician payment has changed from fee-for-service prices similar to prices of most other economic goods and services to complex reimbursement plans based on administrative formulas and negotiation. Increasingly, physicians are involved with managed care plans that pay a **capitation** rate (physicians receive a certain amount per member per month) or **discounted fee schedules** based on **relative value scales.**

3. Most physicians are owners or partners in small businesses rather than employees. They work long hours, but do not face much business risk. On average, **self-employed physicians earned** $195,000 in 1998, while the 40 percent who worked as employees and who were somewhat younger earned $140,000. Physicians who practiced in cognitive and caring specialties (family practice, psychiatry, pediatrics, internal medicine) earned less than those who practiced in procedure-oriented specialties (surgery, obstetrics/gynecology, radiology).

4. The average office medical practice hired **3.5 allied health workers per physician** and had overall expenses equal to 47 percent of gross patient revenues in 2000. While malpractice insurance is the expense category most frequently complained about, **malpractice takes only 3 to 6 percent of gross** revenues for most physician practices.

5. **Uncertainty** creates or exacerbates most of the information problems in medical care. While financial uncertainty due to the random occurrence of illness can be reduced by insurance, uncertainty about the quality of care and outcome of treatment cannot; thus, collective agency mechanisms such as licensure and strong ethical traditions for physicians have been established.

6. **Information asymmetry** arises from the difference between the physician's and the patient's knowledge of medical treatments. Because of this disparity in the cost of knowledge, patients must trust physicians to act as their agents and make decisions on their behalf. In most economic exchanges, the point at which goods and services are transacted is the point at which information cost differentials are lowest. Since a low-cost valuation of well-defined goods is not possible in medicine, a trust relationship of agency has been established to ameliorate this potential market failure.

7. **Licensure** is a collective extension of the doctor-patient relationship of agency. It helps solve the problems caused by uncertainty and information asymmetry. **Licensure increases profits by restricting supply,** thus changing the traditional supply and demand curve analysis. The supply curve is fixed, or vertical, and increases in demand do not result in an increase in quantity, but in increased profits for suppliers known by economists as "rents." **Licensure increases quality** by (a) ensuring that only the best students are selected to enter medical school; (b) mandating that students have three years of medical school, four years of residency, and periodical refresher courses thereafter; and (c) having physicians monitor each other. All these depend on having some excess profits or monopoly rents to serve as an incentive. Licensure is intended both to increase profits and to increase quality. Like any law, it **must satisfy both parties** (physicians and the public/patients) to be a self-enforcing political exchange. The importance of quality concerns is evidenced by comparing the types of care for which licensure is strong (cardiac surgery, chemotherapy) with those for which it is weak (removing corns, prescribing eyeglasses, counseling).

PROBLEMS

1. {*incentives*} Which type of payment gives a physician the most incentive to do the following:
   a. Spend more time with each patient? Spend less?
   b. Provide more laboratory services to each patient? Provide less?
   c. Modify the listing of diagnoses to increase revenues? Be objective?
   d. Reduce hospital utilization? Increase hospital utilization?
   e. Ask patients to return frequently? Try to handle problems once and for all?

2. {*compensation*} Do you believe that radiologists prefer to be compensated in a fee-for-service manner, by relative value scale, on salary, or as part of a capitated rate? Why? Why might practitioners of different specialties prefer different forms of payment?

3. {*organization*} Which organization provides the largest amount of payment to physicians in the United States? How does this organization choose to make these payments? Has the form of payment changed over time? Why?

4. {*earnings differentials*} What are some of the reasons that most pediatricians earn less than most neurosurgeons?

5. {*age earnings profile*} Generally, most physicians' incomes increase as they get older. Is the rate of earnings increase greater for some specialties than others? Why? Do you expect that male and female physicians have the same age-earnings profile? Why or why not?

6. {*earnings differentials*} Would you expect that physicians who earn significantly more than their peers have office practice costs that are above or below average? Are they more or less likely to hire other physicians?

7. {*valuation*} How are the values determined in setting up a relative value scale?

8. {*malpractice*} What are the objectives of the current medical malpractice system in the United States? How well does it work in achieving these objectives?

9. {*uncertainty*} If uncertainty regarding the occurrence of losses can be dealt with through insurance markets, why can't uncertainty regarding the outcome or quality of medical care be similarly priced and transferred?

10. {*agency*} What is an agent? How does employing an agent reduce the costs of making a transaction? Does employing an agent create any problems that would not occur if the consumer acted alone?

11. {*licensure*} Does licensure raise the quality of medical care, or does it raise the profitability of medical practice?

12. {*information asymmetry*} How do agency and information asymmetry lead to licensure? Do agents get more or less of the gains from trade as the degree of information asymmetry increases? Explain why and how the strength of licensure is related to the extent of information asymmetry.

13. {*competition*} Why are the markets for health insurance so much more price competitive than the markets for medical care?

ENDNOTES

1. Eliot Freidson, *Profession of Medicine* (New York: Dodd, Mead, 1970). Victor R. Fuchs, *Who Shall Live? Health, Economics and Social Choice* (New York: Basic Books, 1983).

2. Most of the information here is from surveys done by the American Medical Association and reported in *Socioeconomic Characteristics of Medical Practice*, an annual/biennial monograph. A good sense of the entrepreneurial flavor of medical practice can be obtained by perusing several issues of *Medical Economics,* the "Business Week" of physicians.

3. U.S. National Health Accounts (www.cms.gov/statistics/nhe), see discussion and references in Chapter 1.

4. W. C. Hsiao, P. Braun, D. Dunn, and E. R. Becker, "Resource-Based Relative Values: An Overview," *Journal of the American Medical Association* 260 no. 16 (1988): 2347–2353; William C. Hsiao et al., "Results and Impacts of the Resource-Based Relative Value Scale," *Medical Care* 30, no. 11 Supplement (1992): NS61–79.

5. G. B. Hickson, W. A. Altmeier, and J. M. Perris, "Physician Reimbursement by Salary or Fee-For-Service: Effect on Physician Practice Behavior in a Randomized Prospective Study," *Pediatrics* 80 (1987): 344–350.

6. Medicaid Access Study Group "Access of Medicaid Recipients to Outpatient Care," *New England Journal of Medicine* 330 (May 19, 1994): 1426–1430.

7. Uwe Reinhardt, "A Production Function for Physician Services," *Review of Economics and Statistics* 54, no. 1 (1972): 55–66.

8. Frank A. Sloan, "Physician Supply Behavior in the Short Run," *Industrial and Labor Relations Review,* 28:549-569, July 1975.

9. Mark V. Pauly and Michael Redisch, "The Not-for-Profit Hospital as a Physician Cooperative," *American Economic Review* 63, no. 1 (1973): 87–99.

10. Patricia Danzon, "Liability for Medical Malpractice," *Journal of Economic Perspectives* 5, no. 3 (1991): 51– 69; and "Liability for Medical Practice," in A.J. Culyer and J.P. Newhouse, eds., *Handbook of Health Economics* (Amsterdam: Elsevier, 2000), 1339–1404.

11. Peter A. Glassman, John E. Rolph, Laura P. Petersen, Melissa A. Bradley, and Richard L. Kravitz, "Physician's Personal Malpractice Experiences Are Not Related to Defensive Clinical Practices," *Journal of Health Politics, Policy and Law* 21, no.2 (1996): 219–241.

12. This special economic character of the "trust" relationship with doctors has long been noted, and is discussed in Adam Smith's seminal 1776 treatise, *The Wealth of Nations*.

13. Michael C. Jensen and William H. Meckling, "Agency Costs in the Firm" and "Theory of the Firm: Managerial Behavior, Agency Costs and Ownership Structure," *Journal of Financial Economics* 3 (1976): 305–360. The extensive economic analysis of agency has focused primarily on the manager of a firm who makes decisions on behalf of shareholders. Many of these models are applicable, but since medical outcomes are not as readily measured as the profits of a firm, and since death has even more moral overtones than bankruptcy, the doctor-patient bond has important aspects above and beyond those that characterize the relationships of owner-to-shareholder or supervisor-to-employee. See the books by Gawande and Millenson in Suggestions for Further Reading; and Mark V. Pauly, "Taxation, Health Insurance, and Market Failure in the Medical Economy," *Journal of Economic Literature* 24, no. 2 (1986): 629– 675; Robert L. Kane and Matthew Maciejewski, "The Relationship of Patient Satisfaction with Care and Clinical Outcomes," *Medical Care* 35, no. 7 (1997): 714–730.

14. Kenneth J. Arrow, "Uncertainty and the Welfare Economics of Medical Care," *American Economic Review* 53, no. 3 (1963): 941–973.

15. To give a guarantee means to provide a contract stipulating what you will receive if something goes wrong (replace the item, money back, etc.) What would a "medical guarantee" look like? The broken transmission of a car can be repaired for $900, making money a fully satisfactory replacement. There is no such replacement for health or the pain of disease. Even if we could agree on a monetary amount, it would be different for every illness, different for every person, and different even if it was the same person and illness at a later time of life. There is no way to write a satisfactory contract in advance, hence the need for a substitute form of commercial relationship.

16. Richard Shryock, *Medical Licensing in America, 1650-1965* (Baltimore: Johns Hopkins University Press, 1967).

17. Elton Rayack, *Professional Power and American Medicine: The Economics of the American Medical Association* (Cleveland, Ohio: World Publishing, 1967).

18. U.S. Bureau of Labor Statistics, *Occupational Outlook, BLS Bulletin 2450* (Washington, D.C.: U.S. Government Printing Office, April 1994).

19. Formal licensure actions against physicians are rather infrequent, and usually for misconduct (drug abuse, fraud, sexual advances) rather than poor quality of care, which has led some observers to conclude that the institution of licensure was never intended to improve quality. However, note that revoking of a driver's license is similarly rare. The quality of daily driving is measured by a fifteen-minute test when a person is first licensed, but not thereafter, and revocation of drivers' licenses reflects a similar pattern of egregious personal flaws rather than the traits associated with quality (vision, eye-hand coordination, etc.)

20. Eliot Freidson, *Professional Dominance: The Social Structure of Medical Care* (New York: Atherton, 1970); and *Professional Powers: A Study in the Institutionalization of Formal Knowledge* (Chicago: University of Chicago Press, 1986).

21. Unfortunately, the desire to maintain the value of physician licensure also provides an incentive to cover up cases of poor quality. Admitting that some licensed physicians were actually bad doctors would reduce demand, and thus diminish the value of all licenses. Therefore, sometimes physicians will act to protect their own by hiding evidence of malpractice or other failures even when they strongly disapprove and could get rid of the offender.

22. John Duffy, *From Humors to Medical Science: A History of American Medicine* (Urbana: University of Illinois Press, 1993).

23. *A Consumer Guide to Coronary Artery Bypass Graft Surgery*, Vol. IV, 1993 Data. PHC4 Pennsylvania Health Care Cost Containment Council: Harrisburg, PA, 1995.

CHAPTER 7

MEDICAL EDUCATION, ORGANIZATION, AND BUSINESS PRACTICES

QUESTIONS

1. How much is a year of medical education worth?
2. Are doctors more or less productive than they were twenty years ago?
3. Which controls the supply of physicians, the government or the American Medical Association (AMA)?
4. Why are there more foreign doctors practicing in the United States than U.S. doctors practicing overseas if the needs are much greater there?
5. Can medical groups advertise to attract more patients and increase market power? Are bigger practices more efficient?
6. Is price discrimination legal? Why are some patients charged more for the same service? Why and how are doctors giving discounts on fees?
7. Do physicians trade patients? Are payments between doctors for referrals legal, ethical, or efficient?
8. Are chiropractors a substitute for physicians, or a complement?
9. Who sets the standards of practice to guide clinical decisions?
10. Why do patients in Boston undergo more surgeries than patients in San Francisco?

7.1 MEDICAL EDUCATION

A select and hard-working group of 16,000 students will graduate with doctor of medicine (M.D.) degrees from one of 126 U.S. medical schools this year.[1] For most of them it will be the middle of an arduous process that has taken over most of their lives since high school and will forever change the way they view the world, and how the world views them. Many first thought about becoming doctors in elementary school, but some decided after pursuing other careers. All had to take pre-med courses in chemistry, biology, and so on and did rather well on average—almost half of them had an "A" average as undergraduates (grade point average [GPA] of 3.6 or higher). Getting into medical school was serious business that took substantial effort, and many applied to ten or more schools. Much of the selection, however, was self-selection. Weaker students generally chose not to apply. Less than half of the applicants to medical school were rejected. Of those who were admitted, 98 percent chose to enroll, and of those, 95 percent will graduate, almost all of whom will then enter a hospital-based residency training program lasting three years or more before becoming generalist family practitioners or specialists in one of the other twenty-two recognized areas of medical practice eligible for board certification.

Although much has been made of the cost of medical education, most of that cost is borne indirectly by the government and the health insurance system. Just 4 percent of medical school costs are covered by tuition payments from students, whereas 46 percent comes from patient fees, 30 percent from research, and 20 percent from government appropriations and gifts.[2] Although tuition might run as high as $40,000 per year and most medical students (83 percent) are left with debts from student loans when they graduate, the amount of those loans (which averaged $99,089 in 2001) is not very large in relation to the income a physician can expect, less than 1 percent of lifetime earnings.[3] Far more onerous than the monetary obligations are the years of toil spent in learning the practice of medicine.

Human Capital: Medical Education as Investment

We can use the **human capital** approach to evaluate whether going to medical school is a sacrifice, a sound investment, or both.[4] The returns on medical education are the increased annual earnings, relative to a person's opportunity cost, that flow from the decision to go to medical school. The costs are all the things that are given up, which includes tuition, but mostly the forgone earnings and leisure from working eighty hours a week without pay in medical school or for below-market wages during residency. Before evaluating medical education, let us first consider a hypothetical example, calculating the returns on an undergraduate college education. Bill pays tuition of $5,000 a year. He also gives up a job that would pay him $20,000 a year (forgone wages). He also pays the university $6,000 a year for a dorm room and meal plan, but these costs should not be counted as part of the costs of his education. Thus the total cost of his degree is $(4 \times \$20,000) + (4 \times \$5,000) = \$100,000$. After graduation Bill will be able to earn $28,000 a year instead of $20,000, for a gain of $8,000 a year. We will assume that although his earnings will increase with experience and inflation over time, the real differential will remain approximately the same. The returns on his college education are approximately $\$8,000/\$100,000 = 8\%$. Real returns after adjustment for inflation have historically been about 1 to 3 percent for savings accounts and treasury bonds and 3 to 5 percent for stocks, which are a bit riskier; therefore, the 8 percent return from investing in a college education compares quite favorably.

Empirical studies of rate of return on medical education get considerably more complex in practice, since one must adjust for the superior earning power of above-average students, the costs of the excess hours worked by physicians, and so forth. Also important is the fact that the returns from a medical education are much less risky than from a bachelor of arts (B.A.), master of business administration (M.B.A.), or doctor of law (J.D.) degree, and thus should be adjusted accordingly (see Table 7.1). In addition, becoming a medical doctor confers prestige and other valuable privileges. Empirical studies in labor economics have reached a consensus on some major conclusions, although many details are still subject to disagreement. The return on investment from a college education clearly exceeds the market rate of return on financial assets, and the premium for being a college graduate is rising. The return on investment from graduation from medical school, with real returns of 10 to 20 percent, is higher than that for graduation from college.[5] Returns

TABLE 7.1   Returns to Professional Education

	Business (2 Years)	Law (3 Years)	Dentistry (4 Years)	Primary Medicine (4 Years)	Specialty Medicine (4 Years)
Tuition	$ 34,452	$ 32,317	$ 70,620	$ 74,504	$ 74,504
Annual income (age 40)	$135,579	$139,616	$133,050	$132,592	$219,733
Hours worked (age 40)	2,448	1,959	1,781	2,565	2,707
Internal rate of return	**26%**	**23%**	**22%**	**16%**	**18%**

Source: Weeks and Wallace, 2002.

on other graduate degrees, such as a doctor of philosophy (Ph.D.) degree in biology or sociology, are much lower, and in some fields the returns are effectively zero. Returns on residency training follow incomes: they are high for surgical specialties (20 percent), intermediate for internal medicine (10 percent), and low for pediatrics (2 percent).

7.2   THE ORIGINS OF LICENSURE AND LINKAGE TO MEDICAL EDUCATION

At the time of the American Revolution, there were about 3,500 established medical practitioners in what was to become the United States, but only 400 had received any formal training and fewer than 200 held degrees. The ability to read and quote some Latin and an apprenticeship were considered sufficient qualifications for hanging out a shingle and calling oneself a doctor. As late as 1830, the University of Virginia provided all its students with instruction in medicine. Yet before 1900, there was little scientific basis for the way most doctors practiced medicine, and indeed the treatments prescribed were about as likely to harm health as to improve it. Since there was really no benefit from seeing a trained professional, there was no support for restricting the practice of medicine through licensure. Although state medical associations repeatedly pushed for licensure and were sometimes temporarily successful, the lack of public benefit doomed such efforts. In New Jersey, licensure laws were passed and then repealed at least sixteen times between 1800 and 1900.[6] In other states, licensure laws were on the books, but did not mean much because they were not enforced.

Two major technological breakthroughs radically changed the nature of medicine: anesthesiology (pain killing) and antisepsis (germ killing). Although surgery had been practiced since the dawn of mankind, the lack of anesthesia meant that most operations could last only a few minutes, and even then many patients went into shock and died. The other problem was post-surgical infection, which claimed almost as many lives as the injuries that were treated. Very few of the hundreds of thousands of soldiers who died during the Civil War were actually killed in battle; most died in hospitals days or weeks later. Today, most of those wounded soldiers could easily have been saved. Anesthesia and antiseptics changed surgery from a last resort for the desperate patient who would otherwise die, into a routine procedure used in the treatment of many diseases. The fact that twentieth-century surgery was more effective also paradoxically increased the risks. Patients who never before would have considered letting themselves be cut open went under the knife willingly.

Anesthesia, antiseptics, and a host of other scientific breakthroughs radically changed the promise, and the politics, of medicine. There was no longer any question that doctors must be educated and examined before they were allowed to practice. The Flexner Report of 1910 to the Carnegie Commission, which was supported by the AMA, called for the closure of all medical schools that did not require an undergraduate college degree for admission and provide laboratory training in biology and chemistry, clinical internships, and full-time faculty members. These standards, first viewed as utopian, were implemented with increasing force over the next three decades.

Legal control over physicians resides with state licensure boards, yet supply is actually determined by control over the number of students allowed to enter medical school (and the number of foreign medical graduates allowed to come to the U.S. for training, who often stay to practice). Unlike law school, in which there are many students who fail to graduate, or who graduate and fail the bar exam, or who pass the bar exam and cannot find a job, almost all medical students graduate and practice medicine. There are exams in school and afterward, but almost everyone passes, and the limitation of numbers is sufficient to ensure that everyone who wants to can find a position practicing medicine. By the end of the Depression, the old laissez-faire system of unregulated physician practice with open entry had been entirely replaced by a modern system of medical licensure, with control over supply resting in the hands of the medical schools (which, in turn, were largely controlled by the joint AMA and Association of American Medical Colleges (AAMC) Committee on Medical Education).

A major practical difficulty in implementing licensure was how to handle all the existing physicians then in practice who had not received such an education. Although many were poorly trained and lacked ability, others were good physicians who had the respect of their communities and their colleagues. In order to allow these experienced doctors to continue to practice while upgrading standards for new entrants to the profession, they were "grandfathered" in. That is, a doctor could become licensed either by graduating from an acceptable medical school or by being an accepted member of the county medical society. Over time, the more highly qualified new graduates would replace the older cohort of nonuniversity physicians. Analyzed in terms of property rights, the existing physicians owned the rights to vote on standards. It would not be in their self-interest to vote for higher standards that would put them out of a job, yet a higher quality standard would increase demand and benefit all physicians. The grandfather clause allowed them to reap the rewards from licensure reform and in a sense became a form of payment for their property—control over the future of the profession. As usual, all parties, including the incumbents, must be made better off for a successful political exchange to occur.

AMA Controls Over Physician Supply, 1930–1965

With reform curtailing new entrants and forcing unqualified older practitioners out of business, physician supply declined steadily from its 1900 level of 1.73 M.D.s per 1,000 population to 1.33 M.D.s per 1,000 population in 1930 (Figure 7.1). The supply of physicians held constant at this level for the next thirty-five years. Yet improvements in medicine greatly increased public demand, as did the rise in personal income over these four decades. With supply constant and demand increasing, earnings of physicians rose, as depicted in Figure 6.3. Concern was voiced that not enough physicians were available and that a shortage had arisen.[7]

There are several ways this shortage could have been rectified. The steep price rise that did occur held quantity demanded in check and made physicians happy, but did little for the public. Supply could have been expanded by increasing the productivity of physicians, changing the organization of medical practice, and using more ancillary health workers; some illnesses could have been treated by physician substitutes such as doctors of osteopathy (D.O.s) or chiropractors; or physicians could have been imported from overseas. These alternatives would have undercut organized medicine's control over physician supply and incomes, and were strongly resisted by the AMA. Productivity improvements and lower prices were most strongly identified with prepaid group practices such as the Kaiser Health

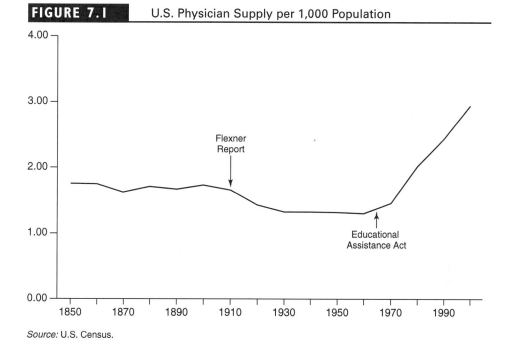

FIGURE 7.1   U.S. Physician Supply per 1,000 Population

Source: U.S. Census.

Plan in California and the Group Health Association in Washington D.C. (see Chapter 10). Concerted opposition by local medical societies led to the expulsion of group practice doctors and an obstinate denial of hospital privileges to physicians who were clearly qualified by education and experience.[8] In 1941, the Washington, D.C., Medical Society and the AMA were indicted, found guilty, and fined by the U.S. Department of Justice for having conspired to monopolize trade in physician services. This is but one of many in a string of cases across the country that left group practices bruised and hampered, but alive. Relations slowly improved, but opposition to prepaid group practice did not end until the 1970s.

The response of organized medicine to substitute providers took two forms: co-opting the competition and all-out war. D.O.s emphasized spinal manipulation in addition to standard medical practices and formed a separate type of care in 1900 with their own D.O. hospitals, but carried out many of the same Flexnerian educational reforms in those transitional years. Over time, M.D. and D.O. cooperation increased through sharing of hospital privileges, enrollment in each other's residency programs, and formation of joint political and social groups.[9] D.O.s were tolerated by the AMA and ultimately brought into the fold as a slightly less polished M.D. Today, the differences between an M.D. and a D.O. degree are almost nonexistent, except that D.O.s are more likely to be general practitioners and do not control any of the high prestige medical schools. In many states a single licensure board covers both types of physicians, and in California the M.D. and D.O. societies merged in 1961, although separate boards were later re-established. Throughout these years, the numbers of D.O.s relative to M.D.s has remained roughly constant at around 5 percent, and hence osteopathy has become more a partner to the AMA in controlling supply rather than a competitive threat.

Chiropractors, who often rely exclusively on spinal manipulation to treat disease and still train some practitioners in for-profit schools, have been severely and relentlessly attacked by the AMA.[10] Licensure acts explicitly exclude chiropractors from the practice of medicine, and this opposition has not changed even though the AMA has not been able to ban chiropractic practice, nor indeed to prevent some of its own members from referring patients to chiropractors. While some of the AMA opposition to chiropractic care is based on the lack of scientific foundation for manipulative treatments, much of it is motivated by economic concerns.

Breaking the Contract: The Great Medical Student Expansion of 1970–1980

Under the control of the AMA and the medical schools, enough new M.D.s and D.O.s were being produced to keep pace with the growth in the U.S. population (about 1 percent a year), but not with the increase in demand due to improved technology or higher disposable incomes. As the benefits of modern medicine became more evident, access to care was increasingly seen as a necessity in the rising American standard of living, one that workers had already paid for through their health insurance premiums. The constraints on supply caused longer waits for an appointment, less time for a patient to talk with an increasingly rushed physician, fewer old-style general practitioners willing to make house calls, and other deteriorations in service. The public was unhappy, and the politicians, who now provided most of the financing for medical schools, were willing to do something to redress the imbalance.

In essence, frustration with the inaction of the AMA led the government to unilaterally disrupt the old system. Congress passed the Health Professions Educational Assistance Act of 1963, forcing medical schools to admit more students and allowing more foreign physicians to immigrate to the United States. In response to the act and subsequent amendments, physician supply rose steadily to 1.61 physicians per 1,000 population in 1970, 2.02 in 1980, 2.44 in 1990, and 2.94 in 2000—more than twice the level of supply that prevailed from 1930 through 1965 (see Figures 7.1 and 7.2). The number of entering students almost doubled in ten years, from 8,759 in 1965 to 15,351 in 1975. The government used two methods to bring about this increase.[11] First, it built more medical schools. Second, it offered additional funding on the condition that existing schools increase the number of students enrolled by at least 5 percent each year. By this time, federal and state funding accounted for 63 percent of medical school financing; hence, the schools were not in a good position to resist, even if they had wanted to. At the same time, changes in immigration rules were made to favor "shortage" occupations, including physicians. Foreign graduates made up just 6 percent of all physicians in practice in 1960, but by 1965 that fraction had doubled to 12 percent and further increased to 17 percent in 1970 and 20 percent in 1980.

Building Pressure: Fixed Domestic Graduation Rates 1980–2002

As the number of residents in training grew rapidly during the 1970s, it began to seem as though there were already plenty of physicians. The AMA complained loudly about a potential surplus, commissioning several studies to show that the United States was training an excess of physicians and that foreign graduates were no longer needed. These arguments were successful in helping the profession reestablish control over supply, and by 1980 the tide of public opinion had turned. The 1981 Report of the Graduate Medical Education National Advisory Committee, widely known as the GMENAC Report, projected a growing surplus, raising the possibility that in the future some physicians would face unemployment.[12] The flow of foreign graduates had already been severely restricted by changes in immigration law included in the Health Professions Educational Assistance Act of 1976. Moves were now made to reduce the rate of growth in the number of U.S. physicians. No more new schools were to be built. Class sizes were fixed at the current level.

FIGURE 7.2   Additions to US Physician Supply, 1950-2002

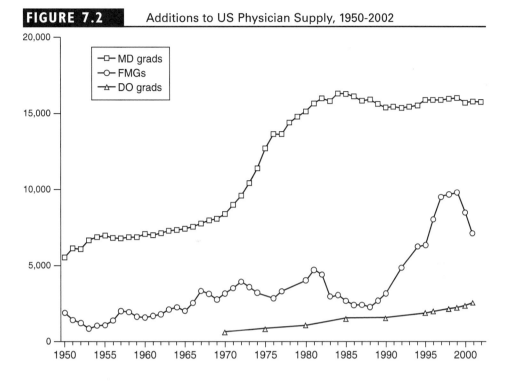

The number of first-year M.D. students peaked at 17,320 in 1981 and has been held below that number since then (16,875 in 2002). Since the number of U.S. medical graduates has not kept pace with the growth in U.S. population, much less the growth in technology and incomes that raised effective demand, all the expansion in supply over the last 20 years has had to come from three other sources: 1) the delayed effect of the 1965–1975 "physician boom," 2) increased immigration of non-U.S. physicians, and 3) increased production of non-M.D. physicians.

7.3   ADJUSTING PHYSICIAN SUPPLY

The Flow of New Entrants and the Stock of Physicians

Although the number of students entering medical school jumped by 50 percent between 1968 and 1973, this had no immediate effect on physician supply because these extra students were still in school for four years. Even then, the sudden increase in the number of new M.D.s caused only a gradual rise in the supply of physicians. To see why, it is necessary to trace the life cycle of work, distinguishing the stock of physicians (the number available at any point in time) from the flow of entrants and retirees into and out of the labor force. Suppose that the average physician began practice at age 33 and retired at age 66. If the same number of physicians started work each year and retired after 33 years, 1/33, or 3 percent, of all the physicians in practice would leave each year and another 3 percent would join. The number of physicians in practice (the physician stock) would stay the same from year to year in this steady state. What would happen if the nation decided to double the physician supply by doubling the number of new graduates each year? In 33 years there would be twice as many, or 100 percent more, practicing physicians, but in the first year there would only be 3 percent more. The number of new additions would be twice as much as before, or 2 × 3% = 6% of the total, and the retirements would be the same, 3 percent, so that net growth would be 3 percent in the first year, 6 percent after two years, 9 percent after three years, and so on. The actual response would be even slower, because there is a lag of eight years from the time new students are admitted until they complete their residencies and become practicing physicians. The full effects of the 1965–1975 "doctor boom" (and subsequent bust) will not be fully realized until this cohort of new physicians has moved through the professional ranks and completed their work lives, some time between the years 2000 and 2025 (see Figure 7.3).

Immigration of International Medical Graduates

The number of foreign medical graduates practicing in the United States doubled in just three years, from 15,154 in 1960 to 30,925 in 1963, with 15,000 more arriving in the next four years. By 1980 there were 97,726 international medical graduates (IMGs) practicing in the United States, 20 percent of the total physician supply. Despite continued restrictions on immigration, the number of IMGs doubled from 1980 to 2000 and now constitute 24 percent of practicing physicians.[13] Although the number of IMGs entering U.S. residency training programs has leveled off at around 6,000 per year since 1995, the effects of the entry bulge from 1988–1995 will continue to expand this component of physician supply for decades to come.

Growth in Non-M.D. Physicians

Although smaller in number, the growth in non-M.D. physicians (primarily D.O.s) has been even more dramatic. In 1970, some 12,600 D.O.s constituted just 4 percent of the total physician supply. Whereas the number of M.D. graduates was essentially held constant at 17,000 from 1980 to 2000, the number of D.O. graduates jumped from 1,059 to 2,304.[14] The number of schools of osteopathy rose from 14 to 19, class size continued to increase, and D.O.s constituted an even larger fraction of the U.S. medical graduates entering residency programs.

FIGURE 7.3   Stock and Flow of Physicians

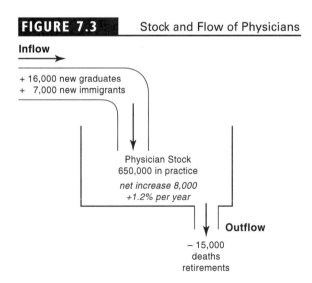

Balancing Supply and Incomes: Tracing the Past and Projecting the Future

The development of scientific medicine created the need for a new type of doctor in the twentieth century, and the history of physician supply and licensure must be interpreted in that context. To raise the quality of the individuals in the profession (as well as their prestige and incomes), the reforms envisioned by AMA leaders and the Flexner report required that most of the inadequately trained practitioners be forced out, thus reducing physician supply from 1900–1930. From then until 1965, the number of new M.D.s graduating each year was held steady at about 4 percent of the total physician stock, numbers just sufficient to offset the 3 percent who retired each year and a 1 percent growth in the U.S. population, so that the physician-to-population ratio remained constant at about 133 per 10,000.

For a professional thinking technically in terms of medical "need" (a specific, fixed number of physicians required to treat a given number of illnesses), a constant physician-to-population ratio was sufficient to meet demand. From an economic perspective emphasizing responsiveness to prices and incomes, it is clear how inadequate both the concept and the numbers used by the medical profession were. Changing expectations, new technology, and a rising standard of living meant that demand was increasing, and the 1 percent growth in physicians set to match the 1 percent increase in population was not enough to forestall market stress and public dissatisfaction.

What evidence does the market provide about the assertions that too many physicians were trained or allowed to immigrate? Pent-up demand kept physician incomes from falling during the 1970s as supply rose. Although real earnings dipped in 1985, and again from 1989–1990, physicians have done much better than the average American worker over the last 15 years. Groups that had to make an extra effort to enter the profession (IMGs, D.O.s) clearly found it worthwhile to do so, and pushed for access in record numbers. Such effort and expansion in auxiliary sources indicates that demand was growing faster than regular domestic supply. However, fewer college students were applying to medical schools. About 2 percent of those admitted to medical school did not attend. While this fraction refusing the opportunity of a medical education was still quite small, it was fourfold above the rate between 1975 and 1985, when just 0.5 percent of those offered a place in medical school turned it down. While projecting the future is always to some extent speculative, it is possible to give a reasonable assessment of the economic situation and prospects of physicians from these trends.[15] Becoming a doctor still offers above-average rates of return on post-college education. However, the very high earnings growth that physicians enjoyed during the 1960s and 1970s were a temporary historical aberration, brought about by rapid growth in demand due to new technology in the context of fixed supply. In the future, doctors will have high, but not such extraordinarily high, earnings. While still doing much better than most graduates from other fields, new physicians will face more competition as they enter the market, and thus will be more likely to become employees holding salaried jobs and to hold on to such positions for longer during their careers. The few who become truly wealthy will be those who have worked their way up the ladder in large health care organizations or who have taken substantial risks as entrepreneurs.

7.4 GROUP PRACTICE: HOW ORGANIZATION AND TECHNOLOGY AFFECT TRANSACTIONS

Physicians who join together in groups have higher net earnings than those who practice alone: $162,000 for solo doctors compared with $199,000 for those in two-physician partnerships, $222,000 for those in three-physician groups, $238,000 for those in groups of four to eight physicians, and $213,000 for those in groups of more than nine (see Table 6.3). Physicians in group practices usually have better life styles: more interaction with colleagues, more support services, and fewer nights spent handling patient emergencies.[16] Economists must ascertain which factors lead to greater efficiency and hence higher incomes for group practice and, conversely, which factors limit the attractiveness of groups so that one-third of all physicians still choose to practice alone. There are fundamentally three ways that group practices serve to increase net income:

- Economies of scale raise the productivity of inputs, and hence lower costs.
- Market gains bring in greater revenues.
- Sharing spreads risk.

What does it mean to have **economies of scale** that make larger practices more efficient in the use of inputs? To a physician owner, it could mean either (a) that the cost of inputs required to produce a given amount of output has been reduced or (b) that the output in visits per hour of physician time has been increased. Analysis of group practice expenditures shows that some of both occurs.[17] Equipment and office space comes in discrete units and therefore is inefficiently used in small practices. An X-ray machine that can handle 10,000 patients may cost only 50 percent more than one that can handle 2,000, and even the smaller one is frequently idle for a doctor practicing alone. A large group can match equipment needs to the total patient volume of the group as a whole, and thereby achieve economies of scale. Similarly, each physician may need from one to four exam rooms at a time to maximize patient flow and from two to six assistants. A solo doctor will compromise by having an office with three exam rooms and four assistants, and thus sometimes the ancillary inputs will be overcrowded and limit productivity, while at other times they sit idle and waste money. A group can plan for an average, since it is unlikely that all the physicians will be busy or inactive at the same time, and thus achieve a better match. Office rent takes up 12 percent of the gross revenues of solo practices, 10 percent of two-physician partnerships, and just 7 percent of large group practices.

On the other hand, labor costs and full-time equivalent (FTE) employees per physician increase as practice size increases. A large group can allow for more specialization in the use of labor, so that a ten-physician group can have a laboratory technician, billing specialists, receptionist, intake nurse, exam room assistant, and so on, while a solo practice must make do with a general-purpose medical assistant or nurse. Increasing the productivity of an input can either decrease or increase its share of total expenditures depending on the elasticity of substitution with other inputs. Office space apparently cannot be substituted for physician time; thus, as it becomes more productive per square foot, it takes up a smaller fraction of total practice expenditures. Ancillary labor can be substituted for physician time, and as this labor becomes more productive, physicians use more employees rather than fewer. It is worth paying more for assistants to save the physicians' time because their net profit per hour of work increases.

Risk sharing across the members of the group also creates economies of scale. Just as random variation in the number of exam rooms required by each doctor can be averaged out in a large group, so can other revenues and expenses, so that the group can collectively enjoy a smoother and more certain income stream. Perhaps even more important, the emergency calls that interrupt the home life of every doctor are much less disruptive when combined and redistributed in a group. A solo practitioner must be "on call" every night, or find someone else who is willing to cover. On Sunday, one emergency call could interrupt a football game, and there could be no more calls until a sleep-shattering call at 3 A.M. For a group, it is usual for each doctor to accept all the calls for a single day. The group doctor might handle seven emergencies on a Sunday, but know that Friday night and

COMPARATIVE ADVANTAGE AND PHYSICIAN ASSISTANTS

The principle that people and firms should produce the things at which they are *relatively* more efficient and use others to produce the things at which they are relatively less efficient is known as **comparative advantage.** There are gains from trade when relative costs differ, even if one party is better at everything. That is why investment bankers let someone else balance their checkbooks, great artists let helpers fill in the background scenery, great athletes let someone else play on punt returns, and even countries where production of everything is inefficient export some goods to get the goods they are inefficient at producing. It makes sense to trade even when you can produce the item for less cost, if doing so frees up time and resources that can be used more valuably elsewhere. For example, suppose that a physician takes 15 minutes to do an intake examination and 5 minutes to do a follow-up. The physician assistant (PA) takes 40 minutes to do an intake examination and 30 minutes to do a follow-up. Even though the PA is less efficient at both tasks, the medical group will use the principal of comparative advantage and make the PAs do intakes, not follow-ups. Why? Because in eight hours a PA could do twelve intakes, freeing up three hours of physician time to do high-value surgery, while having the PA do sixteen follow-ups would free up just 1 hour and 20 minutes of physician time. It is not the "cost" of using the PA to provide services that matters, it is the value of the additional services that the physician can provide. Trade should follow the course of comparative advantage, even though absolute productivity will determine rewards—the physician will earn more per hour than the PA.

It is worth noting how the principle of comparative advantage can work against some of the human traits we value in doctors. Both nurses and doctors can listen and show compassion, and spending more time yields better results. However, the physician can accomplish more high-tech diagnostic procedures per hour than the nurse and will tend to specialize in that direction, at the expense of listening. Even if we tell our doctors that we want them to spend more time with us, and they are very good at listening, they are apt to hire assistants to do so because their comparative advantage lies in the application of medical technology.[18]

Saturday are free, since any patients who need assistance will be handled by one of the partners. The burden of emergencies is not the time spent in caring for patients, but the uneven spacing. This is the risk that is shared, and thus effectively reduced, in a group.

Since it is obviously so much more efficient for a doctor to handle ten patients in one night than one to three patients each night per week, why don't solo doctor's contract with each other to do just that? For that matter, why can't independent physicians arrange to share office space or nurses? To some extent they do, and to that extent, they start to become a group. As the contracts and sharing become more complete and cover more aspects of practice, the doctors who trade with each other become a single firm—that is, a group practice. But, it is difficult to share. All the doctors must agree to standardize certain practices, coordinate efforts, pick a leader, accept the leader's ruling on disputes between them, and so on—in short, to be managed. It means being an employee or partner rather than the boss. Management is costly, and good physician managers, like all good managers, are rare and valuable commodities. Some studies of physician productivity overestimated economies of scale because they did not account for the time physicians must spend in management and how that management time increases as the size of the practice increases.[19] For some physicians, it is cheaper (and more fun) to put up with some inefficiencies and lack of specialized inputs to be their own bosses and not have to listen to, or give orders to, anyone else.

Contracting between many parties and managing larger operations create the costs that limit the attractiveness of group practice. Transaction costs are also the source of the economies of scale in marketing and revenue generation, which are often more important than production cost economies. Consider what happens when a successful older doctor combines his practice with that of a younger physician who is just starting out. The older physician has too many patients, and must turn some away or provide poor service. The young physician has too few patients, and must spend hours waiting for people to show up or moonlighting as an employee in a hospital emergency room. By combining their practices, the successful doctor is, in effect, selling some patients to the younger doctor in return for a part of the younger doctor's income. For such a transfer to occur, patients must be convinced that the junior doctor is as good as the senior one. The senior doctor guarantees the quality of the junior doctor by the act of forming a partnership. In effect, the senior doctor is saying "I trust this doctor; so should you." Transfer is also facilitated by arranging for the junior partner to take a disproportionate share of night emergencies, the new patients who show up at the door for the first time, and those who do not want to wait weeks to see the senior partner. It is the patient's concerns about quality and trust that make the doctor-patient relationship special, and that makes it hard to obtain economies of scale by treating patients en masse. For a group to act as a collective, the guarantee of quality must extend to all the physicians in it. Just as all licensed physicians benefit from monitoring the quality of care provided by the profession and eliminating or reforming bad doctors, a medical group practice benefits from increased demand to the extent that it can closely monitor and control the quality of all its members.[20] The Mayo Clinic is a premier example of a medical group practice that acts as a "brand-name firm" and gains a marketing and revenue advantage from being perceived as a group with identifiable quality rather than just a random collection of individual physicians who happen to work in the same building.[21]

7.5 KICKBACKS, SELF-DEALING, AND SIDE PAYMENTS

"... and if a doctor shall cheat his patient by overcharging for medicaments, then shall a finger of his left hand be cut off."
—*Code of Hammurabi, 2300 B.C.*

From the beginning, the AMA code of medical ethics has dealt with economic issues, rightfully noting that doctors must put the health of patients above profits if people are to trust them. The agency relationship is most threatened in day-to-day business by the practice of paying "referral fees" or **kickbacks.** The agent is supposed to be, and is, paid for acting in the principal's (the patient's) best interest. When doctors accept a fee for referring patients to one hospital rather than another, or for giving a surgical case to Dr. B instead of Dr. A, they may be tempted to go with the one who will pay them the most, not the one who will provide the best care. In ordinary business dealings, such a payment would be termed a bribe or a kickback. Corporate purchasing agents are sometimes caught accepting presents or kickbacks from suppliers in return for steering business their way. For suppliers to pay for business is not bad—they can give rebates or provide customer treats or price discounts. The problem is the distortion caused by directing a payment to the agent who is supposed to be making an objective choice, rather than the principal, who is supposed to get the benefits of any discounts. Before medicine became established as a profession, such practices were common. Surgeons in the large cities would advertise in rural newspapers their willingness to pay $100 or more for each case sent to them. While such behavior seems unthinkable now, kickbacks keep cropping up. What was once the largest chain of psychiatric hospitals was investigated and convicted for paying physicians and social workers who sent in clients. The kickback scheme had become so well established that there was a standard going rate of $70 for each patient day.[22]

Why do kickbacks continue to occur if everyone knows that they are bad and they are condemned by all the official governing organizations? They continue because an agent's control over who gets the business is valuable property. To not make use of that value—that is, to act ethically and follow professional standards which put the interests of patients first—forces a doctor to put aside his or her own narrow self-interest. In the short run, it is easy to profit by betraying a trust to make a dollar. The violator hopes not to get caught. Even if an unethical physician does get caught, much of the punishment actually falls on other doctors, because the profession as a whole gets blamed for a lack of standards and suffers from a reduced demand and falling prices for services. Trust and agency build professional value, and taking a kickback is one way for a member to steal part of that value, benefiting personally while harming others.

One of the major activities of physicians is prescribing drugs. If drug companies made payments to physicians, those dollars could distort the physicians' choices on behalf of their patients, perhaps prescribing a drug that is less effective, or one that is effective but three times as expensive as all the substitute drugs that would work just as well. An even more difficult problem arises when the physician is not just prescribing the drug, but also selling it. Knowing that the patient is in pain and trusts the physician, physicians could fatten their profit margins by overcharging for drugs. That such a problem is not new is evidenced by the quote from the code of Hammurabi at the beginning of this section. The potential for abuse is so high that physicians in this country have been legally prohibited from selling drugs or owning pharmacies since 1934. Even a pharmacy in a medical clinic must be run as a separate business to avoid conflicts of interest. In Japan, where no such law exists, the government sets price controls to keep physicians from overcharging, but that does not stop them from over-prescribing. General-practice physicians in Japan get about a third of their net income from sales of pharmacy items, and their patients are prescribed twice as many drugs as similar patients in the United States.

In the quote from the code of Hammurabi, the prohibition is on overcharging for *medication*. Why isn't overcharging for service similarly condemned? The issue with kickbacks is not price, it is deceit. If Dr. Arnold says, "I am better than the others, and I want $20 more for each visit," that is her privilege. Patients can agree or go somewhere else. There is no fraud. To prescribe a drug and accept a $20 rebate from the manufacturer, or to send a surgical case to Dr. Jones knowing that he will send a case of wine in return, is fraud. The patient is unknowingly paying (somebody has to pay for the wine—to Dr. Jones it is just a cost of doing business that he adds into the overhead for the surgical bill) and has an agent whose decisions may be based on maximizing kickbacks rather than the patient's welfare. If Dr. Arnold and Dr. Jones were partners in a large group practice, a patient would expect to be sent to one of the surgeons in the group (Dr. Jones) and there would be no fraud. Also, Dr. Jones would have expected Dr. Arnold to send the patient to him as a matter of routine, and there would be no kickback payment. The amount of money changing hands in the transaction might be the same, but the ethical and economic considerations are quite different. In essence, a patient of the group is buying "the group" and does not care how Dr. Arnold and Dr. Jones split the money. The patient going to Dr. Arnold, *and unaware that Dr. Arnold has any business arrangement with another doctor,* has a right to expect Dr. Arnold to choose objectively the surgeon who is best and to negotiate the lowest price.

As medicine has become more complex, with more transactions involved in each episode of patient care, it has become even more difficult to avoid conflicts of interest. Of particular concern in recent years have been incidences in which for-profit companies providing ancillary services (e.g., diagnostic radiology, home intravenous therapy) offer physicians "investments" in these businesses in return for sending patients.[23] So many such abuses took place that in 1976 federal anti-kickback laws were passed prohibiting any Medicare or Medicaid payment from companies to physicians based on the volume of patient referrals. The 1989 "Stark law" (named after its sponsor, U.S. Representative Fortney Stark of California) banned physicians from referring patients to clinical laboratories in which they have a financial interest. The 1993 "Stark II" law widened the ban to prohibit self-referrals to hospitals or radiology laboratories in which physicians are invested. The law also prohibits bonus plans within group practices based on the volume of laboratory referrals. Only a minority (less than 10 percent) of physicians invest in businesses that raise conflict of interest issues from self-referral, and only a few engage in profiteering at the expense of the government and patients.[24] Yet the actions of these few are troubling to a public already dismayed over the high cost of health care, and it is likely that further restrictions will be placed on independent diagnostic and therapeutic facilities owned by physicians. Eventually, physician ownership or partnership in ancillary facilities may be banned entirely, as ownership of pharmacies has been.

7.6   PRICE DISCRIMINATION

One of the characteristics of the medical markets first noted by economists was that different patients pay different prices for the same service.[25] Some price differences are attributable to differences in cost or value (e.g., surgery by an experienced board-certified specialist versus a new resident still in training, midnight treatment in the emergency room versus a routine visit to the doctor's office). However, even after these factors are taken into account, there is still a sizable and systematic variation in charges. It is frequently noted that people who are well insured or have high incomes pay more, laboratory and other small ticket items are overpriced, and that services for which patients can "shop around" (e.g., eye exams, normal births, physical therapy) show less price variation than emergency medical care where immediate treatment is required.

A major reason for **price discrimination,** charging different prices for the same service to different types of patients or patients in different types of care, is that it increases total revenue. The change in revenue, marginal revenue, depends on price elasticity as well as price. More formally,

$$\text{Marginal Revenue} = \text{Price} \ (1 + 1/\text{elasticity})$$

To maximize revenues when providing two different types of care, physicians should charge different prices even if their costs are the same for each service and should *charge a higher price where demand is least price sensitive* (i.e., where price elasticity, which is always negative, is smaller in magnitude). Conversely, where demand is very price sensitive, a reduction in price will bring in many more patients and increase revenues (see Figure 7.4). Pain, fear of dying, and wealth all serve to reduce price sensitivity. However, the most important factor making medical consumers less price sensitive is insurance (see Figure 7.5). Therefore, we would generally expect physicians to charge more for those services that are more fully covered by insurance, more life-threatening, more painful, and for which patients have the least ability to shop around. Some ancillary services (lab tests, X-rays, sonograms) are not very price sensitive even when insurance coverage is incomplete,

FIGURE 7.4 Price Discrimination by Patient Type

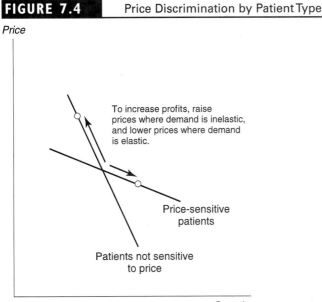

FIGURE 7.5 Price Discrimination by Insurance Status

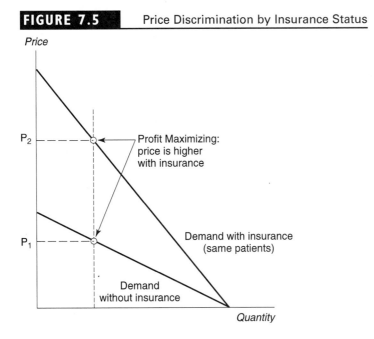

because they are considered secondary and inevitable by-products, and thus rarely receive the kind of scrutiny given an operation or other major expense.[26]

There is an important empirical discrepancy at odds with the revenue maximization model of physician price discrimination: the lower price is sometimes clearly below the cost of providing the service (sometimes care is even free) and, therefore, must decrease rather than increase physician income. Indeed, when queried about differential pricing, some physicians respond angrily to the suggestion that they are maximizing profits and assert that they act from a benevolent impulse, charging high prices to those who can afford to pay (or are well insured) so that they can take care of the destitute. Under closer examination, however, it becomes evident that there is a mixture of motivations that includes both charity and higher incomes in a blend that is not always clearly separable. Charging students less helps out a group that is usually poor and might not get care if they had to pay full price—and brings in more revenue for exactly the same reason. (Why do you think movie theaters and airlines give student discounts—is it a charitable impulse or a smart business practice to raise revenues because they know students have little discretionary money and wouldn't come to the theater or fly as often otherwise?) Price discrimination is pervasive in medicine and well accepted by patients, the government, and insurance companies. If two people come into a shop and one is charged twice as much for oil, food, or rent, the person charged extra will complain or threaten to sue. The unusual willingness of people to accept or even praise price discrimination in medicine is one of the factors that has convinced economists that health care markets differ in significant ways from markets for most other goods and services.

7.7 PRACTICE VARIATIONS

The agency relationship arises because the patient trusts the physician to do what is right. What happens when the physician confronts a lack of information or when medical science provides no clear guidelines on what to do? The professional concept of "need," which assumes there is a right way to treat an illness and hence no necessity for examining trade-offs among costly alternatives, falters if the clinical pathway becomes ambiguous. The fact that some medical practices have been widely used with confidence, only to be later discarded as ineffective or harmful, fosters some doubts about the infallibility of medicine. In a 1934 study, the American Child Health Association chose 1,000 schoolchildren to be examined by physicians to determine whether or not they should have their tonsils removed.[27] Six hundred children had already had the procedure. The remaining 400 were examined, and the physicians recommended that 45 percent of them have a tonsillectomy. Then the 220 not recommended for surgery in the first round were examined by another group of physicians, who recommended that 46 percent of them have their tonsils out. A third exam by another set of physicians on the 118 who were left resulted in recommendations that 44 percent have their tonsils removed. After these three examinations, only 65 of the original 1,000 children were not recommended for a tonsillectomy! From this study, the experimenters concluded that the decision about whether a child needed a tonsillectomy was not primarily based on signs or symptoms or any objective evidence, but on a generally held opinion among the doctors consulted that they should give tonsillectomies to one-third to one-half of all the children they treated in that age range.

Today, tonsillectomy is a much less commonly performed procedure, in part because of these pioneering epidemiological experiments (epidemiology is the study of the distribution of diseases in populations, applying statistical methods to groups rather than studying individual patients). However, the insights regarding the range of uncertainty in common diagnoses were essentially ignored during the glory years of medicine after World War II, when it seemed that science could diagnose and cure every ailment. This optimistic conviction that medical advances would be continuous and consistently beneficial faded as the Vietnam War, the Organization of Petroleum Exporting Countries (OPEC) oil crisis, and rising environmental concerns led to a more cautious and critical assessment of technology. In what was then (in 1973) a little-noticed study,

John Wennberg and colleagues found that the rates of many common types of surgery varied widely across counties in Vermont, with differences as large as six-fold, which were not explainable by differences in insurance, availability of hospitals, or illness rates.[28] For tonsillectomies, the rate varied from as few as eight per 10,000, to as many as sixty per 10,000. In a subsequent study, Wennberg found that the people of Boston, Massachusetts, had more hospital beds, had more employees per bed, and paid 87 percent more on average for hospital care than the people of New Haven, Connecticut, yet in both cities the average health statistics were about the same and most people received high-quality medicine, with many patients treated in academic medical schools. Interestingly, Wennberg found that while the overall rate of surgery was higher in Boston for some conditions, the rate of surgery was significantly higher in New Haven. Thus, it is not simply a question of more or less, but of a large degree of unexplainable variation (see Figure 7.6).

FIGURE 7.6   Variation in age-adjusted rates of hospitalization for different diagnoses and procedures. Each dot represents one hospital market area.

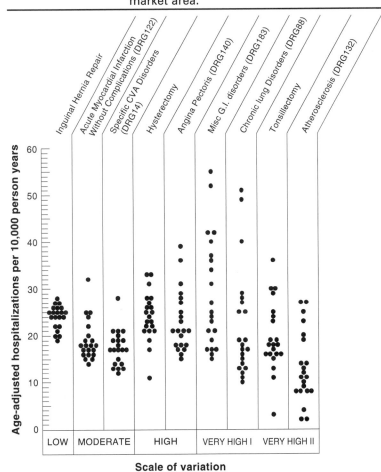

Source: J. Wennberg, K. McPherson, and P. Caper, *New England Journal of Medicine* 311: 298, 1984.

UNCERTAINTY REGARDING HORMONE REPLACEMENT THERAPY

For many years, estrogen and progestin were routinely prescribed for post-menopausal women to replace hormones their bodies could no longer produce in quantity. Clinical judgment suggested that such hormone replacement therapy reduced the risks of heart disease, stroke, and osteoporosis that accompanied aging. Observational studies indicated that risk reductions on the order of 40 percent to 50 percent could be obtained, but there were no randomized studies that established the magnitude of effect with certainty.

The Women's Health Initiative was begun in 1991, and it eventually screened 373,092 women for participation. Of these, 16,608 were enrolled in clinical trials and randomized to receive either hormones or a placebo (inert pill). Participants were to be followed and repeatedly assessed medically for 8.5 years. However, the trial was stopped after just five years of observation because of excess deaths and adverse events among the group receiving the hormones. The negative impact was small but conclusively demonstrated that hormone replacement therapy did not help overall and on average probably harmed those who received it. No single physician, or group of physicians practicing together, would ever have been able see these effects. Among 8,000 women over five years, there were approximately six excess heart attack fatalities and three excess stroke deaths—an annualized difference of just 0.01 percent. Only statistical methods and rigorously planned, carefully recorded observations of thousands of patients at many hospitals and clinics can distinguish effects such as these. In retrospect, the reliance placed on individual judgment and clinical experience resulted in many useless or harmful treatments.[29]

This phenomenon of **practice variation** or **small area variation** has been confirmed by a number of researchers. It suggests that there is a large element of ambiguity that can make widely different treatment choices constitute acceptable medical practice. Conditions in which indications are not so clear, or for which there are good alternative forms of treatment, show large variations (e.g., knee replacement, spinal surgery for back pain, tonsillectomy, treatment of psychoses). However, for conditions in which there are clear indications and a generally accepted treatment, the range of variation is much smaller (e.g., hernia repair, open-heart surgery, lung resection). Work is now under way to develop more formal **clinical pathways,** sets of instructions developed by medical professionals based on verified results of scientifically validated studies. These clinical pathways suggest how a particular illness should be managed, including which tests to perform, which medications to give, how long to wait for symptoms to improve before surgery, and so on. Many doctors denigrate such efforts as "cookbook medicine," while others recognize that clinical pathways, although not able to replace the physician's personal judgment, can help make treatment more efficient. What is important to recognize is that repeated demonstrations of wide variations in practice patterns have called into question the role of the individual doctor as final arbiter of right and wrong treatments. Impetus has been given to examining health policy on the basis of verifiable costs and outcomes of care, rather than accepting current practices as a standard or relying on the opinions expressed by professional associations.

Small area variation is one form of **population medicine,** which uses groups rather than individual patients to define quality of care.[30] Although long used in public health (see Chapter 15), it is only with the spread of managed care contracting for large numbers of people that population medicine has become recognized as a valuable tool for assessing the quality of physician practice. As hospitals become integrated into health care systems to organize and better manage the care they provide to the community, decisions regarding treatment will be shaped more by analysis of statistics on large numbers of patients and less dependent on the experience of a single physician.[31]

NO MORE DR. WELBY

"Marcus Welby, M.D." was one of the most popular shows on the ABC network from 1969 to 1976. Like the earlier Dr. Kildare (played by Joel McCrea in 1937 and Richard Chamberlain in the 1960s), the noble, warm, and caring physician played by Robert Young was everyone's ideal of what a doctor should be. However, like the wise dad Young played in "Father Knows Best," Marcus Welby was a Hollywood fiction that pleased audiences because it conformed to an ideal rather than to reality. When Robert Young died at the age of 91 in 1997, the era of happy TV families and kindly doctors who acted solely out of altruism had already passed.[32]

7.8 INSURANCE, PRICE COMPETITION, AND THE STRUCTURE OF MEDICAL MARKETS

The twinned effects of medical uncertainty, agency, and insurance, are combined in the health care system so that prices are almost uniquely *un*important for consumer behavior or well-being. Licensure and other monitoring procedures try to guarantee that any doctor available to serve you will provide excellent treatment using up-to-date technology, while insurance takes away the impact of cost and any incentive to spend time comparison shopping. Consider how unusual this market is. For cars, clothing, and housing, one expects that better quality will cost more and that only the wealthy will buy the superior brands. Not so for hospitals or surgery. It all costs the same more or less—a small co-payment, a deductible, or nothing. In picking a movie or a pair of shoes consumers assume that they will suffer the consequences of some inevitable bad and poorly informed choices on their part. Not in medical care. It is the doctor's fault, not mine, if the treatment does not fit or does not work properly. Nowhere else is price so irrelevant. Surgeons don't even list their fees, much less put up sale signs offering 40 percent off to increase business. If you buy expensive clothes, you will have to give up your expensive car, or your new apartment, or your tuition for graduate school. But a person can get the best medical care in the world and walk out with their checkbook balance nearly unaffected.

For a patient seeking medical care, quality rather than price is paramount. Medical care must be purchased at the time it is needed, often under great stress. Serious illness may strike at any moment, without warning, or a person may go for years without visiting the doctor or the hospital. Medical services must be performed on the person. The outcome of treatment is uncertain and depends on the quality of care that patients are usually not sufficiently knowledgeable to judge. Even though quality is the most important characteristic, it is hard to measure and even more difficult to translate into dollars to enable the patient to rationally consider whether a highly regarded physician is really worth an extra-high fee. Indeed, in many cases, patients are not even sure exactly what is being done for them; therefore, they can hardly be sure that they're getting their money's worth. Also, if a mistake has been made, no amount of money can readily compensate the patient for having been crippled or killed by poor quality. Experience in purchasing care for one illness may be of little help the next time you get sick, because you may have pneumonia instead of a broken leg.

Although prices do not play a major role in contracting for medical services, health *insurance* markets are very price competitive. Every year, people renew their insurance, and the choice can be planned and researched ahead of time. Insurance is not a direct personal service that must be performed in person; the check can be sent from anywhere. Insurance offers money, an absolutely standard and universal commodity, so that there is little quality variation (friendliness of service and amount of paperwork vary among insurance companies, but these are trivial compared with the variations among good and bad surgeons). If a mistake is made by the insurance company, its effects could be entirely erased by sending another check. Insurance is a regularly purchased routine product that is easy to buy in advance and for which small price differences are meaningful. This is not to say that consumers have no difficulty determining the value of their health insurance coverage and whether they got what they paid for, but that these problems are orders of magnitude less formidable than the problems faced in the purchase of medical care. Furthermore, the actual purchasing of insurance is carried out mostly by the group through a broker or full-time company benefits specialists, whereas consumers must go out and purchase medical care on their own.

While the health insurance market itself is very competitive, *the existence of insurance tends to make price competition more difficult to maintain in the medical care market.* Insurance breaks the linkage between buyer and seller, splitting payment "for" services by patients from payments "for" services to providers. The reimbursement provided by an insurer to a hospital may have almost no relation to the bill the patient receives, or to what the insurer would have reimbursed the patient if the bill were paid out of pocket. In third-party transactions, there is often no longer a single "price" in any meaningful sense, and the role of prices as information is seriously degraded. Prices can no longer communicate to suppliers what the value of services is to consumers, nor do they reflect the costs of inputs in production. By design, insurance removes the burden of medical costs from the patient. There is no longer any need to worry about whether it is worthwhile to go to the doctor or whether an extra visit is worth the additional cost. Insurance acts as a price subsidy by increasing demand and by removing the incentive to use less expensive substitutes. Once the insurance premiums are paid, everything costs the same. Price competition is replaced by quality competition since prices no longer matter.

Insurance tends to distort production behavior as well. Under many reimbursement systems, hospitals and doctors are paid according to the cost of care, rather than the value of services (primarily because value is too difficult to measure). Hence, there is little incentive to work hard for increased efficiency. Some additional costs will be incurred for no reason other than the fact that the insurance will pay for them. With revenues coming from insurance rather than from patients, the connection between consumer service and profits is eroded. It may become easier to make money by providing what the insurance company thinks is important (detailed bills with lots of documentation) rather than providing what patients want or need.

Control over health care is exercised by control over the money that goes to doctors and hospitals. Thus, *insurance and reimbursement rules, rather than legislation, have become the*

WHY THE HEALTH INSURANCE MARKET IS HIGHLY PRICE COMPETITIVE

Unlike medical care, which suffers many market failure problems from lack of consumer knowledge to variable incidence, the market for health insurance meets most of the conditions for purely competitive goods.

- Insurance is a homogenous product. It provides dollars in reimbursement; thus, there is little "quality" variation.
- Insurance can be bought far in advance, when there is no time pressure or illness.
- Insurance can be bought far from home, in a national market.
- Purchasing is done by large and sophisticated buyers (corporate benefits offices, broker agents) who can afford to compare and examine the contracts being offered.

dominant regulatory force in health care. The government does not need to pass a law telling hospitals to do or not to do something. If reimbursement rules are shifted so that only hospitals that meet certain standards get paid, then hospitals will do what the flow of money directs them to do. It is not necessary to exhort doctors to provide examinations. If the money is made available through insurance, the services will appear in the marketplace.

Medicine is a vital service with broad public and professional interest. What that means in practice is that there is often a rhetorical cover blanketing the operation of self-interest by any party. Insurance companies, consumers, and providers all talk about the public interest while trying hard to maintain their own position or to get ahead. Physicians are skilled professionals who care for patients, and as professionals their incomes depend entirely on what can be earned from patients and insurance. Caring is a business, with revenues and expenses, not just a calling. The advice of economists is that following the path of dollars through the system will often tell a student more about what is really going on than listening to the arguments presented in newspapers or on television, or by reviewing the most recent congressional testimony or transcripts from legal cases. Money talks, even to physicians and nonprofit hospitals. For those willing to listen, it speaks loudly and clearly about how the health care system works.

SUGGESTIONS FOR FURTHER READING

Medical Economics (monthly) Medical Economics Publishing, Montvale, New Jersey.

"Medical Education," annual special issue of the *Journal of the American Medical Association.*

Abraham Flexner, *Medical Education in the United States and Canada*, The Carnegie Foundation, 1910 (http://www.carnegiefoundation.org/eLibrary/docs/flexner_report.pdf) excerpt reprinted in the *Bulletin of the World Health Organization* 80, no. 7 (2002): 594–602 (www.who.org).

James Le Fanu, M.D., *The Rise and Fall of Modern Medicine* (New York: Carroll & Graf, 1999).

Gregory C. Pope and Russel T. Burge, "The Marginal Practice Cost of Physicians' Services," *Socio-Economic Planning Science* 29, no. 1 (1995):1–16.

Richard Shryock, *Medical Licensing in America, 1650-1965* (Baltimore: Johns Hopkins University Press, 1967).

Paul Starr, *The Social Transformation of American Medicine* (New York: Basic Books, 1982).

Rosemary Stevens, *American Medicine and the Public Interest* (New Haven, Conn.: Yale University Press, 1971).

John Wennberg and Alan Gittlesohn, "Variations in Medical Care Among Small Areas," *Scientific American* 246 (1982):120–134.

SUMMARY

1. About 16,000 M.D.s graduated from 126 medical schools in the United States in 2002. Since the bulk of the physician supply consists of those who have already been, and will continue to be, in practice for many years, any changes in the number of new graduates will only slowly affect the supply of services. The "physician boom" of the 1970s will move through the health care system creating strains and opportunities until the year 2020. The supply of physicians stayed roughly constant at around 1.4 physicians per 1,000 population from the start of modern medical education in the 1920s until 1965, but has risen rapidly since then to 2.9 physicians per 1,000 population today.

2. Although medical school tuition is expensive, running as much as $40,000 per year, it is still a very good **investment in human capital.** The average medical student will graduate with a debt of about $85,000—but this is less than six months of the average physician's earnings. Overall, taking into account the tuition, years of training, extra hard work, and other factors, going to medical school provides an annual inflation-adjusted return of about 12 percent, three or four times what one could expect if one invested in financial assets rather than education, and about 1.5 to 2 times as much as one gains from most undergraduate and graduate education.

3. **Control over physician supply and licensure in the United States is actually exercised by control over medical education,** a system that grew out of the Flexner Report of 1910 to the Carnegie Commission, supported by the AMA. Three factors contributed to the development of medical licensure based on graduate training at that time: (a) advances in medical technology (surgery, anesthesia, radiology) that were powerful aids to healing, but could also be harmful if used improperly; (b) a scientific knowledge base that gave university-educated physicians a real advantage over physicians who only learned by apprenticeships; and (c) a reformist political climate favoring regulation, combined with evidence that many doctors were not competently trained before entering practice.

4. **Competition** for clients in medical care is dominated by quality, not price. Physicians have used quality concerns and licensure laws to foreclose competition by graduates of foreign medical schools, osteopaths, chiropractors, and other health practitioners.

5. **Control over supply** by professional associations has increased the **profits** of physicians relative to other workers. While the physician-to-population ratio stayed constant from 1930 to 1960, demand was actually increasing due to new medical advances and an increasingly affluent society, creating a physician shortage. The AMA was unwilling to increase the number of physicians (which would have meant lower incomes) but public opinion was sufficiently strong to force the opening of new medical schools and revisions in immigration laws to make it easier for foreign doctors to practice in the United States. As the increase in new graduates during the 1970s and 1980s relieved this pressure, the size of entering medical school classes was reduced and immigration was again restricted. Since 1980, graduate rates have stayed constant even as population and per capita income have grown, increasing demand and pushing physician incomes upward.

6. **Group practice**, increasing the scale of physician operations, requires more coordination and uses more ancillary help, but increases output per physician and uses physicians' informational advantages by having them monitor the quality of one another's practices. The ability to trade patients more efficiently is a major function of such economic organizations. However, such coordination increases transaction costs and limits the autonomy of individual physicians because they must now operate as part of a team.

7. **Price discrimination**, charging higher prices where demand is less elastic (due to insurance, high income, lack of information or alternatives) is common in medicine, although much of the motivation seems to be purely charitable and is officially sanctioned by the public. Even though there are many physicians in a city, each one is unique and patients are reluctant to switch. The reduced price sensitivity that arises from such "monopolistic competition" allows price differentials to endure.

8. The potential for **kickback** payments on referrals and profits from related business may hamper the ability of physicians to act as the patient's **agent.** Ownership of pharmacies and sale of drugs by physicians is prohibited in the United States (but not in Japan, where patients are prescribed more drugs for each visit and many physicians make a third of their income that way). Ownership of laboratories, physical therapy clinics, and diagnostic radiology facilities has been shown to lead to abuses of trust (excessive ordering of tests, excess charges) and is increasingly being discouraged and regulated by government payers.

9. Physicians in some areas perform a specific operation, such as tonsillectomies, at a rate six times that of physicians in another area, even though both areas seem to be similar in all respects. Such unexplained **practice variations** call into question the idea that there is some well-defined need for medical care that can be objectively agreed upon by most physicians. Since such variations have been shown to occur, governments have begun studies to examine more carefully how differences in treatment are related to outcomes, thus developing standard protocols known as **clinical pathways** and **practice standards.**

10. **Markets for health insurance** are more competitive than for the underlying service, medical care, because insurance is a homogenous product (dollars are used to pay bills) with little quality variation, which is bought in advance on a geographically dispersed national market and often purchased by well-informed corporate benefits managers.

11. **Insurance distorts the market for medical care** because use of third-party payment breaks the link between buyer and seller. Insurance acts like a price reduction or subsidy, making consumers less price-sensitive, fostering competition on the basis of quality rather than price, and necessitating special contracts to reimburse providers who do not collect much money directly from the patients they serve. **Insurance rules are the dominant regulatory force in health care because they control the flow of money.**

PROBLEMS

1. {*licensure*} Does licensure raise the quality of medical care, or does it just raise the profitability of medical practice?

2. {*information asymmetry*} How do agency and information asymmetry lead to licensure? Do agents get more or less of the gains from trade as the degree of information asymmetry increases? Explain why and how the strength of licensure is related to the extent of information asymmetry.

3. {*incidence*} Who pays the costs of medical education: the student, the patients, the insurance companies, or the taxpayers?

4. {*annualized returns*} If the rate of return on human capital is 15 percent and the opportunity cost of time for a newly graduated physician is $60,000 per year, how large an incremental increase in annual earnings should the physician expect to obtain from a four-year post-graduate residency?

5. {*demand curves, derived demand*} Draw the demand and supply curves for two medical professions, one with licensure and one without (e.g., physicians compared to hospital administrators).

   a. Which would show the greater percentage increase in incomes for an equivalent shift in demand?

   b. What would be the effect of the government giving scholarships of $10,000 per year to all students entering the licensed profession compared with the effect of giving scholarships to all students entering the unlicensed profession?

   c. What would be the effect of the scholarships on tuition at the licensed and unlicensed professional schools? On the number of students applying?

   d. Would it make a difference if, instead of giving scholarships to everyone, the government gave them to just 5,000 students?

6. {*price controls*} Some states have mandated Medicare "assignment." Assignment means that the doctor agrees to treat a patient and accept the fee Medicare sends as payment in full. Doctors not accepting assignment bill the patient (almost always for more than Medicare would pay) and the patient pays the doctor, sends in the bill, and gets reimbursed by Medicare. Typically 20 percent to 60 percent of physicians in an area accept Medicare assignment because patients prefer it and payment is assured. Other physicians want to bill for the extra money. The number of doctors accepting assignment depends on the rates Medicare is currently paying, local market conditions, how "full" the doctor's practice is, and so on. Draw demand and supply curves to show the effects of passing a state law mandating that all physicians accept Medicare assignment. What happens to price, quantity, demand, and supply? Distinguish between short-term and long-term effects. Describe other effects you might expect.

7. {*competition*} Several politicians have proposed that the United States become more restrictive regarding immigration, allowing fewer foreign-educated physicians to undergo training or establish practices in the United States. Would this increase or decrease the earning power of U.S.-educated physicians? Which specialties would be most affected?

8. {*licensure*} The state of New Jersey was unwilling to allow physicians to become licensed in 1850. Which factors changed to make the state willing to enact and enforce licensure restrictions in 1950?

9. {*licensure, property rights*} How did the reformers in the medical profession who wanted to impose higher standards obtain the consent of physicians who were educated under the old system? Did power get translated into money in the process?

10. {*supply*} What controls the supply of physicians in the United States? Distinguish between short- and long-term and between proximate and fundamental factors (i.e., the actual decision-making individuals and organizations versus the underlying economic and political forces).

11. {*anti-trust*} Has the AMA ever been sued for restraint of trade? Did it win or lose?

12. {*competition*} Are chiropractors substitutes or complements for physicians in the production of medical services? What about podiatrists? Psychologists? Osteopaths? Homeopaths? Which professions are more competitive and which are more cooperative? Why?

13. {*dynamics*} How long does it take to become a doctor? How long does a doctor usually practice medicine? How long does it take for the supply of doctors to adjust to a change in the number of patients or a change in the availability of technology? Is the time required for adjustment different for a city than for a state or the country as a whole? What is the relevant geographic unit for measuring the market for physician services?

14. {*productivity*} Is the productivity of a medical practice determined primarily by the amount of capital employed or the number of people employed?

15. {*trade*} Do physicians pay each other for patients? If so, explain how.

16. {*industrial organization*} Why do physicians choose to practice together in groups? Is assembling physicians into groups any different from assembling employees into a manufacturing firm, or lawyers into a legal firm, or baseball players into a team?

17. {*economies of scale*} What advantages does a large physician group have over a solo physician? What disadvantages?

18. {*input compensation*} Is it possible for a physician to use ancillary inputs to increase profits without paying for those inputs? If so, give several different examples.

19. {*price discrimination*} When physicians choose to give a discount on fees, does it raise or lower their income? Will a profit maximizing physician charge higher prices for services or groups of patients for which demand is more elastic or less elastic? Explain why, providing a numerical calculation to illustrate your point and giving several examples.

20. {*price controls*} Lets assume that the state of Idaho decides that Medicaid will pay only 75 percent of what private insurance pays in order to save money and balance the state budget. Will this cause a shortage ? What kind of evidence would you look for?

21. {*transactions costs*} Why are kickbacks illegal?

22. {*practice variations*} Which factors determine the number of knee surgeries in a state? Will the same factors determine the number of hip surgeries? Colon surgeries? Hospital admissions as a result of asthma?

23. {*price discrimination*} The Saga of the Doctor and the Wannabe:

    a. Dr. Jones is the only doctor in Calexico, a town of Anglos who mostly own farms and local businesses or who work in schools and government and Chicanos who mostly work on the farms growing lettuce. Dr. Jones obviously has a monopoly on medical care in Calexico. Rodrigo is a field worker. Everyone who knows him says he is very smart and muy simpatico (very empathetic) and knows a lot about what makes people sick. His grandmother was a Curandera, or herb doctor, and taught him a lot. He also learned from other native curers and read medical books. He earned straight A's in school until he had to drop out and work in the fields to help support his family. At night and on weekends he acts as the "doctor" to many poor families. He asks them to pay what they can to help him and his invalid mother.

    One day in May a man who was seeing Rodrigo for "faintness" dies. A Chicana who was in labor and being cared for by Dr. Jones also dies. A big fight follows. Rodrigo says, "Dr. Jones gets rich by charging big fees, while he butchers our people." Dr. Jones says, "This illiterate Mexican tries to pass himself off as a doctor and kept this man from coming to me for treatment that could have saved his life." Dr. Jones also states, "I am the greatest friend the Chicano community has. I charge them less than half of what I charge my other patients because I know they can't afford more." *Comment briefly on Dr. Jones's pricing and its relationship to his desire to help Chicanos.*

    b. The fight between Dr. Jones and Rodrigo is getting worse and threatens this once peaceful agricultural community. Anglo and Chicano are openly hostile to each other. But within each camp there is dissension. Some Chicanos say, "Dr. Jones did help a lot of our people, and when they couldn't pay, he didn't send the bill collector or take their car, as the department store or bank would have done. Besides, although the mother died, he saved the baby—if not for him, both could have died." Some Anglos say, "That young upstart Rodrigo may be right. I've been going to Dr. Jones for eight years, he's made a bundle off of me, and my arthritis isn't any better." At the urging of the mayor, Dr. Jones and Rodrigo get together to talk about the problem. Afterward, each has a much different point of view. Rodrigo states, "Dr. Jones is an honest and hardworking doctor who has the best interests of the community at heart. He actually loses money taking care of Chicanos and should be paid more. I will work with him in every case I can." Dr. Jones says, "Rodrigo is an exceptionally talented young man who knows more than any layperson, and even some doctors I have met, about the practice of medicine. We are in complete agreement about the tremendous need for better medical care in Calexico and will work together to solve this problem. Many Chicano patients who cannot afford to see me on a regular basis can be treated just as well by Rodrigo after I have done any initial diagnosis and evaluation, and I will send them to him. Together we can provide better medical care for all." *Explain why this togetherness occurred among two people each of whom had claimed the previous night that the other was a killer. In your answer assume that each was motivated solely by economic considerations. Why does Rodrigo say that Dr. Jones should raise his prices?*

c. One year later, Dr. Jones announces, "Working with Rodrigo has opened my eyes to the plight of Chicanos and the reluctance of Anglos to accept them as equal members of society. Furthermore, as I become older I face the inevitable diminution of my ability to meet the needs of our community, and as a doctor I face the responsibility of ensuring that Calexico can continue to receive good medical care. Therefore, I have formed La Raza de Calexico Scholarship Fund. Rodrigo will work as a staff member at my clinic part time while he completes college and his medical education. He will, of course, continue to help the Chicanos who have always come to him, but he will also treat Anglo patients. This exceptional person should not work as a field hand when he can so ably act to meet the medical needs of all citizens in Calexico. We have just signed a contract that will make him my junior partner the day he graduates from medical school and that will turn over my full practice to him when I retire." *Given that both of them had a good deal with their cooperative arrangement, why take this further step?*

d. In 1994 Rodrigo said, "I can only be grateful to Dr. Jones and his unselfish commitment to helping Chicanos like myself." In 2000, after graduating from medical school, he condemns Dr. Jones as "a racist exploiter who sought to take advantage of me and the whole Chicano community to help himself alone" and seeks to void the 1994 contract and have Dr. Jones expelled from the county medical society. *Why would he do that?*

ENDNOTES

1. Enrollments and other data are taken from the annual "Medical Education" issue of *the Journal of the American Medical Association.*

2. J. Ganem, J. Krakower, and R. Beran, "Review of U.S. Medical School Finances, 1993–994," *Journal of the American Medical Association,* 274, no.9 (September 6, 1995): 723–730.

3. American Association of Medical Colleges, *AAMC Data Book 2002,* tables E1, E4. It is worth noting that while the average doctor under age 35 was at least $200,000 in debt, just 10 percent of that debt was for student loans while 90 percent was for home mortgage, indicating that tuition was not financially burdensome relative to current and expected income; see Lawrence Farber, "How Financially Secure Are Young Doctors?" *Medical Economics* (August 24, 1998): 34–43.

4. Gary S. Becker, *Human Capital* (Cambridge, Mass: Harvard University Press, 1975).

5. William B. Weeks and Amy E. Wallace, "The More Things Change: Revisiting a Comparison of Educational Costs and Incomes of Physicians and Other Professionals," *Academic Medicine* 77, no. 4 (April 2002: 312–319; see also Roger Feldman and Richard Scheffler, "The Supply of Medical School Applicants and the Rate of Return of Training," *Quarterly Review of Economics and Business* (Spring, 1978); W. Lee Hansen, "Shortages and Investment in Health Manpower," in *The Economics of Health and Medical Care* (Ann Arbor, Mich. University of Michigan Press, 1965).

6. Richard Shryock, *Medical Licensing in America, 1650-1965* (Baltimore: Johns Hopkins University Press, 1967); Rosemary Stevens, *American Medicine and the Public Interest* (New Haven, Conn.: Yale University Press, 1971).

7. Rashi Fein, *The Doctor Shortage: An Economic Diagnosis* (Washington: Brookings Institute, 1967).

8. Edward Berkowitz and Wendy Wolf, *Group Health Association: A Portrait of a Health Maintenance Organization* (Philadelphia: Temple University Press, 1988).

9. Erwin Blackstone, "The AMA and the Osteopaths: A Study of the Power of Organized Medicine," *Antitrust Bulletin* (Summer 1977). Jeff Forster, "Remember When Osteopathy was called a cult?" *Medical Economics* (April 27, 1998): 220.

10. Elton Rayack, "The Physicians Service Industry," Chapter 6 in Walter Adams, ed., T*he Structure of American Industry*, 5th edition (New York: Macmillan, 1982): 407–408.

11. U.S. Department of Health and Human Services, *Fifth Report to the President and Congress on the Status of Health Personnel in the United States* (Washington, D.C.: U.S. Government Printing Office, 1984).

12. U.S. Department of Health and Human Services, Office of Graduate Medical Education, *Report of the Graduate Medical Education National Advisory Committee to the Secretary, DHHS*. Pub No. 81–651 (Washington, D.C.: U.S. Government Printing Office, 1981). This became widely known as the "GMENAC Report."

13. American Medical Association, *Physician Characteristics and Distribution in the US, 2002-2003*.

14. *Health, United States, 2002*, Tables 103, 104 (www.cdc.gov/nchs).

15. Richard A. Cooper, Thomas E. Getzen, Healther J. McKee, and Prakash Laud, "Economic and Demographic Trends Signal an Impending Physician Shortage," *Health Affairs* 21, no. 1 , January 20021140– 1154; Richard Cooper, Thomas Getzen, and Prakash Laud, "Economic Expansion is a Major Determinant of Physician Supply and Utilization," *Health Services Research* 38 (forthcoming 2003).

16. Frederick Wolinsky and William Marder, *The Organization of Medical Practice and the Practice of Medicine* (Ann Arbor, Mich.: Health Administration Press, 1985).

17. Uwe Reinhardt, *Physician Productivity and the Demand for Health Manpower* (Cambridge, Mass: Ballinger, 1974).

18. R.A. Cooper et al., "Current and Projected Workforce of Nonphysician Clinicians," *Journal of the American Medical Association* 280, no. 9 (1988): 788–794. B.G. Druss et al, "Trends in Care by Nonphysician Clinicians in the United States," *New England Journal of Medicine* 348, no. 2 (January 9, 2003): 130– 137.

19. Joseph Newhouse, *The Economics of Medical Care* (Reading, Mass: Addison-Wesley, 1978), 40.

20. Thomas Getzen, "A 'Brand Name' Firm Theory of Medical Group Practice," *Journal of Industrial Economics* 33, no. 2 (1984): 199– 215.

21. Helen Clapesattle, *The Doctors Mayo* (Minneapolis: University of Minnesota Press, 1941).

22. Sandy Lutz, "Troubled Times for Psych Hospitals," *Modern Healthcare* 21, no. 50 (December 16, 1991): 26– 27, 30–33; and "NME Totals Costs of Psych Woes" *Modern Healthcare* 23, no. 43 (October 25, 1993): 20.

23. Jean M. Mitchell and Jonathan H. Sunshine, "Consequences of Physician's Ownership of Health Care Facilities—Joint Ventures in Radiology," *New England Journal of Medicine* 327 (1992): 1497–1501.

24. Physicians are allowed to buy stocks and make other forms of investments in laboratories, hospitals and medical businesses, but they cannot be partners or get special treatment different from non-physicians who are not in a position to refer patients.

25. Reuben Kessel, "Price Discrimination in Medicine," *Journal of Law and Economics* 1, no. 2 (October 1958): 20–53.

26. The same process of overcharging for less price-sensitive ancillary items is found when purchasing an automobile, as the dealer puts a larger mark-up on radios, air bags, floor mats, and so on.

27. American Child Health Association, "Physical Defects: The Pathway to Correction, 1934," pp:80-96, as cited in David Eddy, "Variations in Physician Practice: The Role of Uncertainty," *Health Affairs* 3, no. 2 (Summer 1984): 74–89.

28. John Wennberg, J. L. Freeman, and W. J. Culp, "Are Hospital Services Rationed in New Haven or Over-Utilised in Boston?" *Lancet I* (May 23, 1987), : 1185–1188; John Wennberg, Klim McPherson, and Philip Caper, "Will Payment Based on Diagnosis-Related Groups Control Hospital Costs?" *New England Journal of Medicine* 311, no. 5 (1984): 295– 303.

29. Writing Group for the Women's Health Initiative Investigators, "Risks and Benefits of Estrogen Plus Progestin in Healthy Post-menopausal Women." *Journal of the American Medical Association* 288, no. 3 (July 17, 2002): 321–333, (http://jama.ama-assn.org/issues/v288n3/fpdf/joc21036.pdf).

30. David Kindig, *Purchasing Population Health: Paying for Results* (Ann Arbor: University of Michigan Press, 1997).

31. Charles Phelps, "Information Diffusion and Best Practice Adoption," Chapter 5 in A.J. Culyer and J.P. Newhouse, *Handbook of Health Economics* (Elsevier: Amsterdam, 2000), 223–264.

32. David Dranove, *From Marcus Welby to Managed Care, The Economic Evolution of American Health Care* (Princeton, N.J.: Princeton University Press, 2000). Of interest to a health economist, the title of the first Dr. Kildare movie was "Interns Can't Take Money." The young Dr. Kildare saves the life of a gangster, but as a doctor in training, he is not allowed to be paid for his services. The gangster, not bound by social rules, gives him a small fortune ($1,000), which the impoverished young doctor, acting nobly, returns.

CHAPTER **8**

HOSPITALS

QUESTIONS

1. How do hospitals get paid? What do they pay for?
2. Why don't philanthropists donate as much to hospitals as they used to?
3. Does it make a difference to hospitals that 95 percent of their funds come from third-party insurance rather than patients?
4. Who pays for medical research?
5. Does cost-shifting help the poor or the rich?
6. Does tax exemption help hospitals serve the public welfare?
7. Why did hospitals borrow so much and load up their balance sheets with debt during the 1980s?
8. Does reimbursement increase employment? Does it drive up costs?
9. Are hospitals still charitable institutions, or have they become instruments of corporate control?
10. Who owns a nonprofit hospital? Who gets the profits?

8.1 FROM CHARITABLE INSTITUTIONS TO CORPORATE CHAINS: DEVELOPMENT OF THE MODERN HOSPITAL

The hospital as an institution for the care of the sick has a long and noble history. During the twentieth century, the hospital became the dominant organizational force in health care, and the biggest user of health care funds. As the twenty-first century begins, hospitals are being replaced or transformed into larger and more complex "health systems" that encompass different modes of care (inpatient, ambulatory centers, home health, nursing homes) spanning multiple sites.[1]

As long as people have gotten sick, society has needed a place to care for them, both to provide special support and to isolate the ill from the rest of the community. In pre-scientific times, cure was often identified with casting out evil, and hospitals were religious structures. In classical Greece (600 B.C. to 1 A.D.), temples known as *asclepia* took in the sick, especially those who were poor and lacked resources to be cared for at home.[2] Cities used taxes to support hospitals and dispensaries staffed by physicians, who also received fees from those who could afford to pay. The Romans, who created their large-scale hierarchical organizations to rule a vast empire, found it necessary to provide hospitals for the slaves and gladiators who served on plantations or in the military, respectively. The word "hospital" was first used in the twelfth century to refer to a facility run by the church that housed and cared for the sick, the

154

disabled, and the insane, as well as provided lodging for pilgrims and other travelers, orphans, and the poor. Only those who had no homes stayed in hospitals, because everyone else, even if ill, preferred to remain with their families. Economic changes and the great epidemics that came with the expansion of trade greatly increased the need for institutional care. By the end of the thirteenth century, 19,000 hospitals were scattered across Europe. The shift from religious care to scientific cures took place gradually over the next six hundred years, but came even more rapidly toward the end of the nineteenth century. Florence Nightingale's work with injured and sick British soldiers during the Crimean war became the basis for her two books, *Notes on Hospitals* (1858) and *Notes on Nursing* (1859), which significantly changed the shape of the hospital and which are still influential today.[3]

Hospitals were founded in 1527 in Mexico and 1635 in Canada, but it was not until 1751 that a hospital was founded in the American colonies. The Pennsylvania Hospital, still a major hospital today, was created by a bill passed in the Assembly with the support of Benjamin Franklin, which obligated the governor to provide £2,000 to match £2,000 in public donations for construction.[4] Philadelphia already had an almshouse and quarantine hospitals (temporary housing for sailors and others with contagious diseases), but the new building was slated to be a more grand and permanent edifice that would promote science as well as provide care. The six physicians who worked twice a week without pay were selected because they were outstanding and were mostly trained abroad. Other notable early American hospitals were the New York hospital chartered by King George III in 1771 to provide care for the sick poor and instruction to medical students of the Columbia Medical School, and the Massachusetts General Hospital built in 1821 at a cost of more than $100,000, an imposing structure superior to the European hospitals of that time and the first to have indoor plumbing. American hospitals were based on the model of the British and Continental voluntary hospitals. However, the American hospitals were more likely to have paying patients, who tended to be charged extra to subsidize care for the poor.[5]

These three important hospitals still exist, but the economics of hospital operations have changed drastically. In the eighteenth and nineteenth centuries, most funding came from donations, with patient fees playing a minor role, and insurance reimbursement was nonexistent. The major category of expenditure was food, and the work of the staff was supplemented by making patients labor alongside employees cleaning, cooking, and nursing. Today "hotel costs" (room, meals) account for less than 10 percent of hospital expenditures, and it is impossible to imagine making patients work alongside doctors and nurses. The colonial hospitals were similar to most modern hospitals in that they were nonprofit institutions run by volunteer governing boards, with medical care directed and conducted by physician staff members who were not paid by the hospital but were in private practice as independent businesses in the community.

The development of the modern hospital, like the development of medical specialties, was driven by the creation of new technology. With anesthesia and antiseptics making safe surgery possible, a clean and controlled operating suite with skilled assistants became a necessity. The discovery of X-rays made it necessary to acquire access to radiographic equipment. Advances in clinical pathology and chemistry made the laboratory vital for diagnosis. Major capital investment was required to obtain access to all these new technologies. A solo physician practicing alone could not make full use of this new equipment, or manage all the specialized technicians who operated it. It was necessary to bring all the patients of many physicians together under one roof, to obtain funding and make effective use of the new technology, and to hire a manager to coordinate the efforts of medical and ancillary staff. An organizational revolution had to take place.[6] Within the custodial institutions that had existed for centuries serving the disabled poor there arose a new type of hospital, a modern organization with sophisticated and expensive equipment to provide scientific cures where middle-class patients wanted to be treated and were willing to pay. The large and uncertain monetary requirements caused a corresponding financial revolution (insurance reimbursement), which further increased demand and made possible the massive flow of funds required to support a technologically sophisticated system of intensive care costing thousands of dollars for each patient.

8.2 REVENUES: THE FLOW OF FUNDS INTO THE HOSPITAL

From the founding of The Pennsylvania Hospital in 1751 until the beginnings of Blue Cross in 1929, the primary source of hospital funding was philanthropy from the community, supplemented by patient fees. Since 1940, hospital revenues have grown rapidly, but philanthropy and patient fees have decreased drastically as a percentage of the total. Now the largest sources of payment are Medicare, which provides government funding for the 60 percent of patient days used by the elderly, and managed care firms shopping for low prices and good information systems to control costs. Around 1960, the dominant payers were nonprofit Blue Cross plans. At that time, these plans were affiliated with various hospital associations. They were designed to reimburse the full cost of patient care, thus allowing hospitals to break even while taking care of the indigent and undertaking whichever new treatments, diagnostic technology, or research they wanted. By 1995, several Blue Cross plans had fallen into bankruptcy. The survivors all started managed care plans to compete with (or complement) their traditional insurance plans. Some, such as the giant Blue Cross of California, have turned themselves into billion-dollar private for-profit firms.[7]

A new financing system had to be created, and re-created again and again, to provide all the new technology and services that Americans wanted. By 2002, 200 times more money was transferred from the pockets of the public into hospital expenses than had been paid at the end of World War II, with an average increase of more than 10 percent a year. Revenue growth has slowed substantially since 1990 as managed care has taken hold, and more revenues are coming from outside the hospital in the form of outpatient services or new business ventures (ambulance, nutrition counseling, home health care). In 2001, the average community hospital's inpatient revenues were around $50 million, receiving about $7,000 for each patient admitted ($1,400 per day, for an average five-day stay) and another $30 million for outpatient services. Table 8.1 lists the current sources of hospital revenues.[8]

The first thing to note from Table 8.1 is that it is unlikely and implausible that hospital behavior will be significantly shaped by consumers' decisions based on prices in this environment, as they would be in most markets, because more than 95 percent of revenues come from someone other than the recipient of services.[9] The second, perhaps even more important fact to note, is that the "someone else" is likely to be the government, which accounts for 60 percent of all revenues. The next thing to realize is that these are complex contracts for hundreds of thousands, even millions of dollars. Although we may talk about "patient revenues" or the "price" of a laboratory test, to actually bring in revenues, a hospital chief financial officer (CFO) has to enter an intricate legal relationship with Medicare or a joint venture with a group of radiologists, or structure a risk-sharing arrangement with a consortium of community physicians. Such deals are quite different from retail sales added up at the cash register.

TABLE 8.1	Hospital Characteristics, 2001
5,795	Total number of hospitals
169 beds	Average number of beds
12.9 admissions	Per 100 population
5.1 days	Average length of stay
7.2 FTE	FTE employees per patient day
$1,318	Average cost per patient day
44%	Percentage of revenues from outpatients
$ 265	Average cost per outpatient visit
$87 million	Average revenue per hospital
4.9%	Average profit margin

Sources of Funds		Uses of Funds	
Patients self-pay	3%	Labor	53%
Private insurance	32%	Professional Fees	5%
Philanthropy, other private	5%	Supplies, other	34%
Medicare	31%	Depreciation & Int.	8%
Medicaid	17%		100%
Other government	12%		
	100%		

Source: American Hospital Association, *Hospital Statistics 2002.*

Sources of Revenues

Although a complete picture is beyond the scope of this book (and indeed beyond the grasp of most economists and accountants and even experienced hospital financial managers—the details, exceptions, exclusions, covenants, and formulas go on forever), an overview of the major ways in which revenues flow into hospitals is helpful in grasping the financial incentives they face (see Table 8.2).

Philanthropy and Grants   Grants are funds that are donated for a specific purpose: to conduct cancer research, build a new operating pavilion, provide outreach programs for prenatal care, and so on. Donors want to make sure that funds are used for the purpose intended, but there is little direct pressure to compete on price or to control costs. The

TABLE 8.2	Major Types of Hospital Reimbursement
Philanthropy and grants	
Global budgets	
Charges	
Per diem	
Cost reimbursement	
DRGs (per admission)	
Capitation	
Managed care contracts	

program director spends the budget and, if sufficiently good results are achieved in public-relations terms, another grant usually will be forthcoming sometime in the future. This revenue flows from the belief of the donor that the task facing the hospital is important and socially valuable, and is not to make profits or even necessarily to show measurable effects. All nonprofit organizations must begin with a charitable grant. Tax appropriations are a form of grant, with the donor being the government. Tax breaks in the form of relief from property taxes and user fees are even more important to many hospitals these days and have become increasingly controversial.[10]

Global Budgets   A hospital operating under a global budget is getting a grant for all its costs. This form of payment is typical for state mental hospitals, military hospitals, and hospitals run by the Department of Veterans Affairs and other government entities, as well as a few specialized private institutions. Since a global budget is fixed, there are few incentives either to attract more patients or to reduce costs. In Canada, England, and much of the developed world outside the United States, global budgets are the most common form of hospital payment.

Charges   Hospital charges are known as "list prices" in most industries. A hospital, like a flower shop, can set its charges at whatever level it likes. It is rare for a patient, or an insurance company, to actually pay what is "charged." However, these paper charges often form the basis for reimbursement under a system of "discounted charges" (e.g., 60 percent of list price) or under a cost reimbursement system that will be described shortly.

Per Diem   Latin for "per day," per diem payments were common when hospitals originated and are increasingly favored in managed care contracts today. Originally, per diems were charges set by the hospital and usually exceeded costs to help subsidize nonpaying patients. Today per diems are often negotiated with managed care firms under very competitive conditions and are sometimes set below average costs per day in order for a hospital to maintain or increase its market share.

Cost Reimbursement   Cost reimbursement sets the payment level equal to the hospital's audited costs. "Days" and "discharges" are poor measures of the hospital's "product" since they do not account for variations in quality, severity of illness, or use of new technology. Because the hospital's output is so difficult to define and measure, it may be more equitable and easier to reimburse for incurred costs, rather than try to set appropriate prices. The Blue Cross (BC) plans, organized under the aegis of the American Hospital Association, wrote manuals describing how nonprofit hospitals can break even by setting charges to cover costs (including costs for treating nonpaying patients and setting aside money for a prudent reserve) and designed a method of cost reimbursement to break even. This method is known as **ratio of cost to charges applied to charges (RCCAC)**. When Medicare was created in 1965, it adopted the RCCAC methodology; therefore, this form of cost reimbursement became the dominant method by which funds flowed into hospitals from the 1960s until the mid-1980s. The RCCAC methodology is still used to determine most hospital unit costs today. The RCCAC is calculated separately for each revenue-producing department using this formula for BC (Blue Cross) payment:

$$\textit{RCCAC Method} \quad \text{BC payment} = \frac{\text{Total Department Costs}_{\text{all payers}}}{\text{Total Department Charges}_{\text{all payers}}} \times \text{BC Charges}$$

The complicated RCCAC formula is needed because costs must be divided among different payers who are responsible for the costs of different patients. If there were only one payer, it would pay all costs, and cost reimbursement would be like an open-ended grant. With many payers, however, some way must be found to allocate the costs across patients, and the RCCAC method uses the hospital's billed charges to do so. The method worked very well for a number of years to reimburse hospitals for all their costs. Indeed, it worked so well that costs rose explosively. Costs rose so much that cutbacks became inevitable, causing arguments between hospitals and Medicare over money. Medicare removed the return on invested capital as an "allowable cost" for reimbursement. Extra payments to increase nursing employment and wages were dropped. Charity care and bad debts (resulting from patients who were expected to pay but did not) became a source of contention. Medicare initially accommodated the needs of hospitals by covering as a part of overhead the cost of caring for patients who did not pay. In a subsequent interpretation of the rules, Medicare in effect said, "Since we pay all our bills in full and on time, we are not responsible for those who don't." By not counting charity care and bad debt as overhead costs distributed across all payers, these charges get included in the RCCAC formula as if they would be paid by someone. This makes the cost-to-charges ratio smaller so that Medicare pays less. This helps the Medicare budget, but not the hospital, which must then increase charges to other payers to make up the difference.

DRGs—Diagnostically Related Groups   Diagnostically related group (DRG) payments are fixed payments made based on the patient's diagnosis at discharge. DRG payments cover the complete hospital stay, including all ancillary services (but not surgery and other physician fees). To create this prospective payment system for Medicare payments, the government split all illnesses into 473 DRGs and estimated the cost per case within each group (similar to the resource-based relative value scale [RBRVS] payment system for physician services discussed in Chapter 6, Section 6.1). Adjustments are made for these factors: local wages in the area in which the hospital is located, extremely long or short stays, hospitals with large teaching programs, and hospitals with a large proportion of indigent patients. In essence, DRGs are administered prices set by the government at what they believes is a fair rate. It is called a prospective payment system because the DRG rates are set in advance, unlike the previous retrospective cost reimbursement payments that were continually adjusted to match any change in costs so that the final amount was never set until long after the year ended. Under a charge system, the sellers (hospitals) have the power to set rates arbitrarily—subject to the power of the market to refuse to buy. Under a retrospective cost system, there is no set rate, but rather, reimbursement of actual costs incurred, perhaps subject to some review. With a DRG prospective payment system, the buyer (Medicare) has all the rate-setting power. In the first year of operation (1983), Medicare did little to force rates down, but in the years since, reimbursement has become progressively tighter; therefore, Medicare patients have become less and less profitable to treat. Once Medicare's DRG system was in place, it was adopted by many other payers.[11]

Capitation   Capitation payments, previously discussed in Chapter 5, are relatively rare for hospitals, since a large and well-defined number of patients must be pooled to reduce risks and make actuarial projections. Once an organization agrees to accept payment on a capitation basis, it in effect becomes a risk-bearing insurer. Usually, when it is said that a hospital is setting up a capitation arrangement, what is really meant is that some larger organization, such as the corporation that controls a number of hospitals, is creating an

CASE RATES ADJUSTED FOR SPECIAL SITUATIONS*

*This box section on case rate adjustment was prepared by Paul L. Grimaldi, Ph.D. ©2003, health finance consultant and lecturer.

Case-mix classification systems are used to determine the amounts that Medicare pays for the hospital inpatient care its beneficiaries receive. These systems include diagnosis-related groups (DRGs) for acute care hospitals, case-mix groups (CMGs) for inpatient rehabilitation facilities (IRFs), and long-term care (LTC)–DRGs (LTC-DRGs) for long-term care hospitals (LTCHs). Payment rates are established prospectively and are expressed on a case or discharge basis, depending primarily on a patient's diagnoses, procedures, and other clinical indicators. To avoid overpayments that may promote early discharge and underpayments that may jeopardize access, Medicare pays additional or reduced amounts in the following situations:

- Short-stay outliers
- Transfers and readmissions
- Patients who die
- High-cost outliers

The total net payment for these situations is budget-neutral—that is, the net amount for these situations translates into a corresponding decrease in the amount available for care rendered under all other circumstances.

Short-Stay Outliers

Some patients have significantly shorter stays than average for their case mix group. Typically, a short stay costs remarkably less than the corresponding case rate. If the full rate were paid, hospitals would have financial incentives to discharge patients prematurely and would strongly prefer patients who could be discharged quickly to other care settings. In general, Medicare relies on per diem methods to reimburse short stays to align costs and payments more closely. An extra amount may be paid for the first day to acknowledge the disproportionately higher costs associated with the earliest portion of the stay.

For example, for LTCH patients staying no more than five-sixths of the *geometric* average length of stay for the appropriate LTC-DRG, the payment amount equals the lowest of: (1) 120 percent of the estimated cost of the case, (2) 120 percent of the LTC-DRG per diem rate multiplied by the patient's length of stay, or (3) the full LTC-DRG rate. The closer the stay is to the threshold, the more likely the full rate will be the lowest of the three amounts.

For IRF patients who are discharged within three days after being hospitalized, Medicare pays a CMG rate established specifically for short-stay patients. This rate equals about 17 percent of the amount paid for the typical long-stay patient who receives a full course of treatment.

Transfers and Readmissions

A patient may be discharged to another care setting and subsequently readmitted to the discharging hospital. If the intervening period is relatively short and two separate case rates were paid (one each for the discharge and readmission), hospitals would have financial incentives to shift patients around solely to maximize net income. The incentives would be especially alluring if the discharging and receiving facilities were under common ownership or located on the same campus. Medicare makes reduced payments to dilute these incentives.

(Continued)

CASE RATES ADJUSTED FOR SPECIAL SITUATIONS (CONTINUED)

For instance, if an LTCH patient is discharged to an acute care hospital and read-mitted to the discharging hospital within 9 days, the discharge and readmission is defined as one stay and one LTC-DRG rate is paid to the discharging hospital. The threshold is 27 days for IRFs and 45 days for skilled nursing facilities. In addition, there is a 5 percent cap on the proportion of Medicare patients that hospitals within hospitals, distinct-part skilled nursing facilities, and other co-located facilities may discharge and readmit annually. If the cap is exceeded, each corresponding onsite discharge and readmission is paid as one discharge, including those occurring before the cap was surpassed.

Medicare also pays a reduced amount for an IRF patient whose length of stay exceeds three days but is below the average for his or her CMG and who is discharged to another rehabilitation facility. The reduction assumes that care in one inpatient setting is substituted for care in another inpatient setting. No reduction applies, however, if a patient is discharged to a home health agency on the assumption that this pattern represents a normal progression of care. Payment is based on a per diem rate that includes an extra 50 percent for the first day. Thus, if a patient stays 6 days and the applicable per diem rate is $900, the payment would be $5,850 = (6 × $900) + (0.50 × $900).

Patients transferred between acute care hospitals are paid similarly. Medicare pays the transferring hospital on a per diem basis up to the full DRG rate, while the receiving hospital that ultimately discharges the patient is paid the full DRG rate. For 10 specific DRGs, an acute care hospital is paid on a per diem basis up to the full DRG rate for Medicare patients who are transferred to a skilled nursing facility or other post-acute-care setting, including an extra amount for the first hospital day.

Patients Who Die

A reduced amount is paid for certain patients who die while hospitalized. For IRFs, there are four distinct CMGs for Medicare patients who stay longer than three days but die before treatment is completed. The case rate varies with the patient's length of stay and whether he or she was hospitalized for an orthopedic condition. Similarly, Medicare pays acute care hospitals a distinct case rate for neonates who die before discharge or are transferred to another facility.

High-Cost Outliers

Additional payments are made for Medicare patients who are extraordinarily costly to treat. The extra amount is determined by multiplying the excess of the estimated cost of treating the patient over a cost threshold by a marginal cost factor. The cost of treating the patient is estimated by multiplying the amount billed for covered services by the facility's cost-to-charges ratio. The threshold equals the DRG rate plus a predetermined "fixed-loss" amount (e.g., $24,450 for LTCHs and $33,560 for acute care hospitals for fiscal year 2003), which reflects the loss a hospital incurs before outlier payments begin. The marginal cost factor is generally 80 percent. Thus, if a hospital's cost-to-charge ratio is 65 percent and billed charges equal $80,000, the estimated cost would be $52,000 = $80,000 × 0.65. If the cost outlier threshold is $42,000, the outlier payment would be $8,000 = 0.80 × ($52,000 − $42,000). If the DRG rate is $23,000, the total payment would equal $31,000 = $23,000 + $8,000.

insurance company/health maintenance organization (HMO) to provide services on a capitated basis. Once the contract extends to multiple institutions and different kinds of care, the hospital becomes a "health system" rather than a traditional community hospital.

Managed Care Contracts Blue Cross and most private insurance companies are shifting to managed care contracts with hospitals (see Chapter 10). In these arrangements, payment is usually made on the basis of per diems, discounted charges, or a negotiated fee schedule. The crucial difference that sets managed care contracts apart from cost reimbursement or payment of charges is the role of the care manager. Rather than just paying the bills, the insurance company has a specialized **utilization review** nurse or physician critically examine each case to determine, for example, whether hospitalization was justified, a lower cost alternative (such as outpatient surgery) was available, and adequate documentation was provided for all laboratory tests. By negotiating discounts, discouraging use, and denying payment for disallowed or undocumented charges, managed care firms can usually obtain medical care for their clients at a lower cost than traditional indemnity or cost reimbursement insurers and, therefore, are taking over the market. Being constantly questioned and audited has not been easy or pleasant for the doctors who admit patients or for those working in hospital financial departments. Patients also dislike having to justify and obtain approval for every additional service or extra day in the hospital, but are willing to put up with it if premiums are sufficiently reduced.

8.3 COSTS: THE FLOW OF FUNDS OUT OF THE HOSPITAL

Hospitals are personal care institutions, and labor accounts for the bulk of their costs (see Table 8.1). In the early days, food and housing took up most of the hospital's budget, but today such "hotel functions" are relatively minor in comparison with the provision of medical care. Similar to 1750, physician care today is paid for separately and therefore is largely not included in the hospital budget. Few physicians are employees of the hospital, although the services of contracted pathologists, radiologists, and emergency room doctors do show up under the category "professional fees." It might be thought that the acquisition of lithotripters, magnetic resonance imaging (MRI) scanners, and other expensive medical technology would make "equipment" a large category, yet the wages of the skilled people required to operate each new piece of equipment usually runs two or three times the cost of the machinery itself. Much of the category "other" takes the form of services and thus also involves labor hired in the local market. When payroll, professional fees, and local services are added together, about 75 percent of a hospital's costs are labor. This fact makes it politically difficult to cut costs, since the only way to do so is to cut people, by reducing wages or laying off employees. Energy, raw materials, and other goods traded in competitive national and international markets are relatively unimportant in the hospital budget. Access to capital, however, has significantly shaped the growth of health care systems (see Section 8.5).

8.4 FINANCIAL MANAGEMENT AND COST SHIFTING

Revenues must exceed expenses for an organization to survive, but there is no reason that the individuals for whom expenditures are incurred must be the same as the individuals from whom revenues are obtained. While individual matching of benefits and payments is common in most consumer markets, in health care this almost never takes place. For the early hospitals, donations by the wealthy members of the community and general tax funds (paid mostly by landowners) were used to provide services to the sick and poor people with disabilities. Funding and benefits were matched at the level of the community, not the individual. It was considered fair that those who benefited most from the economy should give the most to help those in need. Paying patients who could afford hospitalization were usually charged a bit extra to help support the hospital's charitable mission. In effect, the excess of charges above costs constituted a "hospital tax" on the working-class and upper-class people who happened to get sick.

When hospitals took care of the poor who could not help themselves, it was obvious and necessary that the burden of financing would fall primarily on a different group of people who did have money: philanthropists and taxpayers. As technology advanced and hospital services became more desirable to all people, it was inevitable that there would be a great increase in hospital expenditures and that there would be more overlap between the people who paid and the people who received care. Insurance, pooling funds from the many so that a few could receive care, was a significant extension of financing that furthered the ability of the market to transfer the burden of payment away from the individual who was sick. One of the expenses that was factored into private insurance premiums was charity care; thus, insured patients were also paying for those who had no insurance.

The process of using revenues from one group of clients to subsidize another group is known in health care as **cost shifting.** Under philanthropic funding, all revenues are cost shifted—they are intended as donations to benefit others, not the giver. With insurance and cost reimbursement, the flows are more complex, but it is clear that somebody else is paying for the nonpaying patients (bad debt, charity care) since they do not bring any revenues into the hospital. Several other functions, such as medical education, research, and community outreach, are usually supported through cost shifting, because they bring in very little revenue, certainly less than what they cost to provide.

Financial managers in the early days assumed that the hospital would be a losing proposition and that their job was to find additional revenues from donors, grants, or tax rebates to cover the deficit. Indemnity insurance brought in more funds, but did not change the underlying rules. Hospitals were still nonprofit entities, but many now made an excess that could be used to fund growth or extra services. As cost reimbursement came to dominate payment systems, the financial manager's task became more complex, but easier. A fully reimbursed hospital was guaranteed to break even and thus could do all the research, education, and outreach it wanted because all costs were fully covered retrospectively. Medicare and Medicaid fundamentally changed the economic status of the hospital by providing coverage for what had previously been charity. As of 1970, the typical hospital faced a reimbursement situation similar to this: at the top, commercially insured patients paid full charges, bringing in about 20 percent more revenue per day than the cost-based Blue Cross and Medicare patients; the indigent Medicaid rate was usually lower; and uninsured working patients paid what they could, and charity cases brought in no revenues directly, but did help bolster the hospital's image and its cost reimbursement.

Cost shifting applied to certain services, as well as to certain patient groups. Hospitals needed to perform autopsies to help improve the quality of care, but obviously could not bill the patient. Clinical pathologists found it easy to support this scientific need by charging separately for laboratory tests that previously had been included as part of the regular hospital per diem for services. Billing for lab tests met with so little resistance that charges were pushed up and up, and by the 1970s it was not uncommon for a lab to charge ten times what a test cost and to be a major source of excess revenues for subsidizing other parts of the hospital, such as the emergency room, which was a chronic loser. Research programs must conduct extensive tests, keep patients in the hospital for extra days, and perform experimental surgeries that may turn out to be of no use to perfect techniques and make new discoveries. Since these bills are paid just like any other patient care, research costs are shifted to the insurance company. Also, the bill for a day in the intensive care unit (ICU) is based on the average; thus, the easy cases (since they actually cost less) provide an implicit subsidy for the complex cases and research. Medical education is expensive and usually conducted along with the research that keeps faculties on the cutting edge. Teaching salaries and research equipment are included when calculating the basis for cost reimbursement. Cost per day in a major university hospital is often two to three times that in a small community hospital. Since insurance pays whether the patient gets a broken arm fixed in a local hospital at $800 or a university hospital at $2,000, insurance (or rather the employed workers from whom premiums are taken) are paying for most of the research and education expenses.

Cost shifting and cross subsidies are pervasive and long-standing features of medical care reimbursement. In general, hospitals have had public support for taking revenues from a variety of sources and using them to fund not just basic care, but outreach to indigent people, community prevention programs, research, teaching, and other activities that were seen as being in the public interest. A number of forces have interacted over the past twenty years to cause this consensus on the purpose and funding of hospitals to crumble.

Net income to support research, education, or growth could be obtained either by increasing income or reducing expenses. Growth is difficult to accomplish without increasing expenditures, and thus it is unlikely that managers will concentrate on cuts. Furthermore, there was a general perception in the 1960s and 1970s that health care workers were already underpaid compared with other workers, and there is always a resistance to laying people off. Thus, in the era after 1965, "financial management" came to mean "revenue maximization." The new cost reimbursement rules were very complex and often ambiguous. This left some room for the creative accountant to reclassify, amend, and adjust so that more dollars flowed in. Such financial gamesmanship, along with the inherent expansionary tendencies of cost reimbursement, fueled rapid growth in expenses. Although the number of patients grew only slightly (less than 1 percent a year), the number of employees per patient (full-time equivalent [FTE] per occupied bed) increased from 1.1 in 1960 to 1.4 in 1965, 2.0 in 1970, 3.3 in 1980, and 7.0 in 2002.[12] Cost control was out, and revenue maximization was in.

The tremendous and unanticipated rise in expenditures for Medicare and Medicaid forced the government to try to modify the reimbursement system to cut costs. Payments for returns on equity capital to investors in for-profit hospitals were eliminated, as was a differential payment for nursing and a number of other minor elements. Yet the basic forces that led to explosive cost increases still remained. Also, although the government could change the rules, hospital financial managers had gained experience in working around the rules and could call on the assistance of consultants from major accounting firms to help them find the most remunerative interpretation or allocation basis. After a series of legislative cost controls attempting to maintain the solvency of the Medicare program failed to work, unpopular premium and tax increases had to be pushed through Congress. Medicare, forced into a corner, began to refuse to pay for the cost of charity care. Medicare claimed that it needed to be a "prudent buyer" and therefore reneged on the fundamental cost-shifting premise.

On one hand, Medicare's decision not to fund charity care and bad debt made sense. The bills of all Medicare patients were being paid in full and on time. Acting as an insurer of people 65 and older, this new interpretation certainly fulfilled its financial obligation to hospitals. On the other hand, hospitals had always charged everybody extra to make up for losses on charity care. Furthermore, it appeared that if anyone should be taking responsibility for the poor, it should be the government. Medicare, by taking a narrow interpretation of its contractual responsibilities, broke up the larger social contract based on cost shifting, which had been fundamental to hospitals as caring community institutions. As Medicare ratcheted down its rates, hospitals had to look elsewhere to make up the difference. And so, whereas charges to commercial insurance companies had been 10 to 15 percent above average cost, the breakdown of cost shifting pushed these "overcharges" up to 20 to 30 percent above cost. The private insurance companies howled in protest as they were forced to pick up what previously had been paid for by general tax funds. The university hospitals, with large indigent populations and big research programs, were in even worse shape than the community hospitals. They had a much smaller fraction of revenues coming from commercial insurance and, to make up for losses, had to raise their commercial rates 50 to 100 percent. The federal and state governments argued that the provision of Medicare and Medicaid had reduced the hospitals' burden of bad debt and charity care, but the large number of people seeking care who were still uninsured made hospitals skeptical.

Small price differentials and a shared sense of purpose were sufficient to allow the cross subsidies that made up a social contract for hospitals to continue. Big differentials and a hostile, "I'll pay for mine, and you pay for yours" attitude ruined this consensus. Market forces came into play. The outrageously high prices for tests done in hospital laboratories created a profit opportunity for commercial companies, which started providing services through independent doctor-entrepreneurs, cut prices in half, and still had large profit margins. Specialized psychiatric hospitals that treated only mild cases of mental disorder sprang up, able to make money at a pier diem far below that of the inner city psychiatric wards filled with violent and chronically disturbed individuals and staffed by residents more interested in research and understanding the causes of mental illness than in cost-effectiveness of care. Whenever prices are distorted by cross subsidy, there is an opportunity for a firm to make extraordinary profits by **cream skimming,** providing only the services that are overpriced, not the ones that are more costly and subsidized. Tradition and expressions of disapproval were able to limit the extent to which profits were drained from the system by cream skimming prior to 1970. Since then, however, the margins have become too large, and the ideology of health care too fragmented, to keep the old system afloat.

Founded initially on the premise that government and the wealthy would provide for the poor and support research, the social contract of hospitals was so pervasive and unexamined that it is likely that the people who initially brought it under attack had no idea what those efforts might lead to. However, it has subsequently become clear that hospital financial managers, by taking advantage of the system, and Medicare, by refusing to take responsibility for all of America's needy, contributed to the demise of cost shifting. Rapidly rising per diem costs and distortional cross subsidies eventually led to stringent managed care systems in which an insured employee group contracts to pay only for the services its members use. The public understands that it is not possible to "pay your own way" for hospital care and that risk pooling through insurance is required. The collapse of cost shifting forces us now to confront the question of who will pay for the poor and who will pay for medical research. Although there is a general recognition that caring for the poor and paying for research will cost something, the public seriously underestimates how large that bill will be because of the cost shifting that has gone on for so many years. Most of the income in the United States is earned by employed people between the ages of 30 and 60. This generally healthy group, whose wealth is increasing, makes up less than a third of the population. Paying for the other two-thirds, and for all the medical advances working people want, will require transfers of billions and billions of dollars. We are in the process of giving up on the old system of transferring funds, but have not been able to find and agree on a new one.[13]

8.5 CAPITAL FINANCING

Revenues for an organization must not only exceed current expenses, they must also be sufficiently above operating costs to compensate those who have invested capital. If a hospital borrows $10 million for construction, it must pay back the principal over time and pay interest on the loan each year. For a philanthropist making a donation, the returns on capital take the form of social services rather than interest or dividends. Having a nonprofit organization that is supposed to lose money each year, with the difference made up out of endowment or contributions, tends to blur the line between capital and operating funds. However, the conceptual requirement for a return on capital is clear. The philanthropist could always invest the money in financial assets and make a donation each year from the resulting interest if that is a more efficient way to achieve their charitable purpose than providing a lump-sum capital donation.

The start-up capital for most hospitals came from a combination of philanthropy and local government funds. Land and buildings were often donated. At the beginning of the twentieth century, there were also a number of doctors' hospitals, usually started in a portion of the doctor's house or in a converted dwelling nearby. The capital financing for these small, private hospitals came from the doctor's own savings or from family members. Hospitals grew because they were successful in attracting funds or because they were successful in attracting paying patients and could build up reserves (which would be called "retained earnings" at a for-profit organization). In World War II, millions of servicemen experienced the benefits of modern medical technology firsthand. The power of antibiotics and new surgical techniques to heal impressed many people, especially those from rural areas. This created a desire to spread hospitals across the land.[14] Yet only a few hospitals had been able to build up reserves during the Great Depression or World War II, and organizations that had conserved money wanted to expand their own operations, not help rural communities. The success of the New Deal and the victories of the military made it seem natural to mobilize government resources to meet this need. In 1946 the Hill-Burton Act was passed, making construction funds available to new hospitals in areas that had fewer than four beds per 1,000 people. As a form of repayment, hospitals receiving these funds were to give an equal or greater value in free care to indigent people. City and suburban hospitals were envious of the easy access rural areas had to capital and, because power tends to accrue to those who already have it (i.e., existing hospitals) and not necessarily to those who need it, subsequent changes were made to allow Hill-Burton funds to be used for expansion and renovation projects, as well as new construction.

Hill-Burton, retained earnings, and philanthropic fund drives provided most capital financing until the enactment of Medicare and Medicaid in 1965. Hospitals, which had chronically suffered operating losses, suddenly had steady revenue streams guaranteed by the government. They could meet the demand for new construction by borrowing against that promise, and they proceeded to do so. Borrowing increased from less than $100 million in 1960 to $200 million in 1970, $1,215 million in 1975, and $2.6 billion in 1977.[15] Three factors combined to make debt quickly become the dominant form of hospital capital:

- Guaranteed revenues from Medicare and Medicaid that assured investor repayment
- Tax exemption as municipal bonds made it cheap for nonprofit hospitals to borrow
- Cost reimbursement for interest expenses

Medicare and Medicaid totally changed the financial picture of hospitals, from social organizations that had to beg for money each year, to solidly funded services backed by the government. For a time, it was virtually impossible for most hospitals to go bankrupt and hence for investors not to get repaid. States and localities created "health care financing authorities" that allowed nonprofit hospitals to qualify as municipal borrowers so that investors did not have to pay federal, state, and local taxes on the interest they received. This reduced the cost of borrowing by a third, making it possible for a hospital to issue bonds at 5 percent and invest at 7 percent while waiting to use the money for construction. Such arbitrage generated millions of dollars for astute hospital financial managers before being outlawed. The shift to cost reimbursement also favored borrowing. A hospital that used its own reserves to construct a new building could get reimbursed for depreciation, but the hospital that issued debt to do the same thing got reimbursed for interest expenses as well as depreciation.

In this environment with tax-exempt debt, willing investors, and cost reimbursement, it is not surprising that hospitals went on a borrowing spree, loading up with more than $10 billion in debt by 1980. However, any business that takes on lots of debt is more likely to come under financial pressure. Despite being organized as nonprofit organizations, hospitals were no exception. With millions of dollars of interest payments to make each year, hospital managers had to become more and more bottom-line oriented. As the threat of bankruptcy became more real, the social welfare and community benefit orientation that had prevailed since the turn of the century increasingly gave way to a business orientation.

Hospital borrowing rose so rapidly that it had to lose steam eventually. Too many new beds were added, and debt loads became insupportable. Also, pressures on the Medicare budget led to tighter and tighter reimbursement. In 1985, the first bond defaults began to occur. Investors quickly revised their expectations and treated hospital debt as risky, and hence required a higher rate of interest. Municipalities were less and less pleased about the loss of property and income taxes, and calls were made to limit the use of tax-exempt revenue bonds such as those issued by hospital financing authorities. Access to capital became more difficult. Old and decrepit facilities could not tap the bond market and were acquired by for-profit hospital chains that could use the stock market to quickly raise equity, refurbish the physical plant, and make money. Many towns were willing to sell their hospitals for nothing, even provide special subsidies and tax breaks, rather than let them go bankrupt and disappear. The environment also had changed so that more hospitals felt it necessary to become part of a system covering all types of care over a broad geographic area. To do so, strong hospitals wanted to merge with or buy weaker ones and to buy nursing homes, home health agencies, physician practices, and medical office buildings. In most cases, it was not legal to use tax-exempt debt to do so, nor could the hospitals borrow the hundreds of millions of dollars necessary in the corporate (taxable) market.

The stand-alone community hospital was a good structure for creating a social contract.[18] Business leaders, citizens of the town, and the poor all participated in a visible symbol of community responsibility that was governed by a local board of directors. The move toward larger and more integrated health care systems has shown that this structure is inflexible and increasingly outmoded. People no longer identify primarily with a community or look to voluntary action to provide health care, and the solo hospital has no way to move capital from where the funds are (in wealthy suburbs) to where the needs are (in distressed urban and rural areas, in providing assistance to elderly people with disabilities). Creating a chain of hospitals is one way to regionalize and rationalize the allocation of capital. Recently there has been a spurt of acquisitions and conversions of hospitals to for-profit status, although it is still unclear how far this trend will go and to what extent the government, as the primary payer for hospital care, will let it go. What has become clear is that private equity markets have far outstripped private philanthropy as a source of capital for meeting the demands for new health care services and new health care facility construction in the twenty-first century.

THE ALLEGHENY BANKRUPTCY*

·This section researched and prepared by Patrick M. Bernet, Ph.D. candidate at Temple University.

Allegheny General Hospital was one of the largest hospitals in the Pittsburgh, Pennsylvania area.[16] It provided a broad range of services, had high occupancy and generated large cash flows. In 1987, it merged with the cash-poor Medical College of Pennsylvania in Philadelphia to form Allegheny Health and Education Research Foundation (AHERF). The merger seemed to benefit both organizations: Allegheny General Hospital had the medical school affiliation they needed to enhance their image and the Medical College of Pennsylvania had the cash it needed.

Medical schools represent significant fixed costs however. Shortly after the merger, AHERF began to look to purchase other hospitals in the Philadelphia market over which these fixed costs could be spread. From 1990 to 1996, AHERF went on a hospital-buying spree. They acquired a children's hospital, another Philadelphia medical college, and a number of community hospitals in the Philadelphia and Pittsburgh markets. All along the way, AHERF was leveraging the strong cash flows from its Allegheny General Hospital to buy up financially troubled hospitals.

During the 1990s, many hospitals, fearful of the advent of managed care, began purchasing physician practices to make sure that they would not lose admissions. AHERF was aggressive in doing so, trying to increase market share, and rapidly increasing the price paid for practices in the Philadelphia area. In the end, much money was spent, and few new admissions were gained. Hospitals simply started paying extra for what they had received previously without payment, the doctors' business.

AHERF also began competing aggressively for managed care business during the 1990s, including 'full risk' contracts under which the hospital agrees to take care of all HMO member healthcare needs for a percentage of that member's HMO policy premium. Competition with other hospital networks bid down the prices paid, and inexperience with full-risk management caused expenses to rise, resulting in substantial losses. Yet in the short run these contracts brought in additional cash (as HMO premiums were paid) that could be used for more acquisitions, and only in the long run, as services were paid for, did the losses appear on the balance sheet.

By 1996, AHERF was beginning to suffer on a number of fronts. Economies of scale from owning multiple facilities were not coming to fruition quickly enough since it takes time to consolidate operations. Bidding wars for physician practices resulted in lower returns. Bidding wars for HMO contracts resulted in lower reimbursement rates. To hide poor financial performance, AHERF executives transferred funds from one division to another to make each appear profitable at the time of the division's audit. Some transfers included restricted funds intended for use at one institution only, or for a specific purpose (cancer research, nursing education); such transfers are illegal. Lack of diligence by both AHERF's Board of Directors and auditors left these transfers hidden. Like Enron, this financial shell game eventually came unraveled. In 1997, AHERF became the largest not-for-profit bankruptcy in U.S. history, and its CEO was eventually sent to jail.

Hospital debt was subsequently viewed in the bond market as being much riskier, so all hospitals had to pay higher interest to compensate for the actions of this rogue entrepreneur.[17] Simple, yet powerful economic forces put AHERF in jeopardy. AHERF leadership, through deliberate acts of top executives and passive acceptance by the Board of Directors, compounded the failure.

8.6   ORGANIZATION: WHO CONTROLS THE HOSPITAL AND FOR WHAT ENDS?

The standard model firm in a microeconomics textbook is an organization created by the owners, who invest time and money, to make a profit. To do so, the firm must meet the needs of customers who pay for the firm's products and the needs of employees and other vendors who get paid by the firm to supply inputs. By the fundamental theorem of exchange, each party must benefit for the organization to continue to exist. The customers get consumers' surplus from purchasing products they prefer in terms of price or quality to those of other firms, the employees get jobs they prefer in terms of wages or conditions, and the owners take home as profits the value added by organizing a firm. The owners are known as "residual claimants" because they get what is left over, profits (or losses), a net residual difference between revenues and expenses. A firm operates as a rational economic organization because the owners who make the decisions must bear the consequences, whether good (profits) or bad (losses). The linkages among owners, employees, and customers usually have some slack in the real world, which gets assumed away in textbook models of perfect competition. Corporate "agency theory" deals with the implications of raising capital through the stock market, which separates ownership (stockholders) from control (managers).[19] To the extent that managers are not perfect agents of the owners, they may dissipate or capture some of the firm's profits by purchasing inputs from favored relatives, having big offices, not taking enough risks, or not working hard enough. Such deviations from profit maximization may change the firm's behavior, as can taxes, regulations, social conditions, ideology, culture, and political constraints.

Hospitals differ from the standard firm in three significant ways:

- Patients do not pay because of insurance or charity.
- Ownership is usually unclear because of nonprofit voluntary or governmental organization.
- Medical care is largely controlled by doctors, who neither pay nor receive any money from the hospital and, therefore, have no direct connection from a flow-of-funds perspective.

Doctors are neither customers nor employees nor owners, but in practice they are the dominant voice in hospital operations; therefore, they sometimes look like they are all three. This structure, combining power, money, and service with no direct line of control or financial accountability, is a unique form of economic organization that makes it difficult to model or predict the behavior of hospitals. A hospital does not do anything without directions from a physician; only physicians are allowed to admit patients, perform surgery, or prescribe drugs. The hospital organizes a medical staff, but some claim that the reality is the other way around, that the medical staff organizes a hospital as its workshop. This is the basis of Mark Pauly's model of the hospital as the doctor's workshop, which hypothesizes that the hospital will behave to maximize the profits of the doctors who are on staff, rather than to maximize the profits of the organization (see Chapter 6).[20] Joseph Newhouse has pointed out that hospitals are nonprofit organizations with no owners who can claim the profits, and suggests that hospitals and other nonprofit organizations are run for the benefit of managers.[21] Managers want their hospitals to be the biggest and the best, which, not incidentally, justifies the highest managerial salaries and hence maximizes some combination of quantity and quality of services rather than profits or doctors' incomes. Employees are also important stakeholders, but because their importance derives from being input suppliers, their influence in hospitals is not much different from their influence in other organizations. Most hospital mission statements claim that their primary concern is patient care, yet this sort of general assertion does not address how prices are set, the trade-off between one group of patients and another (e.g., surgery or immunization, abortion or family planning clinics), or the trade-offs between employees and doctors. The American Hospital Association maintains that hospitals are, in essence, public institutions whose purpose is to benefit the community. From a flow-of-funds perspective, this makes sense, because most of the capital investment in a voluntary hospital comes from the community in the form of charitable donations and taxes. The problem is, how is community benefit defined and who, exactly, exercises control?[22] The board, although in theory representing the community, is often deferential to the medical staff and depends on the information provided by the administration to make decisions (see Table 8.3).

Despite a considerable amount of theoretical and empirical work by economists, and a clear recognition that insurance, nonprofit status, and medical control over admissions and treatment make hospitals different, no satisfactory theory of the hospital as a distinct type of organization has been developed. In part, this may result from the fact that competition and the pressure to survive forces a hospital to maximize revenues and minimize costs much like a for-profit firm. The greater the amount of debt, the more pressure a hospital faces, and any deviation from profit-maximizing behavior becomes a threat to survival. Most of the research to date shows little difference between for-profit and not-for-profit hospitals.[23] This might be a result of competitive pressures forcing nonprofits to behave in a profit-maximizing manner, but it might also be a result of social expectations that force for-profit hospitals to meet the standards of community benefit and medical professionalism to attract patients. Most of the differences observed are differences that economic theory leads one to expect. For-profit hospitals are more aggressive in pricing services to maximize revenues and respond more quickly to changes in reimbursement rules that could affect profits. They are sometimes less likely to provide charity care to indigent people, to build in geographic areas of highest need, or to promote immunization, prenatal care, and other uncompensated services. The large hospitals that do most of the teaching and research are almost always nonprofit institutions. Although all general acute hospitals seem to behave in similar ways, it is possible to discern a continuum with for-profits at one end being more aggressive and quick to respond to incentives and with government hospitals at the other end being a bit more inflexible and committed to public service. However, the range of behavior resulting from differences in ownership category does not appear to be very wide and is probably narrowing over time as all hospitals confront rising patient expectations for service and technology, managed care, and reductions in funding due to cost pressures and the federal deficit.

TABLE 8.3

Who Gets the Profits from a Nonprofit Hospital?

Doctors?

Administrators?

Employees?

Patients?

Community?

SUGGESTIONS FOR FURTHER READING

Modern Healthcare and *Hospitals and Health Networks* are biweekly magazines covering the hospital industry in depth.

American Hospital Association, *Hospital Statistics and Hospital Guide* is published annually.

Rosemary Stevens, *In Sickness and In Wealth: American Hospitals in the Twentieth Century* (New York: Basic Books, 1989).

Burton Weisbrod, *The Nonprofit Economy* (Cambridge Mass.: Harvard University Press, 1988), and "Rewarding Performance that is Hard to Measure: The Private Non-Profit Sector," *Science* (May 5, 1989): 541–546.

SUMMARY

1. The Pennsylvania Hospital, founded in 1751, was the first hospital in the United States. Like most **early hospitals,** it was **funded primarily by charitable donations and government** tax appropriations and **housed the sick and poor** people with disabilities, although some paying patients were admitted.

2. The development of **new technology** created the need for a central facility where the **capital cost** of equipment could be shared by many doctors and where dangerous surgical procedures could be performed in a more controlled and supportive environment.

3. More than **95 percent of all hospital revenues come from third parties,** with more than half coming from **government** through the Medicare and Medicaid programs. Patients pay so little of the hospital bill that **charges are virtually irrelevant in decision making.** Although cost-based reimbursement using the ratio-of-cost-to-charges-applied-to-charges RCCAC formula developed by Blue Cross plans under the aegis of the American Hospital Association was the major form of payment from 1965 to 1985, since then the prospective DRG per case payments and a variety of managed care plans have become the main sources of revenues. Approximately one-third of hospital revenues come from outpatient services, and an increasing amount comes from home health, long-term care, and other related services.

4. Hospitals obtain revenues in a variety of ways, including **philanthropy** and grants, **global budgets,** billed **charges, per day** (per diem) payments, DRG per case payments, cost reimbursement, and managed care contracts.

5. **Labor** is the largest category of health care expenditure. When employees of local service firms are included, personnel accounts for more than 75 percent of a hospital's costs. Therefore, the only way to cut costs is to reduce wages or reduce employment, neither of which is politically popular. **Doctors are usually independent contractors** paid separately by the patient or by the patient's insurance and thus do not show up as a large item on hospital budgets, even though they play a dominant role in providing and directing care.

6. **Cost shifting** is the process of charging one group (i.e., commercially insured patients) more to cover the loss due to undercharging another group (indigent patients, Medicaid). The pervasiveness of cost shifting and insurance coverage gave financial managers far more room to raise revenues as a means of supporting the hospital and little incentive to find efficiencies that would reduce costs. **Cream skimming**

is the action of taking on only the profitable patients for whom services are priced considerably above unit costs, while avoiding the loss-making patients with heavy care needs. Changes in Medicare reimbursement and the advent of managed care firms that shop to obtain hospital services at the lowest possible price have eroded the ability of hospitals to cross subsidize and have made it difficult to support research, teaching, and charity care.

7.   Although accounting for just 8 percent of operating costs, **access to capital** has been crucial in shaping the growth of hospitals. Philanthropy was first replaced by government construction grants through the **Hill-Burton** Act of 1946, and subsequently by **tax-exempt municipal revenue bonds** in the 1970s. **Equity** financing through the stock market is becoming increasingly important as hospitals try to acquire nursing homes, physician practices, and other hospitals to form integrated health care systems.

8.   Hospitals differ from most firms in that they are largely paid for by third parties, most commonly **nonprofit organizations** directed by volunteer boards rather than owners and **dominated by doctors, independent professionals** who work for themselves with no direct financial ties to the hospital. Despite much research and lots of theoretical expectations, there appear to be only slight differences among voluntary not-for-profit, government, and private for-profit hospitals. In general, for-profits appear to be somewhat less likely to take on charity care, research, teaching, and outreach and to react more quickly to changes in reimbursement regulations, with government hospitals at the other extreme and voluntary hospitals falling in the middle, but any differences are small and occur only occasionally.

PROBLEMS

1.   {*industrial organization*} Which technological, organizational, and financial innovations caused the rise of hospitals in the twentieth century?

2.   {*incidence*} Who pays for most of the care in hospitals? Are the people who pay the bills the same as the people who receive the care?

3.   {*flow of funds*} Which input accounts for the largest portion of hospital costs? Which input is responsible for most of the growth in hospital cost per patient day?

4.   {*payment methodology*} Both Hospital A and Hospital B are paid by Medicare using the DRG methodology. Assume that the reimbursement for the average Medicare patient (case weight of 1.0) is $2,600. Hospital A has an average case-mix index of 1.32 and admits 24 patients who stay in the hospital a total of 192 days, whereas Hospital B has an average case-mix index of 0.95 and admits 35 patients who stay in the hospital a total of 238 days. Which hospital gets paid more? Which hospital gets paid more per case? Which hospital gets paid more per diem? Which hospital gets paid more for an appendectomy (case weight of 0.85)?

5.   {*flow of funds*} Over the past one hundred years, the major source of hospital revenues has changed three times. Name these types of payments, and explain why each one gave way to the next.

6.   {*payment*} If a hospital decides to raise prices because it needs more money, what effect does this have on the following:

   a.   Patients who pay their own bills
   b.   Patients whose bills are paid by an insurance company

    c.   Insurance contracts reimbursed on the basis of costs

    d.   Previously negotiated per diem contracts with HMOs

7.   {*cost shifting*} Is the mark-up (ratio of prices to direct per-unit costs) relatively constant across different types of hospitals? Are mark-ups the same for different services or departments within a hospital?

8.   {*cost shifting*} How do hospitals pay for medical research?

9.   {*ownership*} Are doctors usually employees, owners, or managers of hospitals?

10.   {*ownership*} Who owns most hospitals? Who gets the profit when a nonprofit hospital makes money? Can nonprofit hospitals be bought and sold?

11.   {*capital financing*} Are the ways in which hospitals obtain capital different from the ways in which doctors obtain capital? Why?

12.   {*rate of return, incidence*} How does a philanthropist who donates funds to a hospital get "returns on capital"? Are these returns measured as a dollar amount, as an annualized percentage rate, or by some other method?

13.   {*ownership, nonprofit, capital financing*} Hospitals received special treatment from the government and were able to borrow subsidized capital using tax-exempt municipal revenue bonds. During the 1970s and 1980s, billions of dollars of tax-free capital flowed into nonprofit hospitals. Did this make them more or less like for-profit firms?

14.   {*financial reporting*} Which is more important in determining the type of financial reports a hospital must prepare, the type of ownership or the major sources of funding? If capital is attracted from different sources, are different types of financial reports required?

15.   {*cost shifting*} What does it mean for Medicare to act as a "prudent buyer" of hospital services? Does doing so strengthen or weaken Medicare as a social insurance program?

16.   {*cost shifting*} What adjustments would a hospital have to make if it began to serve a larger number of indigent patients? Would most of the adjustments come on the revenue side or the expenditure side?

17.   {*cost shifting*} Who benefits from cost shifting, the poor or the rich? Do any health care workers benefit from cost shifting?

ENDNOTES

1.   Paul Starr, *The Social Transformation of American Medicine* (New York: Basic Books, 1992). Rosemary Stevens, *In Sickness and in Wealth: American Hospitals in the Twentieth Century* (New York: Basic Books, 1989).

2.   George Rosen, *A History of Public Health, New York* (New York: MD Publications, 1958)

3.   Florence Nightingale, *Notes on Nursing: What It Is, and What It Is Not* (New York: D. Appleton-Century, 1938).

4.   Charles Lawrence, *History of the Philadelphia Almshouses and Hospitals from the Beginning of the Eighteenth to the Ending of the Nineteenth Centuries* (Philadelphia: C. Lawrence, 1905).

5.   Marshall K. Raffel and Norma K. Raffel, *The U.S. Health System: Origins and Functions*, 4th ed. (Albany, N.Y.: Delmar Publisher, 1994).

6.   An illustrative case study is found in the history of the Mayo clinic. See Helen Clapesattle, *The Doctors Mayo* (Minneapolis: University of Minnesota Press, 1941); Gunther W. Nagel, *The Mayo Legacy* (Springfield, Ill.: Charles C. Thomas, 1966); and compare with an annual report of the Mayo Clinic (now operating in Arizona and Florida as well as Minnesota) in the 1990s.

7.   J. Hermann, "Blue Cross of California goes for the Gold-Wellpoint Health Networks," *Health Systems Review* 26, no.3 (May/June 1993): 14–19; T. Kertesz, "California Blue Cross Tries Again With Bigger Foundation Plan," *Modern Healthcare* 25, no. 16 (April 17, 1995): 2–3.

8. American Hospital Association, Hospital Statistics (Chicago: American Hospital Association, 2002).

9. Prices paid for service by patients are even less important than Table 8.1 would suggest, since much of the 3 percent is actually deductibles, co-payments and other charges that are in effect insurance premiums or taxes and not directly related to the prices of the services chosen.

10. Some legislators argue that hospitals are no longer providing the charitable public services for which they were founded, and hence do not deserve help, and that public funds should be redirected toward community programs or inner-city hospitals. The City of Philadelphia, for example, has forced local hospitals to pay millions of dollars under its PILOTs/SILOTs program (Payments/Services In Lieu of Taxes). A hospital is assessed an amount equal to its tax liability, and then must document provision of services provided without compensation of an equal amount, or pay the city the difference.

11. State Medicaid plans used the DRG system but generally paid fewer dollars for each patient. In time, this underpayment led to complaints, and a series of lawsuits. Temple University Hospital sued the state of Pennsylvania under the "Boren Amendment" to the Social Security Act, which obligated states to make payments sufficient to cover the cost of efficiently provided services. The hospital eventually won—creating a precedent which hospitals around the country quickly followed (and that forced state budgets into deficits). Hence although in concept a charge system gives all the power to the seller, and an administered price system (like DRGs) gives all the power to the buyer, in reality both sides are at least to some extent constrained by the political process and public opinion.

12. American Hospital Association, Hospital Statistics, various years.

13. Henry J. Aaron and Robert D. Reischauer, "The Medicare Reform Debate: What is the Next Step?" *Health Affairs* 14, no. 4 (Winter 1995): 8–30.

14. Odin W. Anderson, *Health Services as a Growth Enterprise in the United States Since 1875*(Ann Arbor, Mich.: Health Administration Press, 1990).

15. Jonathan Betz Brown, *Health Capital Financing* (Ann Arbor, Mich.: Health Administration Press, 1988), 14–18.

16. Cain Brothers, *Strategies in Capital Finance* 27 (Summer 1999): 1–26; Lawton Burns and John Cacciamani, John, "The Fall of the House of AHERF: The Allegheny bankruptcy," *Health Affairs* 19, no. 1 (January/February 2000): 7–42.

17. Jaklevic, Mary Chris, "Pricier, Less Plentiful," *Modern Healthcare* 30, no. 21 (May 22, 2000): 52–56.

18. Robert Sigmond, "From Charity Care to Community Benefit," *Hospitals & Health Services Administration* (Summer 1994).

19. Michael C. Jensen and William H. Meckling, "Theory of the Firm: Managerial Behavior, Agency Costs and Ownership Structure," *Journal of Financial Economics* 3 (1976): 305–360.

20. Mark V. Pauly, *Doctors and Their Workshops: Economic Models of Physician Behavior* (Chicago: University of Chicago Press, 1980).

21. Joseph Newhouse, "How Do Hospitals Make Choices?" in *The Economics of Medical Care* (Reading, Mass.: Addison-Wesley, 1978), 68–73.

22. Robert Sigmond and J. David Seay, "Community Benefit Standards for Hospitals: Perceptions and Performance," in "The Future of Tax-Exempt Status for Hospitals" issue of *Frontiers of Health Services Management* (Spring 1989).

23. E. R. Becker and Frank Sloan, "Hospital Ownership and Performance," *Economic Inquiry* 23, no. 1 (1985): 21–36; Deborah Freund et al., "Analysis of Length-Of-Stay Differences Between Investor-Owned and Voluntary Hospitals," *Inquiry* 22, no. 1 (1985): 33–44; Mark Schlesinger, Theodore Marmor, and R. Smithey, "Non-Profit and For-Profit Medical Care," *Journal of Health Politics, Policy and Law* 12, no. 3 (1987): 427–457.

CHAPTER 9

MANAGEMENT AND REGULATION OF HOSPITAL COSTS

QUESTIONS

1. Why do some hospitals cost more than others?

2. If hospitals are not-for-profit, what do they compete for?

3. The number of patients and the number of days each patient spends in the hospital has gone down. Why have hospital costs continued to increase faster than other health care costs?

4. Are large hospitals expensive because they suffer from diseconomies of scale, or because they admit the most difficult-to-treat patients?

5. Why would a hospital want to buy a new magnetic resonance imaging (MRI) scanner if it expects the MRI to be busy only half the time and the hospital next door already has such a machine?

6. Will computers and other new technology improve efficiency and hence reduce costs, or will they improve quality and hence raise costs?

7. Has regulation cut costs, or cut competition?

9.1 WHY DO SOME HOSPITALS COST MORE THAN OTHERS?

The cost of a day in the hospital can be as little as $300 or more than $1,500. Which factors could account for such a wide variation? It is not surprising if a day in the hospital costs $1,500 for a critically wounded trauma patient in an intensive care unit (ICU) and just $300 for a patient resting after breaking a leg while skiing.[1] The ICU patient is much sicker and requires more complex services. It is also understandable that staying in one of the nation's top research and teaching hospitals under the care of famous doctors can cost more than staying in a small rural facility with limited equipment and staff.[2] The hospital bill can be a misleading guide to costs. One hospital may charge more, but give every patient a discount, while another sticks to list prices. Or, one hospital could charge $400 for the bed, with extra charges for medication, laboratory tests, physical therapy, and so on, while another hospital charges $500 for the bed and all other services, making it less expensive (see Table 9.1).

It is often assumed that a hospital with a lower cost per patient day is more efficient, but such a conclusion is only justified if the comparison hospital provides the same services to similar patients under similar conditions. Unless this *ceteris paribus* (all other things constant) assumption is valid, which it rarely is, efforts must be made to adjust for all the other factors listed in Table 9.1 to compare costs. Of course, patients and their insurance companies prefer a cheaper stay in the hospital to a more expensive stay if all other factors are constant. But when they are not, the more relevant question is: Is a hospital that costs 10 percent more (or 20 percent, or 400 percent) really worth that much more? While this relative value question is more meaningful, it is also much more difficult to answer and the answer depends on the patient's values as well as calculations of technical efficiency. Therefore, it is useful to look first at the simpler and more standard question of variations in costs for the same unit of service.

9.2   HOW MANAGEMENT CONTROLS COSTS

Short-Run Versus Long-Run Cost Functions

What can management do to change the costs of production? If a hospital receives fewer admissions than expected this morning and wants to reduce its costs by the afternoon, not much can be done. People have already shown up for work, meals have been prepared, ambulances and wheelchair transports have been arranged, and so on; therefore, *in the short run almost all costs are fixed*. Any reduction in the number of patients will, therefore, cause the average cost per patient to be higher than usual. If the reduction in admissions continues and management is given enough time to respond, the hospital may shut down a wing, refrain from hiring, and perhaps lay off some employees. This is but one case demonstrating a general rule: as more time is allowed for adjustment, more changes can be made, and as more changes are made, costs per unit become lower.

In the very long run, almost all costs become variable. The director can train new management, hire clinical staff, rewrite treatment protocols, replace the existing building with a new one, pave some grounds for parking, and even move the facility to a more accessible site near a freeway. This ability to plan and choose the optimal scale and combination of inputs allows management to minimize the costs of production for any desired level of output. If management expects to average only 100 patients per day, they would build a smaller hospital, hire fewer people, and incur lower fixed costs. If management expects 175 patients a day, they would build a medium-sized hospital. If 300 patients a day are expected, management would build a large hospital with a dedicated computer system, pneumatic transport tubes to speed laboratory samples between floors, and other equipment (Figure 9.1).

TABLE 9.1   Reasons for Differences in Hospitals Costs
Severity of patient's illness
Quality of care
Intensity of services (e.g., number of nursing hours or lab tests)
Cost shifting to pay for research and teaching
Differences in billing
Prices of labor and other inputs
Efficiency

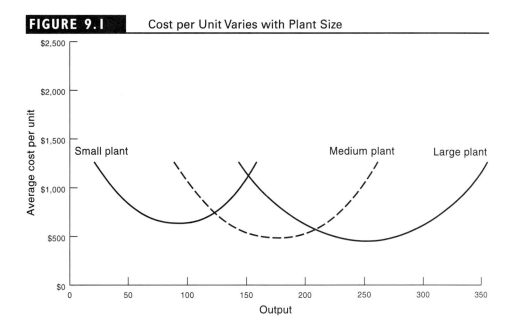

FIGURE 9.1 Cost per Unit Varies with Plant Size

For any expected level of output, management would choose a building size and number of permanent employees that would minimize costs. In geometric terms, the long-run average cost curve (LRAC) is an "envelope" that traces a minimum, just touching all the possible short-run average cost curves (SRAC), as shown in Figure 9.2. No SRAC can fall below the LRAC because if a short-run cost function with lower costs exists, management would choose that production configuration instead and incorporate it into the long-run function. Whether a particular cost is fixed or variable is determined by the time frame for decision making. Decisions regarding temporary agency nurses can be made on a day-to-day basis and thus are fixed for only twenty-four hours or so. Permanent employees take a while to train, or to terminate when no longer needed, and thus are fixed for at least several months. Reducing the number of vice presidents is so traumatic that it may take several years. Construction is a fixed cost once completed, but it is a variable cost during the planning stage.

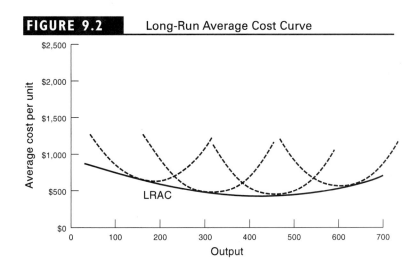

FIGURE 9.2 Long-Run Average Cost Curve

Uncertainty and Budgeting

A manager must deal with two kinds of variation in the level of output: foreseeable and unknown. Expansion to accommodate a growing population in the suburbs, eliminating maternity beds in response to declining fertility, and opening a cardiac rehabilitation unit to serve an aging community are all examples of foreseeable long-run changes. The lower number of hospital admissions on Saturday and Sunday, on Christmas and New Year's day, and during August are examples of foreseeable short-run changes. Adjustment to foreseeable changes can be planned in advance. For example, hiring and training can be accomplished efficiently over a reasonable period of time, and space and building modifications can be accomplished on a schedule, so that the path and pace of adjustment reflect conscious decisions by management to minimize costs. Random variations, on the other hand, must be accommodated in the operations of the organization, but are not known in advance. For example, there may be sixteen admissions on Monday, twelve on Tuesday, twenty-two on Wednesday, thirteen on Thursday, eighteen on Friday, and fifteen on Saturday, and there may be twice as much work for the admitting office to do on Wednesday as on Tuesday, with the same amount of staff and equipment. Staff members are likely to do only what is necessary on a particular day, and perhaps even work late, while putting off until the next day some routine tasks, such as filing charts, checking documentation, and entering data into forms. Long-run unknown changes in output might occur because a new factory is built nearby, resulting in many new families moving to the area; an epidemic such as AIDS increases the demand for care; or a competing hospital is built, reducing demand. Such major changes often force a hospital to change its long-run strategy (see Figure 9.3).

How do managers control costs? Primarily through the use of a budget, a plan stated in dollars.[3] A budget that does not change with volume is called a **fixed budget** (also known as a standard budget), and a budget that changes with volume is called a **flexible budget.** Typically, a hospital or medical group practice creates an **operating budget** that projects all anticipated expenses for the next year. For example, if labor expenses rose 7 percent in 2001 and 9 percent in 2002, management may project an increase of 8 percent in labor costs for 2003. Managers usually define short-run changes as those that occur during the current budget period. Long-run changes and plans are incorporated in a **strategic budget** (also known as a **long-run capital budget**) that focuses on trends in the number of patients and capital renovations and expansions (new buildings and equipment, adding partners). These budgets often are accompanied by *pro forma* **financial statements,** projections of incomes, assets and fund balances for a period of three, five, or even twenty years in summary format. Only infrequently are detailed budgets prepared for more than one year in advance. Most managers define *long-run* changes as those that occur more than one year in the

FIGURE 9.3   How Organizations Deal with Change

	Planned (known)	Random (uncertain)
Short Run	Scheduling Weekly budget Part-timers	Overtime, temps Inventory Maintain excess capacity
Long Run	Capital budgeting Change plant size Facility conversion	Hold financial reserves Encroachment by or on competitors Bankruptcy

future, but some managers designate changes that occur during the next two to five years as *intermediate-run* changes. In any analysis, the terms are relative, making any definition somewhat arbitrary. The important points to gain from economic theory are that short-run adjustment is always more costly than long-run adjustment, and that as the time perspective changes, so does the focus of management attention on cost control.

Known short-run variations are dealt with by making limited changes in the number of staff scheduled. For example, fewer nurses work at 3:00 a.m and on Sundays. However, the percentage change in staff is less than the percentage change in patient load, because all units must still have a head nurse, technical support, and so on, even though they are only partially full. Changes in plant capacity are prohibitively expensive in the short run. Although fifty beds may be empty in the hospital on Sunday night, not all of them would be in unit 7-East. To close that unit down, many patients would have to be transferred out of that unit on Sunday and transferred back in on Monday when patient occupancy increased again. The savings from not having a head nurse on 7-East on Sunday would be more than offset by all the transfers; thus, it would actually cost more to shut down one unit for the sake of "efficiency." Therefore, most units are underutilized on weekends and most staff members usually have an easy day.

A *known long-run change*, such as a declining trend in admissions due to the closure of a local manufacturing plant, calls for a permanent reduction in capacity. Unit 7-East can be converted into storage or nursing home beds, or leased to a group of physical therapists. Furthermore, staffing should be reduced proportionately to the long-run decline in patients, so that every employee carries a regular workload, rather than making partial staff adjustments on nights and weekends.

Random short-run fluctuations are dealt with primarily by building in some excess reserve capacity, making the staff work faster or slower, and allocating less immediate tasks to the slower days. Suppose that admissions are as suggested earlier: Monday sixteen, Tuesday twelve, Wednesday twenty-two, Thursday thirteen, Friday eighteen, and Saturday fifteen. The manager does not care about the cost of care on Monday or Tuesday, but wants to minimize the cost for the week as a whole. There is no reason to reprimand a manager for having too many nurses on duty Thursday, because there was no way to tell whether admissions would be light until the shift started. Also, while management might be able to get staff members to work extra hard and put in overtime on Wednesday to accommodate the influx of patients, they will not stay if they are abused with continual overloads. They will quit and go to work at another hospital, raising labor costs at the first hospital, because the manager would have to use temporary employees and retrain new staff members frequently. If the hospital has a range of ten to twenty-five admissions per day, with an average of sixteen, it can staff for sixteen admissions plus a bit of reserve. However, if another hospital had less random variation and always had fourteen to eighteen admissions per day, it could match staffing more exactly to the number of patients, would need less reserve capacity, and have a lower average cost per unit for the same average number of patients. This is but one example of the general principle that dealing with uncertainty is costly, and the greater the range of uncertainty, the greater the cost.

Unforeseen long-run changes in output really provide the test of the organization's ability to control costs. Here, tactical attention to detail is not enough—the hospital must make a strategic gamble based on a specific expectation of the future (e.g., population will grow older and increase demand, or people will move to Florida, reducing demand; a major competitor will go bankrupt, giving the hospital a great opportunity, or perhaps the competitor will go all out trying to survive by stealing the hospital's patients). The hospital could build in flexibility by making investments to cover both alternatives, but would then incur higher costs per unit, whichever happens.

9.3 CONFLICT BETWEEN ECONOMIC THEORY AND ACCOUNTING MEASURES OF PER UNIT COST

Timing

In Table 9.2, the cost per patient admitted is examined from two perspectives: direct accounting costs and a full economic cost that includes the hidden cost of dealing with disruptions (staff burnout, mistakes, overtime). In this example, the budgeted fixed costs are $5,000 per day and the variable costs are $300 per admission. The direct cost on Monday, when the expected number of patients (16) is admitted, is $5,000 + (16 × $300) = $9,800; therefore, the cost per admission is $9,800 ÷ 16 = $613. On Wednesday, if more patients (22) were admitted than the staff expected, calculated average cost per patient is $11,600 ÷ 22 = $527. It appears that the hospital benefited from its mistake in planning for too small a number of patients. Why not increase the advantage by planning for only 15 admissions instead of 16? Everyone would work even harder and faster, and if that is not good enough, the hospital could just plan for 12 or 10 or 6 admissions and keep pushing the staff to become more and more efficient. Taking the example to an extreme highlights the flaw in the reasoning. The accounting measure does not accurately capture all costs. Let's consider what really happens. To work so hard on Wednesday, the staff must put off some of their routine tasks until Thursday, and they also expect extra consideration from management on Friday when they ask to go home early. Once these costs of catching up afterward are factored in, the surge of patients on Wednesday is seen to have been very costly, not cheap. If everything went according to plan, 16 admissions each day would cost $9,800, for an average cost per admission of $613. Yet extra admissions mean disrupting the plan. To accommodate the costs of making sudden adjustments, an "adjustment cost" must be added into the amount of $100 × (actual-expected admissions)^2, so, for deviating from the plan by one admission, the cost of adjustment is $100; for two, $400; for three, $900; and so on.[4] The actual economic costs (with adjustments) are $15,200 for 22 admissions, an average of $681 per admission rather than $613. Of course, it would be cheaper if a hospital could get patients to come in at evenly spaced intervals, exactly sixteen each day, all between the hours of 9:00 A.M. and 4:00 P.M. so that workload can be exactly matched to staff and equipment. Yet illness does not go according to plan and the flow of admissions is never smooth. Health care managers have learned that such disruptions are costly, that every deviation from the planned level of operation raises costs.

TABLE 9.2	Accounting vs. Economics Costs Per Unit with Short-Run Fluctuations						
	Monday	**Tues**	**Wed**	**Thur**	**Fri**	**Sat**	**Average**
Admissions	16	12	22	13	18	15	16
Direct cost	$9,800	$8,600	$11,600	$8,900	$10,400	$9,500	$9,800
Accounting "cost" per admission	$613	$717	$527	$685	$578	$633	$613
Adjustment cost	$0	$1,600	$3,600	$900	$400	$100	
Total cost	$9,800	$10,200	$15,200	$9,800	$10,400	$9,600	$10,900
Economic "cost" per admission (AC curve)	$613	$850	$691	$754	$600	$640	$681

Note: Accounting per costs per admission are lower for days with many admissions, even though economic costs are higher. In this hypothetical example, a hospital has planned for 16 admissions each day, and has fixed costs of $5,000 plus $300 per admission. Deviations from the plan disrupt operations, reducing efficiency by a cost of $100 × (deviation squared), (i.e., being 1 admission above or below the planned amount reduces efficiency by $100, 2 admissions off by $400, 3 by $900, and so on).

In accountants' terms, the per-unit cost in row three of Table 9.2 is calculated on a cash basis (when spent), rather than allocating costs to different days on an accrual basis (when actually earned or obligated). In practice, accrual and all other adjustments made to the cost accounting system are inevitably incomplete and imperfect. The advantage of using economic theory is that the contradiction of the general principle—short-run costs must logically always exceed long-run costs—let us know immediately that something was wrong with the analysis and, therefore, that these cost-accounting figures, no matter how precise they may have seemed, did not reflect reality. It also explains why the budgeted $613 per admission was less than the actual expenses of $681: random fluctuations forced the payment of overtime, hiring of temps, rush ordering of exhausted supplies, and all other daily crises that managers are hired to work out.

Careful examination of Table 9.2 shows that cost per admission was not minimized on Monday, when the expected number of patients were admitted, but that the cost per admission was actually lower on Friday, when more than the expected number of patients came in, even after including adjustment costs (see Figure 9.4). Why is it not more efficient to increase output or downsize the facility so that the lowest cost per unit comes at the expected level of output? The reason is that the manager must minimize not the cost on the day when output hits the expected level, but the average cost per unit over all the days, with their randomly varying levels of output. If the average number of admissions had been eighteen instead of sixteen, twenty-four admissions might have occurred on the heavy Wednesday, exceeding capacity limits so greatly that an additional $2,800 in costs would have been incurred. Having extra reserve capacity is expensive, but not so expensive as not having it when you need it. In general, managers need to be able to accommodate the usual fluctuations in volume without major disruptions—to have flexibility that minimizes cost over a range. It is possible to have a highly routine production process that is very efficient at a set level of output, but would become very inefficient if it had to be speeded up or slowed down. Such fixed-output mass production may work well for manufacturing cars or light bulbs, but is not well adapted to services such as medical care, where constant adjustments and varying demand are the norm. Managers are willing to pay a bit extra in fixed costs to increase flexibility (see Figure 9.5). Building a facility that is very efficient when exactly the expected number of patients shows up, but that cannot easily accommodate changes in the level of demand (represented by the dark line), is less efficient in the long run than a more flexible facility (represented by the dotted line) that has slightly higher costs at the expected level of output, but is able to maintain average costs per unit at a low level over a wider range.

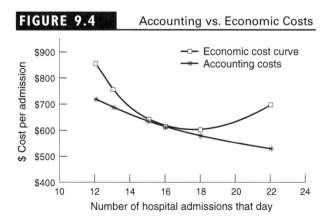

FIGURE 9.4   Accounting vs. Economic Costs

FIGURE 9.5 A specialized plant has lower cost within a narrow range, but the flexible plant has wider range.

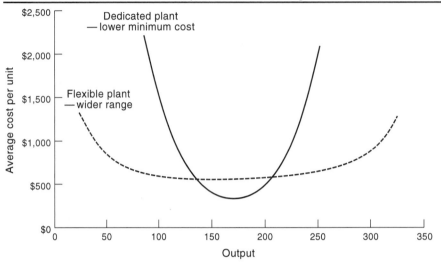

Whose Costs?

The displacement of costs in time is only one accounting mistake that can be made. Attempts to increase efficiency lead to many management practices that are clearly wrong yet persist for years because of an inability to count all costs. For example, many public clinics provide services free to indigent patients. They try hard to produce these services at the lowest cost to maximize the number of clients they can serve (and to keep taxes down). One way public clinics produce services at lower costs is to bring patients in early and keep them waiting so that the doctor's flow of work is never delayed because a patient is late or an appointment is broken. Such "block booking" or "clinic appointments" maximizes the number of patients that can be seen by the physician, but it makes patients unhappy because they have to spend many hours waiting. If the cost of the patient's time is included, it becomes apparent that block booking is not efficient; it only seems so because the clinic budget counts only direct costs.

How can economists tell that block booking is inefficient? Because if block booking were truly efficient, some paying patients would choose to patronize doctors who block booked, putting up with extra long waits to save a little money (i.e., choosing to pay $30 for a block-booked visit rather than $35 for care by appointment). The fact that doctors cannot attract patients by block booking demonstrates that the extra patient waiting time is more valuable than the small $5 savings in the doctor's time. Indigent patients either must put up with inefficiency because they cannot obtain the convenience of an appointment by paying just the marginal $5 cost differential or must forego free care entirely and pay the whole $35 private market price to obtain care by appointment. One might argue that the indigent patient has a lower cost of time and thus is more willing to put up with longer waits than most paying patients; however, the fact that even physicians in low-income neighborhoods have to provide appointments suggests that it is the large gap between marginal amenity cost ($5) and average per visit cost ($35), not lower value per hour of patient time, that allows free clinics to continue block booking.

Time, pain, and other nonmarket costs borne by patients do not show up on the hospital bill. Yet it is precisely these issues—suffering, fear of death, a need for caring and respect—that distinguish the economics of medical care. This is one reason this textbook began with a broader perspective on optimization using the techniques of cost-benefit analysis (Chapter 3) rather than a narrow look at minimizing cash outlays. Some of the common mistakes made in accounting for the true costs of medical care are as follows:

- Provider costs misallocated (displaced in time, overhead, or wrong department)
- Patient costs not counted (wait time, transportation, family care)
- Emotional costs not counted (pride, fear, pain, lack of respect)

9.4 ECONOMIES OF SCALE

Hospitals exist to allow a large number of doctors to share expensive capital equipment and cooperate in the care of many patients. Since many of these costs are fixed, hospitals should show economies of scale (i.e., average cost per patient day falling as more patients are treated).[5] It appears that basic hospital services for routine care are most efficiently delivered when organized and staffed in units of twenty to forty beds, usually known as a floor or wing. The need to accommodate random fluctuations in the number of admissions and to preserve a buffer of empty beds for emergencies creates economies of scale. Admissions to a forty-bed hospital might fluctuate by ±10; therefore, only thirty beds could be occupied on average. In a 400-bed hospital, excess admissions to one unit are likely to offset a lack of admissions in another; therefore, the overall fluctuation might be ±25, which is larger in absolute numbers but much smaller as a percentage. Thus, percentage occupancy rates can be higher, and per unit costs lower, in a large facility that is more able to smooth out patient flow. The greater division of labor in a large hospital that allows staff to become more specialized and efficient at a particular function also creates economies of scale.

There is good evidence that economies of scale are important in hospital services. Hospitals with fewer than one hundred beds are usually too small to offer a full range of services; are unable to fully utilize operating suites, computed tomography (CT) scanners, and other diagnostic equipment; and cannot allow staff to specialize. Very small hospitals clearly have higher costs per day, although this is somewhat obscured because they tend to offer fewer expensive and technologically advanced services. A better indication that hospitals with fewer than one hundred beds suffer from a lack of economies of scale is that a disproportionate number of them have gone bankrupt or been absorbed by larger institutions over the past twenty years. Only in rural areas have small general hospitals been able to thrive, and even their numbers are falling as better highways and helicopter transport have reduced the time required to travel to large urban medical centers.

Diseconomies of scale arise from the difficulties of coordinating and managing a larger and larger institution. Relatively few hospitals have more than 500 beds, evidence that costly administrative and transportation difficulties arise when this number of beds is exceeded. Patients increasingly complain about "getting lost in the system" and being part of a "factory" rather than a caring institution. Table 9.3 shows that costs per day rise long before the 500-bed size limit is reached. How can such large hospitals continue to exist in a competitive environment?

TABLE 9.3	Average Cost per Patient Day by Hospital Size

6–24 beds	$ 896
25–49	891
50–99	744
100–199	925
200–299	1,122
300–399	1,277
400–499	1,353
500 or more	1,468

Source: American Hospital Association, *Hospital Statistics 2002,* table 2.

The Hospital is a Multiproduct Firm

Hospitals are complex institutions, and different parts of a hospital actually produce very different products. The "average" is made up of units for routine care, along with some very specialized units, such as heart transplant, oncology, and respiratory intensive care. Although it might take only twenty beds to create an efficient-size cardiac-care unit, only a large hospital has enough cardiac admissions to fill such a specialized unit. Most 400-bed university hospitals are, in fact, composites, with perhaps one hundred beds providing general care, with twenty dedicated to oncology, fifteen to nephrology and kidney transplant, twenty to cardiology, forty to pediatrics, and so on. Thus, although the efficient size of a unit that produces one product is just twenty beds, the more specialized types of care a hospital provides, the larger it must be to reach efficient scale. Indeed, a hospital large enough to produce heart transplants and nuclear medicine efficiently is too large to produce routine care for broken bones and pneumonia and, therefore, suffers from diseconomies of scale with regard to these less-specialized services.

One solution to the conflict between economies and diseconomies of scale is to treat patients with uncomplicated illnesses at local community hospitals of relatively modest size (100 to 150 beds) with few specialized services, while referring patients whose treatment demands sophisticated technology and expertise to large "tertiary" institutions usually affiliated with universities. However, just as increasing hospital size causes diseconomies of scale by making management communication and coordination more difficult, so does the process of transferring patients back and forth between community and specialty hospitals. The savings from triaging patients so that their illnesses are treated in the most efficient size hospital are to some extent offset and eventually reversed by the increase in the number of transfers required, since each transfer requires some extra documentation, management oversight, duplication of tests, and so on.

Contracting Out

Some services show economies of scale even at sizes far larger than any hospital in existence. Laboratory testing, for example, has become so automated that costs are minimized in facilities that process hundreds of thousands of tests per day. The cost of equipment, information systems, and technical expertise that constitute a good laboratory is largely a fixed cost; therefore, overhead per unit continues to decline even when millions of samples are being processed. To take advantage of such economies of scale, many hospitals are contracting out such services. Rather than having their own laboratories for conducting routine tests, they use a reference laboratory that may service hundreds of hospitals. Food services, security, and even emergency rooms are now contracted out to allow hospitals access to economies of scale through contractual relationships.

9.5   QUALITY AND COST

Technology: Cutting Costs or Enhancing Quality?

What does it mean when someone says that technological improvements have made the production process better? It may mean that the identical product can now be produced at a lower cost per unit. It may also mean that a better product can be produced, regardless of cost. Medicine has been dominated by the latter type of technological change. The tremendous value of any increase in cure rates is one factor biasing researchers toward discoveries that have the effect of increasing costs. Yet quality enhancements have occurred rapidly in other areas of technology, such as computing, while still reducing unit costs. Why have such developments been so notably absent in medicine? Quite simply, it has been much more profitable to discover a new cure than to find a method to cut costs.

Insurance and cost reimbursement virtually eliminated price competition in hospital care. Without it, there was no incentive for research laboratories to seek innovations that reduced costs or for hospitals to switch to cheaper versions of existing equipment. The process of trading off a small reduction in speed or accuracy for a large reduction in price that occurs in most markets has rarely taken place in health care.

Improved Efficiency May Raise Total Spending

It is important to recognize that improved production efficiency always causes the true quality-adjusted cost function to fall, even though the amount spent and cost per unit may rise because high quality is much more affordable than before. This is illustrated in Table 9.4. Suppose, for example, that in 1964 a person had a heart attack (myocardial infarction, or MI) and faced the choice of (a) taking medication costing $150 that gave a 30 percent chance of having a fatal MI within five years (70 percent mortality), or (b) undergoing a new, experimental operation costing $25,000 that gave a slightly better chance of survival, with 68 percent mortality. It would be rational for one to take the medication rather than to give up $24,850 additional dollars for such a slight improvement in one's chances. Let's also suppose that in 2002, much better medication more than doubled the chance of survival, with only 29 percent mortality, and cost only $75. In addition, research and practice improved surgery to the point where it had only a 14 percent five-year mortality and a reduced cost of $15,000. The 2002 option of giving up $14,925 to cut the risk of dying in half is very attractive. Thus, even though technological advances reduced the cost of both options, the amount spent on medical care would rise. Improvements in medical production frequently create this type of response. Even though 1960s medicine can be produced now for less than it cost in 1960, patients choose to spend more to get high-quality modern medicine that would have been impossible or prohibitively expensive to obtain in 1960.

Quality costs money, and the drive for higher quality is one of the defining characteristics of modern medicine. While we cannot always agree on what quality is, we know that more quality is always preferred to less and that the cost-quality trade-off is usually more important in understanding the economics of medical practice than the cost-volume trade-off. Before making a comparison on the basis of cost per unit, it is first

| **TABLE 9.4** | Total Spending May Rise Even as Greater Efficiency Reduces Costs per Unit |

1964	2004

Medication cost $150
  post-MI mortality = 70%
	Medication cost $75
	  post-MI mortality = 29%

Surgery cost $25,000
  post-MI mortality = 68%
	Surgery cost $15,000
	  post-MI mortality = 14%

Decision:
  Take medication for $150
	Decision:
	  Have surgery for $15,000

necessary to ask, "What is the product?" If the product is defined as "a day in the hospital," a top-flight research center may seem very expensive. If the product is "an increase in my chance of survival to age 75," the same institution's $2,500 per day charges might seem like a bargain.

9.6 HOW DO HOSPITALS COMPETE?

The flow of revenues into a hospital follows the flow of patients. In some cases, such as emergency room or outpatient clinic visits, patients themselves decide where to go, and for these types of care, hospitals compete directly by trying to attract patients. However, for most care the decision regarding hospitalization is made by the physician. The agency relationship changes the nature of transaction, so that the patient follows the advice of the physician and, therefore, the hospitals compete for doctors.[6] If the ability to decide on hospitalization is taken out of the doctor's hands by the insurance company, as it increasingly is under managed care (see Chapter 10), then hospitals must compete for contracts and appeal to payers, which usually forces the hospital to put more emphasis on lowering prices. The important point is that the hospital must compete for the contracting party that has the power to make the revenues come to them, not necessarily for the patient.

Quality is the most important aspect of medical care, and hospitals such as Johns Hopkins and Massachusetts General have an edge over the competition because of their reputation for outstanding care and scientific prowess. Regardless of whether the final decision-making power lies in the hands of the patient, the physician, or the payer, all of them must be satisfied, and quality is usually the most important concern. It is difficult to convince patients to go to a hospital they are not familiar with, for doctors to give up control by transferring patients to a specialized facility where they are not on the medical staff, and for insurers to pay extra for admission to a facility where they do not have a contract guaranteeing discounts, yet each of these accommodations becomes easier to make when some accepted expert authority has rated this unfamiliar hospital as "the best."

Competing for Patients

The types of care for which patients make their own decisions are those in which they are able to judge important aspects of quality and in which they pay a large share of cost directly out of their own pockets. Maternity care is a good example. Many mothers want to have their babies close to home, have strong preferences regarding patient services (natural childbirth, religious orientation, attitude of staff), and can get good information for comparing hospitals by talking to other mothers in the neighborhood. Since the need for care is known months in advance, potential parents can do the kind of comparison shopping which is impossible to do after accidents or heart attacks. Also, the fact that births are expected means that they are not "risks" in the insurance sense and, therefore, frequently are reimbursed on a shared or fixed-price basis that leaves much of the marginal cost to the parents. For these reasons, hospitals must actively compete for patients on the basis of price and service. Casual investigation reveals a number of special deals, from free baby clothes, gourmet meals, and a post-partum vacation to cut-rate "fixed-price packages," not unlike the competition for selling cars and houses. Outpatient clinics, where patients are more likely to self-refer and where cost-sharing is usually higher, also use marketing strategies such as nice waiting rooms, receptionists who call to make or remind patients about appointments, free transportation to the clinic, and deductible or co-payment waivers. The rise of "preferred provider" plans (see Chapter 10) that provide full coverage only for a limited group of hospitals has also increased the importance of direct marketing to patients.

Competing for Physicians

The agency relationship and control over admissions means that most hospital competition is over doctors rather than patients. Recruitment incentives are a very visible sign of such competition. Income guarantees (e.g., if you come to hospital X, and your income in the first year is less than $125,000, we will make up the difference), relocation assistance, and promises of referrals from other doctors on the medical staff are common contractual provisions. Sometimes there is even a "signing bonus" similar to what a professional athlete might receive. As Mark Pauly's "doctor's workshop" model suggests, hospitals also compete by helping physicians earn more money in their private practices by providing free or subsidized office space; providing secretarial, phone, and billing services; setting aside ten beds for nephrology or another specialty so that the specialist will always be able to admit a patient; and so on.[7] Reducing practice costs or work effort is a limited competitive tool. Far more important is helping a physician build his or her practice by a hospital's reputation for quality and the technological sophistication of services offered.[8] A cardiologist is able to attract more patients if he or she is the only cardiologist in town who has access to a catheterization lab that does stent, or percutaneous transluminal coronary angioplasty (PTCA), or a newer development in vein obstruction removal. In some instances, such competition can lead to a sort of **"medical arms race,"** in which nearby hospitals each try to be the first with the most, and respond strategically. For example, if one hospital gets an MRI scanner, the other one gets one that is bigger; if one gets a lithotripter, the other gets one that has more settings and finer resolution; and so on. It is possible that competing on the basis of which hospital has the most new technology can lead to inefficiencies and escalating costs, with the two scanners and two lithotripters empty half the time because there are only enough patients in the market to keep one piece of equipment operating at full capacity. This points out one of the major problems of hospital markets structured on the basis of competing for physicians to increase patient flow. A hospital has an incentive to subsidize office space to attract physicians, not to reduce charges to patients, change billing practices, or make trade-offs that lead to overall reductions in the cost of medical care. The competition for physicians does not necessarily push hospitals toward an efficient use of inputs or mix of services.

Competing for Contracts

The scale on which medical practice is conducted is increasing. When organized on the basis of atomistic transactions between individuals, the choice of hospital falls to the doctors acting as agents for the patients under their care. However, it has become more and more common for a payer to make contracts directly with hospitals, negotiating a fixed or discounted price, and limiting patients to hospitals with which the payer has a contract. Payers can direct patient flow even when contracts are not fully binding. Although Medicare has a contract with every hospital, it will allow heart transplants only in certain approved facilities, and in a request for proposals to become an approved provider, price is a factor. Health maintenance organizations (HMOs) can be even more aggressive, sometimes threatening to transfer a large group of patients to a rival facility unless negotiations result in a substantial discount or making approval conditional on assurances that the HMO will receive the lowest price the hospital gives to any contractor.

Although managed care contracting at this level is a relatively recent development, structurally it bears a resemblance to the original social contract between the hospital and the community and to the agreements under which hospitals receive tax subsidies and other favorable treatment from the government. In each of these contracts, there are two parties: the hospital and a representative of consumers as a group (community, insurance plan, taxpayers). Such large-scale arrangements are inevitably less accommodating to the needs of individual patients and the professional autonomy of physicians. However, any attempt to implement public accountability and successful cost control involves compromises. Trade-offs are necessary in any system that takes its broader social responsibilities seriously and are the core concept for creating economic efficiency in health care (see Table 9.5).

Measuring Competitive Success

How can it be determined which hospitals are more successful in the competition for patients? A firm that has failed by going out of business is clearly not successful, and economists have used "survivor analysis" to measure competitive success by counting the number of new entrants or exits (bankruptcy, takeover) within different categories. Survivor analysis has been used to show that hospitals with fewer than 100 or more than 500 beds appear to be inefficient and less able to compete.[9] Such analysis has also shown that for-profit hospitals are not necessarily more efficient or better competitors than nonprofits (the number of for-profit hospitals has fluctuated, but these hospitals accounted for around 10 to 20 percent of total bed supply throughout the twentieth century, indicating competitive performance that is about average). A hospital that has grown relative to its competitors is clearly more successful, and such traditional measures as total assets, market share, and geographic spread have been used as indicators. With 90 percent of hospitals operated by either voluntary (charitable and/or religious) or government organizations, profits are less useful as a measure of success than they are in other industries. However, the excess of revenues over expenditures is available to fund growth and is necessary to avoid bankruptcy, and thus can be a useful indicator. In the current environment, with many hospitals trying to form chains or acquire physician practices to cover a larger area and offer a full line of services for managed care contracting, strong earnings and large financial reserves clearly provide a competitive advantage.

TABLE 9.5	Competition Between Hospitals
Hospitals Compete for:	**On the Basis of Quality and:**
Patients	Amenities, out-of-pocket $$
Doctors	Technology, practice assistance
Contracts	Price, information systems

What has proven almost impossible to measure is the success of a hospital in achieving its goals as a provider of health care to the community. Although charity care, participation in outreach programs, and mortality rates are often monitored and commented on, there is general agreement that these are incomplete and inadequate measures at best, and are frequently misleading. Attempts are being made to assess community benefit in more comprehensive and objective ways, but there is as yet no reason to believe that these will be any more convincing than previous efforts.[10] Economists and other policy makers are in the awkward position of recognizing that they know which dimensions are most important (quality, compassion, technological advances), but they do not know how to gauge them numerically or even how to make a fair comparison between hospitals.

Measuring the Competitiveness of Markets

Competition can be a significant factor in forcing hospitals to become more efficient and provide better services. However, a single hospital in a rural area or a chain that controls almost all the hospitals in an urban market, is not constrained by competition. The potential loss of consumer welfare due to a merger or acquisition that reduces the amount of competition is the central concern of the Federal Trade Commission (FTC) and a source of much litigation under antitrust law. This litigation provides many consulting projects for economists called in to testify as expert witnesses on how competitive a particular market is or will be. Competition is usually measured by the number of hospitals or concentration of market share in a geographic area (e.g., within a 15-mile radius; within a city, county, or metropolitan statistical area) or by the overlap between hospital services (how many patients use several hospitals). Although the complexities of antitrust law and the economic assessment of competition policy are beyond the scope of this text, it is worth noting that all hospitals are multiproduct firms. The relevant market for services such as liver transplant, residential psychiatric care, and abortion, therefore, covers a large area because patients are willing to travel hundreds of miles for treatment, whereas the market for other services such as kidney dialysis, outpatient psychiatry, and prenatal care depend on patients living nearby, and hence are much smaller. After decades of being exempt or ignored, hospitals have come under increasing scrutiny by the FTC, and antitrust enforcement is now considered an important alternative to regulation as a means of controlling costs.

9.7 CONTROLLING HOSPITAL COSTS THROUGH REGULATION

Hospital costs have risen steadily throughout the post–World War II era, from $9 per day in 1946, to $41 in 1965, then rising 600 percent in the next fifteen years to $244 in 1980, to $682 in 1990, and surpassing $1,200 in 2002.[11] Hospital costs have grown about 10 percent a year over the past fifty years. Even after adjusting for inflation, the increase in cost per day is still an astounding 1,790 percent from 1946 to 2002 (an average of 5 percent above inflation each year). By and large, the public has wanted the additional care and new technology and has not been displeased with the billions of dollars expended. However, after the passage of Medicare and Medicaid in 1965, costs became a problem for public policy for two reasons: (1) the influx of government money caused costs to rise much more rapidly than before and (2) the costs were now being paid by the government (i.e., taxpayers) rather than the mutually agreed-upon private transactions of individuals or employer-paid insurance, and thus caused state and federal budget deficits (see Table 9.6 and Figure 9.6).

TABLE 9.6		Hospital Costs per Patient Day 1946-2002
Year	Cost Per Day	Cost Per Day (2002 $$)
1946	$ 9	$ 67
1950	14	89
1955	21	117
1960	29	145
1965	41	191
1970	74	282
1971	83	301
1972	95	330
1973	102	336
1974	113	341
1975	133	367
1976	152	397
1977	173	425
1978	194	445
1979	216	457
1980	244	473
1981	284	504
1982	327	546
1983	368	591
1984	410	635
1985	460	690
1986	499	733
1987	537	766
1988	581	801
1989	631	838
1990	682	872
1991	745	919
1992	816	983
1993	874	1,028
1994	930	1,071
1995	967	1,090
1996	1,005	1,111
1997	1,032	1,119
1998	1,065	1,141
1999	1,101	1,163
2000	1,148	1,188
2001	1,205	1,218
2002	1,266	1,266

Hospital cost per adjusted patient day in nominal current
dollars and inflation adjusted to 2002 dollars using
GDP deflator.

Source: American Hospital Association, *Hospital Statistics,*
various years.

In the immediate postwar period, the Hill-Burton Act of 1946 funded the building of more hospitals, and the Health Professions Educational Assistance Act of 1963 increased the number of doctors. The early 1960s were boom years when it seemed that the economy would continue to grow robustly "forever." This desire to continue spending enabled Congress to create Medicare and Medicaid as entitlement programs in 1965. However, by

| **FIGURE 9.6** | Hospital Costs Per Patient Day 1946–2002 |

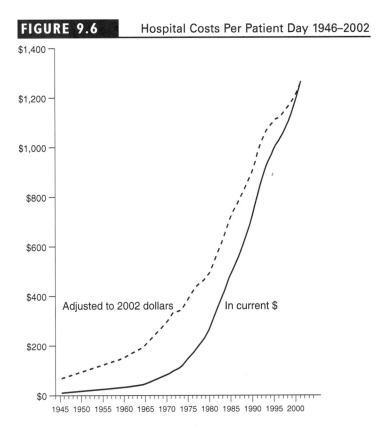

1975, the United States was trapped in a global recession, federal and state expenditures had escalated far beyond even the most outlandish budget projections, and the need for cost-cutting was clear. It was thought that the system efficiencies could be generated through better planning; therefore, a number of initiatives were funded to promote "regional medical programs" and create planning boards for oversight. Evaluations showing that planning alone could not affect costs, and the obvious excess capacity created by the Hill-Burton construction boom, led to the idea that a forced reduction in the growth of hospital beds could reduce the rate of growth in hospital costs.

Certificate-of-need (CON) legislation required that a planning body conduct a study and approve any capital project that would increase the number of hospital beds in the region.[12] In an insightful study of the economics of hospital regulation, David Salkever and Thomas Bice showed that although CON legislation reduced the number of new beds built, hospitals increased the amount of capital equipment for each bed; thus, capital spending continued to rise at the same rate.[13] In discussing their findings, Salkever and Bice argued that "CON regulation is like pushing on a balloon," forcing costs down in one dimension caused them to bulge in another dimension. Similar dynamics have been demonstrated in other studies of many regulatory initiatives over the years; the type of cost subject to regulation declines, but any savings are negated by an overflow in another area so that total health care costs are unchanged (see Table 9.7). An unintended side effect of CON and most other regulations is that they create barriers, making it harder for new organizations to enter the market, thus protecting existing hospitals and retarding the evolution of the health care system toward more efficient configurations. Studies of CON in operation confirmed the economists' version of the golden rule ("them that has the gold makes the rules"): almost every well-established, wealthy, and politically connected hospital that applied for certification eventually got it, while denials fell disproportionately on outsiders that threatened the status quo or weaker institutions that lacked a constituency. The death knell for CON came in the form of a Supreme Court ruling that discriminatory reimbursement of a hospital chain that refused to apply for a CON (which the chain knew would be denied because of opposition from existing local hospitals) constituted an illegal restraint of trade under antitrust laws and harmed consumers by restricting competition.

The attempt to impose controls over other dimensions moved on to utilization review (UR), a process to eliminate unnecessary surgery and other services by having a panel of doctors and nurses in a professional standards review organization (PSRO) review patients' charts to find cases of inappropriate care. The PSRO or other agency would be empowered to order the doctor to change improper behavior and, failing that, to deny payment. In practice, the process proved cumbersome and ineffective, although the current managed care review, which does appear to work better (see Chapter 10), developed from the experience with UR. Rapid inflation and an unwillingness to accept the lessons of history led the Nixon administration to impose **price controls** in 1971. Although removed for most sectors of the economy in 1973, they were maintained in hospitals for an extra year. Rate setting through **budgetary review** was a much more labor-intensive process, involving the line-by-line examination of spending plans. A notable example was the legislation passed in the state of Washington in 1973 when a severe local recession crimped the state's ability to raise tax revenues. The legislation lasted, albeit in weaker and weaker form, for ten years (see Chapter 18, section 4, for more details). Perhaps the most far-reaching cost-control regulation was the replacement of Medicare's open-ended system of retrospective cost reimbursement by the **prospective payment system (PPS)** in 1984, in which **diagnostically related groups (DRGs)** were used for setting federally administered prices per discharge covering the entire patient stay. However, the demonstrable reductions in cost per inpatient admission were more than offset by rapid increases in outpatient charges; therefore, overall Medicare costs have continued to rise as rapidly as before—another example of a regulation pushing on one side of the balloon.

The **Balanced Budget Act of 1997 (BBA)** was much more successful in cutting costs, at least in the short run. It directly reduced Medicare payments to physicians, hospitals and home-health agencies by reducing the hospital update factor (annual base payment increase percentage), reducing payments for graduate medical education, limiting the growth in total Medicare physician payments to a "sustainable growth rate" linked to the annual rate of growth in GDP, establishing a prospective payment system for home-health benefits, and allowing HMOs to compete for Medicare beneficiaries through the "Medicare+Choice" program. Payments for home health care, which had been the most rapidly growing part of Medicare, fell from $16 billion in 1996 to less than $8 billion in 1999.[14] Altogether, these reductions were able to save more than $100 billion over five years. However, as the curbs put in place by BBA really began to bite, protests from hospitals and physician groups have grown louder, and politicians more sympathetic. By early 2003, a consensus had arisen that some release from the stringent constraints imposed on Medicare payment increases would have to be implemented soon.

TABLE 9.7	Types of Regulation to Control Hospital Costs

Certificate of need (CON)
Utilization review (UR, PSRO)
Budgetary review
Price controls (ESPN)
Administered prices (DRGs, PPS, BBA)

The experience with price controls, state rate regulation, and PPS is examined in more detail in Chapter 18, section 4, showing that whatever successes might be attributed to cost-control regulation have been limited and short lived.[15] The failure of this kind of government price regulation to control costs should not come as a surprise since the central difficulty in medical care transactions is the inability to specify what the product is. Special market adaptations, such as nonprofit status and the agency relationships between physicians and patients, are signals that any attempts to set prices or to quantify quality and other important attributes are likely to be exercises in futility. A government official in a state capital, or in Washington, D.C., is not going to be able to specify a detailed contract in advance to purchase something that the participants have trouble measuring even after the fact (e.g., how good the obstetrical care really was for a low-birthweight baby left with disabilities). It would be easy to cut spending on Medicare and Medicaid in a number of ways (set global budget caps, eliminate services, deny eligibility), but there is not sufficient public consensus or political willpower to do so. Managed care and new regulations may bring some relief, but the macroeconomic cost pressures examined in Chapters 14 to 18 will eventually force the public to face these hard choices, and force politicians to deal with the fallout.

SUGGESTIONS FOR FURTHER READING

Healthcare Financial Management, monthly journal of the Healthcare Financial Management Association (www.HFMA.org).

Louis Gapenski, *Healthcare Finance,* 2nd edition (Chicago: Health Administration Press, 2002).

Steven A. Finkler and David M. Ward, *Cost Accounting for Health Care Organizations,* 2nd ed. (Gaithersburg, Md.: Aspen, 1999).

William O. Cleverley and Andrew E. Cameron, *Essentials of Health Care Finance,* 5th ed. (Gaithersburg, Md.: Aspen, 2002).

SUMMARY

1. Managers plan to produce efficiently; therefore, any deviation from the plan (more or fewer patients, shifting wage rates) tends to increase average cost per unit, particularly in the short run. Since management can more fully adapt operations over the long run, the short-run average cost curve always lies at or above the long-run average cost curve. The primary way **managers control hospital costs is through the budget process.** Often extra capacity and flexibility is built in so that uncertainty and changes are not so difficult to deal with.

2. **Economies of scale** are said to exist when increasing the level of output causes the average cost per unit to fall. Gains from the **specialization of labor and spreading the fixed costs of capital equipment** over more volume are the major factors creating economies of scale. **Diseconomies of scale,** in which rising costs per unit eventually set in, are primarily due to the **difficulty of managing and coordinating larger operations.** Hospitals appear to show economies of scale up to a size of about 120 beds and diseconomies of scale after reaching a size of about 500 beds. For simple services, small hospitals appear to be relatively efficient, but only a large hospital has enough patients of a particular type (e.g., brain cancer) to run a specialized service at an efficient volume. Thus, a hospital may be both too big to deliver some services efficiently and too small to deliver others efficiently.

3. **Cost per day in the hospital varies for many reasons:** differences in quality and type of services offered, cost shifting to pay for research and teaching, billing practices, severity of patient illness, prices of labor and other inputs, and differences in

production efficiency. **Hospitals are multiproduct firms,** providing many types of care; thus, comparisons of cost per day or per case may not be very meaningful indicators of how efficiently a hospital is producing care.

4.   **Accounting costs often do not measure true economic costs.** A larger-than-expected number of patients may make average costs appear lower, but actually the overcrowding and staff stress tend to increase costs. Patient time, pain, and worry are other costs often not counted.

5.   **Technology** has tended to increase total spending in health care because generous insurance payments and cost reimbursement have given little incentive to develop cost-reducing techniques or to give up a little quality for a large reduction in cost. An increase in capability to improve health often makes more spending worthwhile.

6.   **Hospitals compete for physicians,** because physicians control the flow of patients (and hence, revenues). Unlike most businesses, hospitals do not compete directly for "customers" because their customers (a) do not pay their own bills and (b) do not make their own choices, but are directed by physicians who act as their agents. Only for some patient-initiated or relatively uninsured services is direct competition important for patients (plastic surgery, childbirth). Larger scale and cost pressures are causing hospitals to compete for contracts, trying to attract employees, HMOs, or insurance companies directly. To do so, they must compete more and more on the basis of price rather than quality.

7.   While able to switch cost from one part of health care to another (pushing on a balloon), **regulation** has not succeeded in controlling the overall cost of health care. CON regulation to control construction and prospective price setting (PPS, DRGs) have forced hospitals to respond in a number of ways, but total spending has continued to soar. Government is responsible for most of a hospital's patients (66 percent of inpatient days are paid for by Medicare and Medicaid), but is unable or unwilling to pay the price, forcing the health care system toward a crisis point. The cost shifting under which the rich cared for the poor and the healthy contributed to pay for the sick has begun to crack under the strain of unequal payments and a burgeoning federal deficit.

PROBLEMS

1.   {*economies of scale*} What major factors create economies of scale in hospitals? Diseconomies of scale? Are most hospitals of optimal size, too small, or too large?

2.   {*case-mix, cost shifting*} Why do university teaching hospitals cost so much more per day of care than local community hospitals?

3.   {*economies of scale*} Misericordia Hospital had a 20 percent increase in admissions from 1995 to 2000. Total patient care costs went from $50 million to $61 million. Does Misericordia show evidence of economies of scale or diseconomies of scale? Could other factors besides the number of admissions affect the costs of care?

4.   {*economies of scale*} The number of patients at Harbordale Hospital increased from 120 to 144 from Monday to Tuesday. The hospital's costs increased $720,000 to $722,000 as temporary nurses were called in to deal with the heavy patient load. Does Harbordale Hospital show economies or diseconomies of scale? Which hospital is better managed for cost control, Harbordale or Misericordia (in problem 3)? Which is more costly, short-run adjustment between Monday and Tuesday or long-run adjustment between 1995 and 2000?

5. {*marginal cost, accounting*} What is the cost of an extra admission to a hospital? Does it make a difference if the admission is for an emergency service or for a scheduled service? Who bears the costs of additional emergency admission? Is there any difference in who bears the cost of a 50 percent increase in emergency room admission in the short run and the long run?

6. {*compensation*} Should hospital managers be rewarded for dealing with random fluctuations in demand, or for dealing with planned changes in demand?

7. {*efficiency, case-mix*} Costs per day are usually lower in community hospitals than in university hospitals. Does this mean that transferring patients from university hospitals to community hospitals would increase efficiency?

8. {*substitution*} Why do people spend so long waiting to be treated in an emergency room? Would it be more efficient if there were sufficient doctors available so that people could be treated right away?

9. {*economies of scale, discrimination*} Many rural counties have fewer hospital beds than urban and suburban counties, even when rural counties experience more accidents and injuries for which immediate access to care is crucial. Does this disparity indicate systematic discrimination against rural counties?

10. {*transactions costs*} Why would a hospital that just expanded its home health care agency to service the patients of other hospitals in the region close down its clinical laboratory and purchase lab services from a neighboring hospital?

11. {*quality*} Why have quality improvements in health care caused costs to rise while quality improvements in computers have caused costs to fall?

12. {*competition*} Wills Eye Hospital in Philadelphia is a 114-bed hospital specializing in ophthalmologic surgery. Who do you think competes with Wills Eye?

13. {*competition*} Describe the factors you would expect to be most important in competition for patients for each of the following services. For which services is price more important? Location? Quality? Would hospitals compete for patients or for doctors?

    a. Heart transplants
    b. Maternity
    c. Immunization
    d. Depression
    e. Chemotherapy
    f. Plastic surgery
    g. AIDS

14. {*technological change*} Automation has vastly increased the efficiency and accuracy of laboratory testing. The cost per test has fallen by more than 75 percent in many cases. Do you think that the total cost of laboratory testing has fallen by more or less than 75 percent? Why?

15. {*price controls*} What would you expect to be the effect of a set of regulations limiting hospital revenues to an increase of 1 percent a year on the following?

    a. Number of nurses hired
    b. Number of doctors
    c. Quality of care
    d. Advertising budgets

    e.   Emergency room staffing

    f.   New construction

    g.   Depreciation

    Would there be a difference if the regulation applied to just one hospital rather than to all hospitals? Would there be a difference between short-run and long-run effects?

16.   *{regulation}* CON regulations effectively limited the number of new hospital beds constructed in a region. Who would favor CON? Who would be against CON? When hospitals in a state with CON regulation renovate old buildings, would you expect the cost per bed to be more or less than in a state without CON regulation?

ENDNOTES

1.   E. R. Becker and B. Steinwald, "The Determinants of Hospital Case-Mix Complexity," *Health Services Research* 16, no. 1 (1981): 439–458.

2.   Frank Sloan, Roger Feldman, and Bruce Steinwald, "The Effects of Teaching on Hospital Costs," *Journal of Health Economics,* 2, no. 1(1983): 1– 28.3. Howard Berman and Louis Weeks, *The Financial Management of Hospitals,* 5th edition (Ann Arbor, Mich.: Health Administration Press, 1990).

4.   The adjustment calculation used here is arbitrary and intended for illustrative purposes only, rather than estimation of actual cost penalties. The important point is that being over or under the optimal level of planned output causes a disproportionate increase in per-unit costs.

5.   T. W. Granneman, R. S. Brown, and M. V. Pauly, "Estimating Hospital Costs: A Multiple-Output Analysis," *Journal of Health Economics,* 5, no. 2 (1986): 107–127; T. G. Cowing, A. G. Holtman, and S. Powers, "Hospital Cost Analysis: A Survey and Evaluation of Recent Studies," *Advances in Health Economics and Health Services Research* 4 (1983) 257–303.

6.   Mark Pauly and Michael Redisch, "The Not-for-profit Hospital as a Physicians Cooperative," *American Economic Review* 63 (1973): 87–99.

7.   Mark V. Pauly, *The Doctor's Workshop* (Philadelphia: University of Pennsylvania Press, 1980).

8.   H. Luft, J. Robinson, D. Garnick, S. Maerki, and S. McPhee, "The Role of Specialized Clinical Services in the Competition Among Hospitals," *Inquiry* 23, no. 1 (1986): 83– 94.

9.   Carson W. Bays, "The Determinants of Hospital Size: A Survivor Analysis," *Applied Economics* 18 (1986): 359–377.

10. Robert Sigmond and J. David Seay, "Community Benefit Standards for Hospitals: Perception and Performance," *Frontiers of Health Services Management* (Spring 1989).

11. American Hospital Association, *Hospital Statistics* (Chicago: American Hospital Association, various years).

12. CON, UR, PSROs, DRGs, and other regulations have all taken many different forms in different state or national programs over time. The brief discussion here refers to general conclusions about that type of regulation, rather than any particular specific program. The interested reader should consult one of the many comprehensive reviews that have been written, such as those in Paul Joskow, *Controlling Hospital Costs: The Role of Government Regulation* (Cambridge, Mass.: MIT Press, 1981); D. Abernathy and D. A. Pearson, *Regulating Hospital Costs: The Development of Public Policy* (Ann Arbor, Mich.: Health Administration Press, 1979); or the relevant chapters of Michael Rosko and Robert W. Broyles, *The Economics of Health Care: A Reference Handbook* (New York: Greenwood Press, 1988); or Sherman Folland, Allen Goodman, and Miron Stano, *The Economics of Health and Health Care* (Upper Saddle River, NJ: Prentice-Hall, 2001).

13. David Salkever and Thomas Bice, *Hospital Certificate-of-Need Controls: Impact on Investment, Costs and Use* (Washington, D.C.: American Enterprise Institute, 1979).

14. Nelda McCall et. al., "Medicare Home Health Before and After the BBS," *Health Affairs* 20, no. 3 (May 2001): 189–198. Charles N. Kahn and Hanns Kuttner, "Budget Bills and Medicare Policy: the Politics of the BBA," *Health Affairs* 18, no. 1 (January 1999): 37– 47.

15. David Dranove and Kenneth Cone, "Do State Rate-Setting Regulations Really Lower Hospital Expenses?" *Journal of Health Economics* 4 (1985): 159–165; C. L. Eby and D. Cohodes, "What Do We Know About Rate-Setting?" *Journal of Health Politics, Policy and Law* 10, no. 2 (1985): 299– 327.

CHAPTER 10

MANAGED CARE

QUESTIONS

1. What flaw in the U.S. health care system forced the development of managed care?
2. How do HMOs use financial contracts to align the interests of patients and doctors?
3. Does managed care reduce individual risks or reduce system-wide average risks?
4. Why do HMOs carve out, or subcapitate, mental health and other special services?
5. Does a physician "gatekeeper" work for or against the patient?
6. How much profit can an HMO make? At whose expense?
7. Does "financial innovation" improve productivity and consumer welfare as technological innovation does?
8. Who are the winners and losers in managed care? Do cost reductions mean that some doctors must earn lower incomes?
9. How are HMO per-member-per-month capitation rates determined?
10. Does a surplus of doctors and hospitals foster or hinder the growth of HMOs?
11. University hospitals seek out the sickest and most demanding patients to practice and improve medical technology. Will HMOs support medical research? Will they seek out those most in need, or try to selectively enroll the healthy to keep costs down?
12. Are HMOs medical care organizations, or financial services companies in the insurance business?

10.1 WHY MANAGED CARE?

The primary impetus behind managed care has been the rise in health care costs, and in particular, the rise in the cost of employee health benefits. Traditional corporate health insurance for employees, Medicare, and Medicaid were open-ended **entitlement** systems. Patients had no reason to worry about costs. Hospitals, doctors, and insurers, being recipients of funds, actually benefited from increased spending. From 1970 to 1980, health care expenditures by businesses rose from 3.1 percent of employee compensation to 4.9 percent. Then, costs grew even more rapidly, and by 1990 these expenditures reached 7.1 percent of

employee compensation.[1] The value of health benefits, equal to 36 percent of after-tax profits in 1970, and 43 percent in 1980, actually exceeded (108 percent) total corporate profits
in 1990. Indemnity insurance premiums for Blue Cross and Blue Shield coverage rose as
much as 30 percent a year in many markets during the early 1980s.

In the face of these large increases, prudence and survival demanded that something
be done to reduce the cost of health care to businesses. The problems of businesses had
actually been made worse by government cost-containment efforts in the 1980s, because
reductions in Medicaid and Medicare rates forced hospitals to shift costs by charging more
to insured patients (see section 8.4 for a discussion of cost shifting). Businesses became
increasingly willing to turn to an outside contractor that could stabilize benefit costs, even
if it meant having to accept some constraints and employee complaints. Health
Maintenance Organization (HMO) contracts and membership exploded, rising from 3
million in 1970 to 9 million in 1980, 36 million in 1990, and 80 million in 2002, with
employer group contracts accounting for 90 percent of total membership.[2]

Costs and Quality

In a system characterized by a lack of financial restraints, it is not surprising that the
United States was spending far more on health care than any other country in the world
(Chapter 17); the surprise was how little health the nation was able to buy with all the extra
money spent. Despite years of insistence by politicians and physicians that the United
States had the best medical care in the world, there is scant evidence that the additional
expenditures led to improvements in longevity, infant mortality, morbidity, or days lost
from work, relative to other countries spending less than half as much per person.[3] What
has become apparent is that the real inflation-adjusted hourly wages of workers have stag-
nated, and even declined, while the cost per hour of employer-provided health benefits has
soared, and that the federal government has been burdened by billions of dollars in deficits
attributable to the soaring cost of Medicare benefits. The nation has searched for an organizational structure that would add the missing elements of planning, coordination, and
control to the health care system to improve efficiency and limit total expenditures.

Management: The Distinctive Feature of Managed Care

The fundamental difference between traditional medical practice under fee-for-service
(FFS) indemnity insurance and managed care is that **a manager** intervenes to monitor and
control the transaction between doctor and patient (Figure 10.1).[4] An outside party, such

---

FIGURE 10.1   The Flow of Funds with Managed Care

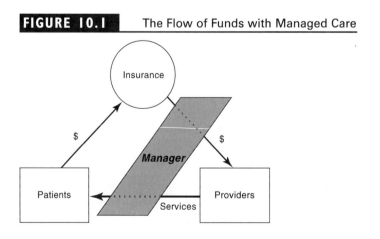

as the plan medical director, a trained utilization review nurse, or a software program, identifies care that is potentially at variance with accepted clinical practice. This may be done through a statistical profile of each physician's practice, assessment of laboratory testing, a review of individual cases, or a combination of techniques. The manager examines the process of care and controls the flow of funds, facilitating payments in some circumstances and holding back in others. Since the **managed care organization** (**MCO**) takes financial responsibility for medical care, it has an incentive to provide care efficiently. To remain viable, it must compete on the basis of both quality and cost. A delicate balance must be maintained between expenditure control, administrative process, and medical uncertainty.

Contractual Reforms to Reduce Costs

Indemnity insurance is a contract to pay for care. The premium must be sufficient to pay for all medical care provided and administrative overhead:

$$\text{Total Premiums} = (\text{Price} \times \text{Quantity}) + \text{Overhead } (load)$$

Total costs can be reduced only by reducing one or more of these three elements. Since a managed care organization adds management, overhead increases. This leaves price and quantity. Of these two, ***prices are the easiest to cut.*** Most of the early successes of managed care plans came from the ability to cut the amounts paid to doctors and hospitals. Sometimes these prices were reduced because of excess supply; sometimes because the MCO became a big buyer and could exercise market power; sometimes the mere threat of taking patients away, or sending more, was sufficient to obtain discounts; and sometimes it was just because no buyer had ever before haggled aggressively in a system that had grown fat and soft. It is worth remembering that during the reign of the indemnity insurance plans, no one, not even the insurance company, stood to gain very much from hard bargaining—so all parties avoided it.

Cutting prices does not change the amount of actual resources used (physician hours, X-ray machines, hospital beds). It simply means one group (buyers) is paying less, and thus another group (sellers) receives less. In economic terms, it is a pure transfer. Presumably buyers are happy to pay less, but sellers are not happy to receive less. Indeed, faced with an onslaught of discounts, hospitals and physicians finally revolted—blaming managed care for all sorts of evil in the service of greed (see "Backlash" in section 10.10). Thus, while price cuts are the most readily used method to reduce costs, and the source of most savings that MCOs have achieved,[5] there are clear limitations to such a strategy.

The second method for reducing costs, cutting the quantity of medical services, has proven to be much more difficult. Despite the rhetoric of "restrictive" managed care plans, the reality is that the total volume of services is rarely reduced by enough to make a substantial difference in total spending. To reduce quantity of services, both the patient and the physician must agree. The initial idea was that medical services that do not have much of an impact on health could be removed without conflict ("cutting out the fat"). Yet whether a service is medically useful has nothing to do with its effect on physician income—both vital and merely marginal services bring in the same fee. Thus, physicians are harmed even if patients are not. Furthermore, while it is relatively easy to discover services that are relatively unimportant ("the need for this service results from a rare side effect"), it is almost impossible to say that such services would never be helpful, that they would not be important in one in a hundred (or one in a million) cases.

What did happen was that the use of services was bent to follow the contract more closely. For example, since many contracts with hospitals specified a set payment per day, the number of days a patient could stay in the hospital was reduced. However, patients still needed the same amount of surgery, after care, drugs, and so on, so the intensity of services was increased—more hours of nursing care and more procedures performed each day. The net result of fewer days and more inputs per day was that the total cost of hospital care was not reduced. As long as more nurses are hired, more drugs are used, and more tests are performed, total expenses cannot fall even though the number of patient days is falling. Over time, the reduction in ALOS (average length of stay = number of days per patient admission) was more than offset by an increase in the cost per day (see Chapters 8 and 9).

The third method for reducing cost was to **substitute cheaper forms of care**—prescribe generic rather than brand name drugs, have patients see a nurse practitioner rather than a doctor, treat patients with medicine rather than surgery, hip replacement rather than long-term nursing home care, and so on. The idea was that a manager could identify an alternate form of care that was just as (or almost as) effective, but significantly less expensive. Substitution has been practiced effectively for pharmaceuticals (see box), but has been less successful for other categories of medical care. Even in pharmaceuticals, the savings from use of cheaper generic substitutes has been more than offset by the rise in the total number of prescriptions and increased use of expensive new compounds so that total drug costs per patient have continued to rise.

Reforming the Organization to Reduce Cost

The rigid equation of Cost = (Price × Quantity + Overhead) holds as long as one considers managed care only as a contractual modification that leaves the underlying organization of medical practice the same. An alternative, more radical, reform is to change the organizational structure. Instead of having an insurance company/MCO that pays bills and having a set of hospitals and physicians that provide care, a single unified organization could integrate both functions. Kaiser, Group Health Cooperative, and others had begun using closed-panel group practice (CPGP) to do so since the 1940s. In a CPGP, the physicians work on salary for the organization, the hospitals are owned by the organization, and the drugs are purchased by the organization. A **single entity combines all the complex functions of providing and paying for medical care.**

Since a CPGP offers a package rather than a set of parts, there are no meaningful prices and quantities, no distinction between insurance overhead and clinical management. It is like getting a package trip to Cancun rather than paying separately for airfare, hotels, meals, excursions, taxis, and a travel agent's fee. This **"fourth way"** of reducing costs was, in fact, the original form of managed care, and the term "HMO" originally applied only to such comprehensive CPGP health plans (since they could presumably save money by maintaining health rather than treating illnesses). (See Table 10.1.) The challenge for an integrated CPGP HMO is to keep premiums low and satisfaction high—the itemized prices and quantities fade out of existence and relevance.

Changing organizational structure offers greater potential for savings, but is harder to bring about, and most CPGPs have rather timidly tried to stay close to "regular" medical practice (see discussion of the Kaiser health plan in section 10.6). The potential for organizational change to reconfigure consumption can perhaps most easily be grasped through a familiar example—music. For 200 years, people have listened to string quartets performing Brahms compositions. To perform a twenty-minute piece, it takes four musicians playing twenty minutes each (and practicing for years) to bring music to the audience. Whether it is 1702 or 2002, it still takes four musicians and twenty minutes. There is little room to cut price (musicians have never been all that well paid), and playing the entire prelude in 15 minutes is not a satisfactory way to achieve efficiency. However, focusing on the needs of the consumers rather than the producers reveals a new way, and a new

TABLE 10.1	How Managed Care Can Reduce Total Costs

Contractual: Reduce Total P × Q by:

1. Reducing prices
2. Reducing quantities
3. Substituting cheaper types
4. **Organizational:** integrate insurance and production in a comprehensive closed-panel group practice (full service package in a single organization, no prices or quantities as such).

organization—a recording company. The performance can be played around the world (OK, so it is not quite as good as being there) for a per person cost that is a fraction of the four musicians' hourly wages. Indeed, once the music is digitized and placed on a compact disc, a person can listen to it at home, in the car, or at a picnic dinner on the beach rather inexpensively. If the revolution in musical consumption seems exceedingly far-fetched as an analogy, consider the health effects of small pox vaccination, sanitation, heart pacemakers, and the Internet on the practice of medicine between 1900 and 2002.

10.2 SOURCES AND USES OF FUNDS

Almost 100 million people, 57 percent of those with private insurance, were in either contractual or organizational HMOs in the year 2000, a tenfold (1,000 percent) increase in just twenty years.[6] Another 12.3 million Medicaid enrollees (49 percent of the total) were in HMOs, as were 6.7 million Medicare enrollees (21 percent). Except for Medicare, the old-style indemnity insurance that paid bills automatically without managerial intervention now accounts for less than 10 percent of private insurance. There has been consolidation in the industry, with the number of operating HMOs dropping to 625 in 2000. By far the largest are the CPGP Kaiser health plans with 9.8 million enrollees. Yet the 86 CPGP/staff model HMOs are outnumbered by the 539 contractual independent practice association (IPA)/network HMOs (see section 10.3 for definitions), which account for 78 percent of total enrollment.

Most contractual HMOs take 15 to 20 percent of the premiums they receive for administration, marketing, and profit,[7] with the bulk of the funds used to pay medical expenses (see Table 10.2). This fraction is known as the "medical loss ratio." The largest expense category is physician services. Although hospitals are the largest expenditure item in the National Health Expenditure accounts, HMOs' tight controls over hospitals and coverage of a generally younger and healthier population, means that less than a third of HMO premiums are used to pay for inpatient hospital services. Some of the HMOs' other expenses are reinsurance (to keep the plan solvent and ensure that patients' bills are paid even if the plan should have a catastrophic loss), taxes, emergency out-of-area services, and certain highly specialized treatments that must be paid for on a FFS basis to noncontracted providers. Over time, the HMO business has become much more price competitive. Administrative expenses and profit margins have been cut as plans become more efficient; therefore, the percentage of total dollars going to treatment (the medical loss ratio) has risen. In earlier years, wide variations of ±25 percent were not uncommon. With more experience and better information, competitive standards have been set so that most HMOs offer a similar price (perhaps ±10 percent) for most benefit packages (see Table 10.2).

TABLE 10.2	HMO Expenses as a % of Premiums

Physician and outpatient	41%	
Inpatient	31%	"Medical Loss Ratio" = 82%
Outside referrals	7%	
Emergency	3%	
Administrative	13%	
Profit	5%	

Source: Hoescht Marion Roussel *Managed Care Digest 1995.*

10.3 THE RANGE OF MANAGED CARE PLANS

The variety and possible configurations of managed care are too diverse for any single definition. It is better to think in terms of a range from unmanaged to tightly managed as illustrated in Figure 10.2. At one end, under FFS medicine with indemnity insurance, the health plan takes all the financial risk but exercises no medical management. Whatever hospitalization, surgery, or drugs any physician decides to order are paid for by the insurance company without question. There is no haggling over prices. Any difference between premiums and expenses becomes a gain or loss to the insurance company, but has no effect on the hospital or physician. The only "control" comes from making the patient pay for some deductibles, coinsurance, or excess over the plan maximums. At the other end is the closed CPGP HMO in which a single organization combines the functions of medical provider and insurance company. It enrolls members; builds hospitals; employs physicians, nurses, and therapists on salary; purchases drugs, beds, cardiac pacemakers, etc.; and controls all finances. Any difference between premiums and expenses is a gain or loss to be shared with the physician group.[8] In between these two ends are a range of contracts that link medicine and insurance, but stop short of combining them into a single organization.

Provider Networks

Under pure indemnity insurance, the contract is solely between the patient and the insurance company. Upon evidence of loss (a bill), the insurance company sends a check to the patient, who is responsible for all relationships with the providers. A managed care organization arises when the insurance company begins to make contracts with physicians and hospitals, forming a network of providers. A **Preferred Provider Organization (PPO)** limits the patient's choice of physicians and hospitals by paying in full (or a larger percentage) only for care received from approved providers within the network. Patients can choose to see a physician outside the plan or to stay in a hospital that is not part of the preferred group if they are willing to pay a larger portion of the bill (see Table 10.3).

A PPO is a contractual intermediary, a corporate entity created by a group of doctors, an entrepreneur, a hospital chain, a union, an employer coalition, or the insurer.[9] It will have procedures to certify providers (valid licenses, meet standards, produce reports and statistics) and a specification for reimbursement (per diems, discounted fees, other), some of which may depend on restrictions ("we get all of your heart surgery") or volume discounts. Contracts may be open or exclusive—a physician may belong to one or many

FIGURE 10.2	The Range of Managed Care Plans

Indemnity FFS	UR	PPO	Open HMO	Closed HMO

No management controls ←————————————→ *Tight management controls*

TABLE 10.3 Hypothetical PPO Payment

	Within Network	Outside Provider
Hospital	100%	80%
Physician	90%	75%
Therapist	90%	50%
Pharmacies	no copay	$10 copay
Drugs		
In formulary	covered	50%
Not in formulary	not covered	not covered

PPOs, an MCO may have one PPO or many, a PPO may contract with one hospital or many, a PPO may contract with one MCO or many. The overlapping contracts and gaps can make the relationships and flow of funds rather complex—and may be one cause of the difficulties currently faced by many MCOs. Usually, the term "HMO" is applied to a plan offering care through a single, fairly limited network. A hybrid HMO-**POS** (**point of service**) allows patients to obtain care cheaply within the HMO network, but also to opt-out "at the point of service" and see any other provider by paying extra. The differences between a PPO, HMO, and an HMO/POS can be subtle, so much so that patients may not even know exactly what type of plan they are covered by unless they examine the contract closely. Many large insurers such as Blue Cross now offer **triple option** plans, in which the enrollee can chose the HMO, the PPO, or indemnity insurance, with the premium increasing in steps as the controls over utilization become weaker.

Gatekeeping

Two restrictions tend to mark the transition from partially managed PPO and POS plans to HMOs: (1) mandatory authorization for hospitalization and (2) primary physicians who act as gatekeepers. Mandatory authorization means that the physician must get on the phone to the health plan and explain why the patient needs hospitalization and document the severity of illness to obtain approval before admitting the patient. Under a **gatekeeper** system, patients must receive all their primary care from a single physician, and any specialist referrals, surgery, prescriptions, and hospitalizations must be approved in advance by the gatekeeper primary physician. In this way, the plan is able to delegate responsibility for cost control and appropriateness to the primary care physician (PCP).

Capitation

Gatekeeper physicians are commonly paid a capitation rate, a fixed amount **per member per month (PMPM)** (currently about $20-$40) for each person enrolled with them.[10] They must provide all primary care for each person and act as a manager by coordinating and approving all other services. Capitation is sometimes used for hospitalization, for laboratory services, and even for certain types of specialty care (heart transplants, oncology, mental health and substance abuse treatment). These are often referred to as "carve-outs" or "subcapitation." Paying for the number of people enrolled rather than the number of services rendered changes the economic incentives from "doing more" (FFS) to "doing less" (capitation). With fixed payments per member made in advance, profits are greater when fewer services are used.

MANAGING PHARMACY COSTS: CARVE-OUTS AND TRIPLE-TIER BENEFITS

In the past, Medicare and most employer indemnity insurance plans did not pay for the cost of pharmaceuticals taken by patients outside the hospital. Outpatient drugs were fairly cheap, billing information was hard to obtain, and therefore benefits were limited. As the cost of pharmaceuticals rose and information systems expanded, it became easier and more valuable to provide prescription coverage. It is now common for employer plans to have a pharmaceutical component, and there is strong political pressure to add drug coverage to Medicare. Yet dispensing prescriptions is sufficiently different from other types of medical services that most insurance companies subcontract with specialized firms called Pharmacy Benefit Managers (PBMs). Thus, it is actually the PBM (not Blue Cross or Aetna) that processes the claims and pays the pharmacy. Drugs have become a carve-out benefit because the PBMs can do the job better, at lower cost.

How do PBMs manage care to save costs? First, they obtain **price discounts** and rebates. PBMs are large, handling millions of prescriptions a year, and can use their market power at both ends: manufacturing (pharmaceutical companies) and retail (pharmacy chains). Second, they can use **substitution.** A recent study showed that mandatory generic substitution (MGS) reduced average costs by 8 percent.[11] In such a contract, the insurance only pays for the generic version of a drug if the Food and Drug Administration (FDA) has deemed it equivalent to the more expensive brand-name version, regardless of how the prescription is written. While 8 percent may not seem like a lot, it is larger than the profit margins in most retail businesses.

More sophisticated contracts divide drugs into tiers to provide incentives for patients to actively cooperate in **reducing the use** of expensive drugs. In the sample three-tier plan shown here, the most favored tier 1 drugs have only a $2 co-payment. These are generic versions of expensive brand-name drugs or brands for which the PBM has negotiated a large discount or rebate. Tier 2, with $10 co-payments, is made up of drugs on an approved list (formulary)—drugs with no generic equivalent, drugs with small discounts, and the like. Tier 3, in which patients face a hefty $30 co-payment, is reserved for the expensive brand name drugs that have a generic equivalent in tier 1, drugs of limited usefulness or drugs that are frequently prescribed for off-label (i.e., not approved by the FDA) purposes, or expensive drugs whose benefits seem relatively minor (Viagra, Cox-2 inhibitor, and low-dose antihistamines might fall into this tier).

Sample Triple-Tier Drug Benefit Plan

Category	Patient Co-pay	Types of Drugs
Tier 1	$2	generics, sole source
Tier 2	$10	approved formulary
Tier 3	$30	off-patent brands, lifestyle

Tiered pharmacy benefit plans were relatively rare a decade ago, but are now found in 85 percent of large employee health insurance plans.12 They have been shown to reduce total costs by increasing rates of generic substitution and by (slightly) reducing the number of prescriptions filled. What may be even more important to employers, though, is that they provide a relatively simple way of shifting more of the cost to the employee (all those co-payments add up). Indeed, dissatisfaction with large and repeated co-payments make the integrated CPGP-HMO solution, in which the HMO has an in-house pharmacy and uses salaried pharmacists to distribute drugs, look more attractive—and is one reason for the sudden influx of veterans who have other insurance plans moving into the Department of Veterans Affairs (VA) health system.

What, then, keeps the HMO from doing less and less until it maximizes profits by providing no services at all? Quite simply, the need to attract new members and keep the old ones. Competition and the potential loss of enrollment makes HMOs strive to maintain quality and patient satisfaction. In FFS, profits increase as more is done. What keeps a surgeon from performing an unnecessary operation in order to make more money? Control over excessive surgery under FFS is largely a matter of professional ethics and disapproval by peers, since there is no external reporting and no manager who intervenes to question the appropriateness of treatment.

Withholds

All HMOs must use FFS payment for some types of care, especially for specialty services in which use by enrollees is rare and unpredictable. **Withholds** are a way of incorporating part of the cost-control incentive of capitation into FFS payment. An HMO specialty referral withhold plan might work as follows: Each specialist receives 80 percent of the agreed amount at the time the patient is treated. The other 20 percent goes into the withhold pool. The HMO projects a total dollar expenditure for specialty referral services for the year. If the total of referral bills from all specialists is at or below that amount at the end of the year, the withhold pool is distributed in accordance with the amounts billed. In this case, the specialist receives 100 percent of the amount billed, but has to wait until the end of the year to receive the last 20 percent. However, if the total billings are more than 20 percent above the projected total, the HMO keeps the withhold pool to help pay for the unanticipated extra volume. In this way, part of the risk of overutilization is shared with the specialists. If the total bills are more than 100 percent of the projected total, but less than 120 percent, the specialists and the HMO split the withhold pool at the end of the year.

Utilization Review

Some of the other management interventions used to control cost and utilization include the following:

- **Second opinion**—A second doctor must review the record and concur with the initial doctor's recommendation before surgery is performed.
- **Precertification**—Approval must be obtained in advance from the insurance company before elective surgery is performed.
- **Pre-admission testing**—A requirement that many tests be performed in advance on an outpatient basis so that the patient spends fewer days in the hospital.
- **Concurrent review**—Regular evaluations are made by a case control nurse to authorize a continued stay in the hospital or additional procedures.
- **Database profiling**—Graphs and charts indicating the number of services used per 1,000 patients by each doctor or hospital are maintained to identify abnormally high or low patterns of utilization.
- **Intensive case management**—A nurse in the insurance company follows and manages any case expected to cost more than $10,000.
- **Generic substitution**—A prescription for a brand-name drug is filled with a cheaper generic version if the two are deemed equivalent by the FDA.
- **Discharge planning**—A social worker meets with the patient and family early to facilitate rapid transfer back home or to a nursing home.

- **Retrospective review**—An evaluation is conducted after the patient is discharged from the hospital to deny payment for any medically unnecessary services.

- **Audits**—An insurance company representative ensures that all services billed for were actually performed.

10.4 HOW CARE IS MANAGED: A MENTAL HEALTH EXAMPLE

To illustrate how care is managed, some typical procedures in **managed behavioral health (MBH)**—managed care subcapitated carve-out plans for mental health and substance abuse treatment—are presented here and contrasted with FFS indemnity practice.[13] An insured person might seek help for a behavioral problem by calling a specialist (usually a psychiatrist or psychologist) or might have a behavioral problem noted by a physician during a medical visit ("Gee, Mr. X, as your doctor I would like to suggest that having five drinks after dinner every night may have something to do with your chronic fatigue and stomach pains."). Or the problem may not get noticed until a crisis occurs. Many times an FFS physician with a patient who has a behavioral problem will suspect that substance abuse is a primary or contributing factor, yet because the patient is in denial or is afraid of stigmatization, the physician will continue treatment using a nondescriptive diagnosis (stomach pain, anxiety) or make a referral to a psychiatrist. This leads to costly and ineffective treatment.

Talking with a psychiatrist while under the influence of drugs is a great way to waste $125 an hour. Often the real problem is not treated until it erupts and requires emergency attention (nervous breakdown, paranoia, abuse of family members, arrest for driving under the influence of alcohol or drugs). Unfortunately, the closest hospital emergency room is not the best place for drug detoxification or treatment of a mental health problem, yet under indemnity insurance, Mr. X is likely to be taken there. He might then be sent to a psychiatric hospital, where he will be kept for 28 days. Why 28? Because that is the standard FFS insurance benefit for alcohol treatment. After discharge, Mr. X may repeat the cycle of crisis and hospital admission. Eventually, he will either get better, or lose his job and his insurance.

With MBH, Mr. X is more likely to receive treatment prior to crisis. His employer will have an employee assistance program (EAP) with a confidential toll-free number that he, his physician, a family member, or his supervisor may call. An appointment will be made for an initial discussion with a trained counselor (CAC, M.S.W, Ph.D., M.D., or other certification) employed by the MBH or a practice that performs evaluations under a high-volume, low-cost ($30 to $75) contract. Evaluations are usually done within 72 hours, with immediate arrangements made for the appropriate form of therapy.

Waiting until crisis hits means lost wages and lost productivity for the employer and costly ($20,000 or more) inpatient hospitalization. The MBH evaluator can often place the employee in less costly and confining intensive outpatient programs or halfway houses that allow people to continue to work while being treated, which are less disruptive to personal and family life and tend to decrease the chance of relapse. Once Mr. X is alcohol free and can benefit from psychological therapy, he will receive it. In severe cases, the counselor will make a referral directly to residential programs that specialize in "dual-diagnosis" (i.e., mental illness with substance abuse) treatment. The coordinated treatment of mental health and substance abuse in MBH illustrates two principles: substitution (use the less expensive mode of treatment) and appropriateness (reduce length of treatment by more precise matching of services to the patient's needs). Substitution and appropriate treatment are primary methods used by managed care to achieve cost reductions.

Even if the diagnosis is made during a crisis admission, MBH is apt to handle it more efficiently. Under FFS, an emergency psychiatric patient is often admitted for an inpatient stay at the receiving hospital. Emergency admissions often take place at inner-city hospitals, where research-oriented university facilities geared toward complex cases costing more than $1,000 a day are common, and where the clinical professors may have little interest in treating another routine alcohol abuse case. A Friday-night admission to a teaching facility may mean the postponement of a definitive diagnosis until Monday or Tuesday.

In contrast, receiving an HMO MBH patient obligates the emergency room staff to contact the managed care plan before admission. The patient may be transported to a more appropriate facility costing only one-half or one-third as much per day, and a treatment plan including provisions for discharge and community services must be filed within twenty-four hours in order for the bills to be paid. Once the patient is admitted, the case manager will authorize an expected number of days for treatment in consultation with the attending physician. Then, every day, the case manager will call the facility to conduct **concurrent review,** checking on the patient's progress, determining whether additional days are needed or if early discharge is possible, and arranging for post-hospitalization services and community support. The medicine may be similar, but the management is quite different.

Bulk contracting allows the MBH to insist on uniform reporting to better monitor the quality of care. Building a provider network by negotiating standard contractual agreements with mental health and substance abuse treatment providers is a crucial task for determining the efficiency of the managed care plan. With a network in place, the MBH can create statistical profiles to determine which therapists tend to take longer to complete treatment, or whose patients are most likely to be readmitted or suffer other problems.

Profiling illustrates the difference between managed care and FFS approaches to quality. In managed care, quality is defined by the experience of the group, on how well most patients do relative to what can be expected. Only a large plan with a comprehensive and uniform information system can do the profiling necessary to measure quality in this way. While the individual examination of a single FFS case might appear to be more detailed, it is methodologically flawed because it lacks a standard and is subject to random variation. Consider how foolish it would be to assert that skydiving is safer than walking just because I survived ten parachute jumps while my friend got killed the first time he went for a hike. Thinking in terms of the group and making comparisons to a standard based on large numbers of cases are the basic tools that make quality assurance under managed care more effective than individual efforts under FFS.

Capitation gives the MBH firm an incentive to control costs, but direct financial incentives play a relatively minor role in the management of care. Most of the time, just knowing that costs are being monitored and that additional resource use must be justified and documented is sufficient to make providers work more efficiently. A therapist feels embarrassed being called to task for violating what he or she knows to be the principles of quality care, and that concern may eliminate the biggest sources of waste—admissions made without any thought given to a treatment plan, heavy medications used to keep a patient in a holding pattern, weekend days in idle observation, and failure to consider discharge and community support services.

Behavioral health is the area in which management has proven most effective at reducing cost while raising quality and patient satisfaction.[14] Why? In part because mental health and substance abuse are difficult to define objectively, hence subject to significant moral hazard and even fraud. During the 1980s, admitting patients for inpatient psychiatric care had become so profitable that many hospitals aggressively sought extra patients, with some stepping over the line by paying kickbacks for referrals or by holding patients much longer than necessary (sometimes even against the wishes of patients and family members). Abuses by one psychiatric hospital chain were so widespread that the company was taken to court and fined $400 million.[15] Although the outright fraud and profiteering that characterized the worst part of the FFS psychiatric industry were relatively rare, they tainted the entire industry and indicated a lack of concern with the cost to the patient, the employer, and the government, which demanded a concerted response.

Capitation and case management allowed doctors to provide better care and still reduce mental health and substance abuse treatment costs by 50 percent or more, significantly greater than the 10 to 25 percent savings achieved elsewhere in medicine. Another reason management was so successful in reforming behavioral health care was the expanding availability of a competent non-M.D. workforce and clear benefit from specialization. Certified Alcoholism Counselors paid $25 per hour were as effective, or more effective, than M.D.s costing many times more. Residential rehabilitation facilities could be run with nurses and psychologists for $180 per day rather than the $1,250 per day paid for emergency admission to an urban teaching hospital. Social workers could be trained to deal with eating disorders, grief, and family violence so that M.D. physicians' time was spent on acute treatment and prescription of appropriate medication. In no other area of medicine were strides made so quickly to comprehensively change the structure of the system in a way that provided more personalized care, more patient satisfaction, and lower costs.

10.5 INDIVIDUAL AND SYSTEM RISKS IN HEALTH CARE

It is important to distinguish between the variation in individual medical costs and variation in system costs. The variation between individuals regarding medical costs is very great, more than a thousand to one. A fair number of individuals have minimal costs, while some unfortunate few face bills of hundreds of thousands of dollars in the absence of health insurance. However, by placing everyone into a single insurance pool, individual risk is diversified away: each person can cover his or her expected losses by paying a modest premium in advance. A group of 10,000 people has reasonably predictable health care costs, and a group of 100,000 has negligible variation in average costs due to the random variation among the individuals who make up the group. To the individual, even substantial differences in average costs mean very little. For two people worried about medical bills, it is the one who gets most ill who will spend more, not the one who belongs to the more expensive health care system. On the other hand, at the aggregate level, random individual variation averages out and systematic differences dominate. Comparisons among small areas within the United States (see section 7.5) and among countries (chapter 19) reveal major differences in the average level of spending that are not explainable by differences in health status or random variation (Figure 10.3). Managed care seeks to capitalize on these systematic differences in the average level of health care costs among groups.[16] Whereas an insurer pools risks so that the individual can cover losses with an actuarially fair premium equal to the average, the managed care organization seeks to reduce the average. Since it deals in large groups, the managed care organization must take on the function of an insurer as it tries to reduce costs, but those insurance functions are, in a sense, incidental to the central purpose of managing care: controlling costs while maintaining quality.

The **business risks** to an HMO should be distinguished from the risks to participating physicians, hospitals, and patients (see Figure 10.4). The major risks to the individual, random variation in illness or health status, are diversified away for any HMO with a large number of members. The more relevant individual (client) risks to an HMO are related to marketing: selection and volume. An HMO attracting a larger proportion of seriously ill

FIGURE 10.3   Financial Risks in Health Care

Cost Variability	=	**Health Variability**	+	**Resource Use Variability**
		(individual 1,000:1)		5:1 between small areas (Wennberg)
		(group, diversified away)		4:1 between countries (OECD comparisons)

people will suffer financially from adverse selection as much as any other insurer.[17] The more serious marketing risk is the inability to attract a sufficient number of clients. To break even, a certain volume must be attained, and growth is a primary determinant of profitability. In this case, HMOs are similar to most other businesses. Indeed, the primary risks an investor must evaluate in considering HMO profitability are standard business risks: pricing (capitation rate); input prices (e.g., per diem hospital costs, cost of referrals); and productivity (how much labor and capital it takes to run the HMO).[18] The "core competency" of an HMO is identified in Figure 10.4 as allocative efficiency, the ability of an HMO to match patient needs to care providers to reduce costs while maintaining or increasing satisfaction.

The willingness to moderate and, when necessary, override the provisions in the financial contracts is essential for managed care operations. Although most patients fall within the normal range, there are some exceptional cases, and the manager maintains the morale and motivation of the provider network by making appropriate exceptions. Just as government intervention is required to blunt raw market forces to put a kind face on capitalism, the manager is required to judiciously consider medical realities and put a kind face on the HMO contract. If all contracts were perfectly self-enforcing and there were no need for human intervention, then "managed care" would disappear and a legalistic software program could run the system. Rules are necessary, but analysts err when they identify managed care with the contracts that constitute the legal definition of the plan. In the real world, it takes people to deal with people, and often a physician to deal with other physicians. Two HMOs may have identical contracts and one could be very successful while the other fails, and the reason for the difference is management. There is

FIGURE 10.4   Capitated Provider's Business Risks

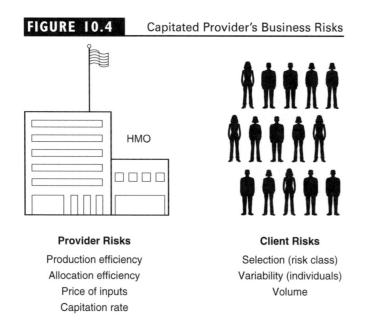

Provider Risks	**Client Risks**
Production efficiency	Selection (risk class)
Allocation efficiency	Variability (individuals)
Price of inputs	Volume
Capitation rate	

good management and bad management, just as there are good surgeons and bad surgeons. Education and intelligence make a difference, but in the end there is an undefinable quality that separates the winners from the losers. A major function of the market is to practice what Joseph Schumpeter called the "creative destruction" of capitalism, rewarding managers who come up with new ideas and organizations that meet consumers' needs, and allowing better organizations to grow by displacing firms whose structure is out of date or whose management is bad.[19]

10.6 KAISER: THE EVOLUTION OF AN HMO

Kaiser Health Plan, with more than 9.8 million members, is the largest HMO in the United States, and one of the largest medical delivery systems in the world. Its origins lie in the efforts of a young surgeon, Sydney R. Garfield, to find a place to practice when he completed residency at Los Angeles County Hospital in 1933.[20] The disastrous economy of the Depression made it impossible to open up a new solo FFS practice in Los Angeles as he wished to do, so Dr. Garfield reluctantly began looking for a salaried job to tide him over until times improved. The Metropolitan Water District was building an aqueduct from the Colorado River to Los Angeles and was looking for a physician to staff a small clinic to treat construction workers in the desert. Garfield thought the salary they offered, $125 a month, was too little for someone as well trained as himself. With the support of a local doctor as partner, he decided to open his own hospital at Desert Center. The construction companies were very anxious to have a doctor for their workers and agreed to help Garfield and send all their industrial medicine cases insured under the new workers' compensation plan to his facility. Garfield opened a top-notch hospital, complete with modern operating facilities and air conditioning, an unheard of luxury for industrial workers at that time.

The injured workers and the construction companies loved the facility, but two financial problems quickly arose. The workers' compensation insurance companies thought Garfield treated the workers too well, and they argued over many of the bills submitted. Garfield also treated the men for non-industrial illnesses, but few could afford to pay private practice fees for extended hospital stays or major surgery, even though Garfield felt obligated to treat them. Garfield threatened to close the hospital unless he could obtain a steady source of funding. The foundations of a major innovation in health care financing were laid when an executive of the major workers' compensation insurance companies suggested that they pre-pay Garfield by giving him one-eighth of the worker's compensation insurance premium, which amounted to $1.50 per month for each of the 5,000 construction workers on the project, and for workers to voluntarily pre-pay an additional $1.50 per month to cover all non-industrial accidents and illnesses.[21] Garfield's experiment in prepaid HMO medicine was very successful. He added two more hospitals; at the end of five years, as construction slowed and the hospitals began to close, Garfield had made a net profit of more than $250,000 (equivalent to $3 million after adjustment for inflation to 2002).

Although Garfield intended to take his profits and set up a private practice in Los Angeles, he was lured north to open another prepaid workers' clinic by one of the aqueduct contractors, Henry J. Kaiser, who had just made a deal to complete the Grand Coulee Dam in Oregon. Kaiser was impressed by the efficiency and high quality of Garfield's operation in the desert and felt that establishing a similar facility would help him attract workers to another remote construction site. At Grand Coulee, SR Garfield & Associates provided twenty-four-hour medical coverage to 15,000 workers and family members in a modernized and, once again, air-conditioned hospital with a group of five physicians and six nurses. Garfield himself, however, remained in Los Angeles undergoing more medical training and looking after business interests, flying to Grand Coulee and working in the clinic only once every six weeks. It was as a manager that Garfield made the health plan successful, while his status as a physician gave him a special connection with the professionals who worked under his direction. He was, in the words of one of the physicians who worked for him, "a genius at keeping salaries and expenses down."

With Grand Coulee nearing completion and Garfield ordered up for service in the Army Medical Corps during World War II, it appeared that his days as an entrepreneur were over. However, Kaiser had just been given a new contract to construct sixty freighters at a hastily organized shipyard in Richmond, near San Francisco, and he wanted Garfield to provide the medical care for his wartime crew. Within a year, Garfield built a hospital and was caring for 90,000 workers. His commitment to staying at the forefront of medical practice is evidenced by the establishment of a research program and a new journal, the *Permanente* (Kaiser) *Foundation Medical Bulletin*, in 1943. By 1944, Garfield had a hundred doctors working for him to care for more than 200,000 workers and dependents. Although his first recruits were outstanding doctors from Stanford University, the University of Southern California, and other leading medical schools who wished to join a prepaid group practice, others were hired only because they were unfit for military service and needed a job. From them, Garfield learned an important management lesson, which he later stated as, "No matter how the principles of our plan are meant, if you don't have the physician group who have it in their hearts and who believe in prepaid practice, it won't work," emphasizing that it is the culture and the people even more than the financial contracts that define a successful HMO.[22]

As fast as the war had created a need for the Kaiser medical plan, the end of the war took it away. The only clinic not to suffer a major enrollment decline was the one at the new Kaiser steel mill in Fontana, in the desert outside Los Angeles. The Alameda County and San Francisco medical societies, tolerant during the war emergency, grew openly hostile. Kaiser doctors were denied medical society membership, and hence could not join hospital medical staffs or participate in many forms of professional advancement. Yet Garfield, Kaiser, and many of their closest associates, including health economist Avram Yedidia, decided that the appropriate course of action was to regroup and expand their visionary health plan rather than shut it down. In the immediate postwar period, enrollment stabilized at fewer than 20,000. By 1948, it had rebounded to 60,000, with much of the growth coming from marketing to unions and firms whose employees would join as a group.

Yet the pressures of fluctuating enrollment, requirements for capital, and a need for clearer lines of authority made the entrepreneurial organization, with Sydney Garfield alone in charge of all the Kaiser health facilities, untenable. The new structure had three entities: a charitable corporation for the hospitals, a nonprofit foundation for the health plan, and a private for-profit partnership for the physician group. Garfield was paid $257,000 for his interest in the hospitals, and subsequently gave up his interest in the partnership, so that by 1949 he was just an employee, albeit a very important one. By 1952, enrollment reached 250,000, but the organizational difficulties were not over, and financial disputes between the health plan and the physician groups had become serious. In 1955, Garfield resigned his post as executive director, and a new profit-sharing plan for the physician group was drafted. The medical group was to be paid on a capitation basis, have a pension plan, and get half of all revenues in excess of the funds needed for expenses, capital replacement, and reserves for distribution as bonuses. This financial agreement between Kaiser Health Plan and the Permanente Medical Group has continued essentially unchanged for the past fifty years.

In 1962, enrollment exceeded 1 million subscribers and dependents, 2.5 million in 1972, and 10 million in 2002. Kaiser health plans have maintained an enviable record of growth over forty years, more than doubling in most decades. Although Kaiser remains strongest in its initial market areas around San Francisco, Los Angeles, and Portland, it has expanded to Hawaii, Colorado, Connecticut, North Carolina, and Washington, D.C. Yet even as the forces of managed care began to revolutionize the U.S. health care system, Kaiser, the exemplar of prepaid organized medical practice, had begun to falter.[23] The Kaiser plan established in Hartford, Connecticut, was unable to grow past 30,000 members after ten years, below break-even size. To penetrate the competitive Washington, D.C., and North Carolina markets, Kaiser departed from its traditional closed-staff model and set up open, IPA HMOs contracting with already-established local physicians. Despite—or because of—these changes, Kaiser in 1994 suffered its first enrollment decline in fifty years. A once-dominant and innovative organization had drifted, giving up its core competency to imitate the newer IPA HMOs that could grow rapidly by just signing contracts. After losing hundreds of millions of dollars, Kaiser finally regrouped and recovered in the year 2000. When the federal HMO Act was passed in 1973, Kaiser accounted for more than 2 million of the 3 million total HMO enrollees in the United States, a market share of 70 percent. By 2002, although still the largest HMO, Kaiser's 10 million enrollees represented less than a 10 percent market share.

10.7 OWNERSHIP AND CAPITAL MARKETS: SIGNS OF FAILURE

The Kaiser Health Plan operated as a nonprofit foundation; thus, there were no stockholders or individual owners who stood to gain by expanding into new markets. To some extent, it might seem as though the physicians were shareholders, but in one important way they clearly were not owners. When each new region got started, it took capital from the existing Kaiser foundation. However, once the region was up and running, no "returns" were paid back. The physicians who had given up some current income to enable the new offshoot to grow gained nothing. Thus, it is not surprising that Kaiser plans grew robustly where they were already established (since that medical group stood to benefit), but had difficulty obtaining the resources to move into new areas. Garfield built Kaiser single-handedly, but after 1949, he held no legal ownership interest, and in 1955 he was forced out. Garfield was apparently willing to do it for the glory, but the fact is that someone of his talent and training would surely have ended up a wealthier man if he had stuck with his original plan to open an FFS surgical practice in Los Angeles. The incomplete and complex ownership structure was not able to protect his interest, nor was it able to maximize the potential of the Kaiser Health Plan.

GHA: A Consumer Co-op Gets Bought Out by a Franchise Chain

The history of another of the first HMOs makes a similar point regarding ownership. Group Health Association (GHA) of Washington, D.C., was founded in 1937 as a consumer's cooperative to provide physician services to its members, largely federal employees. The physicians were employees, not partners. The American Medical Association and the D.C. medical society sought to put GHA out of business, and GHA's victorious antitrust suit, which was affirmed by the U.S. Supreme Court in 1943, was considered crucial to the survival and growth of all HMOs, including Kaiser. Yet ten years later, GHA still had fewer than 20,000 members. The cooperative structure legally made every subscriber an owner. Some existing members were ambivalent about letting large unions join, since it would change the dynamics of control. A basic management function, marketing, was the subject of great ideological debates rather than concerted action. GHA did become more solidly established after becoming an option in the Federal Employees Health Benefits Program, reaching 50,000 members in 1962 and 100,000 in 1975. An attempt by the physicians to set up a medical group partnership similar to that at Kaiser met with resistance from GHA members and their elected board. As a chronicle of GHA observes, the physicians "failed to comprehend GHA's special environment, in which the members instinctively reacted against the notion of a profit motive."[24] Unable to form a corporate medical group, GHA's physicians formed a union in 1977 and went on strike in April 1978. GHA continued to suffer financial reversals and labor disagreements. The nurses and physical therapists went on strike in 1982, and the physicians struck again in 1986. GHA weathered the storm, but continued to struggle. Enrollment reached 150,000 in 1986 and 200,000 in 1992. In 1994, unable to persevere in an increasingly competitive market, GHA was acquired by Humana. Thus, an organization that had begun as a consumer cooperative became part of a for-profit chain, one of whose founders had honed his business skills developing the Colonel Sanders Kentucky Fried Chicken franchise.

The rapid expansion of HMOs from 10 million enrollees in 1980 to 100 million in 2002 occurred mostly within the corporate for-profit structure. Many HMOs that started as nonprofits switched to for-profit to take better advantage of their market opportunities. Why have for-profit firms been more successful, and why didn't they emerge earlier? Sydney Garfield dreamed of "one organized integrality" that encompassed all of medicine as a business, including hospitals, laboratories, physicians, financing, and marketing under one roof. He was able to maintain unified control by force of personality during Kaiser's formative years, but lost control when confronted by these vital questions: Who can borrow enough money to build a hospital? How are wages to be set once profits start rolling in? How can one physician single-handedly manage a group of doctors too large for all of them to be personal friends? The common answer to all of these questions lay in the "corporatization" of health care organizations.[25]

Corporate Advantage

In a corporation, control is more clearly defined. The board of directors has the power to appoint senior management, which, in turn, has the power to hire and fire employees, purchase assets, and borrow money. The stockholders have a clear right to the profits. However, being numerous and diffuse, these stockholders usually have little control over the management of operations. The corporate structure is able to delegate authority and establish accountability reasonably well. Opponents of for-profit health care might argue that nonprofit organizations can be very well managed. In fact, nonprofit and for-profit hospitals both have boards of directors and suites full of administrators who seem to look and act similar in most ways. The difference is the nonprofit organization's lack of direct ownership. No one in a nonprofit organization has the incentive, or the power, to take a big risk in the hope of achieving a large capital gain. Furthermore, the lack of unified control makes it hard for any one person to make rapid and risky decisions on behalf of the whole organization in times of turbulent change and emerging opportunity.

A nonprofit structure with diffuse ownership may actually be an advantage when leadership requires achieving a consensus among a large number of stakeholder groups. Such a situation was characteristic for most community hospitals from 1950 to 1980. Yet when profits and survival depend on hard bargaining, innovation and quick commitments to capture opportunities that expand and disappear in a moment, the diffuse voluntary structure is overwhelmed. It is simply harder for an entrepreneur to work in a nonprofit structure or to take the organization he or she has built and sell it for a large capital gain.

U.S. Healthcare: A Profitable Growth Company

U.S. Healthcare, founded by Leonard Abramson in 1975, is a good example of the new for-profit HMO firms that are coming to dominate the market. Abramson was from a South Philadelphia family of modest means and had driven a taxi to put himself through pharmacy school. After working as a detailer calling on physicians for a pharmaceutical firm (see chapter 12), six years in retail pharmacy, and participation in equipment leasing and other health care businesses, Abramson was astounded by the freedom of doctors and hospitals to raise prices whenever they wanted. "It was a blank check," he said in a 1985 interview.[26] Abramson was much taken with the promise of HMOs to bring business methods to health care and knew a number of physicians who shared his enthusiasm. Taking advantage of the government loans made available by the HMO Act of 1973, the Health Maintenance Organization of Pennsylvania was incorporated as a nonprofit prepaid health plan in January 1975, obtained a state HMO license in 1976, and was designated as a federally qualified HMO in 1977.[27] Operations started in April 1977 by taking over the assets of an existing prepaid health plan, Family Medical Care. HMO/PA began enrolling members and grew rapidly. In 1981, U.S. Healthcare went private, using venture capital from Warburg, Pincus and Company, paying back a $2.5 million loan to the federal government. Its initial public offering of stock came in 1983, as did its expansion into New Jersey.

The Philadelphia market of the 1980s was old-style traditional medicine: lots of specialists, lots of hospital beds, and FFS indemnity insurance. With changing medical trends and the advent of Medicare's prospective payment by DRG (see Chapter 8), it was becoming clear that there was a surplus of hospitals in the area and that even good specialists were having some trouble attracting all the patients they wanted. There was room for an entrepreneur who could cut premiums by contracting in advance for surgery and beds at a discount. Abramson was a sharp negotiator. It often seemed that he came into a bargaining session knowing more about a hospital's operations and finances than its administrators. Discounts of 20 percent, 30 percent, or more were often won. Abramson made information a weapon in the fight for market share and low prices, and honed it to a fine edge in repeated competitive encounters.

Not everyone was enamored of U.S. Healthcare's tactics. Some hospitals were terrified that they would lose so much revenue that they might go out of business, and the Philadelphia Blue Cross plan was furious that an upstart was trying to invade its market by cutting prices.[28] The acrimony spilled over into name calling, then full-page attack advertisements in the newspapers, and finally a series of lawsuits charging libel and unfair trading on both sides (most of which were settled or won by U.S. Healthcare, although bad feelings between the two companies continued to run high). By 1985 U.S. Healthcare, with more than 500,000 enrollees, was the sixth-largest HMO in the nation, and probably the most profitable. Its medical loss ratio was only 75 percent, whereas the average was closer to 80 percent, and Kaiser was above 95 percent.[29] The formula of aggressive contracting, meticulous claims review, and conscientious client service made the company successful and financially sound, although with less than a 20 percent market share it was far from dominant and was not universally loved.

Abramson was not content to let the company rest on its laurels and pile up profits. He made a strategic decision to emphasize quality. Whereas most primary care physician incentive payments in the original HMO/PA reimbursement plan were cost controls dependent on reductions in the quantity of referrals and other services used, the Quality Care Compensation System (QCCS) for primary physicians, inaugurated in 1987, based 40 percent of practice bonuses on quality and consumer satisfaction measures. The 1992 QCCS revision raised the bar further, making 82 percent of incentives reliant on medical chart review, availability of evening hours, retention of existing patients, ability to attract new members, and ratings on questionnaires mailed to patients, with only 18 percent related to reductions in utilization.[30] For hospitals, the CapTainer™ payment system introduced in 1992 paid a quality- and diagnosis-adjusted per diem rate. Quality incentive plans were introduced for obstetrician/gynecologists in 1994 and for other referral specialists in 1996.[31] However, the most important part of the new strategy was the development of a new corporate subsidiary in 1990, USQA, devoted solely to quality measurement. USQA created databanks based on millions of patient records, consumer surveys, pathology reports, and laboratory tests. The physician-information scientists working at USQA published significant studies on the cost-effectiveness of laparascopic cholecystectomy, asthma treatment, influenza immunization, and autologous bone marrow transplantation for treatment of breast cancer. It used $2 million to fund a fellowship in Managed Care and Quality Assessment at Jefferson Medical College. In 1993, U.S. Healthcare was the first HMO to release the full 1992 Health Employer Data and Information Set (HEDIS) report and, in 1994, the first to provide members with a detailed report card on each participating physician.[32] U.S. Healthcare had clearly gone far beyond compliance and established a leading presence in the quality assurance and health care information field.[33]

Growth continued to climb, reaching 1 million members in 1989 and 2 million members in 1995. In the face of such rising demand, Abramson's announcement that he would cut premiums in order to build market share came as quite a surprise.[34] Publicly traded HMO stocks fell by as much as 16 percent the following day. Yet the strategy of favoring long-term growth over short-term profitability was sound, and share prices soon recovered. U.S. Healthcare ended the year trading at 46_, with a total market capitalization of $7.1 billion. In April 1996, Aetna Life & Casualty declared that it would acquire Abramson's company.[35] The information and quality assurance systems of USQA would now be deployed to serve 14 million members, reaching roughly one out of every twelve people with health insurance in the United States.

Why did Abramson decide to sell if U.S. Healthcare was such a successful company? Although any analysis of internal motivations and assessments is largely speculative, some plausible reasons do appear upon reflection. Although U.S. Healthcare had created startups and/or joint ventures in Florida, Illinois, Delaware, and Maryland, as well as ten other states and even in Europe, by 1996 it was becoming more difficult to maintain the 10 to 20 percent growth rates it had enjoyed. Every major market now had an established HMO, often several, and the indemnity insurers such as Blue Cross, CIGNA, and New York Life had developed their own HMO plans; therefore, signing up each additional employer group was a struggle. Merger with Aetna meant that U.S. Healthcare's 11 million (mostly indemnity) members could be transferred over rather than fought for. Tremendous economies of scale in the use of USQA's software and statistical profiles could be immediately obtained. In 1992, heady with success, the management of U.S. Healthcare envisioned that USQA would attract other HMOs as clients, and that soon it would be spun off as a separate company, perhaps growing larger than its parent. Later, it became clear that such a strategy was not viable—monitoring quality and developing information systems is so intimately intertwined with the core business of an HMO that it would never allow a competing entity to participate in that task or to access such sensitive data. Hence, USQA technology could only be used in-house or sold only in regions (such as England) where U.S. Healthcare could never be a competitive threat.

In the end, it may have been Abramson himself who was the most compelling reason for selling the company. U.S. Healthcare never developed a faceless corporate style—it was always Leonard Abramson's company, where he personally made most of the important decisions. Although he had groomed several of his children for leadership roles and brought in a number of senior executives, there was no clear successor in sight.[36] The genius and prime mover of the company was now sixty-three. He sold the company—at the peak, for $8 billion.

Even though U.S. Healthcare was bought by Aetna, the smaller company, U.S. Healthcare, was supposed to colonize the larger old-line insurer from within, with its executives taking leading roles and spreading the managed care and quality measurement techniques to transform the older indemnity insurer. How well did the deal work? It vaulted Abramson into the role of leading philanthropist, and threw Aetna/UShealthcare into a tailspin from which it still has not recovered. Most of the U.S. Healthcare executives targeted to lead the combined firm drifted away or were let go. An Aetna insurance executive took the reins, tightened controls, cut payments—and drove the hospitals and physicians into revolt. The market had changed and providers were no longer willing to do anything and make sacrifices to get an HMO contract. Providers threatened to pull out—and Aetna had to pull back. Finally, a new CEO, a doctor from academia with almost no insurance experience was brought in to restore confidence and rebuild relationships. Marginal lines of business were cut or sold. Today, Aetna/UShealthcare is no longer the largest health insurer in the United States. It is losing money, and after five years its total market capitalization has fallen below $6 billion—less than it paid for U.S. Healthcare.

10.8 THE ENTHOVEN "MANAGED COMPETITION" PLAN

Economist Alain Enthoven published a provocative proposal for a Consumer Choice Health Plan in the *New England Journal of Medicine* in 1978, envisioning a future in which managed care was the norm and FFS was the secondary alternative.[37] It was based on a recognition that consumers, confronted with thousands of possible illnesses, millions of possible prices, and indemnity coverage that was (a) difficult to understand and (b) comprehensive enough to make the effort of comparing costs not worthwhile, actually made decisions that were very remote from the market in which suppliers operated. Consumers looked for plans with low co-payments, or coverage of eyeglasses and orthodontics, or benefit maximums set at reassuringly astronomical amounts—factors that had nothing to do with the average total cost of most medical care or the rising premiums that employers had to pay each year, which were reducing profits and wages. In contrast, "consumer choice" as presented by Enthoven was based on making a choice between two or three competing plans, each with a price that was known in advance and for which the consumer would have to pay the full difference between the low-cost plan and the high-cost plan if they preferred to obtain greater choice, more coverage, or higher quality. Far from being an intellectual abstraction, Enthoven's proposal was based on successful experiences of the Federal Employees Health Benefits Plan, which had worked well for 25 years offering federal employees a choice from a menu of HMO and indemnity plans in each area.[38]

Although by 2000 it was evident that managed care would indeed push indemnity FFS into a small corner, few of the specifics of the Enthoven proposal came to pass. No universal guarantee of basic care for all Americans has been made, employer tax subsidies still favor more expensive plans, and most HMOs do not compete on the basis of care (since they have overlapping lists of hospitals and physicians) but rather on minor contractual stipulations regarding co-payments, dental benefits, referral procedures, and extent of coinsurance

10.9 IS MANAGED CARE THE SOLUTION TO RISING COSTS?

Evidence on Cost Reductions

A large number of studies in many markets over many years have consistently shown that medical care managed and financed through an HMO costs 10 to 20 percent less than under indemnity insurance.[39] Most of the savings come from two factors: the ability to obtain lower prices by contracting for large volumes of hospital, physician, laboratory, and pharmacy services, and a substantial reduction in the number of hospital days per 1,000 enrollees. This reduction in hospital days is somewhat offset by a greater use of ambulatory physician services and outpatient surgery among HMOs, but since these substitutes are less expensive than inpatient services, overall dollar savings are realized even when the quantity of services used stays the same or increases. The following questions have arisen regarding this record of HMO cost reductions:

- Are some of the apparent savings overstated because HMOs enroll people who are at lower risk to begin with?
- Is the quality of care as good when costs are lowered?
- Can newer forms of managed care (IPAs, PPOs) reduce costs as much as closed HMOs can?
- Will cost reductions be offset by higher administrative costs and profits?
- Does the switch to managed care give just a one-time 20 percent reduction in health care costs, or can it slow the rate of price increases?
- If most patients and payers are winners, are there also some people who stand to lose from the spread of managed care?

Risk Selection

Most companies adding an HMO option have found that the older and sicker employees stayed with the indemnity plan. Such adverse selection occurs because young, healthy couples are attracted to the free or low-cost preventive, prenatal, and baby visits offered by the HMO, while older and sicker employees are more likely to have become attached to a particular physician, are thus unwilling to accept an HMO that limits their choice of doctors, and are more likely to want "the best" care at famous (and expensive) academic research hospitals rather than be limited to the providers within the HMO network.[40] However, there are also some reasons that sicker people might prefer the HMO: better coverage of pharmaceuticals, lower co-payments, and no deductible. Evaluation results have consistently shown that HMOs do tend to have a more favorable risk selection. Estimates of the net effects have been mixed, but it appears that after adjusting for differences in age, sex, prior hospitalizations, and other factors, average total group costs (HMO and indemnity) usually decline a bit for employee groups, but may actually be higher for the elderly in Medicare.

Quality of Care

From the time prepaid medical plans were first developed, they have been attacked for providing incentives to reduce services and hence to reduce quality. However, decades of research show that on average, the quality of care in HMOs is comparable to or better than that provided under indemnity insurance.[41] In particular, HMO patients are more likely to receive preventive services, see physicians more often, receive coordinated care from a variety of providers, use primary physicians rather than emergency rooms for acute illnesses, and be subjected to less unnecessary surgery. On the other hand, HMO patients are less likely to receive treatment for some disorders such as depression and back pain. Also, HMOs use less aggressive therapy and thus more frequently err on the side of doing too little surgery rather than too much. Surveys of consumer satisfaction show mixed results. Patients are usually more satisfied with the financial aspects of an HMO than an indemnity insurance plan (no paperwork and billing hassles, no deductibles). However, patients may be less satisfied with service and amenities, particularly when they feel forced to accept an HMO option, even though extensive research has shown little difference in morbidity, mortality, or extent of functional recovery from accidents and chronic illness.[42] The net effect is that quality is roughly comparable in the two sectors, a little better in the HMO for some things, a little better under FFS for others.[43]

Costs Reductions in IPA HMOs, PPOs, and POS Plans

The more open and less restrictive a managed care plan is, the more acceptable it is to new enrollees who are accustomed to FFS care. That is why the great expansion of HMO membership in the 1980s and 1990s occurred in IPA HMOs, PPOs, and POS plans. These less tightly managed plans are able to obtain volume discounts, but are only able to change provider behavior when they adopt stringent UR procedures, carefully assess each day of hospitalization, aggressively substitute less costly drugs and therapies and, in general, tighten up the management of care to a degree equivalent to that of the closed HMO.[44] When HMO enrollment accounts for less than a quarter of a physician's practice, his or her behavior shows little change. When most of a physician's patients are in a single HMO, he or she begins to act much more like a physician in a closed HMO, with lower rates of hospitalization, more careful attention to administrative procedures, awareness of drug and laboratory reimbursement limits, and so on. In short, to get something (cost control), something must be given up (freedom of choice and clinical autonomy).

Administrative Costs and Profits

Some commentators have worried that reductions in the cost of medical care do not benefit consumers, but are taken up by the higher administrative costs required to manage care and by the profits that for-profit HMO companies pay to shareholders as dividends. Since 20 percent of the premiums HMOs receive go toward administrative costs and profit, the reason for concern is evident. However, management is a cost of doing business, a cost that has increased over time as business has become more complex and more efficient. Douglass North, who received the 1994 Nobel Prize for his work in cliometrics (the use of statistical measures to study economic history), estimated that in 1800 less than 10 percent of the gross domestic product of a largely rural U.S. economy went to transaction costs, but that by 1970, more than 50 percent of economic activity was accounted for by managers, salespeople, consultants, accountants, telecommunications and other administrative costs.[45] The production of high-technology equipment and services requires more of the "management" input than input of raw materials, unskilled labor, and the like. It was sensible for solo physicians of the 1950s to do their own billing, office maintenance, and record-keeping; it is not very efficient in 2002 when the treatment of any serious illness usually requires the services of a dozen doctors and hundreds of ancillary personnel, and when most patients seek information about therapeutic options over the Internet.

Without profits, there is no clear signal of which firms are most efficient or which firms produce services of greatest value to consumers. Some well-managed HMOs do a better job of quality control and negotiation with 11 percent of premiums than others do with 15 or 20 percent. As HMOs became more able to control where patients received care, they improved efficiency and, more significantly, were able to take some of the profits that previously had been received by hospitals and physicians. This made shareholders happy, but not the hospitals and physicians, who quite rightly resented being managed and having some of "their" producer's surplus taken away. Over time, competition among HMOs will transfer that surplus to employers (who will pay lower premiums) and ultimately to workers (who will receive higher wages as health benefit costs decline).[46]

One-Time Savings?

Will the search by HMOs for market share and greater profits revolutionize U.S. health care or just enrich a few owners and shareholders? In most evaluations so far, only one-time savings have been demonstrated (Figure 10.5).[47] Even Kaiser's premiums, although consistently lower than Blue Cross premiums, have grown at about the same annual percentage rate over the past fifty years. Managed care may prove to have started a revolution that brought price sensitivity and continuous quality improvement to health care, or prove to be just another management fad that held the attention of politicians and health care administrators for a few decades.

10.10 BACKLASH: ARE THERE LOSERS AS WELL AS WINNERS?

By 2001, there was a tremendous backlash against managed care, with HMOs attacked as villains in the Hollywood movies *As Good As It Gets* and *John Q*. Despite Hollywood's spin, the major victims of managed care were hospitals and doctors, not patients—it is just harder to sell a story about how HMOs cut surgical fees or prevent psychiatric hospitals from holding troubled adolescents a few more days to collect additional revenue. The MCO emphasis on preventive services and case management has been notably successful in achieving better outcomes for children with asthma (the illness of Helen Hunt's young

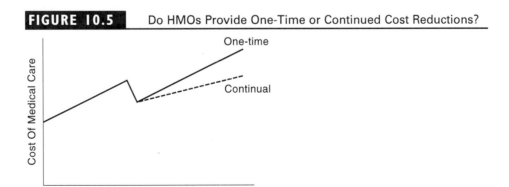

FIGURE 10.5   Do HMOs Provide One-Time or Continued Cost Reductions?

son in *As Good As It Gets*) and in reducing expenses while maintaining equivalent survival rates for cardiac care (the crisis confronting Denzel Washington's son in *John Q*).

Most of the opposition to managed care has come from the traditional powers on the supply side of medicine, licensed professionals, and nonprofit hospitals, which clearly stand to lose money as costs are cut.[48] Yet it is on the demand side that the weakness of managed care as a strategy for controlling cost is revealed. The problem is that the rather small groups of people who need a lot of care (e.g., the chronically ill, children with HIV/AIDS, the frail elderly) are quite separate from those who can afford to pay for care (the employed).

Surely employees will take care of each other, from president to parking lot attendant. But will working people willingly pay for treatment of AIDS in intravenous drug abusers, or for the years of therapy needed by a child born with Down's syndrome to a single unemployed mother, or for treatment during the final years of decline in a patient with Alzheimer's disease? For a hundred years, the U.S. health care system has funded care of the indigent, chronic disease treatment, and medical research through cost shifting (see Chapter 8 section 4). Managed care seeks lower costs for the group of patients being managed and roots out costs that belong to others. When an intoxicated patient is shifted from a university hospital psychiatric unit costing $1,200 a day to a community hospital costing $400 a day, and then to a halfway house costing $80 per day, the health plan not only saves money by using more appropriate services, it avoids the cost of teaching residents in the university hospital, the cost of uncompensated care, and the cost of medical research. Shifting patients who need coronary-artery bypass grafts to efficient high-volume providers means that those fees can no longer be used to subsidize organ transplants. The profit margins in HMOs are around 5 percent. Managers are constantly searching for an extra 0.5 percent. Avoiding enrollment of the seriously ill, or even reducing the number slightly, usually reduces costs by more than that. Managed care gives an incentive for efficiency, but it gives an even bigger incentive for exclusion of expensive cases. In this way, it may act to further separate those who are well off from those who are needy.[49]

SUGGESTIONS FOR FURTHER READING

Association of American Health Plans, *HMO Performance Report* (annual).

David M. Cutler, Mark McClellan, and Joseph P. Newhouse. "How does managed care do it?" *RAND Journal of Economics* 31, no. 3 (Autumn 2000): 526–548.

Alain Enthoven, *Theory and Practice of Managed Competition in Health Care Finance* (Amsterdam: North-Holland, 1988).

Marsha Gold et al. "A National Survey of the Arrangements Managed Care Plans Make With Physicians," *New England Journal of Medicine* 333 (1995): 1678–1683.

Interstudy, *The Interstudy Edge,* Excelsior, Minn. (annual).

Peter R. Kongstvedt, *The Managed Care Handbook,* 4th edition (Aspen: Gaithersburg, Md., 2001).

Managed Care Digest (annual), (www.managedcaredigest.com).

Robert H. Miller and Harold Luft, "Managed Care Plan Performance Since 1980: A Literature Analysis," *Journal of the American Medical Association* 271, no. 19 (1994): 1512– 1519.

John G. Smillie, M.D. *Can Physicians Manage the Quality and Costs of Health Care: The Story of the Permanente Medical Group* (New York: McGraw-Hill, 1991).

Charles W. Wrightson, *HMO Rate Setting and Financial Strategy* (Ann Arbor, Mich.: Health Administration Press, 1990).

SUMMARY

1.   The **escalation in costs** under open-ended entitlement financing from Medicare, Medicaid, and employer-provided health insurance has been the primary force driving the development of managed care.

2. **Managed care** is a diverse set of contractual and management methods used to arrange the financing and delivery of medical services. Its distinctive feature is that *a manager* intervenes to monitor and control the transaction between doctor and patient. Traditional insurance provides value through risk pooling so that medical expenses can be covered by an actuarially fair premium equal to the expected average loss. Managed care adds value by systematically **reducing the average** loss through utilization review, preauthorization, formularies, case management, statistical profiling, and other process controls.

3. HMOs **reduce costs by** saving money on both the demand and the supply side. They obtain **discounts** by contracting in volume with physicians and hospitals, **substitute** less expensive services (e.g., home care instead of hospital stays), and **control utilization** through the approval process. HMOs may use one-third to two-thirds fewer inpatient hospital days per thousand people than traditional fee-for-service insurance, although they often use more ambulatory services.

4. With **indemnity FFS** health financing, **hospitals and physicians profit by seeing more patients** and the risk of excess utilization is borne by the insurance company, which passes it on to the employer or government in the form of higher premiums. **In managed care, the HMO forces the physicians and hospitals to bear some of the risks** for excess utilization, provides incentives to use fewer services by paying a fixed amount per month, and controls total premium expense by using withholds and other financial arrangements.

5. A **pharmacy formulary** limiting payment to those drugs listed, a **preferred provider network** that makes patients pay extra for using hospitals and physicians not on the list, **capitation,** primary care **gatekeepers,** and **utilization review** are some of the ways that managed care firms control costs. However, simple **price cuts** obtained through hard bargaining appear to be the major source of savings. Managed care has made many doctors bitter since these savings reduce the income and professional autonomy of physicians.

6. About **80 percent of HMO premiums go to pay hospitals, physicians, and other providers.** This fraction is known as the medical loss ratio. About 10 to 20 percent is used for administrative and marketing expenses, leaving up to 10 percent for profit.

7. Division of labor is practiced by HMOs that **carve out** and **subcapitate** a particular service (such as mental health treatment), letting another firm that specializes in that area bear the risk, contracting with providers, and using its expertise in managing that aspect of the care process.

8. Most HMOs started as nonprofit organizations. Some were explicitly collectivist and anti-capitalist in origin, but have become increasingly businesslike. **Kaiser,** founded just after World War II, is **the largest HMO** with more than 10 million members. However, the lack of a clearly defined ownership structure, limited access to capital, and resistance to capital mobility between regions have been major impediments to further growth. Over time, the more rapid **growth of for-profit firms** has led them to dominate the industry, and now even many nonprofit HMOs have for-profit subsidiaries.

9. Managed care attempts to create a much greater degree of **vertical and horizontal integration** in a medical system that has resisted organizational change. Changes in telecommunications and **information technology** make it possible for management to practice utilization review and monitor quality of care at dispersed sites around the country.

10. Managed care has been shown to **reduce costs,** but is probably not the answer to all of America's health care problems. Some HMOs have made money by **risk selection,** accepting mostly healthier patients. Other HMOs **may find it hard to maintain quality of care** once the easy savings from discounting and substitution have been taken, and thus may be tempted to reduce services in precisely those areas where patients, hampered by information asymmetry, depend most on professionals for monitoring quality. Extending coverage to the homeless, those with birth defects, the disenfranchised, and the chronically ill will provide the true test of managed care as a strategy for universal cost control.

PROBLEMS

1. {*incentives*} Which surgeons are more subject to financial incentives when deciding between alternative courses of therapy, FFS physicians who own their own practices or salaried physicians working for an HMO?

2. {*industrial organization*} If an HMO reduces the patient's marginal cost of surgery, hospitalization, chemotherapy, and other expensive items to zero, how can it provide incentives for reduced utilization?

3. {*information systems*} In contracting for hip replacements, who would have an incentive to contract on a line-item basis and who would have more incentive to contract on a bundled basis, an insurance company serving as a third-party administrator for a self-insured employer, or an HMO offering community rated plans to employers?

4. {*industrial organization*} Is an HMO able to obtain the biggest discounts where it has a large market share or where it has a smaller market share?

5. {*transactions costs*} Since managed care firms must hire managers to review all hospitalizations and surgeries, isn't managed care necessarily more expensive than unmanaged FFS care due to this extra administrative cost?

6. {*incidence*} If ABC corporation shifts from an indemnity plan to an HMO plan that lowers its cost of employee benefits by 35 percent over three years, who benefits? Who loses?

7. {*dynamics*} Does a surplus of hospital beds in an area make it easier or harder to start an HMO? Does a surplus of doctors? Does a surplus of insurance companies?

8. {*selection bias*} If a company offers both an HMO and indemnity plan, which employees will choose which?

9. {*selection*} Would an HMO entering the Medicare market expect to experience favorable or adverse selection? Would the magnitude of the selection bias be larger or smaller for an HMO entering the commercial employee benefit market? The Medicaid market?

10. {*costs*} What are the three main ways HMOs act to reduce the cost of care?

11. {*dynamics*} Will a contract that lowers the amount an HMO pays providers be more important with regard to short-run or long-run profitability? Why?

12. {*information*} In what ways can an HMO use information to increase profits? As information technology has become more efficient and cheaper to use, have health care firms invested more or less in computers?

13. {*distribution*} Why do "star" surgeons rarely work for HMOs, even the largest and wealthiest ones?

14. {*physician behavior*} What is the purpose of a withhold fund? Do HMOs have substitutes for financial incentives in controlling physician behavior? What factors make these substitutes more or less effective?

15. {*property rights*} What are the advantages and disadvantages of (a) nonprofit status and (b) publicly traded stock that provides incentives to physicians?

16. {*property rights*} Who owns Kaiser Permanente? Is there stock? Have ownership rights ever been sold?

17. {*property rights*} Why were HMOs formed in the 1930s often collectives attracting physicians with liberal or socialist leanings, while today HMOs are most often formed by entrepreneurs with capitalist ideals?

18. {*pricing*} How did Sydney Garfield set the monthly premiums for his first prepaid health plan? How are premiums set for Kaiser today?

19. {*regulation*} Did the HMO Act of 1973 affect competition and capital expenditure in a manner similar to the certificate of need (CON) acts passed during the same period?

20. {*dynamics*} What technological change has been most important in fostering the growth of managed care?

21. {*selection*} Is a person who is chronically ill and has a long-term relationship with a physician more likely to choose an HMO, PPO, or indemnity plan? How will this affect HMO capitation rates?

22. {*incentives*} What incentives does a capitated physician have to keep his patients happy? What incentive does an FFS physician have? If Mr. Jones is a cranky old man who smokes and drinks so much that his liver and other organs are going downhill, which payment system provides more incentive to keep Mr. Jones satisfied? Which provides the most incentive to render extra care? Which provides the most incentive to make sure that the level of care is optimized?

23. {*marginal cost*} Suppose a family physician has HMO patients who are capitated for primary care, HMO patients who are capitated with a withhold for hospital care, and FFS patients. For which patients is the marginal cost of doing additional laboratory services highest? For which patients is the marginal cost of admitting them to the hospital the highest?

24. {*aggregation*} What do HMOs reduce more, individual risks or system risks? (*Think* about this. Definitions are important, and relative risks are different from absolute risks.)

25. {*incidence*} Which groups tend to win by a general move toward capitated managed care? Which groups tend to lose?

ENDNOTES

1. The U.S. Bureau of Labor Statistics Employee Compensation measures have varied over the years and the various issues of the *BLS Handbook of Methods* should be examined to understand the vagaries of comparison (www.bls.gov). Braden, Bradley R. and Stephanie L. Hyland "Cost of Employee Compensation in Public and Private Sectors," *Monthly Labor Review* 116, no. 5 (May 1993): 14–21.

2. *2001 HMO-PPO/Medicare-Medicaid Digest*, Aventis Pharmaceuticals, (www.managedcaredigest.com). This is a standard compilation of HMO statistics that has been published for a number of years under various titles and corporate sponsors.

3. The United States ranked 26th in male life expectancy among 191 nations in 2000 (28th for females), a bit behind most other developed countries. The risk of dying between ages 15-59, a perhaps more significant measure, was even worse (36th for males, 38th for females). Overall, the World Health Organization ranked performance of the U.S. health system 37th, *World Health Report 2000* (www.who.int/whr). See also Victor Fuchs, "The Best Health Care System in the World?" *Journal of the American Medical Association* 268, no. 7 (1992):916–917; Jack Hadley, *More Medical Care, Better Health?* (Washington, D.C.: The Urban Institute Press, 1982); OECD, *OECD Health Data: Comparative Analysis of Health Systems* (Paris: Organization for Economic Cooperation and Development, 2002).

4. Neelam K. Sekhri, "Managed Care: the U.S. Experience," *Bulletin of the World Health Organization* 78, no. 6 (2000): 830–844 (www.who.org or www.who.int).

5. David M. Cutler, Mark McClellan, and Joseph P. Newhouse. "How Does Managed Care Do It?" *RAND Journal of Economics* 31, no. 3 (Autumn 2000): 526–548; Daniel Alman, Richard Zeckhauser, and David M. Cutler, "Enrollee Mix, Treatment Intensity and Cost in Competing Indemnity and HMO Plans. NBER working paper No. 7832, August 2000 (www.nber.org). Ann Barry Flood et al, "How do HMOs achieve savings?" *Health Services Research* 33, no. 1 (April 1998): 79–99.

6. *Managed Care Digest 2001*, www.managedcaredigest.com; Robert H. Miller and Harold Luft, "Managed Care Plans: Characteristics, Growth and Premium Performance," *Annual Review of Public Health* 15 (1994): 437–59.

7. *Managed Care Digest: HMO-PPO Digest 1995* (Kansas City, Mo.: Hoechst Marion Roussel, 1995). In an integrated CPGP HMO, administrative and medical expenses all occur within the same organization and cannot meaningfully be separated. In reports, Kaiser or Group Health often say their administrative expenses are very low, 2 percent or so, but this low figure comes from counting only the central office staff, and not all the clerks, secretaries, medical directors, information specialists, etc., who are at work in the clinics.

8. In principle, an integrated closed HMO could be run as a for-profit corporation benefiting stockholders, a division of a voluntary hospital chain, or a consumer co-op with all profits used to increase community benefits. In practice, the residual ownership interest has *de facto* resided primarily with the senior physician group, even when they are technically employees of the HMO.

9. The term "PPO" is commonly used to refer to two things: an insurance plan and a corporate entity. The two are distinct. Your "PPO" insurance may actually have contracts with a dozen PPO organizations. Conversely, a single PPO organization with 50 physicians may have contracts with more than one insurance company (and at different prices).

10. Marsha Gold et al., "A National Survey of the Arrangements Managed-Care Plans Make With Physicians," *New England Journal of Medicine* 333 (1995):1678–1683; Gerard Anderson et al., "Setting Payment Rates for Capitated Systems: A Comparison of Various Alternatives" *Inquiry* 27, no. 3 (1990): 225–233.

11. Geoffrey F. Joyce, Jose J. Escarce, Matthew D. Solomon, and Dana Goldman, "Employer Drug Benefit Plans and Spending on Prescription Drugs," *Journal of the American Medical Association* 288, no. 14 (October 9, 2002): 1733–1739.. See also the comment on the article by Donald M. Steinwachs "Pharmacy Benefit Plans and Prescription Drug Spending," on pages 1773–1774.

12. Kaiser Family Foundation and HRET, Employee Health Benefits, 2002 Annual Survey, Chart #12 "Percentage of Covered Workers Facing Different Cost Sharing Formulas for Prescription Drugs: 2000, 2001, 2002," (www.kff.org/content/2002/20020905a).

13. Norman Winegar, *The Clinician's Guide to Managed Mental Health Care* (New York: Haworth Press, 1992). John K. Iglehart, "Managed Care and Mental Health," *New England Journal of Medicine* 334, no. 2 (1996): 131–135. The monthly publications *Open Minds* and *Behavioral Health Management* are also useful sources of current information on managed behavioral health care.

14. William Goldman, Joyce McCulloch, and Roland Sturm. "Costs and Use of Mental Health Services Before and After Managed Care," *Health Affairs* 17, no. 2 (March 1998): 40–52; Ma, Ching-to Albert and Thomas G. McGuire, "Costs and Incentives in a Behavioral Health Carve-Out," *Health Affairs* 17, no. 2 (March 1998): 53–69.

15. Sandy Lutz, "NME Totals Costs of Psych Woes," *Modern Healthcare* 23, no. 43 (October 25, 1993): 20.

16. M. Chassin et al., "Does Inappropriate Use Explain Geographic Variations in the Use of Health Care Services? A Study of Three Procedures," *Journal of the American Medical Association* 256 (1987): 2533–2537.

17. Charles Wrightson, "Selection Bias and Premium Rate Setting," in *HMO Rate Setting and Financial Strategy* (Ann Arbor, Mich.: Health Administration Press, 1990), 245–292.

18. The term "risk" is used to mean many different things. The technical definition frequently used in finance is "random variation over which managers have no control" and is equated with the *standard deviation* of some statistical series. Most businesspeople use "risk" to mean something such as "all of the things that can happen." In health care, "taking on risk" means accepting capitation—and taking a fixed monthly payment would be seen by most businesses as getting rid of the risk from an uneven flow of FFS payments. A leading healthcare business consultant said, "What cannot be controlled, should not be assumed as risk,"

(Joseph Coyne, *Healthcare Financial Management*, August 1994, p.33). This definition, relying on managerial control over clinical processes, is quite at odds with the definition of risk used by currency and bond traders, who strive to make money contracting strictly for things they cannot control.

19. Joseph Schumpeter, *History of Economic Analysis* (New York: Oxford University Press, 1954). For an application of Schumpeter's ideas to health care, see L. D. Brown, "Policy Reform as Creative Destruction: Political and Administrative Challenges in Preserving the Public-Private Mix," *Inquiry* 29, no. 2 (1992): 188– 202.

20. Much of the information in this section comes from John G. Smillie, M.D. *Can Physicians Manage the Quality and Costs of Health Care: The Story of the Permanente Medical Group* (New York: McGraw-Hill, 1991); and Paul de Kruif, *Kaiser Wakes the Doctors* (New York: Harcourt, Brace & Co. 1943).

21. Prepaid medical group practice had existed in America since at least 1790, when such a plan was used at the Boston Dispensary. The innovative prepayment contract between The City of Los Angeles Department of Water and Power and Drs. Ross and Loos to provide all medical services to 12,000 employees and 25,000 dependents for $2 per month (excluding hospitalization) was a more proximate example that probably influenced Garfield.

22. Quoted on page 55 of John G. Smillie, M.D., *Can Physicians Manage the Quality and Costs of Health Care: The Story of the Permanente Medical Group* (New York, McGraw-Hill, 1991).

23. Louise Kertesz, "Kaiser Retools to Fight for Lost Ground," *Modern Healthcare* (July 17, 1995): 34–40.

24. Edward D. Berkowitz and Wendy Wolff, *Group Health Association: A Portrait of a Health Maintenance Organization* (Philadelphia: Temple University Press, 1988), 144.

25. Paul Starr, *The Social Transformation of American Medicine* (New York: Basic Books, 1982).

26. As quoted in Gilbert Gaul, "U.S. Healthcare's Abramson: Dedicated, Perhaps Ruthless," *The Philadelphia Inquirer,* April 2, 1996, sec. A, p. 5.

27. Much of the information in this case study comes from interviews with Sandra Harmon-Weiss, M.D., Medical Director of U.S. Healthcare, and other executives, "A Brief Overview: U.S. Healthcare" by Hyman R. Kahn, M.D. (mimeo, November 28, 1994), and annual financial reports of U.S. Healthcare.

28. In the words of Pulitzer-Prize-winning journalist Gilbert Gaul, "For years, some of the most prestigious hospitals in Philadelphia refused to sign contracts with U.S. Healthcare. Those that did often complained bitterly about the hard-line negotiating style of Abramson and his colleagues, which resulted in lower reimbursement rates for the hospitals." in "U.S. Healthcare's Abramson: Dedicated, Perhaps Ruthless," *The Philadelphia Inquirer,* April 2, 1996, sec. A, page 5.

29. Accounting practices are significantly different in the nonprofit Kaiser plan, so the figures are not entirely comparable. It is, however, generally accepted that of the major HMOs, Kaiser probably has the highest percentage of premiums going to medical costs, while U.S. Healthcare had among the lowest.

30. Neil Schlackman, "Evolution of a Quality-Based Compensation Model: The Third Generation," *American Journal of Medical Quality* 8, no. 2 (1993): 103–110.

31. Nicholas Hanchak, Neil Schlackman, and Sandra Harmon-Weiss, *U.S. Healthcare's Quality-Based Compensation Model,* 32 pages (mimeo) (Blue Bell, Pa.: U.S. Healthcare, 1996).

32. Paul Kenkel, "U.S. Healthcare 'Report Cards' Expanded to Primary-Care Docs," *Modern Healthcare* (April 11, 1994).

33. Eleanor H. Kerns, health care analyst for Alex Brown & Sons, a leading investment banking firm, has opined publicly that U.S. Healthcare's information systems are superior to those of competitors: see Marian Uhlman and Andrea Knox, "Aetna, U.S. Healthcare Plan Merger," *The Philadelphia Inquirer* (April 2, 1996): A1, A5.

34. George Anders and Ron Winslow, "HMO Stocks Skid on U.S. Healthcare Announcement," *The Wall Street Journal,* April 20, 1995.

35. Leslie Scism and Steven Lipin, "Aetna Near $8 Billion Deal to Acquire U.S. Healthcare," *The Wall Street Journal,* April 1, 1996, sec. a, p. 3.

36. Gilbert Gaul, "U.S. Healthcare's Abramson: Dedicated, Perhaps Ruthless," *The Philadelphia Inquirer,* April 2, 1996, sec. A, p. 5.

37. Alain Enthoven, "Consumer Choice Health Plan," *New England Journal of Medicine* 298 (1978): 650–658, 709–720; and *Theory and Practice of Managed Competition in Health Care Finance* (Amsterdam: North-Holland, 1988).

38. Alain Enthoven, "Management of Competition in the FEHPB," *Health Affairs* 8, no. 3 (1989): 33–50.

39. Harold Luft, *Health Maintenance Organizations: Dimensions of Performance* (New York: John Wiley & Sons, 1981); Robert H. Miller and Harold Luft, "Managed Care Plan Performance Since 1980: A Literature Analysis," *Journal of the American Medical Association,* 271, no. 19 (1994): 1512–1519; J. Hill et al., *The Impact of the Medicare Risk Program on the Use of Services and Costs to Medicare* (Princeton, N.J.: Mathematica Policy Research, 1992); D. K. Freeborn and C. R. Pope, *Promise and Performance in Managed Care: The Prepaid Group Practice Model* (Baltimore: Johns Hopkins University Press, 1994).

40. Gail Wilensky and Louis Rossiter, "Patient Self-Selection in HMOs," *Health Affairs* 5, no. 4 (1986): 66– 80; S. E. Berki and M. L. Ashcraft, "HMO Enrollment: Who Joins and Why: A Review of the Literature," *Milbank*

Memorial Fund Quarterly 58 (1980): 588–632; Kyle Grazier, William Richardson, Diane Martin, et al; "Factors Affecting Choice of Health Care Plans," *Health Services Research* 20, no. 6 (1986): 659–682.

41. S. M. Retchin and B. Brown, "The Quality of Ambulatory Care in Medicare Health Maintenance Organizations," *American Journal of Public Health,* 80 (1990): 411–415; I.S. Udvarhely et al., "Comparison of the Quality of Ambulatory Care for Fee-For-Service and Prepaid Patients," *Annals of Internal Medicine* 327 (1991): 424–429; J. E. Ware et al., "Comparison of Health Outcomes at a Health Maintenance Organization With Those of Fee-For-Service Care," *Lancet* (1986, I):130–136. Maggie Mahar, "Time for A Checkup: HMOs Must Now Prove That They are Providing Quality Care," *Barron's* (March 4, 1996): 29–35.. Ray Robinson, "Managed Care in the United States: A Dilemma for Evidence-Based Policy?" *Health Economics* 9, no. 1 (January 2000): 1–7.

42. Karen Davis, Karen Scott Collins, Cathy Schoen, and Cynthia Morris, "Choice Matters: Enrollees' Views of Their Health Plans," *Health Affairs,* 14, no. 2 (1995): 99–112; H. R. Rubin et al., "Patients Ratings of Outpatient Visits in Different Practice Settings: Results from the Medical Outcomes Study," *Journal of the American Medical Association,* 262 (1989): 57–63.

43. Robert Hurley, Deborah Freund, and John Paul, *Managed Care in Medicaid: Lessons for Policy and Program Design* (Ann Arbor, Mich.: Health Administration Press, 1993).

44. Robert H. Miller and Harold Luft, "Managed Care Plans: Characteristics, Growth and Premium Performance," *Annual Review of Public Health* 15 (1994): 437–459. Laurence C. Baker, "Managed Care Technology Adoption in Health Care: Evidence From Magnetic Resonance Imaging," *Journal of Health Economics* 20, no. 3 (2001): 395–421.

45. John J. Wallis and Douglass C. North, "Measuring the Transaction Sector in the American Economy, 1870–1970," pp 95–161 in Stanley L. Engerman and Robert E. Gallman, *Long Term Factors in American Economic Growth,* NBER Studies in Income and Wealth, #51 (Chicago: University of Chicago Press, 1986).

46. While this is probably true in the long run, in the short run the managers of many firms push to capture as much as possible of the surplus for themselves. Such efforts may transcend regular or even aggressive business practices and pass over into accounting distortions, mis-statement of reserves, and fraud. Virtually all of the rapidly expanding HMOs fell into financial problems, and several flirted with insolvency during the 1990s.

47. Robert H. Miller and Harold Luft, "Managed Care Plan Performance Since 1980: A Literature Analysis," *Journal of the American Medical Association,* 271, no. 19 (1994): 1512–1519.

48. Council on Ethical and Judicial Affairs, American Medical Association, "Ethical Issues in Managed Care," *Journal of the American Medical Association,* 273, no. 4 (1995): 330–335; Ezekiel Emanuel and Nancy Dubler, "Preserving the Physician-Patient Relationship in the Era of Managed Care," *Journal of the American Medical Association,* 273, no. 4 (1995): 323– 329; Marc Rodwin, "Conflicts in Managed Care," *New England Journal of Medicine,* 332, no. 9 (1995): 605–607.

49. See Julie Rovner, "The Safety Net: What's Happening to Health Care of Last Resort?" and Howard Larkin, "Employed but Uninsured: Why Business is Cutting Back on Health Insurance," in *Advances,* quarterly newsletter of the Robert Wood Johnson Foundation, Princeton, N.J., Issue 1, 1996.

CHAPTER 11

LONG-TERM CARE

QUESTIONS

1. Do the elderly pay to be cured, or to be cared for?

2. Who provides most long-term care for the disabled elderly? Who is the largest insurer?

3. What do nursing home owners compete for? Do they want patients who are more or less ill?

4. How can substituting nursing homes for hospitals increase the total cost of care if the cost per day is lower at nursing homes?

5. Have government payments and regulations raised or lowered the quality of care?

6. How can Medicaid payments create an excess and a shortage of patients at the same time?

7. Do certificate-of-need (CON) rules reduce costs or reduce access?

8. Are retirement communities "managed care" for the aging? Is there "managed death"?

9. As people live longer, does that mean that they are healthier, and thus spend less on medical care, or more disabled, and spend more?

Of the $144 billion paid for long-term care (LTC) in 2002, most is spent for institutional services in nursing homes. Yet for every person in a nursing home, there are two equally disabled people living in the community who are cared for by family and friends. Hence, more care comes from unpaid labor and acts of obligation and love, rather than patient fees or third-party payments.[1] **LTC** revolves around *care* rather than cure, around quality of life rather than treatment of disease. LTC needs are defined by a person's ability to function, the ability to conduct activities of daily life. Most LTC patients continue to require assistance for the rest of their lives. Food, housing, comfort, and social relationships are more important than diagnostic tests and surgical procedures. Although doctors, hospitals, nurses, drugs, and all the other elements of modern medicine are employed in LTC, they are actively involved in only a small portion of the care that patients receive, and LTC is not "medical" in the same way that most acute care is. These differences—long-term chronic disabilities rather than short-term diseases capable of being cured, predominantly human caring rather than medical science, and a reliance on unpaid acts of love and obligation rather than services purchased in the market—tend to make LTC transactions quite different from acute medical care transactions and from the ordinary two-party transactions for most economic goods and services.

The challenge of meeting both medical and social needs has left LTC public policy in a confused state, with legislators uncertain about which aspects of care should be funded through social welfare programs and which should be funded as part of the health care system. The response to people with chronic illness and disability is an LTC system in which boundaries are often unclear and many fundamental issues are unresolved. This chapter presents a few aspects of the many and multifaceted economic entities that make up the fragmented LTC sector.

11.1 DEVELOPMENT OF THE LONG-TERM CARE MARKET

The original hospitals were LTC facilities. They served destitute patients who could not work and could no longer live at home. Most people had family members who took care of them at home when they became sick, old, or infirm, and the wealthy called upon the services of paid home nurses; therefore, only a small group of disabled and indigent paupers were forced to reside in hospitals. However, after the scientific revolutions of the nineteenth century, curative medicine was increasingly separated from caring for the disabled. By the start of World War II, the distinction between acute medical care and LTC was clearly demarcated in the minds of the public and in the flow of funds. It was hoped that poorhouses and "almshouse hospitality" would disappear as infectious diseases were cured and the desperately poor were elevated by a rising economy. To a large extent, sanitation and Social Security did cause the old system to fade, but some problems were troublingly persistent. No cure was found for mental illness and more people were confined to state hospitals. These institutions made limited attempts at cure, but often served more to relieve the community of a burden rather than to improve the patients' quality of life. Rising incomes meant that fewer and fewer elderly people were left truly destitute, but there were always some who had no friends, no family, and no place to go except to a county "home" once they could no longer work. Although people with severe mental illness and homeless elderly people had persistent needs, they were small in number and almost ignored in planning for the overall health care system. In 1940, nursing home expenditures constituted less than 1 percent of the nation's total health spending.

The number of elderly people rose rapidly in the postwar era, from 10 million in 1940 to 17 million in 1965 and 35 million in 2002. This burgeoning group of elderly Americans is relatively healthy, thanks to years of good nutrition and sanitation, and relatively wealthy, thanks to pensions and years of saving. After the 1960s, a sizable population could look forward to living for many years after working, with no need to depend on their children for financial support. This emerging group of retirees constituted a distinct market. They wanted to enjoy their "golden years" and often looked to each other for social activity. Retirement communities sprang up in Florida, California, and Arizona that catered to this growing group of middle-class elderly people. Retirement communities were specially designed to appeal to the elderly, featuring single-story dwellings without steps, limited traffic, and social centers for bridge games, dancing, and crafts. Many of these communities discouraged or excluded families with children. This market response to the special needs of the elderly occurred without any reference to medicine or LTC.

Nursing home patients constituted another small group within the elderly population that was destined to grow rapidly during the postwar era. The fraction of total health expenditures devoted to nursing homes, which was less than 1 percent in 1940, more than doubled by 1950, doubled again by 1960, and nearly doubled again by 1970, but was increasingly constrained after that (see Table 11.1). The fraction of total health spending devoted to nursing homes peaked at 8 percent around 1980 and has held steady since then, while the number of active retirees living in segregated housing with special amenities continues to soar. Distinguishing the active senior citizens from the institutionalized patients is easy at the extremes, but there is a range in between for which neat separation is impossible. The simple dichotomy of "at home" versus "in a nursing home" has been replaced by a range of organizational settings, from high-intensity facilities that are almost like hospitals, to a variety of intermediate care and assisted-living facilities, to houses identical to those occupied by young families. The picture is further clouded by the provision of visiting nurse services, Meals on Wheels, home intravenous (IV) and physical therapy, and other supplemental services that make it possible to provide a wide range of care where people live before they become disabled.

Although some disabled younger people receive LTC, the majority of people who receive LTC are above age 65, and the rate of institutionalization increases with advancing age (see Table 11.2). Residents in nursing homes are disproportionately female (74 percent) and poor. Older males who are disabled are more likely to be married and hence receive assistance from a spouse or adult child. Traditionally, care of disabled elders has been provided by adult daughters who were expected to take on the task of caring for one or more parents or parents-in-law after their own children were raised. This informal system was adequate in the 1950s, when most women married and had children early, and did not have careers. In the 1990s, with the majority of women in the labor force, and child-bearing frequently delayed so that children did not leave home until the mother was in her fifties, finding time to care for a 78-year-old parent was much more difficult. The "shadow price" (forgone wage opportunity) of unpaid middle-aged females has become much greater. At the same time, demand has risen. In the immediate postwar 1950s era, fewer parents lived past age 70. In addition, families were larger; therefore, middle-aged women were likely to have several sisters to help share the burden. As family size shrank and longevity increased, there were more elderly disabled parents per potential caregiver daughter. The stress and family complications became greater. As the supply of unpaid labor fell and demand rose, what formerly had been care provided within the household became care purchased in the marketplace.[2]

The services provided by family members are invisible in the national income (gross domestic product GDP) accounts: no one is billed, no one is paid, and from one point of view, no transaction has taken place. Yet from another point of view, one that pre-dates the existence of money, the obligations of parents to care for children, of neighbors to care for the sick, and of any person present to ease the pain of dying, are fundamental transactions that define society. In LTC, the boundary between market and nonmarket activities is blurred. The fact that nursing home admissions or expenditures double does not mean that twice as many disabled people are getting care or that they are getting more or better services. Some of that increase is simply the movement from the realm of household production and family obligation into monetarized commerce.

TABLE 11.1	Changes in the LTC Market						
	1940	**1950**	**1960**	**1970**	**1980**	**1990**	**2000**
People aged 65+	9,540,000	12,400,000	16,600,000	20,100,000	25,710,000	30,390,000	34,778,000
% of population	7.2%	8.1%	9.2%	9.8%	11.3%	12.2%	12.6%
Nursing home $ (millions)	$28	$178	$980	$4,687	$19,989	$54,810	$92,947
% of Total health $	0.7%	1.5%	3.6%	6.5%	8.0%	7.9%	7.1%
Home health $ (millions)	–	–	$37	$143	$1,347	$11,056	$32,426
% of Total health	–	–	0.1%	0.2%	0.5%	1.2%	2.4%

TABLE 11.2

Percentage of Population in
Nursing Home by Age

Under 65	0.1%
65–74	1.1%
75–84	4.3%
85+	18.3%

Source: CDC,
NCHS, *Health
United States, 2002.*

11.2 DEFINING LTC: TYPES OF CARE

A person's potential need for LTC can be analyzed as occurring in three dimensions: physical illness (medical diagnoses), functional disability (ability to perform activities of daily living [ADLs] and instrumental activities of daily living [IADLs] (see Section 11.5), and psycho-socioeconomic deficits (family support, see Table 11.3). LTC can be provided either at home or in an institutional setting. Institutional settings can be ranked by the intensity of medical intervention: acute hospitals, long-term hospitals providing rehabilitation and psychiatric treatment, nursing homes (skilled, intermediate), and assisted living or board-and-care homes. Placement depends on the interaction among medical, social, economic, and functional needs rather than any single dimension. A postoperative patient who only needs regular bathing and hourly medication could be cared for at home if there is sufficient support from the family. A patient without actively involved family members may be a candidate for nursing home placement, and if there are no available nursing home beds, the patient might continue to stay in the hospital for many days.[3]

Home health care is growing rapidly in two different directions.[4] On the one hand, medical treatments that used to be performed in the hospital are being performed in the patient's home, paralleling the trend away from the hospital evidenced by shorter lengths of stay, the growth of ambulatory surgery, and the development of outpatient rehabilitation. For home medical care to be effective, the physician and nurse must be able to count on a high degree of family support to assist in monitoring the patient, administering medication, and performing basic nursing functions such as feeding, bathing, and changing clothes. In contrast, personal home care is provided to otherwise healthy but homebound individuals whose lack of relatives at home is compensated for by having unskilled aides do ordinary cleaning, cooking, and other household tasks. Meals on Wheels, a publicly funded program that delivers hot meals to the homebound, is a good example. Although the services are quite different, the terminology and provision can become confusing, since a single provider may do both. A visiting nurse could stop at one house to change an IV antibiotic and proceed to the next house where the only service provided is to help someone into a wheelchair.

TABLE 11.3   Dimensions of LTC Need

	Medical Need	Functional Need	Social Need
Acute hospital	********	--	--
Rehab hospital	***	***	--
Nursing home	*	********	********
CCRC	--	--	*
Skilled home care	********	***	*
Personal home care	*	***	***
Family/community	*	*	*

******** High
*** Medium
* Low
-- Varies or not applicable

A person who has good friends, good health, and no functional limitations can have an active life in the community. As elderly people begin to need more care and protection, their likelihood of being placed in a nursing home depends most of all on the presence of social support. For example, most married people with Alzheimer's disease can continue to live at home and be cared for by their spouses at least through the early phases of the disease. Those who have children, but no spouse, are less likely to be able to remain at home, and those with no family nearby are likely to be institutionalized. The extent of disability is the second most important factor. Eventually, almost every family who cares for a person with Alzheimer's becomes overwhelmed by the necessity to provide constant attention, as well as by the pain and alienation of caring for someone who may not know or appreciate any of the things being done. Mental dysfunction is a significant cause in more than half of all LTC institutionalization. Medical needs, while often critical in precipitating a crisis, are relatively less important than social, housing, and functional needs in determining the use of LTC.

The goal of acute care is to increase the level of functioning and reduce the risk of dying. In contrast, most LTC is supportive. Attempts are made to slow the patient's decline and stabilize functioning, but only rarely is an attempt made to achieve a definitive cure, and it is expected that the person will remain dependent. Since acute medical care is focused on cure, the quality of the meals, the room, and social functions are incidentals and contribute little to the total cost of a hospital stay. Most of the cost of LTC, on the other hand, is for helping people with their daily lives, not treatment. Drugs are supposed to help the patient get through the day, not to get better, and curative procedures account for a relatively minor fraction of total expenditures. A physician may show up at a nursing home only once a month. In studies of nursing home costs, physician services account for only 1 percent of costs, as do drugs, while wages, salaries, and benefits, mostly for unskilled labor, account for 69 percent. A breakdown of nursing home inputs by category (see Table 11.4) shows that most LTC expenses result from providing supported living rather than medical care.

11.3 MEDICAID: NURSING HOMES AS A TWO-PART MARKET

TABLE 11.4

Breakdown of Nursing Home Costs

Physician services	1%
RNs (estimated)	9%
Other wages & salaries	53%
Employee benefits	7%
Food	10%
Fuel	4%
Drugs	1%
Other supplies	3%
Insurance	2%
Taxes	2%
Rent, debt, service, profit, etc.	8%

Source: HCFA detailed breakdown of Nursing Home Input Price Index Weightings, BLS Employment Statistics Survey.

The nursing home market was radically transformed, almost created anew, by the passage of Medicare, Title XVII, and Medicaid, Title XIX, of the Social Security Amendments of 1965. When Medicare was drafted to provide health insurance for the elderly, Medicaid was somewhat of an afterthought. Medicare explicitly did not pay for the kind of supportive care provided by most nursing homes.[5] It was presumed that housing, nutrition, and personal assistance were individual or family responsibilities. Inability to provide for oneself indicated a need for charity or welfare assistance, not medical insurance.[6] Medicaid was originally intended mostly to expand and consolidate insurance coverage of medical services for indigent women and children who received Aid to Families with Dependent Children (AFDC—now TANF, Temporary Assistance to Needy Families). Since it was directed toward a dependent indigent population, Medicaid did pay for social support such as that provided in nursing homes. Therefore, elderly people who were poor, or who could become poor after "spending down" or giving away their savings, could obtain government insurance payments for institutional LTC. Soon Medicaid was funneling billions of dollars each year into nursing homes. Medicaid now accounts for 52 percent of total nursing home funding, with Medicare paying 8 percent (mostly for skilled medical nursing care and therapy), as illustrated in Figure 11.1. Medicaid is a joint state/federal program, with poor states getting as much as 80 percent of their total Medicaid funding from the federal government, while wealthy states get only 50 percent. States are required to cover basic medical services for people who are on public assistance and/or who meet federal poverty definitions, but have discretion to increase benefits and eligibility above these limits. (Please note that any brief description of Medicaid must be qualified, because there are more than fifty state Medicaid payment systems with numerous clauses, exceptions, and special programs.)

Although nursing homes were only a minor consideration in the creation of the Medicaid program, LTC payments soared out of control, more than doubling every five years. Governors and state budget officials discovered that Medicaid, even with federal matching funds, was an onerous financial burden. In most years since 1965, Medicaid has been the most rapidly growing category of state spending. The surge of Medicaid money into what had been a tiny market caused a rapid increase in prices and a shortage of spaces for millions of new patients. As prices rose, state financial burdens increased. Any new nursing homes built were quickly filled with more of the waiting Medicaid-eligible people, adding millions to state budget outlays. States responded to this financial drain in two ways: capping the price they would pay for each day of nursing home care and halting the construction of new nursing homes. The methods of price control varied, but usually regulations were based on costs incurred or on a set percentage increase over prior years (see Section 11.5). Control over the number of beds was established by requiring that nursing home owners obtain a certificate of need (CON) before building or expanding facilities (see Section 11.4 and discussion of hospital CONs in Chapter 9, Section 7).

FIGURE 11.1   Nursing Home Sources and Uses of Funds

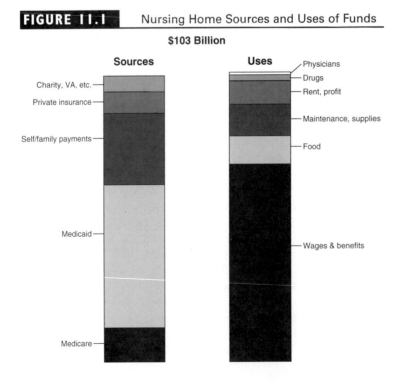

With these two moves, price controls and capacity constraints, government created a unique market for nursing home beds. This market's distinctive feature is a constant excess demand, but an excess of below-market-price Medicaid patients only. Consider Figure 11.2. On the upper-left side is private market demand, with a normal, downward-sloping demand schedule. The upper-right panel shows Medicaid demand. Since price is fixed by government regulation, there is no change in price as quantity increases; therefore, the demand "curve" is a right angle. Nursing homes can get as many patients as they want at the state-regulated price, until there are no more Medicaid-eligible patients in the area. The lower-left panel shows the combined private and Medicaid demand. Only private-pay patients can be served above the fixed Medicaid price; thus, the initial portion of the demand curve is composed solely of private patients and is downward sloping. Once the Medicaid price is reached, the demand curve flattens out, because the nursing home can get more patients without reducing price. If a nursing home gets too large, it would eventually exhaust the excess Medicaid demand and have to attract additional private patients with even lower prices, as shown by the bottom third, downward-sloping segment. Increasing the number of beds sufficient to force nursing home owners to dip into the demand of those only willing to pay an amount less than Medicaid pays is usually unintentional, since expansion typically ceases before all Medicaid patients are served. The two-part market faced by the nursing home owner is shown in more detail in the lower-right panel of Figure 11.2.[7] The vertical line represents the total bed capacity of the nursing home, the maximum number of patients that can be cared for. To maximize profits, the owner first sets a price for private-pay patients (P_{pp}) that maximizes the total amount of excess revenues above the Medicaid rate (i.e., the dotted rectangle $Q_{pp} \times [P_{pp} - P_{medicaid}]$)

FIGURE 11.2   Two-Part Nursing Home Market

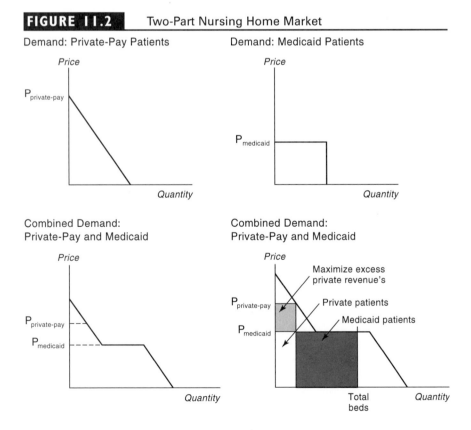

and then fills the remaining beds from the waiting list of Medicaid patients who pay the state-regulated price $P_{Medicaid}$ (the shaded rectangle $[Q_{max} - Q_{pp}] \times P_{Medicaid}$).

The two-part market structure causes nursing home utilization to have an unusual U-shaped relationship to income. Although most normal goods show demand steadily rising as income rises, in this market, utilization is high at low incomes (where patients readily qualify for Medicaid), drops for middle incomes (where lack of coverage reduces demand), and rises at high incomes (where wealthy people can afford $30,000 or more per year for care).

The real world is, of course, more complicated than the straight lines drawn in Figure 11.2. Often a nursing home will only admit private-pay patients. Many patients come into a nursing home with considerable assets, but over the years **spend down** all their savings by paying for care, and only then become poor enough to be eligible for Medicaid.[8] There are stories of couples becoming divorced solely to allow the spouse who is disabled to qualify for Medicaid so that the one who is still living at home can keep the savings accounts. Elderly couples are protected to some extent by federal guidelines that allow the spouse at home to keep the house, car, and some additional assets. Elderly single people may give their assets to their children in anticipation of entering a nursing home. This must be planned with care, however, since most states include recently transferred assets as part of personal funds to be used before Medicaid reimbursement is allowed. Families that would never consider "going on welfare" use asset transfers to make aging parents dependent on state funds as indigents. With 50 percent of all nursing home bills paid for by Medicaid, the conclusion that many middle-class and wealthy people are benefiting from a program designed for the poor is inescapable.[9] The fact that a certain amount of subterfuge is required ("convenience" divorces, paper-only transfer of ownership of cars and land, "giving" money to children that the parent still controls) only makes this process more distasteful and morally undermining.[10] Medicaid is an entrenched part of the nursing home market, but it is not well liked by taxpayers or beneficiaries, and it is difficult to justify Medicaid as being either equitable or ethical.

11.4 CERTIFICATE OF NEED: WHOSE NEEDS?

It is important to understand the implications of regulatory constraints on the LTC market and to examine whose interests are served by creating a situation of chronic excess demand in which frail and sick patients must wait months for a bed. For example, the surge of Medicaid money into nursing home care after 1965 meant that there would be a shortage of beds for the years it would take until the market could catch up. In addition, imposing a construction moratorium through the CON process increased the shortage and made it permanent.

Money and Quality

It would seem that pushing more money into nursing homes during the late 1960s would have improved the quality of care provided. However, for perfectly reasonable economic reasons, conditions actually became worse in most nursing homes. For instance, a nursing home owner does not choose furniture or service based on what can be afforded, but on what will maximize profits. With a long line of Medicaid patients waiting to get in, it was not necessary to keep up the appearance of the nursing home to attract new patients, nor was it necessary to provide good nursing service or good food to keep patients there. Since every bed was always filled from the waiting list, profits were maximized by reducing costs (e.g., providing fewer hours of nursing, employing less-skilled nurses, providing less maintenance, no new furniture). The flood of Medicaid money washed away any incentive to provide high-quality care to attract more patients.

Competing for Certificates of Need, Not for Patients

With chronic excess demand guaranteeing full occupancy from the first day, new nursing homes were sure money-makers. If placed in nice locations to attract a sizable share of private-pay patients, even more money could be made. CON regulations slowed, but did not entirely stop, the construction of new nursing homes. Since a CON was now required, what would determine who got to build these facilities and where they would be placed? State officials faced a dilemma. If the beds were built in a nice area, they would generate higher profits and would not cost the state as much money, since only a few beds would be taken by Medicaid patients. On the other hand, placing a nursing home in a poorer area of high need would do more to relieve the shortage of Medicaid beds, but cost the state more money. The conflict between patient needs and state budget pressures made it necessary to compromise. It is unlikely that CON regulation actually did much to change or improve the location of new nursing home beds.

Who gets to build?   Certainly the state might favor faith-based groups that donated money to help care for patients. However, being political, the state might favor nursing home owners who donated money to help elect a congressperson or senator. With chronic excess demand, the CON itself became valuable property. In effect, one could "buy" patients by obtaining a CON from the government. Once a nursing home owner had a CON, the supply of Medicaid patients was ensured and the owner would not have to do any marketing or make any quality improvements to attract patients. Competition was thus shifted away from the market and into the political regulatory arena.

Windfall profits accrued to anyone who was able to obtain a CON for new construction or who already owned a nursing home. This does not mean that the next owner would make excess profits. When the facility was sold, the new owner had to pay for the building and implicitly for the CON—a piece of paper whose value was roughly equal to the expected future profits of the facility. The new owner, after paying $10 million for a $5 million building to get the CON, would have high fixed costs and find it hard to make a profit unless he or she reduced operating costs and hence reduced quality.

Who Pays?   CON restrictions succeeded in reducing state Medicaid budgets and providing excess profits to nursing home owners. So the question then became, if both owners and regulators benefited, who got hurt? The answer is that patients and their families paid, directly or indirectly, to generate those financial gains. Without competition, patients were often forced to take whatever bed they could get. Instead of conducting market research to meet patient needs, nursing home operators sensibly devoted their dollars to lobbying for continued regulation. Restrictions on supply also meant higher prices for private-pay patients. The biggest cost of CON regulation is all the hours of unpaid labor and disruption imposed on families who could not get their loved ones into a needed nursing home bed, or who had to wait months to do so. In the highest need category (people with dementia, people with multiple impairments in performing ADLs), more than 90 percent are in nursing homes in states where there is no shortage of beds, but only 50 percent of similarly impaired patients are in nursing homes in states that continue to impose tight limits on bed supply.[11] What happens to the other 40 percent? Who cares for them and at what personal sacrifice? Just because family labor and unnecessary declines in quality of life are not charged for in the market does not make them less costly.

Evidence on the Effects of CON

The primary purpose of CON from the beginning has been to limit the growth of states' Medicaid expenditures. The crisis atmosphere generated after Medicaid suddenly flooded the market has eased over time and, with it, the reflexive need to use regulations to impose order on a market out of control faded. The shortage of beds created by restricting supply became more of an issue. Long waiting lists and the protests of families whose lives were disrupted by having to provide unpaid caregiving put pressure on states to relax or eliminate their CON rules. The differences between states that have continued to use CON and those that have stopped illustrate some of the effects of artificial controls on supply. The length of time a patient has to wait for a bed has fallen in states where CON has been repealed. Also, the large disparity in waiting time between private-pay and Medicaid patients has been reduced or eliminated as shortages have disappeared. It often has been assumed that nursing homes with a high percentage of Medicaid patients are less successful in attracting private-pay patients and are thus of lower-than-average quality. A study comparing states with and without CON showed that higher percentages of Medicaid reimbursement were indeed associated with lower quality in states where CON caused a chronic shortage of beds.[12] However, this was not the case in the states without CON. As free entry made more beds available, nursing homes had to compete for Medicaid patients by providing better quality. Since 1990, the supply situation has continued to ease, and more and more states show declines in occupancy. With empty beds, competition for all types of patients has intensified.

11.5 CASE-MIX REIMBURSEMENT

Even with an adequate supply of beds, the fact that the state pays only a single fixed rate per day for nursing home care means that some patients may be denied care. A patient who is very sick or whose disruptive mental condition requires frequent attention costs more than a patient who is healthy and lucid. With revenue per day fixed, a nursing home can increase profits by accepting only less costly patients who need very little care. To provide nursing homes with incentives to admit more severely ill patients, some states have developed **case-mix reimbursement** systems that increase payments based on an index of need. Whereas the starting point for acute medical case-mix reimbursement is the diagnosis (see Chapter 8, Section 2, for a discussion of diagnostically related group [DRG] reimbursement in hospitals), in LTC the starting point is the patient's level of functioning. Most frequently, this is measured in terms of the number of **ADLs** for which the individual needs assistance (dressing, grooming, bathing, eating, mobility, transferring, walking, toileting, see Table 11.5) as well as the level of assistance required.[13] In New York state, the association between number of ADLs and cost of care was used to create a number of **resource utilization groups** (**RUGS**).

The U.S. General Accounting Office issued a report in 1990 showing that the problem that "heavy care" patients have in obtaining a nursing home bed is substantially reduced in states with systems that adjust reimbursement according to case mix. However, the adjustment is always imperfect, and even with differential payment rates, nursing homes may find it profitable to accept some patients while turning others away.[14] Minnesota created a system with eleven levels of reimbursement from A (patients with 0 to 3 ADLs and no special problems) to K (patients with 7 to 8 ADLs who require special nursing). To the extent that differences in payment rate correctly adjust for differences in cost, a nursing home would have no reason to selectively admit one group rather than another. However, researchers at the University of Minnesota estimated that categories H and J were significantly overcompensated, while categories C and F were significantly undercompensated.[15] The total number of days of care remained basically the same from 1986 (the first year of the case-mix reimbursement system) to 1990, but nursing homes admitted more patients in the overcompensated categories over time and admitted fewer

---

TABLE 11.5   Activities of Daily Living (ADL) Evaluation Form

For each area of functioning listed below, check the description that applies (The word *assistance* means supervision, direction, or personal assistance).

Bathing—either sponge bath, tub bath, or shower

☐ | ☐ | ☐

| Receives no assistance (gets in and out of tub by self if tub is usual means of bathing) | Receives assistance in bathing only one part of the body (such as the back or a leg) | Receives assistance in bathing more than one part of the body (or not bathed) |

Dressing—gets clothes from closets and drawers, including underclothes, outer garments, and using fasteners (including braces, if worn)

☐ | ☐ | ☐

| Gets clothes and gets completely dressed without assistance | Gets clothes and gets dressed without assistance except for assistance in tying shoes | Receives assistance in getting clothes or in getting dressed, or stays partly or completely undressed |

Toileting—going to the "toilet room" for bowel and urine elimination; cleaning self after elimination and arranging clothes

☐ | ☐ | ☐

| Goes to "toilet room," cleans self, and arranges clothes without assistance (may use object for support such as cane, walker, or wheelchair) | Receives assistance in going to "toilet room" or in cleansing self or in arranging clothes after elimination or in use of night bed pan or commode | Doesn't go to room termed "toilet" for the elimination process |

Transfer—

☐ | ☐ | ☐

| Moves in and out of bed as well as in and out of chair without assistance | Moves in and out of bed or chair with assistance | Doesn't get out of bed |

Continence—

☐ | ☐ | ☐

| Controls urination and bowel movement completely by self | Has occasional "accidents" | Supervision helps keep urine or bowel control; catheter is used or is incontinent |

Feeding—

☐ | ☐ | ☐

| Feeds self without assistance | Feeds self except for getting assistance in cutting meat or buttering bread | Receives assistance in feeding or is fed partly or completely by using tubes or intravenous fluids |

Source: Adapted from Katz et al., "Studies of Illness in the Aged. The Index of ADL: A Standardized Measure of Biological and Psychosocial Function" *Journal of the American Medical Association,* 185:94ff. 1963.

patients in the undercompensated categories (see Table 11.6). Even though some of the change may have been due to "gaming" of the regulatory system by reclassifying patients into more profitable categories, part of the change appears to have been a result of selective admissions policies. The lesson of this study is that nursing homes, even nonprofit nursing homes, will respond to any remaining inaccuracies in case-mix reimbursement.

11.6 SUBSTITUTION

The lack of extra payment for patients who need extra care may mean that they cannot be transferred to a nursing home and hence must remain in a high-cost acute hospital bed for additional administratively necessary days (ANDs). Some hospitals have even purchased nursing homes primarily to make it easier to discharge their post-acute patients. Yet opportunities for system-wide savings are often passed up because different parties are paying different bills. For instance, Medicare (federal) pays most hospital bills, while Medicaid (state) pays most nursing home bills. A state may be unwilling to pay for additional nursing home days, even though each additional hospital day is much more expensive, because the cost of hospital days is borne by the federal government, not the state.

A larger and more general problem in trying to use service substitution to reduce costs is controlling who gets the additional days of nursing home care. Increased bed supply and changes in reimbursement that make it easier to transfer patients from hospitals to nursing homes also make it easier for new patients to obtain care. The cost of providing care to these new patients tends to outweigh the savings obtained by switching some patients from hospitals to nursing homes. A large experiment attempted to demonstrate cost savings by "channeling" patients at high risk for repeat hospitalization into less expensive nursing homes, home health care, and social services.[16] The channeling project was not able to

| **TABLE 11.6** | Nursing Homes Admit More of the Patients that are Relatively More Profitable | | | | | | |

	(care level)	Case Index	Revenue	Estimated Cost	Profit	Days of Care 1986	Days of Care 1990	Change %
A	(0–3 ADLs)	1.00	$47.50	$43.64	9%	3,008,098	2,781,037	–8%
B	(0–3 ADLs with behavior problem)	1.30	$51.40	$55.31	–7%	1,236,058	1,066,884	–14%
C	(0–3 ADLs with special nursing)	1.64	$55.83	$68.09	–18%	193,084	76,229	–61%
D	(4–6 ADLs)	1.95	$59.86	$66.96	–11%	1,466,417	1,457,940	–1%
E	(4–6 ADLs and behavior problem)	2.27	$64.01	$61.40	4%	1,252,917	1,071,265	–14%
F	(4–6 ADLs and special nursing)	2.29	$64.28	$89.53	–28%	249,083	105,049	–58%
G	(7–8 ADLs and heavy feeding)	2.56	$67.79	$66.00	3%	1,791,836	2,471,990	38%
H	(7–8 ADLs, heavy feeding & behavior)	3.07	$74.42	$60.66	23%	1,225,666	1,370,201	12%
I	(7–8 ADLs and very heavy feeding)	3.25	$76.76	$79.85	–4%	1,812,752	954,488	–19%
J	(7–8 ADLs, feeding & severe neurology)	3.53	$80.39	$62.79	28%	1,688,881	2,345,085	39%
K	(7–8 ADLs and special nursing)	4.12	$88.06	$89.86	–2%	1,364,042	835,112	–39%
Average			$66.39	$67.64	–0.3%	14,658,834	14,535,280	–0.8%

Source: J. A. Nyman and R. A. Connor, "Do Case-Mix Adjusted Nursing Home Reimbursements Actually Reflect Costs? Minnesota's Experience," *Journal of Health Economics* 13, no. 2 (1994): 145–162.

generate savings because only a few hospitalizations could be avoided. Counseling patients was itself expensive and, for the most part, resulted in new patients using additional services rather than moving old patients from hospitals to cheaper LTC substitutes.

It was once thought that expanded home health care and ambulatory surgery would save money for Medicare by reducing hospitalization. Part A (hospital) expenses have indeed declined in recent years, but Part B (professional services) expenses have increased by a much greater amount. For example, cataract surgery, IV antibiotics, and physical therapy are cheaper when performed on an outpatient basis, but once the need for a hospital admission was eliminated, so many new patients utilized these services that the total cost of treatment more than doubled.

11.7 FINANCIAL REIMBURSEMENT CYCLES

There is a recurrent cycle of scarcity, generosity, and abuse that occurs in the financing of medical services. This is well illustrated by home health care, which just moved through a surge of uncontrolled spending and is now being restrained. There are typically four stages of reimbursement, beginning with charitable assistance, moving through cost reimbursement and complex administered price systems, and ending with firm controls over total budgets (see Table 11.7). This extended cycle is seen in the development of financing for hospitals, ambulatory surgery, nursing homes and, most recently, home health care. Before the spread of insurance coverage, most medical organizations were nonprofit and the need for more services (and more funding) was broadly recognized. Requests for payment were based on trust. It was assumed that the fees were less than the cost of care or that any excess was being used to subsidize needy people. The amount of funding was limited primarily by the availability of donors. For home health care, this situation held for a number of years. The dominant providers were community and regional visiting nurse services, charitable agencies that employed salaried nurses to visit the disabled homebound. As such, home health care was a minor and unprofitable niche within the health care system, accounting for less than 0.3 percent of national medical expenditures.

As the length of stay in hospitals began to shorten, patients were discharged "quicker and sicker," raising the need for skilled assistance at home. Reimbursement on the traditional "what you ask for" basis was made, mostly to visiting nurse services. Soon, Medicare was paying 25 to 30 percent of the bills, with Medicaid picking up another 5 to 10 percent. Entrepreneurs spotted a new guaranteed stream of funding and developed for-profit businesses that were tightly managed, paid nurses well (and made them see more patients per hour), and raised charges to build the bottom line and expand rapidly. By 1980, home health care had become a $2 billion business, accounting for about 1 percent of total health expenditures, rising to $10 billion (1.6 percent of national health expenditures by 1989).

TABLE 11.7	The Reimbursement Cycle
Stage 1	**"What you ask for"**—Trusting charity providers
Stage 2	**Cost reimbursement**—Leads to expansion, manipulation of cost reports
Stage 3	**Complex administered prices**—PPSs put in place to reduce costs get "gamed" by providers seeking even more reimbursement
Stage 4	**Global budget control**—Set reimbursement increases to match increases in tax base

The second stage of the reimbursement cycle commences when the payer attempts to replace traditional fees with a more precise determination of what services actually cost. This impulse is driven by two opposing claims: (1) from the providers, that the existing payments are not sufficient to cover their costs and will not allow expansion to provide services to all patients who need care, and (2) from the payers, a suspicion that fees are too large and provide excess profits and incentive to create new providers where none are needed. So begins the debate and the implementation of reimbursement based on costs, rather than fees.

Cost reimbursement appears simple—and then the accountants move in. What exactly is "cost" anyway? Should owners be paid more for the use of their buildings and other capital and not just for operating expenses? Is it important to pay owners extra to ensure that patients who are more difficult to treat (those with dementia or AIDS) are able to obtain service? Should every new home health care agency that opens receive enough cost reimbursement to make sure that it stays in operation? While these positions are defensible, such cost reimbursement is much different from the way capital markets respond to investors opening new restaurants (which are frequently allowed to fail) and predictably leads to a massive increase in capacity. The facile comment regarding accountants should not be taken as disparaging. The accountants who work for health care providers are doing their jobs—which in this situation is to maximize reimbursement so that providers can grow and do more. Over time, the accounting system becomes more highly regulated and more complex, but no more satisfactory. No matter how costs are counted, there always will be disputes (overtime wages, capital arbitrage, sunk costs) and continual expansion (since more costs mean more reimbursement). Eventually, the cost reimbursement system becomes unsustainable, and the era of cost-control arrives. For home health care, this turning point was reached in the early 1990s.

After the pathologies of open-ended cost reimbursement have become apparent, attempts are made to set payment limits in advance, usually based on an objective indicator such as patient diagnosis. This method was adopted by hospitals (via DRGs), physicians (via resource-based relative value scale [RBRVS]), and nursing homes (via RUGS). These payments were more difficult to arrange in home health care because the extent of disability and social isolation, not medical need, drives care. Also, unlike surgery or nursing home admission, home health visits were actively welcomed by the homebound elderly and even by elderly people who just needed someone to change their sheets, make a meal, and chat for a while. In some cases, agencies appear to have driven demand by calling elderly patients and asking "Would you like someone to visit you at home? Medicare will pay for it." Abuse of the system became rampant. Payments, which rose 17 percent a year from 1980 to 1989, rose by 40 percent in 1990, 35 percent in 1991, and 37 percent in 1992. This exploitation of the system was unsustainable and led to the inevitable retrenchment with multimillion dollar lawsuits for fraudulent billing and improper referrals.[17] Several years were required to bring the system under control. In 1996, Medicare and Medicaid were still paying $20 billion for home health care, more than half of all home health care expenses. While Medicaid expenditures continued to rise slightly, by 2000 Medicare had cut payments by 50 percent to just $9 billion. Forcing patients and private insurance to pay directly for more visits restored some balance to the system.

October 2000 marked the implementation of the newest Medicare home health financing reform, a fixed predetermined payment rate per 60-day episode.[18] The payment rate depends on an assessment of the patient's overall need for care as classified into one of 80 home health resource groups (HHRGs). Doctors must certify (and recertify) a patient as qualifying for care when the first visit is made, but the number of visits made within a 60-day episode has no effect on total payments. It appears that home health care reimbursement has entered the third stage of the reimbursement cycle, because it is semi-fixed and largely divorced from the cost accounting procedures of providers.

The endpoint of cost-control comes when the payer decides to match payments to the availability of funding, not to the number of patients or visits, or to diagnoses. This has already happened for Medicare payment of physicians under the rubric of sustainable growth rate (SGR), a mechanism for linking the increase in total payments each year to the increase in gross domestic product (and hence to the tax revenues available). Such a rigid and mechanical approach to funding, of course, brings its own problems, leading to further amendments, enlargements, reforms, and revolutions. In this regard, it is not so much the end as the start of a new cycle. What is important in this discussion is not so much the specifics of home health care or federal payment regulations, but the idea of payment as a strategic game between payers and providers. One side wants to control costs, while the other side wants to increase revenues. The rules are not abstract truths or arbitrary legal dictums written in stone, but are themselves part of the game. Expanded funding in a new area, such as home health care, inevitably means excesses and a certain amount of fraud. Such excesses will, to a greater or lesser extent, be corrected over time.

11.8 CONTINUING CARE RETIREMENT COMMUNITIES AND THE WEALTHY ELDERLY

Elderly people with enough money to afford LTC insurance have not been particularly interested in purchasing it. However, the wealthy elderly have flocked to retirement communities and other market alternatives. Among the most successful have been life care communities or continuing care retirement communities (CCRCs). In essence, these residential developments combine an LTC insurance health maintenance organization (HMO) with a retirement community, guaranteeing people a pleasant place to live and nursing care for the remainder of their lives.[19] In most retirement communities, new entrants (usually married couples in their 70s) pay a substantial fixed fee upon entry ($75,000 to $250,000) for their apartments, and then a monthly fee ($600 to $2000 a month) for maintenance, housekeeping, social services, and some or all meals. Home health nurses are provided when needed. As a person becomes disabled, he or she can enter a nursing home on the premises. Residents do not own their apartments, but do have the right to live in them until they die or are admitted to the nursing facility. Major advantages of CCRCs are the controlled environment geared toward the elderly, the possibilities of creating a new circle of friends even as health declines, and the ability to continue seeing these friends daily even after entering the nursing facility. CCRCs range from modestly nice to quite luxurious. The nursing facilities tend to be less institutional than those in most nursing homes. Even severely impaired people may still have table linens, candles with dinner, and a homelike atmosphere.

The large entry fee and sizable monthly payments generate two problems: (1) the possibility of bankruptcy or fraud on the part of the owner and (2) lack of affordability. The first CCRCs depended almost entirely on entry fees, and had very low monthly rates. Many were "sponsored" but not financially supported by religious denominations. After taking the up-front fee (sometimes, the entire savings and estate of the couple), CCRCs were obligated to provide care for life. They should have invested the money wisely so that interest income could have been used to pay for maintenance and nursing home care. Unfortunately, the actuarial estimates were often quite far from the mark. Financial projections assumed that apartments could be turned over and resold every ten years or so, but the people who chose to enter lived much longer than usual for their ages (a form of adverse selection). In many cases, the husband began to need nursing home care (which cost extra) while the wife continued to live for many years (occupying a large apartment that could not be resold). Some religious leaders were uncomfortable about raising monthly fees when millions of dollars in investments were in the bank, even though the future obligations for nursing home care and maintenance were greater than what could be covered by the interest. Necessary financial reserves were depleted over time when monthly rates were not raised promptly. These factors alone would have been sufficient to cause problems, but were compounded in case after case when unscrupulous CCRC operators paid themselves excessive sales fees or salaries, or simply embezzled funds. Immediately after a facility opened, there would be millions of dollars in entry fees in the bank. The loss or mismanagement of these funds would not become evident until years later, when buildings needed repair or residents needed nursing home care. By then, the money was sometimes literally out of the country. Numerous reforms have been instituted to maintain the financial integrity of CCRCs. Now, if a religious denomination agrees to sponsor a facility, it must legally guarantee future expenses. Reserves must be routinely reported and financial viability, including coverage of medical and nursing home expenses, must be demonstrated. The risky "pay everything up front" financing has been supplanted so that more costs are covered by monthly fees, and often the nursing home care component is paid for separately and subject to standard underwriting practices (e.g., waiting periods, extra fees, exclusions for those entering with preexisting conditions such as cancer or Alzheimer's disease).

More and more elderly people can afford the cost of entering a CCRC. Definitions of "wealthy" are to some extent always subjective, but by any measure, the wealth of the elderly has risen dramatically both in absolute terms and relative to the wealth of the younger population. In the 1950s, many elderly were poor, still struggling with the aftermath of the Depression. In contrast, young families faced bright economic prospects, and relatively few children lived in poverty. By 1990, Social Security, marital patterns, and other factors had reversed the incidence of poverty. The elderly were much better off than their children. Favorable tax and transfer treatment, along with years of savings, have made people 55 to 64 the wealthiest group in America, with a net worth of $727,000 in 2001, and people 65 to 74 almost equal in net worth at $673,800 (see Table 11.8).[20] This does not mean that there are no sub-groups of the elderly with high poverty rates (the single black elderly are notably poor, as are the oldest old, above age 85), but it does mean that many can afford to buy care and protection in the market using their own substantial assets rather than depending on government programs. Married couples reaching age 65 have higher average incomes than the rest of the population, and twice as many financial assets. At least half of them can readily afford a CCRC or other market-based LTC financing mechanism. Public protection of the poor will always be necessary. What is important to change is the perception that all or even most of the elderly are "poor."

Medicare Catastrophic Coverage Act of 1988 and the Taxpayer Revolt

Policies designed without regard to the diversity in wealth among the elderly may be seriously flawed and are apt to be rejected in the marketplace. A prime example is the Medicare Catastrophic Coverage Act (MCCA) passed by Congress in 1988—and repealed in 1989. The act was intended to extend Medicare coverage by reducing co-pays, deductibles, and limits; adding a pharmaceutical benefit; and making other benefit increases. It appeared that the MCCA would be quite popular, because many of the elderly had been buying Medigap insurance at far greater cost, pharmaceuticals were a major

TABLE 11.8	Average Income and Wealth for Different Age Categories			
	Income		Wealth	
	Median	**Average**	**Median**	**Average**
All Families	$39,900	$68,000	$ 86,100	$395,500
Under 35	33,400	44,200	11,600	90,700
35–44	51,400	77,100	77,600	259,500
45–54	54,500	93,200	132,000	485,600
55–64	45,200	86,900	181,500	727,000
65–74	27,800	58,100	176,300	673,800
75 and older	22,400	36,700	151,400	465,900

Source: Federal Reserve Bulletin, page 1–32, January 2003.

source of out-of-pocket expenditures, and the largest lobbying group for the elderly, AARP (formerly the American Association of Retired Persons), strongly supported passage of the bill. The problem came in designing a payment mechanism. MCCA was intended to be "**budget neutral,**" in that additional premiums and taxes would pay for the cost of the new benefits. Unlike Medicare Part B premiums, which are the same for all participants, MCCA premiums increased with income. The poor elderly would not have to pay anything. To subsidize the poor elderly, the higher income elderly would have to pay as much as $800 per year, more than the expected value of the additional benefits. Although perhaps willing to vote for higher taxes (which mostly fell on younger working people), the wealthy elderly were outraged at being forced to pay extra to cover the poor. Legislators visiting their local districts expecting accolades were pelted with questions and complaints. Angry older people blocked cars in protest, wrote letters, and swore revenge. In short order, the biggest extension of Medicare since 1965 had to be repealed. Although it benefited most elderly people, MCCA was not financially beneficial to the upper-income elderly, and it is this group that is most politically active.[21]

Similar tensions characterize the current debate on adding prescription benefits to Medicare. Both parties agree that coverage should be extended, but differ on how to do so in ways that have predictable economic effects. Republicans favor various tax subsidies to allow the elderly to buy their own pharmaceutical insurance, which favors those who pay more taxes (the rich) and creates a divided market dominated by private insurance companies. The various Democratic plans place drug coverage within the existing Medicare program, spreading costs and benefits widely and uniformly through a national government program, thus favoring poorer Americans who tend to pay fewer taxes and are less likely to have retirement health benefits.

11.9 THE EFFECTS OF AGING ON COST AND UTILIZATION

Defining Boundaries: Is Long-Term Care "Medical"?

The Medicare program is immensely popular (and immensely expensive) because it serves every elderly person regardless of need and, therefore, provides an upper-middle-class standard of care to all by using taxpayers' money. Attempts to forge an equally popular LTC program have failed. While numerous cultural and political factors are involved, a major reason is that most of the features that characterize medical care (randomly occurring illness, reliance on physicians when quality can be a life-and-death issue, rapid technological innovation) are missing in LTC. Instead, much of the cost of LTC is for housing, food, social amenities—things normally identified as personal responsibilities or life style choices rather than medical care. The boundaries between medical care, social services, and living expenses often become ambiguous. Distinctions between professional services and unpaid family help are often similarly unclear. The divergence between medical care and LTC suggests that the types of health insurance financing developed for medical care may not be appropriate for financing the costs of assisted daily living characteristic of most LTC.

What difference does it make if LTC is called *medical* or not? In a word, money. Distinguishing services as *medical* makes it more likely that they will be covered by insurance, more likely that the people providing services will be licensed, and more likely that quality will be regulated and that choices by consumers in the marketplace will be supplanted by professional standards. LTC has more in common with social insurance programs such as disability, workers' compensation, pensions, and Social Security. Yet the tremendous cost of expanding entitlements and the lack of taxpayer support has caused many advocates to try to find ways to "medicalize" LTC to increase the flow of funds to professionals and institutions.

LTC Insurance

Although most medical care is paid for through third-party insurance, private LTC insurance did not even come into existence until the 1980s, and still pays for less than 3 percent of nursing home and home health care bills. There are several major reasons LTC insurance is not as attractive to consumers as insurance for acute medical care, which are summarized in Table 11.9. The incidence of disability requiring LTC is not so much random, as delayed. If we live long enough, almost all of us will need some form of LTC. Yet if we wait until age 70 to purchase LTC insurance, the premiums will be very high, since the likelihood of loss is so great. A more prudent course would be to plan in advance. However, people who purchase LTC insurance at age 40 will have to wait many years to obtain benefits. Financially, they may do almost as well if they put aside savings to be used for LTC if the need arises, letting interest accrue over the intervening years. In addition, people may die without entering a nursing home, and hence the money used for LTC premiums could instead be passed on to their heirs. If one did end up needing a lot of LTC and ran out of savings, there would always be Medicaid to fall back on. Why should people pay premiums for thirty years when the government would pay if they really needed help?

A final barrier to LTC insurance is the nature of the benefit: payment for a nursing home stay. Unlike payment for acute medical treatment, which is expected to improve health or reduce the risk of premature death, payment for nursing home care just makes it easier to be taken from home and be placed in an institution. It is hard to get excited about paying thousands of dollars to merely slow the rate of decline and extend the number of

TABLE 11.9   Reasons LTC Insurance is Not Popular

1. Incidence of LTC is less random than acute illness.
2. Insurance must be purchased so far in advance of anticipated need that savings become a good alternative to insurance.
3. Medicaid is always there, providing a stop-loss against large expenditures.
4. To get benefits paid, purchaser must be admitted to nursing home. Unlike treatment for acute illness, the person would usually rather make treatment more rather than less difficult to obtain.
5. Benefits mostly reduce expenditures by heirs and Medicaid, rather than helping the patients who pay the premiums.

years spent living with disability. Upon reflection, it becomes clear that the greatest bene-ficiaries of LTC insurance are not the patients, but their children and the Medicaid pro-gram. Children benefit because they may find it easier to send a disabled parent to a nursing home if the charges are paid for by insurance. In addition, children protect their inheritance by having the risk of caring for a disabled parent insured. Medicaid also ben-efits because nursing home charges are paid for by premiums rather than state and federal tax monies. Expansion of private LTC insurance will be limited until (a) benefits are mod-ified so that they help patients continue to live at home rather than making it easier to be admitted to a nursing home; (b) payments are made in advance with favorable tax treat-ment by employers, as is the case with most group medical insurance; and (c) policies are coordinated with Medicaid so that they yield financial benefits to patients, their spouses, and heirs, instead of offsetting government expenditures.

The Effects of Aging

It is widely assumed that aging increases the need for, and the use of, medical services. This assumption, at least in its simplest form, is not well supported. As an economist, you would quickly point out the constraints imposed by a limited life span. Treating disease in a patient who is expected to die of other causes within five years is less valuable than treat-ing a young patient likely to live another fifty years. When scarce medical resources have to be allocated, most people, even the elderly, support favoring the young. Scarcity imposes another constraint that may limit use: elderly people who cannot afford care. In 1953, older people in the United States spent about 1.5 times as much ($435 versus $341) on medical care as the middle-aged.[22] More, but not a lot more. With the advent of Medicare, older people spent about two times as much on medical care as the middle-aged in 1970, four times as much in 1987, and five times as much in 1998 (see Table 11.10 and Figure 11.3).[23] The reason so much more money is spent on medical care for the elderly today than 50 years ago is because the system has made more money available, not because today's elderly are sicker. Comparisons made with other countries confirm that income and insurance, not aging, have caused expenditures to rise.[24]

Close examination of data show that today's elderly are healthier and less likely to be disabled than in prior years. Much of the growth in spending has been for the oldest old, and for LTC rather than for curative medicine or surgery.[25] The data suggest that the number of elderly is growing, and cumulative disability is increasing, but that health sta-tus at age 65, at age 75, and even at age 85, is markedly improving. Spending on medical care is significantly higher for the last year of life—but that final year, by definition, only occurs once in each lifetime. Furthermore, heroic efforts to save life that seem necessary at age 30, and perhaps justified at age 70, look intrusive and wasteful at age 90. Thus, the actual pattern of spending for medical intervention peaks at about age 75 and begins to decline after that as family and physicians become more willing to accept the dictates of

TABLE 11.10	Health Care Spending of Young and Old, 1953–1998						
	1953	**1963**	**1966**	**1970**	**1977**	**1987**	**1995**
All people	$ 88	$141	$182	$292	$ 658	$1,776	$2,884
Under age 65	85	135	155	236	512	1,287	1,946
Age 65 and older	108	191	445	799	1,856	5,360	8,953
Ratio: over/under	1.28	1.41	2.87	3.39	3.63	4.16	4.60

Source: Cutler and Meara, 1997, Lubitz et al., 2001.

FIGURE 11.3   Health Care Spending in the Old and Young, 1953 - 1995

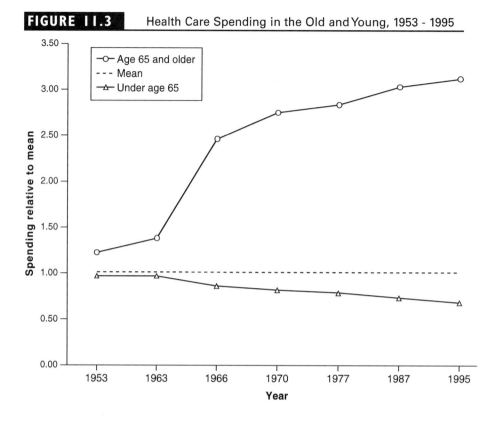

nature. Total health spending continues to rise with advancing age only because more is spent for nursing home, hospice, home health, and related supportive care.

The market for supportive services among the elderly is affected not only by demand, but also by supply. In this regard, it is important to remember that most care is actually provided by unpaid family and friends. New estimates by Darius Lakdawalla and Tomas Philipson suggest that the increase in the number of healthy older people able to care for others, and particularly the increase in the percentage of the elderly who are male (and thus likely to be married to the more numerous females), will reduce the number of elderly people placed in institutions.[26] It is the lack of someone at home to care for you, not just disability, which drives up the rate of nursing home admissions.

SUGGESTIONS FOR FURTHER READING

National Institute on Aging "An Aging World: 2001," (www.census.gov/prod/2001pubs/p95-01-1.pdf).

National Center for Health Statistics, "Trends in Health and Aging," (www.nchs.cdc.gov),

AARP (www.aarp.org).

Urban Institute, "Long-Term Care: Consumers, Providers and Financing," a chartbook,(www.urban.org/pdfs /LTC_Chartbook.pdf).

Connie J. Evashwick, ed. *The Continuum of Long-Term Care* (Albany, N.Y.: Delmar Publishers, 1996).

William Scanlon, "A Theory of the Nursing Home Market," *Inquiry* 17, no. 1 (1980): 25–41.

US General Accounting Office, *Nursing Homes: Admission Problems for Medicaid Recipients and Attempts to Solve Them,* GAO report #GAO/HRD-90-135 (September 1990).

Darius Lakdawalla and Tomas Philipson, "The rise in old-age longevity and the market for long-term care." *American Economic Review* 92, no. 1 (March 2002): 295–306.

SUMMARY

1. Most LTC expenditures are for nursing home care, but most care of the disabled elderly is **provided by unpaid family members** and friends.

2. As the number of elderly rose, and the **shadow price of labor** by adult daughters increased, more and more LTC was shifted from unpaid household production to commercial market purchases of care.

3. Nursing home economics is dominated by a **split two-part market.** Private-pay patients tend to pay more and sometimes receive better care. Medicaid patients must demonstrate to the state that they qualify by being poor. The state pays their bills, but will not pay as much; therefore, there is a chronic excess of Medicaid patients trying to get into beds that nursing home owners would prefer to fill with private-pay patients.

4. CON **regulations** were intended to halt the construction of new nursing homes after the passage of Medicaid in 1965 greatly increased demand and hence the tax burden on the states. CON has exacerbated the shortage of nursing homes and caused patients to wait months for a bed. **Competing for CONs** has helped regulators and nursing home owners, but has not helped the patients who are forced to wait months for a bed or accept substandard care.

5. In a shortage situation, patients most in need of nursing home care are more likely to be denied a bed, because their care tends to be more costly. To alleviate this problem, some states have replaced the flat-rate per diem with a rate that is **case-mix adjusted** for differences in need. Such systems help match reimbursement with cost, but can never be perfect.

6. **Substituting** lower-cost LTC for hospital care (or home health care for nursing home care) sounds good, but usually increases total system costs because so many new patients are brought in.

7. The expansion of home health care, like that of most other medical services, was financed by a system of payments that proceeded through four stages:
   a. **Fees** paid to trusted voluntary organizations
   b. **Cost reimbursements**
   c. Complex **administered prices**
   d. Total cost control through global **budgets** adjusted to match growth in GDP
   This reimbursement cycle is driven by the strategic behavior of providers who push the boundaries and "game" the system to maximize revenues.

8. LTC primarily provides assistance to people with disabilities to help them perform activities of daily living, and financing is appropriately done through social insurance. "**Medicalizing**" LTC enables providers to tap new sources of funding, allows workers to justify licensure, probably increases quality, and clearly increases total costs. It has become clear that **increases in income and insurance,** not increases in disease and disability, **have allowed medical care expenditures to rise.** The cost of medical care for the elderly is now five times higher than the cost of medical care for the middle-aged, whereas in 1950 the cost of medical care for the elderly was less than two times the cost of medical care for the middle-aged.

9. People in the United States are living longer. While this means that there will be more and **more elderly people,** the average person age 75 **will be healthier,** more

likely to live at home, and more likely to be able to care for a spouse or friend so that he or she too can live at home rather than being admitted to a nursing home.

PROBLEMS

1. {*utilization, cost*} How much is the average cost per day of a nursing home day? On a typical day in the United States, are there more patients in hospitals or nursing homes? Which type of care is growing more rapidly? What is the most rapidly growing form of LTC?

2. {*incidence, social insurance*} Who provides most of the care for elderly people who need assistance with the daily tasks of living? How do these helpers get paid?

3. {*case-mix selection*} Does the administrator of a hospital want to admit patients who are more sick than average or less sick than average? Does the administrator of an LTC facility want to admit patients who are sicker than average or healthier than average? Why do LTC administrators face financial incentives that are different from those that hospital administrators face?

4. {*competition*} Hospitals compete for doctors and the newest technology. How do nursing homes compete? Does price play more, or less, of a role? What about technology?

5. {*supply controls*} Draw a set of supply and demand diagrams illustrating how CON legislation could cause waiting lists and increase the price of care.

6. {*labor markets*} Several major trends have characterized labor markets in the United States over the past 80 years: wages have increased, life expectancy has increased, and female labor force participation has increased. Discuss how each of these has affected the market for LTC services. Which has been more important in determining the shape of LTC markets, changes in labor market factors or changes in medical technology?

7. {*substitution*} Use supply and demand diagrams to show what would happen if additional LTC insurance allows more substitution of nursing home care for hospital care. According to your diagram, do LTC expenditures increase or decrease? Do hospital expenditures increase or decrease? Do total expenditures (LTC + hospital) increase or decrease?

8. {*rent seeking*} If there is competition for CONs, what is the price of a CON? Who gets paid? Is the CON worth more than is paid for it? If so, who obtains these gains from trade?

9. {*shortages, discrimination*} Would a shortage of beds created by regulation make it easier or more difficult for a nursing home administrator to racially discriminate among patients for admission? Draw supply and demand graphs to illustrate.

10. {*risk*} Are the risks born in LTC insurance different from the risks in hospital insurance?

11. {*substitution*} Does the federal/state-funded Medicaid program expand or contract the market for private LTC insurance? Who would benefit from a federal subsidy of private LTC insurance plans?

12. {*productivity, outcomes*} To measure the productivity of medical care, economists attempt to measure outcomes of treatment: increases in longevity, fewer sick days, increased earnings. Which measures would you use to compare the productivity of two nursing homes?

13. {*Medicaid, two-part market, tax incidence*} If you were elderly, would you be in favor of or against a proposal to increase the amount paid per day under Medicaid? Which factors would your response depend on?

14. {*management, vertical integration*} In what ways is a CCRC like an HMO? In what ways is a CCRC different? Are payments made on a similar or different basis? Which is more subject to adverse selection? To moral hazard? Which relies most on gate-keepers? On financial incentives to physicians?

15. {*incidence*} Which socioeconomic groups in the United States benefit most from extensive government funding of LTC? Is the flow of funds progressive or regressive?

16. {*risk aversion, Medigap insurance*} Virtually all elderly people in the United States qual-ify for Medicare. Almost 70 percent also purchase Medigap insurance, which covers co-payments, deductibles, and often home health care and pharmaceuticals. Which insur-ance, Medicare or Medigap, provides the largest "welfare gain from risk pooling" (see Chapters 4 and 5). Does Medigap insurance increase or decrease the cost of Medicare?

ENDNOTES

1. Peter S. Arno, Carol Levine, and Margaret M. Memmott, "The Economic Value of Informal Caregiving," *Health Affairs* 18, no. 2 (March 1999): 182–188.

2. A. E. Benjamin, "An Historical Perspective on Home Care," *Milbank Quarterly* 71, no. 1 (1993): 129–166.

3. Robert L. Kane, Joseph G. Ouslander, and Itamar B. Abras, *Essentials of Clinical Geriatrics* (New York: McGraw-Hill, 1989), 30–44.

4. Susan Hughes, "Home Health Care" in Connie J. Evashwick, ed., *The Continuum of Long-Term Care* (Albany, N.Y.: Delmar Publishers, 1996), 61–81.

5. Brian Burwell, William H. Crown, Carol O'Shaunessy, and Richard Price, "Financing Long-Term Care," Chapter 13 in Connie Evashwick, ed., *The Continuum of Long-Term Care* (Albany, N.Y.: Delmar Publishers, 1996), 199.

6. William Aaronson, "Financing the Continuum of Care: A Disintegrating Past and an Integrating Future," Chapter 14 in Connie Evashwick, ed., *The Continuum of Long-Term Care* (Albany, N.Y.: Delmar Publishers, 1996), 225.

7. William P. Scanlon, "A Theory of the Nursing Home Market," *Inquiry* 17, no. 1 (1980): 25–41.

8. Korbin Liu, Pamela Doty, and Kenneth Manton, "Medicaid Spend-down in Nursing Homes," *The Gerontologist* 30, no. 10 (1990): 7; H. Temkin-Greener, M. Meiner, E. Petty, and J. Szydlowski, "Spending Down to Medicaid in the Nursing Home and in the Community," *Medical Care* 31, no. 8 (1993): 663–679.

9. Brian Burwell, *Middle-Class Welfare: Medicaid Estate Planning for Long-Term Care Coverage* (Lexington, Mass.: Systemetrics, 1991).

10. S. Moses, "The Fallacy of Impoverishment," *The Gerontologist* 30, no. 1 (1990): 21–25.

11. U.S. General Accounting Office, *Nursing Homes: Admission Problems for Medicaid Recipients and Attempts to Solve Them*, GAO Report #GAO/HRD-90-135, September 1990.

12. John Nyman, "The Demand for nursing Home Care," *Journal of Health Economics* 8, no. 2 (1989); and "Excess Demand, the Percentage of Nursing Home Patients, and the Quality of Nursing Home Care," *Journal of Human Resources* 23, no. 1 (1988): 76–92.. 13. S. Katz, A. B. Ford, R. W. Moskowitz, B. A. Jackson, and M. W. Jaffee, "Studies of Illness in the Aged. The Index of ADL: A Standardized Measure of Biological and Psychosocial Function," *Journal of the American Medical Association* 185 (1963): 94ff.

14. U.S. General Accounting Office, *op. cit.*

15. J. A. Nyman and R. A. Connor, "Do Case-Mix Adjusted Nursing Home Reimbursements Actually Reflect Costs? Minnesota's Experience." *Journal of Health Economics* 13, no. 2 (1994): 145–162.

16. P. Kemper, "The Evaluation of the National Long-Term Care Demonstration," *Health Services Research* 23, no. 1 (special issue) (1988).

17. George Anders and Laurie McGinley. "How Do You Tame a Wild U.S. Program? Slowly and Reluctantly. Medicare Home Health Visits Are a Boon for Entrepreneurs; Costs Explode 30% a Year." *Wall Street Journal*, March 6, 1996, sec. A, p. 1ff.

18. Paul L. Grimaldi, "Medicare's New Home Health Prospective Payment System Explained," *Health Care Financial Management* 11 (November 2000): 46–56.

19. H. S. Ruchlin, "Continuing Care Retirement Communities: An Analysis of Financial Viability and Health Care Coverage," *The Gerontologist* 28, no. 2 (1988): 156–162.

20. Ana M. Aizcorbe, Arthur Kennickell, and Kevin B. Moore, "Recent Changes in U.S. Family Finances: Evidence from the 1998 and 2001 Survey of Consumer Finances," *Federal Reserve Bulletin* 89, no. 1 (January 2003): 1–32.

21. William Aaronson, Jacqueline Zinn, and Michael Rosko, "The Success and Repeal of the Medicare Catastrophic Coverage Act: A Paradoxical Lesson for Health Care Reform," *Journal of Health Politics, Policy & Law* 19, no. 4 (1994): 753–771.

22. David M. Cutler and Ellen Meara, "The Medical Costs of the Young and Old: a Forty-year Perspective." National Bureau of Economic Research Working Paper #6114, Cambridge, Mass. (July 1997).

23. James Lubitz et. al. "Three decades of Health Care Use By the Ederly, 1965-1998." *Health Affairs* 20, no. 2 (March 2001): 19–21.

24. Thomas E. Getzen, "Population Aging and the Growth of Health Expenditures," *Journal of Gerontology: Social Sciences* 47, no. 3 (1992): S98–104.

25. Brenda C. Spillman and James Lubitz, "The Effect of Longevity on Spending for Zcute and Long-term Care," *New England Journal of Medicine* 342 (May 11, 2000): 1409–1415.

26. Darius Lakdawalla and Tomas Philipson, "The Rise in Old-age Longevity and the Market for Long-term Care." *American Economic Review* 92, no. 1 (March 2002): 295–306.

CHAPTER 12

PHARMACEUTICALS

QUESTIONS

1. Which are most important in the pharmaceutical industry, fixed costs or variable costs?
2. How many drugs do Americans take? Who pays for them?
3. What events led to the regulation of prescription drugs by the Food and Drug Administration (FDA)?
4. Are patents a cost or an asset?
5. Why is so much more spent on marketing drugs than on marketing surgery or psychotherapy?
6. How profitable is the drug industry?
7. Do patents raise or lower the productivity of research?
8. Do generic drugs replace or compete with brand name drugs?
9. How are prescription costs "managed" by insurance companies?
10. Do pharmaceutical companies compete for patients, prescriptions, or payments?

In any given week, more than 80 percent of U.S. adults use some form of medication, with 50 percent taking a drug prescribed by a doctor.[1*] Eleven prescriptions per year are filled for the average American. It is this "ethical" prescription pharmaceutical market that is examined in this chapter. Sales of creams, ointments, vitamins, herbal supplements, headache pills, digestive aids, and other over-the-counter (OTC) medications, which can be obtained without a prescription, amount to around $30 billion; a large sum, but only a fraction of the $161 billion spent on prescription drugs in 2002.[2] Pharmaceuticals are a physical product; they can be packaged, stored, and shipped, a primary reason this part of health production is truly international. U.S. companies make more than a third of their sales overseas, and several major U.S. suppliers are based in Europe and Asia.

Drugs account for 10 percent of national health expenditures, but are a much larger part of the free cash flow in health care because the pharmaceutical industry is so concentrated and profitable. With many prices far above marginal cost, drug companies are vulnerable to criticism, and repeated calls have been made for price controls. However, it is evident even to critics that pharmaceuticals have been one of the major technological success stories of the twentieth century, with new drugs extending life span and

---

*The first edition version of this chapter was prepared with the assistance of Thomas Abbott, Ph.D., Senior Economist, Outcomes Research Management, Merck & Co. Major revisions have been made for this edition, and the responsibility for all representations, opinions, and statistics rests with the primary textbook author, T.E. Getzen.

productivity at much lower cost than surgery and hospitalization. The profits earned by shareholders, while perhaps excessive in some cases, have been the incentive for expanding corporate research and development (R&D), which has increased from $2 billion in 1980 to more than $30 billion in 2000. The gains in health directly attributable to profit-driven pharmaceutical innovation are collectively worth far more than all sunk costs and shareholder dividends.

12.1 HOW FUNDS FLOW IN

As with all health care services, funding for pharmaceutical products comes from a variety of sources, including patients, employers and private insurance, and federal and state governments (see Table 12.1). The process of obtaining a drug begins with the patient visiting a physician. After making a diagnosis, the physician may give the patient a prescription for a specific drug and directions for its use. Although all drugs are approved for sale by the **Food and Drug Administration (FDA)** based on specific indications, physicians can prescribe drugs as they think appropriate. Moreover, when writing a prescription, physicians do not have to provide a specific indication for the medication, although some exceptions occur in managed care plans. The prescription may be written using the scientific name of the drug or a brand name made up by the manufacturer that first patented the drug.

Usually the patient takes the prescription to the local pharmacy, where a licensed pharmacist fills the prescription. Pharmacists provide additional information about how to take the drug and its potential side effects. If the drug has been in use for a long time, the original patent period may have expired and there is apt to be a chemically and biologically equivalent FDA-approved **generic** version that is cheaper than the original brand name version. The pharmacist will usually substitute the cheaper version unless the prescription explicitly requires the brand name (47 percent of all prescriptions were filled with generics in 2001). The average prescription has a retail cost of about $50—$70 for brand names and $23 for generics (see Table 12.2).[3]

Most patients have insurance and pay only the co-payment, which currently averages $6 for generics and $12 for brand names. Some insurance plans require the patient to pay a percentage of the price (coinsurance) rather than a specified amount, and other insurance plans require the patient to pay in full when the prescription is filled and send a copy of the bill for full or partial reimbursement later. These alternatives are more confusing and more cumbersome, which is one reason the market has shifted over time to the co-payment system run by carve-out managed care organizations called **pharmacy benefit managers (PBMs)**. PBMs are invisible to patients. They are subcontractors chosen by insurance companies to develop benefit plans, administer claims, and manage relationships with pharmaceutical companies (manufacturers) and retail pharmacies. PBMs do not have any direct control over physicians' prescribing behavior. However, by creating a

TABLE 12.1	Sources of Funds for Pharmaceutical Products
Total	$536 per person, 10% of National health expenditures

Out-of-pocket	32%
Private insurance	46%
Medicare	2%
Medicaid	17%
Other public programs	3%

Source: CMS National Health Accounts.

TABLE 12.2				Pharmaceutical Sales, R&D and Profits		

Major Brand Pharmaceutical Manufacturers	Total 2001 Revenues	U.S.	R&D	Profit	A Major Drug	U.S. Sales
Pfizer	$32,084	$ 17,631	$4,847	$7,752	Lipitor	$4,423
GlaxoSmithKline	29,847	15,474	5,496	4,498	Flonase	na
Merck	47,716	12,519	2,456	7,282	Zocor	4,690
Johnson & Johnson	33,004	10,922	3,591	5,668	Procrit	2,335
Bristol-Myers Squibb	19,423	10,505	2,259	2,570	Glucophage	2,655
Lilly	11,543	7,627	2,235	2,809	Prozac	1,659
Wyeth	14,129	6,983	1,869	2,285	Effexor	1,098
Pharmacia	19,302	6,512	2,949	1,291	Celebrex	2,447
Schering-Plough	9,802	5,059	1,312	1,943	Claritin	2,716
Abbott	16,285	3,770	1,578	1,550	Depakote	869
Total U.S. sales, including generics		175,000 ($millions)				

Generic Manufacturers

Teva	$2,077			$278	Fluoxetine (Prozac)	
Ivax Corp.	1,215			236	Onxol (Taxol)	
Watson Pharmaceuticals	1,161			116	Diliatizem (Cardizem)	
Andrx	740			73	Loratadine (Claritin)	
Barr	510			63	Oral contraceptives	

Biotechnology Firms

Amgen	$4,016		$967	$1,120	Epogen	$2,109
Biogen	1,043		366	273	Avonex	972
Genentech	2,082		613	404	Humulin	1,061
Incyte	219		183	(188)		
Millenium	246		510	(192)		

Source: Standard & Poors *Industry Profile, Pharmaceuticals 2002;* CMS *Health Care Industry Update—Pharmaceuticals, 2003.*

formulary (list of preferred drugs) and setting differential co-payments (see discussion of three-tiered benefits in Chapter 10, section 3), PBMs indirectly influence physicians' choices through patients' pocketbooks. In addition, PBMs have become sophisticated about calling physicians and suggesting product substitutions.

In 1970, 82 percent of all drug costs were paid by patients out of pocket. The little bit of drug insurance that was available operated retrospectively through "major medical" benefits, requiring the patient to submit bills and wait for payment, or through government programs for the indigent. This situation was totally reversed by 1999, when only 33 percent of prescription costs were paid out of pocket. Shifting payments to insurance and providing a "drug card" that could be used at the local pharmacy required the development of a new form of contractual intermediary—the PBM, which took care of all claims and rebates that had to be processed. PBMs expanded rapidly and were responsible for more than half of all prescriptions filled in 2002.

Medicare and Medicaid

Unlike the rest of the health care system, in which Medicare is a dominant payer, Medicare is a minor source of funds for pharmaceuticals—accounting for less than 2 percent.

Because the elderly do not obtain insurance for pharmaceuticals under Medicare, most purchase supplemental "Medigap" plans or join Medicare health maintenance organizations (HMOs) to obtain drug coverage (see Chapter 5). Medicaid, in contrast, is a major factor in the pharmaceutical market, accounting for 19 percent of expenditures overall and for more than half of expenditures for some specific drugs. In most Medicaid plans, patients pay nothing or a small co-payment (perhaps $2) once they obtain a drug card. The pharmacy bills the Medicaid program (or its PBM) directly for the cost of the drug, plus a dispensing charge (about $5). State Medicaid agencies keep track of the drugs purchased through their programs and obtain rebates from manufacturers of single source (i.e., only one manufacturer) drugs.

Inpatient Pharmaceuticals

The process of receiving a drug as an inpatient in a hospital differs significantly from the process used for outpatients. Again, it begins with a physician writing a prescription, but the prescription goes directly to the hospital pharmacy. The prescription is filled by the staff pharmacist and administered to the patient by the nursing staff. All medications are carefully noted on the patient's hospital chart.

Payment for an inpatient's drug depends on how the hospital is reimbursed for its services. Under Medicare, the hospital receives a flat, fixed payment based on patient diagnosis and the average cost of treating a patient with that diagnosis (DRG, as described in Chapter 8, section 2). A component of this payment is based on average drug utilization, but the hospital does not receive payment linked directly to drug utilization. A number of states have adopted all-payer DRG reimbursements that extend this form of payment to all patients. If the hospital is being paid on a per diem rate, average drug utilization generally is incorporated into the daily rate. Again, the hospital does not receive any payment directly associated with drug utilization. Only in cases where the hospital is paid on a "charges" basis is drug utilization itemized and billed directly to the patient or third-party payer. Thus, in many cases, the hospital bears the full marginal cost of the drug.

Because hospitals often bear the marginal cost of the drugs they administer to patients, they have a strong financial incentive to minimize the overall pharmaceutical budget. In pursuit of this objective, hospitals often establish their own formulary of drugs they keep in stock and from which physicians may prescribe. By negotiating with pharmaceutical companies over including particular drugs in the formulary, hospitals are able to utilize their market power to obtain discounts on drugs that have close competitors. However, a hospital must balance these economic decisions against antagonizing the physicians on the hospital medical staff, on whom the hospital must rely for admissions.

12.2 USES OF FUNDS

When a person goes to a local pharmacy to fill a prescription, the retailer gets 20 to 25 percent of the $70 (average price) total to cover the costs of labor, overhead, and profit.[4] Most of the remainder, 70 to 80 percent, goes to the pharmaceutical company that manufactured the drug. A small amount, 2 to 3 percent, goes to a wholesaler that obtains drugs from many manufacturers, and warehouses and delivers them to a variety of retail pharmacies. The flow of funds is complicated because most payments come from insurance companies (which must be compensated for risk bearing) and go through PBMs (which must get compensated for claims processing and negotiating). This flow of funds also depends in part on the negotiating power of each party. A diagram of this flow is presented in Figure

12.1, which has been simplified to reduce clutter and make the flow of funds more understandable. In addition, the amounts are approximate because only partial or incomplete survey estimates are available for many aspects of the industry. Patients using their own money are not involved in this complex set of transfers—and they lose! Patients without insurance pay list rather than discounted prices, which are 5 percent to 45 percent higher than what HMOs, insurance companies, and Medicaid plans pay for the identical prescription filled at the same pharmacy.[5]

Retail Pharmacies

There are 52,000 local pharmacies, with more than a third in five large chains (CVS, Walgreens, Rite-Aid, Eckerd, Wal-Mart).[6] Increased competitive pressure and the need for sophisticated information systems for insurance billing, ordering, marketing to consumers, and preventing drug interactions have caused the number of pharmacies to fall and an increasing number of them to be in chains. Patients with chronic illnesses who take large quantities of medicines on a continuing basis have increasingly turned to mail-order and Internet pharmacies with even lower prices and distribution costs. Mail-order now accounts for about 15 percent of retail drug sales. Most retail pharmacies purchase inventories from

FIGURE 12.1   Flow of Funds in the Pharmaceutical Market

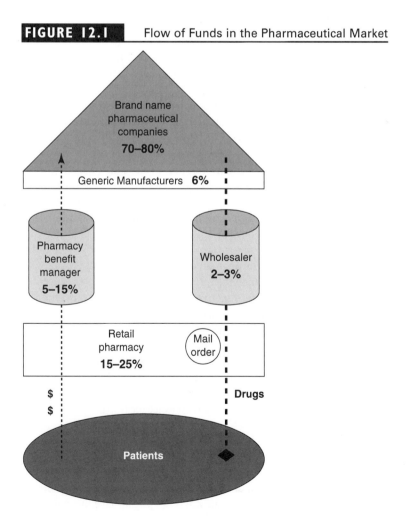

wholesalers that buy both generic and brand name drugs from the manufacturers. Because of the many drugs available, most local pharmacies do not carry a large inventory of each drug but rely on computerized inventory systems to get deliveries from the wholesaler daily. Wholesalers and pharmacists usually cannot switch patients from one product to another (except for generic products). As a result, they are unable to exert market power against the manufacturer, but instead must pay the full, list price of the drug—often called the **average wholesale price (AWP)**. Hospitals purchasing drugs for inpatient use may buy directly from the manufacturers, but usually purchase from wholesalers.

Wholesalers

Three companies (McKesson HBOC, Bergen Brunswick, Cardinal Health) account for more than 60 percent of the wholesaling business.[7] Their jobs are limited to warehousing and distribution—they play no role in the acquisition of patients or insurance financing. Thus, the physical movement of drugs—buying and selling on the wholesale side—is totally separate from the complex flow of funds on the patient/retail side. As such, moving drugs is fairly cheap and accounts for only a fraction of total costs despite the large volume of items being shipped around.

Insurance Companies and PBMs

The financial side of the pharmaceutical business is made up of insurance companies and PBMs, some of which may not be entirely distinguishable from one another because large insurers (Aetna, CIGNA, Wellpoint) have their own PBMs. Managed care has had a major impact on the way the pharmaceutical industry conducts business. PBMs consolidate the purchasing power of multiple insurance companies and employer health benefits plans covering millions of people, and thus can force manufacturers to give sizable discounts. The three big PBMs (Express Scripts, Merck-Medco, AdvancePCS) have a majority of the business and are relatively independent, although they have equity ties both to insurance entities and to pharmaceutical manufacturers. More than half of the total pharmaceutical dollars now flow through PBMs, leaving perhaps one-quarter to one-sixth still flowing through unmanaged insurance payment systems.

The PBM gets fees from the insurance company for handling claims (and may even be a capitated, risk-bearing provider of benefits), but gets most of its funding from pharmaceutical manufacturer discounts. Aggregate purchasing power is exercised in the form of mandatory rebates. Although the prescription passes through the wholesaler at list (AWP) price with a retail markup, the PBM negotiates with the manufacturer, and a rebate of 5 to 15 percent is paid directly to the PBM. Medicaid gets a special superdiscount of 15.1 percent based on the best available price given to any nongovernment buyer, which returned $5 billion to state budgets in 2002.[8] The various transfers and rebates make it difficult to determine exactly who gets what in dollar terms. Health insurance premiums paid by employers and patients include prescription coverage, but the amount attributable to pharmaceuticals (with or without overhead) cannot be determined without using a set of arbitrary allocations. Rebates should be counted as revenue to the PBM, but are not routinely reported. Thus, the percentages in Figure 12.1 should be considered approximations rather than exact measures.

Pharmaceutical Firms

About $120 billion dollars in 2002 went to the pharmaceutical manufacturing companies, accounting for the bulk (70 to 80 percent) of all drug costs. The top brand name blockbuster drugs (e.g., Celebrex, Claritin, Lipitor, Prilosec, Prozac, Zocor, Zyprexa) have more than $2 billion in annual sales, and a single drug can make or break a company (see Table 12.2). The largest pharmaceutical companies (Merck, Johnson & Johnson, Pfizer, GlaxoSmithKline) each have more than $30 billion in sales, and the top ten pharmaceutical companies account for 68 percent of all prescription dollars.[9]* Conversely, while generics account for 47 percent of all prescription volume and are four of the ten most frequently prescribed drugs in terms of units, they account for only 18 percent of total sales in dollars. Only one generic firm, Teva, had prescription sales of $2 billion or more.

Funds that flow into pharmaceutical firms are used in a variety of ways. For example, they are used to support R&D efforts as firms seek to develop newer and better drugs before their competitors. These funds are also used to support the marketing and promotional efforts needed to get physicians to prescribe their drug rather than a competitor's drug. In addition, some of these funds are used to cover the costs of manufacturing, distribution, and administration that go along with any production process, and a portion of these funds are profits, which are either given to stockholders in the form of dividends or reinvested in the company in the form of retained earnings. A breakout of the uses of funds is shown in Table 12.3.

Manufacturing the drugs takes about one-quarter of pharmaceutical companies' resources. Most studies have shown that there are constant returns to scale in the manufacturing of pharmaceutical products; that is, the average manufacturing cost is independent of the amount produced. In part this is because most drugs are manufactured in small batches rather than in a continual process. Production in small batches is a result of the need to maintain high quality standards. Although large batches are generally more economical to manufacture, there is a greater variance in the quality of the product and a greater chance that some of the units will have either too much or too little of the active ingredients. With pharmaceutical products, such deviations could be deadly; hence, small manufacturing batches are the norm. However, the initial development of the sophisticated extraction and production process is itself very costly and constitutes a large fixed (sunk) cost, which gives rise to economies of scale.

Advertising and promotional activities account for 20 to 35 percent of the pharmaceutical dollar. These activities primarily consist of detailing, sampling, and journal advertising. Of these, detailing and sampling are the most important. Detailing involves a representative of the pharmaceutical firm calling on an individual physician. During this meeting, the representative will discuss one or two products with the physician. For each drug discussed, the representative gives the physician the results of recent tests, explains how the drug works, what the potential side effects are, and discusses the advantages of this drug over competitors' drugs. The representative may give the physician literature on the drug, as well as free samples to pass on to patients. In addition, the detailer answers questions the physician might have about the drug or its use. The information presented and literature given to the physician must meet with strict FDA guidelines. Empirical studies have shown that detailing can have a large impact on a physician's prescribing behavior and on the elasticity of demand for individual products. As a result of these studies, a number of politicians have charged that the promotional activities of the industry are wasteful and excessive and have called for increased regulation of the industry. Whether such actions are justified, and the overall social impact of such actions, are the subject of ongoing research and debate.

TABLE 12.3

Uses of Funds for
Pharmaceutical Products

Cost of goods	30%
Research & development	13%
Sales, marketing, admin.	31%
Taxes	6%
Net income	20%

Source: CMS *Health Care Industry Update—Pharmaceuticals, 2003.*

---

*Standard & Poor's Corporation generously made available access to a number of its proprietary industry reports.

R&D accounts for 10 to 25 percent of the total pharmaceutical dollar. Viewing R&D in this manner, however, is somewhat inappropriate because it gives the impression that R&D activities are funded by current sales, a notion perpetuated by current accounting practices and the drug industry itself. It is more appropriate to view R&D expenditures as investments in intangible capital rather than a current period expense. Viewing R&D in this manner reveals that current cash flows are the result of past R&D expenditures and that the primary incentive for current R&D efforts is the future cash flows expected from these investments. When viewed this way, it is clear that policies and environmental changes that jeopardize future cash flows adversely affect current R&D incentives.

Profits account for 10 to 25 percent of the pharmaceutical dollar. Pharmaceutical firms are consistently ranked as the most profitable industry by *Fortune* magazine, and have been for many years. In 2002, profitability was reported as 18.5 percent of sales. Banking was ranked as the second most profitable industry at 13.5 percent of sales. The median profitability of all industries was reported to be 3.3 percent.[10] Looking at the profits per dollar of sales, however, may not be the correct way to examine the issue. It is necessary to examine the implied rate of return on capital invested in the pharmaceutical industry to determine whether returns are excessive. Doing so requires a complicated set of adjustments, in part because of the need to capitalize R&D expenditures. Depending on how R&D is treated, on the cost of capital used for the industry, and on the time period examined, researchers have reached various conclusions.

Cost Structure

The economics of the pharmaceutical industry are dominated by fixed costs. Discovery, R&D, regulatory approval, and market introduction all are sunk costs when the first pill is sold. The cost of manufacturing an additional unit is a fraction of the price, usually less than 20 percent, and sometimes amounts to mere pennies on the dollar. After fixed costs are recovered, each additional unit sold is almost pure profit. This makes it worthwhile to put millions, even billions, into marketing. The pharmaceutical industry is an exemplar of the post-modern "information economy," where a label is worth much more than the cost of the product on which it is placed. Other industries where most costs are fixed, such as information technology (software, Web sites), media (movies, CDs, books), and luxury goods (clothes, perfume) tend to use mega-marketing techniques for the same reason— the gross margins (revenue-variable cost) are so attractive.[11]

Such a disproportionate cost structure does not apply to the other parts of the pharmacy industry: retail drug stores, wholesalers, insurance companies and PBMs. While there are some economies of scale, costs rise almost proportionately (perhaps 80 percent) with volume. Since there are substantial incremental variable costs per unit, it is not worth pushing so hard for more sales or putting so much money into marketing. Hence, behavior in these parts of the industry resembles that of more traditional firms.

12.3 HISTORY AND REGULATION OF PHARMACEUTICALS

The pharmaceutical industry has existed in its current form since the 1930s. Before then, local pharmacists (or chemists) mixed potions and elixirs from bulk chemicals using either standardized formulas or their own concoctions. Today, the modern U.S. pharmaceutical industry comprises more than 1,200 firms that produce a wide range of products for disease treatment and prevention, although the industry is dominated by a much smaller number (about 20) of very large firms. Recently, the pharmaceutical industry has drawn considerable attention for its pricing and promotional policies. Some politicians have alleged that the industry charges excessive prices and spends too much money promoting products to physicians. These allegations have resulted in calls to regulate prices in the pharmaceutical industry.

The regulation of the pharmaceutical industry and its products evolved during the twentieth century in response to increased potency, effectiveness, and toxicity of drugs. Until the late 1800s, most "pharmaceutical preparations" had an immediate effect of making the patient feel better, although in most instances they did little to cure the underlying disease. This meant that patients could directly evaluate the benefits of the drug and did not need extensive guidance from health care professionals in choosing which products to use.

The first "modern" pharmaceutical product, diphtheria antitoxin, was developed in the mid-1890s and dramatically reduced the incidence of diphtheria. However, because this new drug did not have an immediate effect on the patient or make them fell better (it just prevented the person from becoming sick), it was much more difficult for the patient to see and evaluate the benefit. Although the benefits were not readily apparent to the patient, some of the dangerous side effects were all too obvious. Thus, health care professionals with specialized knowledge about drugs became involved in helping patients decide which products to use.

The first regulation of pharmaceutical products was the Biologics Control Act of 1902. This legislation was a direct response to contaminated diphtheria antitoxin that fatally infected thirteen children. This incident contributed to overall concerns about the safety of the food and drug supply that were being raised in the popular press and in books, such as Upton Sinclair's *The Jungle*. These events were quickly followed by the passage of the Pure Food and Drug Act of 1906. Although the act focused primarily on the food supply, it required drug manufacturers to provide adequate labeling. The manufacturers either had to use a standardized formula for making the product or provide a complete list of its' contents.

These companies were not producing pharmaceuticals the way today's integrated firms do. Mostly, they were producing bulk and specialty chemicals for sale to packaging firms and local pharmacies. They were contract producers, with firms providing similar lists of products and competing on the basis of price and service, not science.[12] Moreover, despite producing many "drugs," few diseases could actually be cured or controlled by drugs. The 1902 and 1906 acts reduced the number of competitors, making the remaining firms larger and more profitable. Then the start of World War I brought an unexpected and inadvertent windfall. Germany, at that time the leader in chemical and pharmaceutical research, held most scientific and process patents. U.S. firms paid license fees for use of these patents, but rarely did their own research. When the United States entered the war against Germany, the existing patents were voided or transferred to U.S. firms, and the production of specialty chemicals greatly increased (because obviously the nation could not depend on an enemy to provide medications). U.S. firms came out of the war flush with profits, with a portfolio of patents taken from German firms such as Bayer and IG Farben, and vastly increased their technological capabilities. During the 1920s and 1930s, pharmaceutical firms built a new strategy, forging alliances with physicians and being identified with "ethical" (prescribed) medications rather than industrial chemical suppliers and secret tonics for home use.[13] Prior to 1930, most drug profits came from these "patent medicines" (which did not really have a patent) using secret formulas (usually heavy on alcohol and opiates) with fancy names and labels (Lydia's Little Liquid Drops, Dr. Johnson's Miracle Feelgood) marketed to people at "medicine shows" held in rural areas or general stores in towns. After 1940, profits increasingly came from purified medicines, made under strict supervision using scientific methods, prescribed and administered by doctors.

In 1931, the regulatory aspects of the Federal Bureau of Chemistry became known as the FDA, which today is responsible for evaluating new products and overseeing their manufacture (see Table 12.4). In this era before antibiotics, the discovery of broad-spectrum sulfa drugs was a major breakthrough. While saving many lives, however, they also precipitated a major public disaster. Produced as a yellow powder, sulfa was awkward to ingest in large quantities. The Massengill Company decided to provide a liquid formulation, but the powder would not dissolve in water or alcohol. Eventually the company produced Elixir Sulfanilamide by dissolving sulfa in ethylene glycol. This solvent, however, commonly referred to as antifreeze, is quite poisonous. More than a hundred people who drank the new product convulsed from pain and suffered agonizing deaths. Outraged, the public called for sanctions—but could find no law the company had broken. Massengil, an old and proud company, was mortified and anxious to make amends. Killing people with a toxic product was not yet against the law; therefore, the company pled guilty to "mislabeling" (technically "elixir" was supposed to mean "in alcohol") and paid a fine of $26,100, the largest such fine ever paid. Reaction to the incident led to major legislation.[14]

The Food, Drug, and Cosmetics Act of 1938 established several important provisions. First, it required pre-registration of all new drugs with the FDA, giving the agency the opportunity to test the drug before marketing. The act also gave the FDA the mandate of preventing unsafe drugs from *entering* the market. The new law, however, specifically excluded drugs that were administered by "trained professionals" for testing purposes. Second, it increased the amount of information that had to be included on the label of any drug sold without a prescription. This information included statements of recommended uses and potential dangers. Drugs sold by "prescription only" were not held to these same labeling standards.

Through these labeling provisions, the Food, Drug, and Cosmetics Act created the first real distinction between prescription and over-the-counter (OTC) drugs. Although previously any nonnarcotic could be sold as either prescription or OTC, after 1938 nearly all new drugs were classified as prescription only. This was an unintended effect of the law; the original intent was not to restrict self-medication, but simply place the use of the most dangerous drugs under professional supervision. Manufacturers, however, soon realized that *restricting sales of a product to prescription only reduced the elasticity of demand,* since the physician writing the prescription was not directly paying for the drug and the patient paying for the drug rarely challenged the physician's authority. The lower price elasticity, in turn, allowed the firm to charge a higher price, since the patient and pharmacist could not substitute a cheaper product once the prescription was written. Moreover, requiring a prescription gave the appearance that the drug was more potent or effective. Finally, the medical profession strongly supported these restrictions, in part, because the profession directly benefited from forcing patients to see a physician before receiving treatment.

TABLE 12.4	Major Legislation Affecting Pharmaceuticals
1902	Biologics Control Act
1906	Pure Food and Drug Act
1938	Food, Drugs, and Cosmetics Act
1962	Harris-Kefauver Drug Act Amendments
1984	Hatch-Waxman Drug Price Competition and Patent Restoration Act
1992	Prescription Drug User Fee Act
2001	TRIPS: Agreement on Trade-Related Aspects of Intellectual Property Rights (World Trade Organization)

During the 1940s, three key changes dramatically altered the pharmaceutical industry. First, new techniques for discovering and isolating potentially beneficial substances were developed in the process of discovering streptomycin. Second, the U.S. Patent Office ruled that the chemical modifications made to streptomycin, which enabled it to be isolated and purified, created a new product. Moreover, the process that developed this product and the product itself were patentable. Third, instead of licensing patents to competitors, as had been done in the past, pharmaceutical firms began to exercise their patent rights to control the production, distribution, and price of the product. Together, these changes ushered in the era of the modern pharmaceutical firm. These firms are R&D driven and use patents to maintain prices above short-run marginal cost and reap the rewards of R&D activities.

The 1950s and early 1960s represented a heyday of drug development, as one firm after another introduced "wonder drugs." Many states passed "anti-substitution" laws, which further reduced the elasticity of demand by requiring pharmacists to fill the prescriptions as written rather than substituting cheaper generic products. However, questions began to arise about the effectiveness of some of these new drugs and whether the prices were too high.

In 1959, Senator Estes Kefauver's Antitrust and Monopoly Subcommittee began hearings on whether too many drugs that were minor variations of existing drugs were being introduced to extend the patent life of a product line, a concern that has a familiar ring today. However, it was the Thalidomide incident in 1961-1962 that triggered passage of the 1962 Harris-Kefauver Drug Amendments and brought this heyday of drug development to a screeching halt.

Thalidomide was a drug used to treat nausea during pregnancy. Although it had not yet received FDA approval, it was being widely distributed to physicians for "experimental purposes" when it was discovered that it caused major birth defects in some babies of women who had taken the drug. This inflamed the fears that drug companies, in their rush to market new drugs and earn large profits, were "egregiously exposing humans to potentially harmful drugs during clinical trials."[15] As a result of this fear, Congress passed legislation that greatly increased the burden on pharmaceutical firms not only to show that their products were safe, but also to show that they were effective when used in the manner directed. In addition, the testing procedures used to establish these results were put under the oversight of the FDA. The 1962 amendments also required pharmaceutical firms to follow "good manufacturing and laboratory practices," as defined by the FDA, and gave the FDA the authority to inspect manufacturing plants. Finally, the 1962 amendments extended these testing requirements to both generic (identical) and similar (me-too) drugs. Previously, these drugs could avoid pre-market testing through certification from the FDA that they were in effect the same as the original drug.

These amendments dramatically increased the costs of and time required for new drug development and, as a result, slowed the rate of new drug introductions. The average number of new drug introductions fell from fifty-one per year between 1956 and 1961, to only twenty per year between 1962 and 1967. Although these restrictions increased the development cost for pioneering drug firms, they also reduced competition once patents expired, by creating larger barriers to entry for the producers of generic products. Thus, over the years, considerable debate erupted over whether these restrictions were excessive, whether they increased or decreased consumer welfare, and whether they increased or decreased the profitability of pharmaceutical firms. What is clear, however, is that after the passage of the 1962 amendments, the length of time between the discovery or synthesis of a new drug and its market introduction increased dramatically. In 1960, the average drug development time was 35 months; by 1980 this had increased to 145 months. These amendments also had a chilling effect on the introduction of generic products, since generic manufacturers had to duplicate all the research conducted by the pioneering firm to gain approval for their own new drug application.

In 1984, Congress passed the Drug Price Competition and Patent Term Restoration Act (known as the Hatch-Waxman Act after its sponsors), which attempted to remedy some of the problems created by the 1962 amendments. First, the act established the Abbreviated New Drug Application (ANDA), which allowed a generic manufacturer to show that its drug was "bioequivalent" to the pioneer manufacturer's product, rather than repeat all the safety and efficacy studies. Since 1984, hundreds of products have been introduced under the ANDA provisions. Second, the act established a formula for increasing the patent life of a new product to restore some of the time (up to five years) lost due to the pre-market regulatory process.

The 1997 FDA Modernization Act made a number of changes to speed the approval of new drugs. It also allowed seriously ill patients easier access to experimental compounds, provided new incentives for development of pediatric medicines, and expanded the ability of pharmaceutical companies to provide information about off-label (unapproved) uses of drugs.

The World Trade Organization (WTO) brought drug patents into the global trading system through the Agreement on Trade-Related Aspects of Intellectual Property Rights (TRIPS) adopted at the November 2001 meeting in Doha, Qatar. The TRIPS agreement establishes minimum international obligations, including a patent term of 20 years and a period of exclusivity for clinical data. This agreement has been adopted by 140 countries and represents a major step forward. In negotiations, exceptions were provided to allow countries to take special measures to protect public health, thus creating special mechanisms to provide AIDS medications to developing countries at low cost.

Regulation of the pharmaceutical industry has evolved over the past hundred years by responding to the perceived needs for consumer protection and industry development, attempting to balance the benefits and costs of regulation. What began as a requirement for adequate labeling, ensuring that the public was protected from adulterated or misrepresented products, grew into a system where consumers no longer make choices about the drugs they receive, but rely on their physicians (and sometimes even third-party payers) to make these choices for them. Along the way, the entire industry was transformed from one that simply manufactured bulk products to one that spent $30 billion dollars actively searching for new products in 2002.

12.4 RESEARCH AND DEVELOPMENT

The pharmaceutical industry consists of many small companies, each producing only one or two products, and about twenty-five global corporations that have broader product lines. Even in the largest corporations, however, one or two blockbuster drugs are responsible for most revenues. Competition for the development of these key products, through R&D activities, is fierce. The success or failure of even a single product could mean the success or failure of the corporation. As a result, R&D activities drive competition in the pharmaceutical industry. The cost of developing a new drug ranges from $150 million to $1.5 billion, and the process can take up to ten years. Once developed, patents protect the new product from competition. Patents give the innovator the exclusive right to manufacture and sell that product, once approved, for up to twenty-two years from the time of discovery. Pharmaceutical firms spent an amount equal to 17.7 percent of sales on R&D in 2001, more than four times the 4 percent of sales spent by the average nonpharmaceutical firm and significantly more than the 11.9 percent pharmaceutical companies spent on R&D in

1980.[16] To understand competition in this industry, one must be familiar with the R&D process and its role in the industry.

The R&D of a new product takes place in several distinct steps, with the pharmaceutical company making decisions on whether to continue the project or abandon it at each step. The first step is either the discovery stage or the synthesis stage, reflecting two very different approaches to new drug development. In the discovery stage, natural chemical compounds having desirable properties are isolated from biological samples. Alternatively, in the synthesis stage, a new synthetic compound is created in the laboratory based on the results of previous research or computer models. Once the new compound has been isolated, regardless of its source, it is generally immediately patented and then screened for pharmacological activity and toxicity, first *in vitro* (i.e., in test tubes with tissue cultures) and then in animals. This preclinical phase can take up to three years, and literally thousands of compounds are examined and rejected for each one that moves on to the next stage of testing. Once a promising compound has been found, the firm files an **Investigational New Drug (IND)** application with the FDA and, unless rejected, the firm can begin testing in humans within thirty days of filing the application. There were 1,817 INDs filed in 2001, somewhat below the average for the previous decade.[17]

Clinical trials (i.e., human testing) are generally conducted in three distinct phases (see Figure 12.2). **Phase I** testing is usually performed on a small number of healthy patients, although cancer drugs are typically tested on patients who are terminally ill because a high level of toxicity is generally necessary to kill the cancer cells. The objective of these studies is to obtain preliminary information on the toxicity and tolerable dosage range in humans. Generally, the drug is given sequentially to sets of three patients at each dosage level until a preset toxicity threshold is crossed (the acceptable toxicity level depends greatly on the nature of the disease the drug is intended to treat and the availability of alternative therapies) or until a predetermined dose is reached. During Phase I trials, data are also collected on the drug's absorption, metabolic effects, and how the body eliminates the drug. These trials generally last slightly more than a year. Although signs of efficacy are always encouraging, they are not necessary for moving on to the Phase II trials because the sample size is so small.

In **Phase II,** the drug is administered to a limited number of patients whom the drug is intended to benefit (generally 30-300 patients). The first evidence of efficacy is obtained

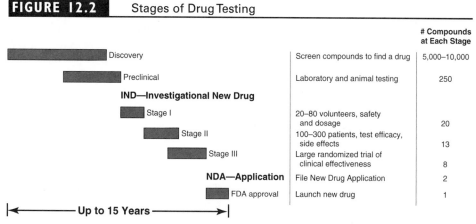

FIGURE 12.2   Stages of Drug Testing

		# Compounds at Each Stage
Discovery	Screen compounds to find a drug	5,000–10,000
Preclinical	Laboratory and animal testing	250
IND—Investigational New Drug		
Stage I	20–80 volunteers, safety and dosage	20
Stage II	100–300 patients, test efficacy, side effects	13
Stage III	Large randomized trial of clinical effectiveness	8
NDA—Application	File New Drug Application	2
FDA approval	Launch new drug	1

◄———— Up to 15 Years ————►

Total: 3–15 years, cost of $100M–$1,500M to bring one new drug to market.

at this stage, even though the general focus of the trial is still on safety. The trial also begins to examine the cumulative effects of the drug. On average, these trials last about two years. If the safety profile continues to look good and there are signs of beneficial effects, the drug is moved into the final stage of human testing.

The final stage of clinical testing, the **Phase III** trials, are intended to establish the efficacy claims of the manufacturer. Large samples, frequently thousands of patients, are exposed to the new drug. Often, these trials are double blind, where neither the patient nor the treating physician knows whether a specific patient is taking the experimental drug or the control drug (perhaps a placebo). In addition to looking for evidence of efficacy, researchers continue to look at the safety profile of the drug and begin to look for potential adverse reactions to the drug.[18] To obtain information on the long-term effects of the drug, these Phase III clinical trials can go on for several years and on average last nearly three years.

When the clinical trials are under way, pharmaceutical firms typically continue their long-term animal testing, looking for possible adverse genetic and/or reproductive effects. Once the firm believes that it has sufficient information to show that the product is both safe and effective, it files a **New Drug Application (NDA)** with the FDA. Once the NDA is filed, the FDA has sixty days to determine whether there is sufficient information in the NDA for the agency to conduct a substantive review. Although the FDA is supposed to render a decision within six months, the Office of Technology Assessment estimated that for drugs approved in 1990, the average time from application to approval was nearly thirty months. Part of this delay was the result of additional testing required by the FDA before granting approval. A section of the FDA Modernization Act of 1997 extended the 1993 Prescription Drug User Fee Act allowing the FDA to charge companies for applications and to use the money (more than $100 million per year) to hire extra personnel. This reduced the time required for approval to 16 months in 2001.

On average, only one out of five drugs for which an IND is filed with the FDA ultimately obtains FDA approval for use. As a result of the lengthy testing and approval process, a total of more than ten years generally elapses from the time the firm first began spending money on researching a new product until a successful drug is introduced to the market. Because of this lengthy period of time, it is very important to take into account the opportunity cost of these expenditures when assessing the costs of drug development. In perhaps the most comprehensive analysis to date, DiMasi et al. estimated that the capitalized out-of-pocket costs to pharmaceutical firms at the point of market approval averaged $231 million (1987 pre-tax dollars).[19] This figure includes the cost of projects abandoned along the way. Thus, each individual marketed drug represents a substantial investment of resources for the firm. These investments are made in the anticipation of obtaining future profits on the manufacture and sale of the drug. The estimated average cost of a drug development project in 2002 was approximately $800 million. Others have examined the profitability of these investments, and one study found that only the top 20 percent of the drugs tested had large enough returns to cover the cost of R&D.[20]

A portfolio of patents, and the creativity and expertise of the scientists that generated them, are major assets to the pharmaceutical firm. Mergers are often carried out to obtain a set of patents, to fill out a product line, or to create synergies in research. While marketing benefits from increased size, it appears that economies of scale and scope are quite limited in research.[21] Indeed, some of the most innovative work is performed in small boutique biotechnology firms composed of a few scientists moonlighting from a university laboratory, suggesting diseconomies of scale. The causes and antecedents of successful research are difficult to determine. It does appear, however, that some firms and research groups are just better at it than others, and obtain more new products and conceptual breakthroughs with the same level of resources.

12.5 PHARMACOECONOMICS AND OUTCOMES RESEARCH

Are new drugs worth the high prices drug companies charge to cover their R&D and marketing costs? Drug discovery in general is obviously beneficial, but should we really pay $2 per pill (or $250 or $1,500 per prescription) for a particular drug? Could the company get by with charging only $1.50 per pill? Conversely, from the company's point of view, since blockbuster drugs are rare and must cover the cost of many failed R&D efforts, could the company reasonably charge $2.50 per pill? An entire discipline with its own scientific journals, conferences, and university professorships has developed to answer these questions. Known variously as "pharmacoeconomics," "disease management," and "outcomes research," this discipline attempts to determine the following:

- How much of a gain in health (outcome) will this drug provide?
- How much will people value that gain?
- Do other drugs provide similar effectiveness in treating this disease?
- How many people will benefit from this drug?
- Will some benefit more than others?
- Will some value the drug more than others?

These questions have become increasingly pressing as the cost of pharmaceuticals has soared. Australia, Canada, Sweden, and other countries with national health systems have created expert panels of health economists to advise governments on whether a new drug should be added to the national health insurance plan and on the maximum amount that should be paid per treatment. Even in the United States, where administrative price controls do not exist, drug companies have found it useful to employ health economists to estimate the potential size of the market for a new drug and to create an economic justification to help sell the drug to price-conscious buyers with limited budgets (Medicaid, hospital pharmacies, and increasingly, PBMs). Indeed, so many economists are looking at the value of drugs that many doctors and pharmacists think that this is all there is to health economics, and use the term "health economics" as a synonym for pharmacy value studies without considering all the other issues covered in the chapters of this textbook.

Most health economists in pharmaceutical companies are employed in the marketing department. Even though committed to objective social and medical science, their job is to sell drugs and to help the company sell the largest amount of drugs at the highest price possible (actually, to maximize the present value of future revenues, which is a bit more complex). To obtain greater expertise and credibility, corporate health economists often work with or fund studies conducted at universities. However, as most economists would predict, studies funded by pharmaceutical companies are consistently more favorable to the products of those companies (and unfavorable to competitors) than those done independently, leading to increased calls that all conflicts of interest be publicly identified.[22] It is not realistic to expect that funding will have no effect on judgment, even for scientists.

12.6 INDUSTRY STRUCTURE AND COMPETITION

The market for pharmaceutical products can be divided into three segments based on the type of buyer: **individual** patients, **group** purchasers (hospitals, PBMs), and **government.** In the traditional retail market, physicians prescribe drugs and consumers and/or insurers pay for them. Because these actions are separate, individual patients have little influence over what the physician prescribes and, as a result, this market segment is not very price sensitive. The second market segment, which has been growing in importance, is the group purchasers. In this market, drugs are purchased directly by PBMs and hospitals, and a physician's choice of which drug to use is constrained by the use of a formulary and ordering directives. Because PBMs and hospitals can shift a large number of patients from one product to another, they have some market power, and are more sensitive to prices. Exercising this market power enables discounts to be obtained from drug manufacturers. The third market segment consists of the largest purchasers of pharmaceutical products: state and federal government. Governments make and interpret the rules, potentially giving them absolute control over the market.

Market Segmentation: Types of Buyers

Competition for sales differs significantly across these segments. In the traditional retail market for individual patients, where consumers (patients) are price insensitive, competition takes place among products on the basis of product quality and detailing in which the salesperson provides a physician with detailed information on approved uses. Even though much of the demand for a product may be for treating a disease for which the drug is not yet (or ever) approved by the FDA, detailers are prohibited from discussing such **off-label** uses of the product.[23] Studies have consistently shown that detailers greatly influence a physician's choice of drugs. Moreover, once a physician becomes familiar with a particular product, its method of action, and its potential side effects, he or she may be reluctant to try a new product unless it offers either a substantial advantage in efficacy or a decrease in side effects. Price tends not to be an important criterion for consumers.[24] Thus, competition in this market is usually based on product quality, effectiveness, and detailing, hence generics have not been able to make significant inroads in this market.

To date, government purchasers have chosen not to exercise fully their monopsony-market power on a drug-by-drug basis, but instead have adopted a standardized discount policy that pharmaceutical firms can either accept or reject. Under this policy, the government is rebated an amount equal to 15.2 percent of the average wholesale price for Medicaid purchases, or equal to the best deal given by the drug company on a particular product. Similar provisions have been established for other government contracts. In exchange for agreeing to these discounts, Medicaid agreed not to establish restrictive formularies. Thus, although pharmaceutical firms must cut their prices to sell to this market, they are essentially free to detail physicians on their products and do not face stiff competition from generic products.

The growth, and most of the change, has come in the "managed" segment. HMOs, PBMs, and hospitals paying directly for drugs can influence physicians' prescribing patterns through a formulary. These group purchasers are the ones most interested in, and able to assess, price and cost-effectiveness. This is the segment in which generics have had the most impact, because they are chemically identical to brand name products and sold at a much lower price (up to 60 percent less). When the patent expired on Eli Lilly's blockbuster drug Prozac, 70 percent of prescriptions were switched to generic substitutes within a single month.[25] Unless a drug has demonstrated clear superiority through health economics outcomes research studies, price-sensitive managers choose the cheaper product. Most large pharmaceutical companies have developed sales, marketing, and research groups aimed at addressing the concerns of the managed market. In addition, pharmaceutical companies are beginning to explore new contractual relationships to increase sales and lock in specific customers.

Contractual Responses to Pharmacy Benefits Management

Managed care greatly increases the elasticity of demand. Organized payers with sophisticated information and outcome assessment methods are able to switch large numbers of patients from one drug to another in response to small changes in relative prices. Pharmaceutical firms can respond in several ways to this shift in market power.

The first response is by making **price reductions.** Pharmaceutical firms can compete with one another through successive reductions in the prices of their competing products. Since much of the costs of drug development and manufacturing are sunk, short-term competition can significantly reduce prices. During the past few years there has been increased price competition, particularly in pharmaceutical categories in which several branded products exist, such as antihypertensives and cholesterol reducers. Price reductions reduce profitability and thus are not popular with pharmaceutical firms. These firms argue that continued reductions would reduce funding for research and eventually lead to fewer new drugs.

A second response to the increased elasticity of demand is the development of new ways to establish **product differentiation.** Outcomes research, pharmacoeconomics, and disease management are several ways pharmaceutical firms try to differentiate their products from their competitors and develop "value" messages about their products. Fundamentally, these are attempts by the industry not only to demonstrate the safety and efficacy of their products, but also to translate the efficacy of treatment into measures that consumers value. For example, rather than simply showing that a cholesterol drug can reduce LDL cholesterol by x percent, pharmaceutical firms have undertaken studies to show what that percent reduction means in terms of reduced coronary events (e.g., heart attacks, strokes) and to show that reducing these events reduces future health care expenditures and improves the quality of patients' lives. New metrics, such as cost per life year saved and cost per quality adjusted life year (QALY) saved have been developed to provide more descriptive information to physicians and consumers to help them make decisions (see Chapter 3). Nearly every major pharmaceutical firm has begun to develop expertise in this area, and several new scientific journals have been founded to publish the results of these kinds of studies.

A third response involves developing **contractual relationships** that serve to "lock in" customers to a specific product line. These are often called "disease management programs." Possible arrangements include the following:

- Providing discounts for specific drugs based on specific performance measures (i.e., reduced prices, but only if purchaser provides manufacturer with increased market share)
- Establishing cost-sharing arrangements or warranties on specific products
- Developing capitated contracts, whereby a pharmaceutical company agrees to provide all the drugs needed for a fixed (per member per month) charge for a managed care population (e.g., specific drugs, drug classes, or even large bundles of drugs)
- Developing complete disease management programs, whereby the pharmaceutical firm assumes some of the financial risk for the total costs of treatment, not just the pharmaceutical costs

Value and Cost

The structure of the pharmaceutical industry is dictated by a single fact: the large and important costs are all sunk costs. The value of a drug depends on how useful it is in treating disease, not how many years it took to conduct clinical trials or perfect the production process, nor on the number of failed projects the company had to fund in order to get a winner. Research and testing to bring the pill to market costs so much more than manufacturing that there is essentially no rational connection between price and cost, however measured. Instead, value and price depend on therapeutic effectiveness.[26]

Medical "value" is worthless economically unless potential buyers know how effective a drug is. Treatment capability must be turned into effective demand. This means marketing. Given the large gross margin (profit per unit) caused by the combination of high sunk research costs and low per unit variable production costs, it is inevitable that marketing will be much more important and expensive than physical distribution—as it is for products with a similar cost structure such as software, movies, CDs, and perfume. Most of this marketing is directed toward doctors, since they are the ones who write prescriptions. For each practicing physician, pharmaceutical companies spent more than $2,500 on meals, events, and scientific meetings (some conducted in very nice resorts).[27] Spending on personal visits by industry representatives and free samples was more than $10,000 per doctor. The size of the expenditure on marketing indicates how valuable the power to influence doctors is in terms of company profits.

Marketing creates additional divergence between price and "unit cost" because the value of each pill increases as it becomes better and better known as a brand name drug. While clinical value may not depend on marketing, economic value does. Once the drug is launched in the market, any distinction between the value added from increased therapeutic effectiveness and the value added from increased marketing is not meaningful. (How much of a film's profit is derived from star power? From plot? From the cool thirty-second video advertisement that drew everyone into standing in line to see it the first weekend?) Even the drastic difference in price between brand name and generic versions (20, 40, 50, or even 80 percent) probably underestimates the value added by marketing. Perfectly good drugs have languished almost unused for years because they were not being advertised and detailed to doctors.

Once marketing launches a drug, the brand name is worth something even if the drug has been superceded by superior competitors (kind of like old sports stars still being used to sell athletic shoes). The brand-name version will often continue to sell at the old high price even after the patent has expired in order to capture the consumer surplus of customers who are not price sensitive. Also, competition from generic manufacturers has created incentives for research-based brand name companies to introduce and subsequently patent minor changes in their most important products. These changes might include introducing a sustained release or once-a-day formulation, or changing the route of administration from injection to inhaler or pill. AstraZeneca made such an effort to shift users of Prilosec, its blockbuster antiulcer drug, to a new improved version, Nexium, which retained the distinctive purple coloration of the original and incorporated minor modifications protected by new patents to limit the impact from generic competitors.

The Prilosec/Nexium example illustrates an important aspect of the pharmaceutical market: competition is between treatments for a specific disease (in this case, ulcers). Most drugs do not compete with one another because they are used for different illnesses. The real market is "treatments for disease X" and thus is much narrower than "all prescription drugs." Firms focus their research and marketing efforts on a particular set of diseases (cardiovascular, neurological, gastric), making the effective market share (and market power) of the top firm, or top three firms, more concentrated than it appears to be when reviewing industrywide statistics.

CLARITIN: DIRECT-TO-CONSUMER ADVERTISING, OVER-THE-COUNTER MEDICATION, AND PRICING

Claritin had a tortuous transition from laboratory to market. Schering-Plough submitted a new drug application (NDA) for the compound (scientific name, loratadine) in 1980, but did not obtain approval until 1993, by which time there were only five years left on the basic patent.[28] The FDA felt little pressure to approve what was classified as a "me-too" drug promising little clinical advance over existing prescription and OTC antihistamine remedies for allergy and hay fever. However, when FDA rules regarding **direct to consumers (DTC)** advertising were relaxed in 1997, Schering-Plough put $322 million promoting Claritin to the public. Ads featuring clear skies and happy faces (with pollen carrying flowers in the background) were seen on TV shows, billboards, bus stops and leaflets handed out on street corners. Sales of Claritin ballooned to more than $2.6 billion in 2000.

In clinical trials, 46 percent of allergy sufferers showed improvement with Claritin, compared with 35 percent who showed improvement when given a placebo. Tests indicated that Schering-Plough's old drug, Chlor-Trimeton, now sold cheaply over the counter, was equally or perhaps more effective in relieving symptoms—and may not have been much more sleep-inducing when used in a low dose. Was it really worth paying six times as much for the new version? The question rarely arose because prescriptions were covered by insurance. Wellpoint, a large health insurance company, sued in 1998 to force Claritin and similar allergy drugs to be sold over-the-counter without prescription, claiming that they clearly were safer than the existing OTC medications such as Chlor-Trimeton. If Claritin were declared safe enough to be used without a prescription, then it would no longer qualify for insurance reimbursement, consumers would have to pay out-of-pocket, and demand would become much more price-sensitive. Despite concerted efforts by Schering-Plough and other pharmaceutical firms, the insurance companies made a persuasive case. In November 2002 the FDA approved Claritin for OTC use. Schering-Plough's stock dropped precipitously as the price of Claritin had to be cut, and cut again, to compete in the more wide-open OTC market, and as Johnson & Johnson and Wyeth geared up production of generic versions of loratadine to sell at less than $20.

The Role of Middlemen: Distribution Versus Marketing

Wholesalers distribute drugs. They buy in bulk from pharmaceutical manufacturers and distribute on demand to retail pharmacies and hospitals. The customer is not involved in this back-office physical distribution network, and it is a commodity business with low margins. Conversely, the PBM never touches the physical product, but controls the flow of customers and money, and for performing this market aggregating function, is paid handsomely. The essential element here is control. Assume that a drug cures a horrible disease and thus is worth more than $1,000 to the patient, but production cost is only $1. This difference is up for grabs. If there is lots of competition, prices may get forced down toward $1.50, providing just enough for the costs of manufacture, distribution, and small profits. If patents or market power keep competition out, then profits of $100 or $500 or even $999 per customer are possible. It is that possibility which makes marketing so valuable.

Consider how different the case of diamonds is. The product itself (not the label) is valuable; therefore, anyone involved in transport and transfer must be trustworthy and highly compensated—it is worth a lot of money to keep from losing a few diamonds. Jewelry stores can advise, but they cannot prescribe, 2 carats, extremely fine yellow-white, or Lucida™ cut. Thus, in the case of diamonds, wholesaling and physical distribution is relatively profitable, and although marketing is a decent business, the large number of competitors keeps margins small relative to the cost of operating a jewelry store.

The essential question is control—who "owns" the business. To a large extent, the business of patients is controlled (owned) by the doctors who write the prescriptions for them. However, these doctors are prohibited by law and ethics from taking any of that $999 in surplus value. If there is only one treatment for an illness, and it is protected by a patent, the company with the patent in effect "owns" the business. The main question becomes how much business (total sales) there will be. A company will detail doctors to push them to prescribe more, but they do not have to worry about competing drugs. If there are two or more treatments for an illness, the situation becomes more complex. In theory, the choice should be made by the patient, balancing therapeutic effectiveness, cost, and side effects. In this case, marketing will focus directly on the patient (**direct-to-consumer [DTC]** advertising). However, patients often do not have enough information or confidence to make complex choices and tend to rely on their doctors to advise them. Thus, the marketing effort (detailing, scientific meetings at nice resorts) is directed at the doctor.

Insurance companies pay for most drugs, and they may be able to induce some patients to switch from treatment A to treatment B by making the co-payment for brand name A much larger, or even insisting on providing reimbursement only for treatment B if it is a chemically equivalent generic version. In this case, the insurer/PBM captures some of the surplus. Notice how little market power and how little excess profit the pharmacy is able to get. Even though pharmacies are the point of contact where the patient obtains the drug, they have to fill the prescription as written by the doctor or as modified by the insurer (generic substitution, tiered co-payments) and are not allowed to try to shift patients from A to B. Pharmacies are almost as neutral and powerless as wholesalers—they simply distribute pills from manufacturer to patient. It is much more difficult and costly at the individual retail end, which is why retail accounts for 20 to 25 percent of costs and wholesale only 2 to 3 percent, but there is not a lot of excess profit to be obtained here. Actually, one of the most lucrative parts of the retail pharmacy business is all the other stuff (candy, bandages), which pharmacies sell at above-average markups to people who come in to fill their prescriptions. That is, the pharmacy does not "own" the prescription business (because there are so many retail pharmacy competitors and wholesale prices are fixed), but it does own the idle shopping time of the patient who is waiting to have his or her prescription filled—and can exploit that to sell high-markup magazines, mints, and other items.

Research Productivity

Research is a sunk cost for drugs already on the market. These drugs would still be manufactured even if prices were reduced to the level of marginal cost, but then no new research would be undertaken. The high prices are the incentives for investing millions of dollars in the hope of making a discovery. Almost every economist and politician accepts this simple premise connecting research expenditures and innovation to the promise of future profits. However, some issues remain. How much profit is necessary to provide an incentive? If a company can make $1 billion on a new drug at a price of $30, will allowing the company to make $2 billion at a price of $60 double the productivity of its research labs—or increase it only by 10 percent? While there is no question that higher profits lead to more research, the magnitude of the gains and the real importance to patients is still an open and relevant issue. Research indicates that increases and decreases in R&D funding are more tied to short-run changes in past profits rather than changes in expected future profits which theory would predict.[29] More disturbing, it is not clear whether more R&D spending leads to the development of more innovative new drugs. Much of the expenditure goes for imitative "me-too" drugs to fight off the competitive threat from generics and chemically related drugs that other companies have made sufficiently different (by adding some side molecules or by using a new production process) to engineer around existing patents and claim their own brand names. Whereas 46 percent of all new drug approvals in 1991 were for new molecular entities (NMEs), by 2001, only 35 percent of approvals were for new molecules. Furthermore, only seven of these twenty-four NMEs were ranked by the FDA as priority drugs promising important advances entitled to expedited review, compared with 19 in 1999.[30] During the 1990s, research spending grew from $10 billion to $30 billion, yet the number of important new drugs brought to market fell, and the number of INDs submitted by pharmaceutical companies to the FDA declined from 2,116 to 1,872. Investment banking firm Lehman Brothers expected global drug firms to launch only 47 new drugs in 2002, down a third from 1997.[31] *The Wall Street Journal,* Standard and Poor's industry surveys, *Modern Healthcare* magazine**,** and most reputable analysts agree that the major financial problem facing the industry is a lack of important new drugs in the pipeline.[32] More than 10 years of increased R&D spending have not provided impressive results, making it hard to argue that having a bit more profit to pour into laboratories would make a big difference in the rate of therapeutic advances or drug discovery.

It may be that research productivity is in a stage of secular decline. Some analysts suggest that "discovery" methods have been played out, with most significant compounds already investigated and under patent, so that any surge of new drugs will have to come from "synthesis" and rational drug design, perhaps following from the increased understanding of fundamental disease processes brought about by deciphering the human genome. Most analysts opine that a real therapeutic benefit from such breakthroughs is at least 10 (maybe 15, or 25, or 35?) years in the future. Someday there will be designer drugs customized for each patient—not a pill for high cholesterol and another for gastric reflux, but a pill for the current health condition (and preventive needs) of Mr. ABC at age 36, who has decided to run a marathon and move to Tampa. The gains from that set of advances will be amazing—and a long time in coming.

12.7 TRENDS: FORM FOLLOWS FUNCTION (AND MONEY)

The structure of the pharmaceutical market is wondrously strange and revealing. It was an unintended consequence of the labeling provision in the Food, Drug, and Cosmetics Act of 1938 that made "prescription" drugs so inelastic with respect to price, adding to the power of physicians and the profits of pharmaceutical companies. This triangle (patient as payer, physician as prescriber, pharmaceutical company as producer) was first strengthened, then undermined, by the expansion of insurance. At first, prices became even more irrelevant with third-party payment. Pharmaceutical profits soared, making still more expensive physician detailing worthwhile. Then the vast sums of money being spent made it worthwhile for insurers to set up sophisticated systems to (a) save more by increasing price elasticity with formularies and differential co-payments and (b) use this countervailing market power to extract discounts from producers. As the prescribing power of physicians and the pricing power of drug companies declined, the gap was filled with appeals to patients through DTC marketing, empowering them to ask for a new drug by name. Claritin was the drug made famous (and its parent company Schering-Plough rich) through advertising. The revenge of the payer came when insurance companies made the case that if consumers could be trusted to use advertising information to ask for a drug, they could be trusted to choose it over the counter without a prescription. Empowered consumers, acting on their own—and with their own dollars at stake—drove prices rapidly downward.

Research creates a wedge between price and marginal cost, but it is marketing that consolidates big margins. With regard to pricing power, the demand side may prove more powerful than supply. Strategic growth and mergers have made market share more concentrated within each therapeutic category, despite the limited evidence for economies of scale in research. Moreover, it appears that much of the significant research in the coming decades will be conducted within small biotech firms. Changes in legal structures have played a role in this, as the courts have ruled that new organisms created in the laboratory may be patented. Much of the most basic research has shifted from the large firms in the industry to smaller, high-risk ventures. As these products move out of the laboratory and into clinical testing, biotech firms usually take on partners from the traditional pharmaceutical industry, are bought out by established firms, or develop licensing agreements. The growing split between discovery and development/marketing may presage a growing split in the sources of capital: venture capital for high-risk discovery in biotech firms, and reliance on the vast pools of equity capital extracted from the success of old drugs for the financing of methodical development, approval, and marketing efforts.

The structure of the pharmaceutical industry is so shaped by historical accident, so unbalanced, and so subject to repeated changes over the last century, that stability would be strange. A continued shift in organizational relationships and contracts, twisting and diverting the flow of funds in more new (and old) ways, seems inevitable. As health care in America continues to evolve, the pharmaceutical industry has begun to evolve in response to these changes. These responses have taken several directions, including shifts in the focus of R&D activities, consolidation of the industry, new measures of product value, and new contractual relationships between the industry and managed care providers.

SUGGESTIONS FOR FURTHER READING

2002 Industry Profile. PhRMA (Pharmaceutical Research and Manufacturers of America), (www.phrma.org).

T. A. Abbott, "Regulating Pharmaceutical Prices," in *Health Care Policy and Regulation* (Boston, Mass.: Kluwer Academic Press, 1995), 105–34.

Iain M. Cockburn and Rebecca M. Henderson, "Scale and Scope in Drug Development: Unpack the Advantages of Size in Pharmaceutical Research. *Journal of Health Economics* 20, no. 6 (November 2001): 1003–1057.

David H. Kreling, David A. Mott, and Joseph P. Wiederholt. "Prescription Drug Trends, a Chartbook Update" (November, 2001); and "Prescription Drug Trends" (September 2000), Kaiser Family Foundation, (www.kff.org).

S. Peltzman, "An Evaluation of Consumer Protection Legislation: The 1962 Drug Amendments," *Journal of Political Economy* (September 1973), 1049–1091.

Standard & Poor's Industry Surveys—Healthcare: Pharmaceuticals (June 27, 2002) Standard & Poor's (www.standardandpoors.com).

P. Temin, *Taking Your Medicine: Drug Regulation in the United States* (Cambridge, Mass.: Harvard University Press, 1980).

SUMMARY

1. The average American fills eleven prescriptions a year. Pharmaceuticals were a **$161 billion industry** in 2002, for which government and private insurance paid two-thirds of the bill. Of all the funds flowing in, about 70 percent go to pharmaceutical companies, 20 percent to retail pharmacies, and 10 percent to PBMs and insurers—much of that in the form of rebates from manufacturers.

2. Once an industry that made most of its profits from household potions and elixirs, the pharmaceutical industry has been revolutionized by **science, regulation,** and **insurance.** Pharmacology is among the most successful of technologies, having greatly improved human welfare and generated enormous profits—18.7 percent of sales in 2001, more than any other industry in the Fortune 500. A single successful drug can earn more than $5 billion in a year, and make or break the company.

3. R&D of new products is a risky, lengthy, and costly process. Only one in a thousand compounds initially studied eventually makes it to the market. On average, the time from discovery to successful market introduction is more than ten years, at a total cost of $800 million. The most costly part of the process is the clinical trials needed to establish safety and efficacy claims, which can take up to five years and involve thousands of patients.

4. **Patent protection** means that the price of a drug is determined by its value to consumers, not the cost of production. The hope of making large profits from discovering the next blockbuster product keeps pharmaceutical firms investing in R&D and fuels progress in the pharmaceutical industry.

5. The **dominant** economic feature of the pharmaceutical industry is the large **sunk costs,** first for R&D and then for the physician detailing and marketing blitz required to launch sales. The marginal cost of producing additional pills is small, therefore, most of the price is pure profit once these large fixed costs are covered. The ability to control the flow of funds determines who will hold onto most of these profits; the brand name manufacturer with a patent, the generic competitor, the government, the physician, the PBM, the insurance company, or the patient.

6. **Generics** (chemically identical compounds made by other firms) have increased in importance since the legal changes in 1984 enabled easier approval. Generic drugs sell for much less than branded products ($25 versus $75) and have been increasingly successful as the **price-sensitive** managed care PBM market has grown.

7. Pharmaceutical manufacturers have begun to respond to changes in their markets brought about by managed care and generic competition. These changes include the use of discounts, development of **pharmacoeconomics** and disease management, and the development of various forms of risk-sharing contracts.

PROBLEMS

1. What determines the price of a drug?

2. Why are fixed costs more important for pharmaceuticals than physical therapy? How does this affect marketing expenditures?

3. What events led to the formation of the FDA? Does regulation change because of successes or because of failures?

4. Do patents raise or lower the productivity of research?

5. How are prescription costs "managed" by insurance companies?

6. {*flow of funds*} What fraction of the total cost of pharmaceuticals is paid for directly by patients? Does this mean that price is more, or less, important than for other types of medical care?

7. {*research, incidence*} How is most pharmaceutical research paid for? What is the most costly aspect of pharmaceutical research?

8. {*market segmentation*} How many distinct market segments exist in the pharmaceutical industry? How do these segments differ?

9. {*competition*} On what basis do pharmaceutical firms compete in each market segment? Is price a more important factor for the choice of which doctor to see, or for which drug is prescribed?

10. {*insurance coverage*} The major form of health insurance coverage for the elderly is Medicare, and the elderly are much heavier users of pharmaceuticals than other groups. It would seem reasonable to expect that Medicare is the largest source of payment for drugs. Is it?

11. {*marginal costs, revenues*} Do hospitals have more of an incentive to control the costs of surgical implants, anesthesiologists' fees, or pharmaceuticals? In which case do they bear the highest fraction of marginal cost? In which case do they receive the highest fraction of marginal revenue?

12. {*patents*} How would a change in the length of the patent period affect the structure of the pharmaceutical industry?

13. {*competition*} Marketing accounts for a much larger portion of the cost of pharmaceuticals than the cost of other forms of care. Why? To whom are most pharmaceutical marketing efforts targeted?

14. {*capital investment*} If $50 million is invested in a drug that subsequently fails to gain approval from the FDA, what is the rate of return on this investment? Are pharmaceutical firms more, or less, capital intensive than hospitals? Than doctor's office practices?

15. {*anti-trust*} Since FDA regulations limit the entry of new drugs into the market, do they constitute an "unfair restraint of trade" that reduces competition and raises prices to consumers?

16. {*price elasticity*} When a brand name drug loses patent protection after seventeen years and competing generic products enter the market, will the price of the brand name drug increase or decrease? (Hint: what changes occur in the brand name drug's demand curve?)

17. {*risk*} Which form of investment is more risky, developing a new drug or building a new nursing home? Which type of publicly traded for-profit firm would you expect to show greater variability in earnings, a pharmaceutical firm or a nursing home chain?

ENDNOTES

1. David W. Kaufman et al., "Recent Patterns of Medication Use in the Ambulatory Adult Population of the United States," *Journal of the American Medical Association* 287, no. 3 (January 16, 2002): 337–344.

2. "Drugs," *The Economist* (June 3, 2000), 106. 3. David H. Kreling, David A. Mott, and Joseph P. Wiederholt, *Prescription Drug Trends, a Chartbook Update* (November, 2001); and *Prescription Drug Trends* (September 2000), Kaiser Family Foundation. (www.kff.org).

4. "Prescription Drug Trends," Exhibit 3.2.

5. John K. Iglehart, "Medicare and Prescription Drugs," *New England Journal of Medicine* 344, no. 13 (March 29, 2001): 1010-1015; *Prescription Drug Trends*, Exhibit 1.4.

6. *Prescription Drug Trends*, 2000, Exhibit 4.13, 4.15.

7. *Prescription Drug Trends*, 2000, Exhibit 4.9.

8. *2002 Industry Profile*. PhRMA (Pharmaceutical Research and Manufacturers of America), (www.phrma.org). Estimate projected from 1999 PhRMA estimate for 1999 increased by the percentage increase in pharmaceutical spending from 1999 to 2002 from U.S. National Health Accounts.

9. *Standard & Poor's Industry Surveys—Healthcare: Pharmaceuticals* (June 27, 2002) Standard & Poor's (www.standardandpoors.com).

10. "Industry Rankings," *Fortune* (April 15, 2002), F26.

11. "The prize for finding a blockbuster luxury product is much the same as in the pharmaceuticals industry, magical margins(quote from) "Luxury Goods," *The Economist* (March 23, 2002), 65.

12. Jonathan Leibenau, *Medical Science and Medical Industry: The Formation of the American Pharmaceutical Industry* (London: Macmillan, 1987), 34, 79.

13. Edward Kremers and George Urdang, *History of Pharmacy*, 2nd ed. (Philadelphia: Lippincott, 1951).

14. Peter Temin, *Taking Your Medicine: Drug Regulation in the U.S.* (Boston: Harvard University Press, 1980).

15. Peltzman, "An Evaluation of Consumer Protection Legislation: The 1962 Drug Amendments," *Journal of Political Economy* (September 1973), 1050–1051.

16. *Standard & Poor's Industry Surveys: Health–Pharmaceuticals* (June 27, 2002), Standard & Poor's (www.standardandpoors.com).

17. *Standard & Poor's*, 5.

18. Despite the relatively large sample sizes, many important adverse reactions can be missed during the phase III studies because they have a low probability of occurring. For example, a 1:10,000 adverse reaction causing death could easily go unnoticed in a phase III trial on several thousand patients, even though it could cause 30,000 deaths if the drug were released to all 300 million citizens. As a result, when a new drug is released, the FDA requires the pharmaceutical firm to conduct extensive post-marketing surveillance for any adverse reactions and to immediately report all deaths of people taking the drug, regardless of whether there appears to be a direct link between the death and the drug usage.

19. J. A. DiMasi, R. W. Hansen, H. G. Grabowski, and L. Lasagna, "Cost of Innovation in the Pharmaceutical Industry," *Journal of Health Economics* 10 (1991): 107–42.

20. Henry J. Grabowski and John Vernon, "A New Look at the Returns and Risks to Pharmaceutical R&D," *Management Science* 36 (July 1990): 804–821.

21. Iain M. Cockburn and Rebecca M. Henderson, "Scale and Scope in Drug Development: Unpack the Advantages of Size in Pharmaceutical Research," *Journal of Health Economics* 20, no. 6 (November 2001): 1033–1057.

22. Nitessh K. Choudhry, Henry Thomas Stelfox, and Allan S. Detsky, "Relationships Between Authors of Clinical Practice Guidelines and the Pharmaceutical Industry," *Journal of the American Medical Association* 287, no. 5 (February 6, 2002): 612–617; H.T. Stelfox, G. Chua, K. O'Rourke, A.S. Detsky, "Conflict of Interest in the Debate Over Calcium Channel Antagonists," *New England Journal of Medicine* 338 (1998): 101–106; F Davidoff et al., "Sponsorship, Authorship, and Accountability," *Journal of the American Medical Association* 286, no. 10 (September 12, 2001): 1232–1234.

23. As discussed earlier, although a product is approved by the Food and Drug Administration for a specific use or indication and some drugs may have multiple indications, physicians are permitted to prescribe the

product as they see fit. At the same time, physicians and drug companies are always exploring potentially new (or related) uses for the drug. The results of these studies are often published in the literature long before a new indication is obtained from the FDA. As a result of these publications, many drugs are prescribed for conditions outside of their indications. This practice is called off-label prescribing.

24. Alan T. Sorenson, "An Empirical Model of Heterogenous Consumer Search for Retail Prescription Drugs," NBER working paper 8548, National Bureau of Economic Research: Cambridge, Mass. (www.nber.org).

25. Cinda Becker, "Drugmakers Fight for Good Name," *Modern Healthcare* (August 27, 2001): 28–33; Standard & Poor's, op. cit., 3.

26. Z. John Lu, and William S. Comanor, "Strategic Pricing of New Pharmaceuticals," *The Review of Economics and Statistics* (1998): 108–118.

27. Scott Hensley, "AMA, Prescription Drug Makers Agree Ethics Policy Needs Better Implementation." *The Wall Street Journal* (January 21, 2002).

28. Stephen S. Hall, "The Claritin Effect: Prescription for Profit," *New York Times*, Magazine Section (March 11, 2001), 40ff. Laura Benko, "Ugly wait at the Counter: Insurer Pushes to Make Allergy Drugs Nonprescription," *Modern Healthcare* (August 6, 2001), 22–23.

29. F.M. Scherer, "The Link Between Gross Profitability and Pharmaceutical R&D Spending," *Health Affairs* 20, no. 5 (September 2001): 216–221.

30. Standard & Poor's, *op. cit.*, pages 3, 5.

31. "Bloom and Blight," *The Economist* (October 26, 2002), 60. 32. Gardner Harris, "For Drug Makers, Good Times Yield to a New Profit Crunch," *The Wall Street Journal* (April 18, 2002), sec. A, p.1; Standard & Poor's, op. cit.

CHAPTER 13

INTRODUCTION TO THE MACROECONOMICS OF HEALTH

QUESTIONS

1. Why abstract from reality if you want to study trading in the real world?
2. What is the "fallacy of composition"?
3. How should the wealth of a community be measured?
4. What determines how many people in a society are rich? How rich the richest 1 percent are? How poor the poorest 20 percent are?
5. Why does size make a difference?
6. Are prices the essence of trade or just one aspect?
7. Does cheating hurt the individual or the system?
8. Who makes the rules that govern the economy? Who challenges them?
9. Is community health the same as individual health?
10. Are questions better answered by comparisons over time, or by comparisons among people and places?

13.1 WHAT IS MACRO HEALTH ECONOMICS?

Macro means large. Macroeconomics deals with large-scale properties and institutions that characterize the system as a whole. Individuals become an economic system only when they start to trade with one another. In doing so, they create a whole that is larger than the sum of its parts, develop a government to set the rules under which trade will occur, and create a special medium, money, for conducting trade.[1] Macroeconomics evaluates gross domestic product (GDP) as a measure of national economic activity, whether growing (expansion) or falling (recession), and the dynamics of the process by which change occurs (investment, trade, unemployment, bankruptcy). Rather than investigating the income of a particular individual or firm, macroeconomics investigates growth and distribution of income. Macroeconomics seeks to determine how many people are rich, how many people are poor, whether the same people always make up the same groups over time, and whether the gap is widening or narrowing toward more economic equality.

Macroeconomic (system) Properties

Growth

Dynamics

Distribution

Macro (system) Institutions

Government

Money

The macroeconomics of health is concerned with a parallel set of large-scale system issues concerning (a) spending, employment, and other aspects of health as a part of the economy and (b) the biological health status of the population as a whole and its relation to economic changes. Thus, it must address how GDP growth affects the number and income of physicians as well as how GDP growth affects the health (longevity, morbidity) of the population and, consequently, how an increase in longevity affects both spending on medical care and growth in overall GDP.

Health System Properties

Economic	Biologic
Spending	Longevity
Employment	Fertility
Prices	Productivity

Health (system) Institutions

Medical professions

Hospitals and caring organizations

Financing (insurance and reimbursement) structure

13.2 PROPERTIES OF THE INDIVIDUAL VERSUS PROPERTIES OF THE SYSTEM

Microeconomics examines how individuals choose—how they minimize costs or maximize profits (or wealth or utility) within a given trading system, subject to a set of rules and prices. Microeconomists examine how individual choices are altered when prices change or when rules change. Macroeconomics, on the other hand, examines the properties of the system as a whole (growth, unemployment, inflation) and how the system changes over time as people modify the rules to better satisfy their needs. One could say that microeconomics is about how the game is played, and macroeconomics is about how the rules of the game are changed to make it better, more fair, or to favor one group over another, as well as the keeping of statistics on league standings.

Systems may behave differently than individuals, even when exposed to the same forces. For example, if the government makes a mistake and sends me a $100,000 tax refund, I am much richer and can buy a fancy new car. What would happen if the government sent everyone a check for $100,000? There would be no extra production; therefore, as a society, we would not be any richer. What would happen is that a burst of inflation would disrupt prices and everyone's savings plans so that we would all be made worse off by this massive mistake. The difference between individual and system impact is known as

the fallacy of composition. Other examples are as follows: If I push my way to the front of the line at a dentist's office, I get served quicker. If everyone pushes, it will take longer for all of us to get served. If I cheat on my health insurance, I am better off. If everyone cheats, premiums, waste, and administrative overhead will rise, making us all worse off.

There is an anecdote among business journalists, "If everyone I know is working, we are in an expansion. If my neighbor is unemployed, we are in a recession. If I become unemployed, we are in a depression." An individual is either working or not, but the rate of unemployment is a characteristic of the system as a whole. The rate affects what the individual does (if unemployment is high, I will always be polite to my boss, not grumble about overtime, and think about joining the Army when I graduate). However, rates are systemwide properties and must be measured at the level of the system as a whole. Similarly, a particular individual might be saving to buy a car or borrowing to make a purchase, but it is the aggregate actions of all individuals that determine the interest rate. Inflation is perhaps the best example of a system property. Every individual consumer and firm reacts to and sets prices, but it is the flow of money into the system, and the degree of public confidence in the value of that money, which determines how fast the average price will rise.[2] Regarding health, an individual is either dead or alive. Yet for the system as a whole, averages (mortality rates, longevity) become useful measures of system performance.

In moving toward a larger perspective, it is important to remember that all macro phenomena arise from individual maximizing behavior. The system exists to serve the people, not the other way around. Government, credit cards, and bankruptcy laws may be inconvenient for me, but they make the economy as a whole function better. Similarly, all the special features of medical care such as insurance, licensure, and so on are ultimately justifiable on a micro level as being results of choices people have made to make themselves better off. Adam Smith's 1776 book *The Wealth of Nations* expressed a fundamental insight into system behavior and individual motivation that has come to be known as the "invisible hand" of the market—that people make others better off not so much because they want to, or out of altruism, but because going to work, obeying the law, and discovering a cure for arthritis is profitable.[3] The primary way to make oneself better off in a society is to do something for someone else. However, those who have the power to write the rules often bend them in their own favor, and such individual maximization can lead to adverse social consequences. Inflation, unemployment, and war all occur because somebody benefits.

13.3 DYNAMICS: CHANGE OVER TIME

It takes much less time to make a deal than to change the way deals are made. Some of the confusion between individual and systematic responses arises because it takes longer for the system to respond. If we all get checks in the mail, it will take a while for prices to rise and eliminate this apparent windfall gain. Similarly, if a terminally ill person with AIDS charges a lot of fancy gifts on his credit cards before dying to repay the friends who took care of him, he may seem to be making his community better off, but such behavior will, if it becomes prevalent in the long run, mean that no one with AIDS can get credit. Standard supply and demand analysis uses "comparative statics" to study the change between one set of equilibrium conditions and another, asking only what the result was, not how the system got there or how long it took. A question regarding the effects of a change (e.g., Will expansion of the hospital cause nurses' wages to rise?) is microeconomic in scope. A macro perspective must also address the **dynamics** or process of change, why and how growth occurred, how long it took, and what things had to happen (bankruptcy, unemployment, war) before a new equilibrium was reached. A recession does not occur because GDP is $5 billion, or $500 trillion, or $990 quadrillion, but because GDP is falling or is lower than expected.

Microeconomists can make comparisons between individuals at a particular point in time and test their theories using **cross-sectional analysis.** Macroeconomists usually cannot. They must look at the economy as a whole and see how it has changed from one year to the next as the money supply rose or the population got older. Even if macroeconomists were not interested in dynamics, they would be forced to use longitudinal **time series** methods to test their theories by observing the same groups or individuals at different points in time. When economists make comparisons between the economies of different nations, often there are so few observations and so many differences in government and culture that any conclusions regarding the effects of money supply, age, education, and other variables must be very tentative.

The fallacy of composition operates over time as well. Perfect efficiency right now implies that all current waste be eliminated. Excess staff members sitting at their desks wondering what to do, indulgently impractical research schemes, half-baked management reorganization projects, and so on must be cut to minimize costs. Yet it is precisely from such waste and indulgent impracticalities that the creative energy for new technology and new managerial structures arise. To change and grow over time, every organization in the economy must "waste" some resources trying out new ideas that don't work or don't yet work very well.[4] Dynamic efficiency, optimizing economic output over time, requires that there be some activities that look wasteful from a static perspective, which considers current costs and benefits only.

13.4 ABSTRACTIONS AND COMPLICATIONS

While the terms micro and macro can be applied to purely individual and purely systematic effects, respectively, most of reality occurs between these extremes. Figure 13.1 provides a conceptual map of the different levels at which an economic question can be addressed.

The simplest form of trade occurs on a spot market. A one-dimensional good is traded, at a single point in time, for a specified amount of money (the price). A transaction, whether going to the supermarket for groceries or being admitted to the hospital for gall bladder surgery, is an event that may involve a number of goods and take some time. Exchange is a broader concept that brings in the notion of reciprocity and balance, that all parties be satisfied with what they get from trading. Thus, an exchange may include a third

FIGURE 13.1   The Context of Trade

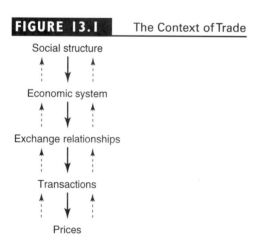

party (patients pay insurance companies that pay doctors) and involve relationships of long duration (my employer owes me something for my years of loyal service). Exchange takes place within a trading system (economy) that specifies ownership and the rules of exchange. There is an understanding on everyone's part about what you can and cannot do, what you should expect, and how a fair price is determined—even when the unexpected happens, such as a facial scar that results from a surgeon's mistake. In the current U.S. economic system, the patient might sue for malpractice and take the doctor to court. In another economy, the doctor who blundered might not get paid or might get beaten up. Finally, the economy exists within a social structure that expresses our collective sense of who we are and how we live together (Figure 13.1). Even before considering the terms of trade, it is necessary to determine who gets to have what and how much can be traded away. Are you supposed to beg, or pay, for something you need? Who gets to order whom about, and how much do they have to pay? Is cheating allowed? If not, how much will it cost me if I get caught? Whose desires count the most? Should we treat outsiders as customers or enemies to be looted? Creating the best set of institutions (government, laws, markets, nonprofit organizations) for satisfying people's wants is what politics and philosophy and economics is all about. More realistically, we try to make small improvements in the system we have without destroying all the benefits of the traditions that have developed over time.

To simplify economics and make it amenable to abstract mathematical formulation, a neoclassical approach makes a sharp distinction between properties of the system (macroeconomics) and individual trades and traders (microeconomics). Then the complex sets of relations involved in trade are collapsed into one bare essential—price. Governments, laws, institutions, reputations, and other complex structures that arise in the attempt to organize trade in the face of uncertainty and costly information are assumed away so that the workings of supply and demand are more clearly revealed. In terms of Figure 13.1, neoclassical economics ignores social structure and only considers elements of the economic system that are common to all economies as the appropriate focus of macroeconomics. More precisely, neoclassical economics considers the social and cultural context for trade that prevails in global markets and in Western democracies, so that this set of institutions forms a sort of unconscious assumption. These simplifications, that macroeconomics is divorced from social and cultural context and that supply and demand are separate domains communicating solely through prices, are extremely powerful and useful—yet, like all intellectual tools, they have a cost as well as a benefit. This abstract representation is much closer to reality for some economic transactions (timber, steel, retail food) than for others (art, insurance, medicine). We might be lured into the error of the motorist who spent the night searching the street for his lost car keys. The police asked why he spent so much time looking in the street, when he had probably lost the keys while walking through the bushes. He replied, "Because it was dark, and the light was much better in the street." Similarly, we may be tempted to look in the well-lit neoclassical street of clearly separated supply and demand divorced from social and systematic complications because the concepts are much clearer there than in the dimly lit reaches where each transaction depends on tradition and trust as well as price. Yet already, in previous chapters, we have been forced to talk about the rules of the system and how these institutions (professional licensure, insurance, regulation) change to apply the concepts of supply and demand to medicine. Consider how quickly a simple question such as "What is the price of an abortion?" shreds the orderly neatness of monetary exchange between firms and households. The complicated features of medical markets do not come from a desire to make this textbook longer, but because the trades organized by doctors and hospitals are not simple. These exchanges do not merely touch, but often must define difficult social issues, such as what it means to be alive or to be human. The special institutions of medicine are there to make people better off; they come from the complex nature of the good to be traded (medical care) and the shaping of the rules by the groups that have the power to do so in their own interest, subject to the controls of economic and political competition.

13.5 THE ROLE OF GOVERNMENT (OVERVIEW OF CHAPTERS 14–18)

Governments attempt to develop rules so that individuals' incentives are in line with the good of society as a whole. Thus, we have laws against stealing, a social consensus to prevent people from standing in their seats at a ball game, the National Institutes of Health to conduct medical research, and a central bank to offset fluctuations in aggregate demand. One of the most difficult tasks of a government is to determine which activities are best left for people to work out for themselves (what to eat, who to marry, what to wear, where to worship) and which activities require government control (what you can own, when to fight, who to protect). Health touches some controversial areas in which agreement over what is a public responsibility and what is private is difficult to reach (which drugs you can take, how and with whom you can have sex, whether you can take your own life).

The remaining chapters examine the role of government in health from a macro perspective. Chapter 14 analyzes market failure and the role of governments in health. Chapter 15 considers "public goods," which can be provided efficiently on a collective basis only (national defense, air traffic control, securities regulation, control of infectious disease). Chapter 16 discusses the historical relationship between economic growth and health status, and uses demographic tools to determine how much of the great increase in life expectancy is attributable to public health activities, private medical care, or improvements in the prevailing standards of housing, education, nutrition, and other aspects of general economic well-being.

International comparisons of health systems in countries as varied as Kenya and Japan are presented in Chapter 17. These comparisons provide several lessons, notably that life expectancy and the amount spent on medical care are more related to economic development and per capita income than to any other factor. This sets the stage for Chapter 18, where the reaction of public and private health care spending to changes in GDP is addressed. Adjustment dynamics and the use of regulation as a form of health care cost control are related to standard macroeconomic concerns regarding business cycles, inflation and employment. Chapter 19 presents projections for the future, identifying economic issues likely to be contentious as the health care system in the twenty-first century takes shape.

SUGGESTIONS FOR FURTHER READING

James S. Coleman, *Foundations of Social Theory* (Cambridge, Mass.: Harvard University Press, 1990).
Mervyn Susser, "The Logic in Ecological," *American Journal of Public Health*, 84, no. 5 (1994): 825–835.
Oliver E. Williamson, *The Economic Institutions of Capitalism: Firms, Markets, Relations* (New York: Free Press, 1985).

PROBLEMS

1. {*aggregation*} Macroeconomics analyzes the large-scale aggregate effects of many micro decisions made by individuals. Is it possible to simply add up the behavior of all individuals, or to multiply the behavior of the average individual by the total number of people, to determine system behavior?

2.   {*fallacy of composition*} Give two examples of the fallacy of composition that are plausible enough to fool some newspaper readers. Give an example that illustrates the fallacy of projecting micro behavior on the basis of macro changes and one that shows the fallacy of projecting macro behavior on the basis of individual decisions.

3.   {*competition, welfare maximization*} Does the "invisible hand" work in health care markets? Give an example that clearly illustrates the welfare-maximizing effects of self-interested competition and one that calls self-interested competition into question. Is health care more, or less, nonprofit than other types of human productivity and exchange?

4.   {*dynamics*} Explain the difference between the comparative statics and dynamics of a market, such as physician services and long-term care.

5.   {*transactions costs*} Do all economic exchanges have a monetary price? How would a politician pay the price of changing insurance legislation to cover hospital-sponsored health maintenance organizations (HMOs)? To whom would the price be paid? Do laws regulating exchange make trade more expensive or less expensive?

ENDNOTES

1.   This chapter borrows selectively from a number of authors, including James S. Coleman, *Foundations of Social Theory* (Cambridge, Mass.: Harvard University Press, 1990); Douglass North, *Structure and Change in Economic History* (New York: W. W. Norton, 1981); and Oliver Williamson, *Markets and Hierarchies* (New York: The Free Press, 1975).

2.   Mervyn Susser, "The Logic in Ecological," *American Journal of Public Health* 84, no. 5 (1994): 825–835.

3.   Adam Smith, *An Inquiry Into the Nature and Causes of the Wealth of Nations* (1776, reprinted by Random House: New York, 1985).

4.   Consider the similarities with the role of "excess" profits in pharmaceutical innovation. Since research is a sunk cost, setting price just equal to marginal cost would still allow firms to produce drugs, but there would be no capital to build laboratories, investigate the human genome, or track potential side effects.

CHAPTER 14

THE ROLE OF GOVERNMENT

"To do for the people what needs to be done, but which they cannot, by individual effort, do at all, or do so well, for themselves."

— *Abraham Lincoln*

"In the evolution of economic enterprise, the things which could be produced and sold for a price were taken over by private producers. Those that were not, but which were in the end no less urgent for that reason, remained with the state."

— *John Kenneth Galbraith*

QUESTIONS

1. Is competition better than regulation?
2. Which parts of the health care system are paid for, or controlled, by government? Why?
3. Why is Medicare so much more popular than Medicaid?
4. Does the Food and Drug Administration, or any other agency that regulates health, operate in the interest of the public, in the interest of the people who work there, or for the special-interest lobbies?
5. Is it because health is "priceless" that medical markets are so heavily regulated?
6. Do people vote for what is good for society or what is good for themselves?

14.1 THE FLOW OF GOVERNMENT HEALTH FUNDS

State, federal, and local government accounted for almost half of all health spending (45 percent) in 2002. However, most "government" health care is actually third-party insurance payment to the highly regulated private health care industry composed of independent physicians, hospitals, nursing homes, and so on. More than 90 percent goes to such providers of personal health care services, and less than 10 percent goes to core government functions such as medical research, infectious disease control, collection of national health statistics, and public health. Government's share of the rapidly growing health care sector tripled from 14 percent in 1929 to 45 percent in 2002. In earlier years, state and local governments were larger sources of funding than the federal government. In 1965, the biggest single category of government spending was state and local hospitals, institutions providing care for both general medical conditions and chronic mental illness. Since then, Medicare and Medicaid have become much larger, and in 2002 they accounted for more than two-thirds of all government spending on health care.

The bulk of the $697,100,000,000 in 2002 government funds came from general tax revenues. Premiums paid by enrollees for supplemental Medicare insurance (set originally to pay a quarter of costs) brought in $21 billion, and the designated Medicare Hospital Insurance tax of 2.9 percent on the wages and self-employment income of all workers brought in another $130 billion. These funding schemes shift the incidence of the tax burden, but do not change the total amount. Ultimately, all government spending must come at the expense of private consumption and investment.

Although the U.S. government provides the largest flow of funds into health care services, it has remained relatively passive. Both Medicare and Medicaid are **entitlement** programs, open-ended commitments for government to pay the bills incurred by any eligible patient (i.e., age 65 or over or indigent, respectively). Unlike budgeted programs, in which a fixed dollar amount is appropriated each year, there is no limit on the amount that can be spent on Medicaid and Medicare. Explosive growth in expenditures is a major cause of deficits in state and federal budgets and "crowds out" spending on vital public health activities. From 1965 to 2002, the share of federal government health care dollars devoted to public health declined from 4.6 percent to 1.2 percent, and spending for medical research to discover new therapies and diagnostics fell from 26.8 percent to 4.8 percent. The future health of the U.S. population is being compromised to pay for uncontrolled and excessive use of resources (see Table 14.1 and Figure 14.1).

14.2 THE ROLES OF GOVERNMENT

Government is Necessary, Even for Private Exchange

As people go about their daily activities, trying to stay happy and healthy and save a few dollars, they are usually not aware of government intrusion. Suppose that you get a headache and go to the drugstore for some aspirin. You are making that choice individually, as a

TABLE 14.1	Distribution of Government Funds	
	2002	**1965**
Total (millions)	$697,100	$10,799
Medicare	38%	–
Medicaid	35%	20%
Veterans/DOD	5%	18%
Worker's compensation	4%	8%
Maternal/child health	1%	2%
State/local hospitals	3%	22%
Public health	8%	8%
Research	4%	12%
Construction	1%	7%
Other	1%	3%

Medicaid category includes general assistance (welfare) payments for health care, and in 1965 is composed of a variety of medical care programs for the indigent, as Medicaid was not yet enacted.

Source: CMS National Health Accounts.

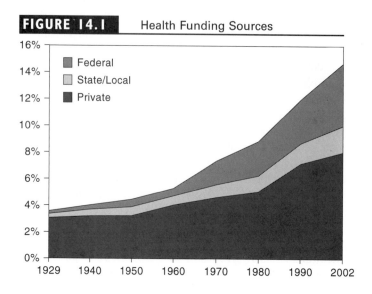

FIGURE 14.1   Health Funding Sources

private citizen, and buying from a private company. Yet this simple transaction could not take place unless a government had already done many things to prepare for the welfare of you and the company. To begin with, government provides a medium of exchange (money) and maintains its value. Without money you would have to engage in barter and search for someone who wanted you to cut their lawn, or care for their children, or whatever, in exchange for the aspirin. Not only is the value of money determined by the government, so are the measurements of what you buy. You don't ask for "some" or a scoop of aspirin, but for 100 250-milligram tablets. Furthermore, without government policing, you could not be sure whether the white pills were made of aspirin instead of sugar or flour, or some noxious chemical. In fact, you depend on your government to keep your local store from selling you anything that could kill you when ingested. Without this form of consumer protection, you would have to spend a lot of time and money making sure that the drugs you bought were safe. All the government activities that make exchange easy and inexpensive are going on almost without notice.[1]

   To make any transaction, you must be able to say, "I own this, and I will give it to you in exchange for that." The most fundamental function of government is to maintain law and order. Unless we can define and enforce rights, including property rights, there is no way for people to cooperate and move beyond the law of the jungle—each person for himself or herself alone. Being killed because somebody wants your house or your cow or your mate is the most basic of threats to your health. In response to such threats government arose. Families banded together into tribes to protect one another. To do so, they had to agree on how to work together—who would farm and who would fight, who would lead, and when it was OK to disagree with the leader. Douglass North, the 1993 Nobel Laureate in economics, defines the state as "an organization with a comparative advantage in violence, extending over a geographic area whose boundaries are determined by its power to tax constituents."[2] The state monopoly on violence makes it less costly for citizens to defend themselves and their property. Government is there to produce those goods and services that it can provide more efficiently than the market. When we say *efficient*, we do not mean that government has no waste, or makes no mistakes, only that it does the job on the whole better than private action—or competing governments.

Efficiency of Markets Under Conditions of Perfect Competition

The best way to run the economy is usually to let people work, play, and consume what they want without restriction. This interaction of supply and demand in the market leads to an equilibrium at the point where marginal benefits equal marginal costs. The prices that arise direct people to (a) work at the jobs where their skills provide the most value to society, (b) find the most efficient means of production, (c) limit the consumption of goods that are most scarce, and (d) save and invest for the future. If there were no special problems or difficulties, the entire economy could be coordinated without any central control or direction from the government. The power of market prices to organize production and consumption to maximize welfare is expressed in the two fundamental theorems of welfare economics: under "perfect" conditions (1) competitive markets will always lead to an efficient allocation of resources for production and consumption and (2) *any* efficient allocation can be obtained through a market system without any central government control by adjusting initial distribution.[3] These theoretical results emerged from a continuing debate among economists and politicians of all persuasions, from conservative to liberal to Marxist, during the early twentieth century. They provide the prime intellectual underpinning for advocating the use of markets rather than government intervention to solve economic problems.

Economists' most frequent criticism of government intervention is that it distorts prices so that marginal costs and marginal benefits are no longer equated at the margin. In trying to make things better, government gives up some efficiency, and often makes things worse. Governments also inevitably tend to favor certain politically powerful interest groups (e.g., tobacco producers, the military-industrial complex, sons and daughters of senators), and by helping them, harm the rest of society and reduce the overall efficiency of the economy. Yet recognizing that government action is sometimes wrong or self-serving does not mean that it is not necessary. Conditions are not always perfect, and there are things that only government can do. Carefully examining the conditions of theoretically perfect competition (i.e., many buyers and sellers, all fully informed; costless transactions, with free entry and exit into the market) provides some insight into the roles of government in the real world. **Market failures** necessitating corrective government intervention arise if (a) there is a **monopoly** in the market because there is only one (or just a few) buyers or sellers, (b) access to **information** is restricted or prohibitively costly to obtain by certain participants, (c) **transactions costs** are so high that many potentially beneficial agreements cannot be negotiated, or (d) the market is closed by constraints of technology, morality, or law. Sometimes the problems with competition are so extreme that they preclude a market from developing at all, making it necessary for government to create one. In the case of **public goods** (Chapter 15), the technology is such that only the government can act as a buyer or seller. Finally, the second theorem of welfare economics states only that the desired outcome "could in principle" be achieved if income were initially distributed in a particular way—which it is not. Governments must actively intervene if **redistribution** is desired.

Government in a Mixed Economy

Government has four primary tasks in all economies:

- Maintain law and order
- Provide public goods
- Deal with market failures
- Redistribute income

To achieve these goals, a government may (a) *produce* services, (b) *finance* services that are provided by private contractors, or (c) *regulate* the private market. In practice, programs usually serve several functions and use a combination of methods. The Medicare program, for example, deals with market failure due to adverse selection and redistributes income to the sick elderly. While mainly functioning as a financing mechanism, Medicare also uses regulation to enforce compliance and participation. In the face of such complexity, a simplified conceptual framework helps organize the analysis and make the fundamental economic forces more evident.

14.3 LAW AND ORDER

National defense and its complex domestic version—law and order—are the most fundamental tasks of governance. Without protection of life and property, society could not exist. A uniform interpretation of the law and a system of taxation must be enforced by the police and the courts. If the law applies to some and not to others, people are split into two different societies, even if they are nominally within the same nation. Coercive powers of taxation and law enforcement are freely given to the state by the citizens—we agree to have the government take our money and punish us if we break the law because we are better off that way. Each of us fighting our own battles is more expensive than all the taxes, parking fines, and so on that we love to complain about. Government is expensive, but anarchy, while it doesn't cost anything, is ruinous.

Getting people to agree that there should be law and order is much easier than reaching agreement on exactly what those laws should be, who pays how much tax, and so on. The philosopher John Rawls, in his book *A Theory of Justice*, suggests a useful way of looking at the problem of reaching a social consensus.[4] Rawls argues that much of the conflict over what is right and wrong is due not to differences in beliefs, but to differences in the positions that people are coming from. Older people want government to provide nursing home insurance, while young families believe that better schools are more important. The rich want taxes to be kept low, while the poor (who hope to benefit from redistribution and government aid) want taxes to be higher. People with AIDS favor a national health insurance system that insures everyone, while healthy workers tend to favor higher take-home pay and insurance premiums based on expected costs. In each case, the supporters tend to be those who can expect to benefit, while the critics tend to be those who stand to lose (through higher taxation, less service, or loss of preference).

Consider the formation of policy on disability. It is expensive to provide home care, prostheses, therapy, and building modifications. Including students with disabilities in regular classrooms (mainstreaming) helps them become integrated into society, but imposes costs on the other students in the diversion of teachers' attention, pacing of lectures, disruption, and so on. If everything that can possibly benefit the disabled students is done, it will cost too much. Yet providing only those benefits that reduce costs (e.g., a prostheses to help someone return to work) is not enough. Whether people primarily focus on the costs or emphasize the benefits depends mainly on whether they are disabled or whether they care deeply about a child, parent, or friend who is. However, even people who are healthy recognize that there is some chance that they might become disabled in the future (e.g., after an automobile accident) and switch their focus. Rawls defines justice as a set of policies people would vote for "behind the veil of ignorance" (i.e., what people would consider an optimal balance of costs and benefits if they did not know whether they were disabled or healthy, or gay or straight, or young or old). Formally, Rawls' notion is a lot like insurance, where people willingly contribute to an insurance plan to spread the risk and cover their expected losses. Most health care, disability, and pension financing systems in Europe and Asia are considered "social insurance" operating under principles of fairness and solidarity rather than private actuarial principles (such as rating and payment according to risk category) used in commercial insurance.

Justice is more than an abstract notion; it is necessary for the operation of society. Unless people believe that the system is fair and serves their needs, they will not trust the government, and it becomes prohibitively costly to force them to behave according to the rules. Pervasive cheating will cause the whole system to break down. If members of a group think they are not being treated fairly, the group will lose respect for the law. At the extreme, they will revolt and perhaps set up a separate government that conforms more closely to their ideal of a fair system.

14.4 PUBLIC GOODS AND EXTERNALITIES

A public good is something that everyone consumes collectively. National defense is a public good. So is clean air, the discovery of penicillin, and the publication of national health statistics. Public goods have two distinguishing properties. First, they are *inexhaustible*; therefore, once produced, there is no additional cost for having additional people use them (i.e., marginal cost of additional users is $0). Second, they are *nonexclusive*; therefore, people cannot be stopped from using a public good once it is there. Private goods are exhaustible and get used up by consumption (a pill, an hour of a doctor's time), while public goods (the formula for the pill, the discovery that eating foods rich in vitamin C reduces certain diseases, clean air) do not. If one patient uses a doctor's time, another patient cannot. Yet if one patient uses a formula, clean air, or nutritional advice, the amount available for someone else is not reduced. Private goods are *exclusive*; thus, if one person uses them, another person cannot. This makes it easy to charge consumers for using a private good and to pay the costs of production. Public goods tend to be nonexclusive and indivisible; thus, if anyone gets the benefits, everyone does. Since no one can be prevented from using a public good like clean air, no one has any incentive to pay for it. Selfishly, it makes sense for me to wait for someone else to clean up the air, discover a cure for AIDS, or build the Internet, because whether I contribute or not will make little difference. This is known as the **free-rider** problem. If no one is charged for public goods and no one voluntarily contributes, there is no way to conduct medical research, reduce pollution, or build highways. Therefore, governments are allowed to force everyone to "donate" taxes to pay for public goods.

Many goods are not purely private or purely public, but somewhere in between, and the extent of "publicness" may change with market conditions. For people in an isolated rural area, building and staffing a hospital is mostly a public good. Without the hospital, they have no medical care, but once it is built, anyone who wants to can use the hospital without displacing or reducing anyone else's consumption because there is plenty of excess capacity (i.e., marginal cost of additional patients is near $0). However, if population increases and the hospital becomes full, each additional patient displaces someone else who might have received care, and care becomes more like a private good (and marginal cost rises to approximately equal the average cost per unit). Highways, parks, and movie theaters show similar congestion effects, being almost pure public goods when they are mostly empty and more like private goods once they fill up.

Externalities

The production or consumption of a private good may have social consequences because it affects other people. A firm that produces cars may not pay for the exhaust they emit, an airport may not compensate residents in neighboring houses for the disruption caused by jets taking off at night, a student who cheats may not compensate classmates for the inconvenience caused by new test-taking rules, and a student who comes to class with a cold to take an exam may not compensate classmates for exposing them to illness. Externalities exist whenever a transaction affects an uncompensated party. The term *"public good"* focuses attention on the collective concerns that face all of us: a need for consensus, government control, and a universal tax system. The term *"externalities"* focuses attention on concerns in which the costs and benefits of actions are borne by different people, making private and social costs diverge. Whether considering public goods such as national defense and scientific research, or externalities such as infection control and pollution, we end up with the same issue—how to design appropriate institutions and government rules to align individual incentives with social welfare.

There are positive as well as negative externalities. Governments subsidize schools and colleges because they think that educated people will become better citizens (and able to pay more taxes). A person who fixes up an old house increases the value of all houses in the neighborhood, a cook who washes his hands reduces the risk of spreading infection, and a technological discovery that allows more efficient production by one firm creates external benefits for other firms that copy it. However, that same technology may create negative externalities for some corporations and people, because it puts an obsolete factory out of business and causes workers to lose their jobs. In fact, whether an externality is positive or negative depends on the perspective from which it is viewed. The cook may have thought that he was doing his patrons a favor by washing his hands. The patrons may have thought that being clean is part of his job and that not washing his hands was an unwarranted burden to impose on them. This mirror-image aspect, that an action may be considered either a negative cost reduction or a positive benefit increase leads to an important insight.

The Coase Theorem: Transaction Costs and Property Rights

If transacting were indeed costless, as is assumed under perfect competition, a factory would pay a fee for the smoke it emits, a cook with dirty hands would pay a fee to customers who became ill, and a student with the flu would not show up for an exam unless he or she was willing to pay each classmate $20 for exposing them to airborne viruses. These externalities would then be internalized by market transactions. If only one or two people are affected by an externality, individual transactions can be used to deal with it. For example, a person who dumps dirt in a neighbor's yard or who breaks a neighbor's window, or a doctor who negligently causes a leg fracture, will pay for it. If many people are affected by an externality, the cost of arranging thousands of individually negotiated transactions becomes prohibitive and **property rights** (who controls what, who must pay whom to use it) become unclear. No market develops to handle externalities at this scale. Therefore, government must act on behalf of many people by creating rules and regulations. It is cheaper to deal with a problem once and for all, despite some inefficiencies, than to make thousands of individual transactions with everyone who might be affected by the problem (e.g., pollution, infection, air traffic control).

Suppose that the socially optimal decision, in which marginal costs equal marginal benefits, is to force factories to reduce the pollution emitted from their smokestacks by 80 percent. The **Coase Theorem** asserts that there is *no difference* in outcome whether the factory has a right to pollute or the people have a right to clean air.[5] As long as all rights are well-defined, there are no transacting costs (a big if), and income distribution effects are ignored, the result will be the same. If a factory has the right to pollute, its neighbors will pay the company a fee to install smokestack scrubbers until pollution has been reduced to 20 percent. If the neighbors have a right to clean air, the factory will pay each resident a fee to allow discharge of 20 percent of the smoke and will buy scrubbers to clean up the rest. Either way, the result will be the same: air that is 80 percent cleaner. The ability to make mutually beneficial trades through the market guarantees that whoever values air quality more, whether positively or negatively, will "buy" it from the other party. The Coase Theorem is important, not because outcomes would be the same under some hypothetically perfect conditions, but because it shows how transaction costs and assignment of property rights affect distribution and efficiency in the real world, and how distortions and difficulties increase to the extent that the characteristics of a good are more public than private.

Politicians: Entrepreneurs Who Try to Get Votes

Markets operate through voluntary exchange, whereas public goods can be provided only through political intervention. You cannot go to the store and buy more clean air, better schools, or safer highways. We depend on politicians to act as entrepreneurs, to propose a plan of action that appeals to us so that we will put them in positions of power. Like all entrepreneurs, politicians expect to be paid for their efforts, extracting "rents" in the form of influence, prestige, perquisites, and salary. To an extent, the political arena can be viewed as a market, with people "spending" votes or influence. However, the correspondence is very imperfect—people are not allowed to buy and sell votes, borrow votes by paying interest, or trade votes by setting up joint-stock corporations. The property rights to votes are much less well defined and enforceable, and thus the transactions costs are very high.

Because it is difficult to make a political bargain, a lot of the effort and money must be wasted. Millions of dollars are used to win support or to keep a wavering supporter in line. Formally, economists talk about the problems of "rent capture." If ordinary entrepreneurs have a good idea, they can trade the idea to a firm for money. For example, inventors, biochemists, and screenwriters avoid the hassles of marketing and production by licensing the rights to their ideas and obtaining royalty payments in return. These profits are called **rents** because once the entrepreneur has the idea, no more work needs to be done to get the money. It is similar to collecting rent on a piece of land. Also, like land, the rent depends entirely on the demand. A good idea (Mickey Mouse, penicillin, mobile phones) is valuable the way land in downtown Tokyo is valuable; bad ideas are like acreage in the Gobi Desert.

Rents and rent seeking are major obstacles to providing an optimal level of investment in public health. Many good ideas (well-child care, genetic counseling for expectant parents, dietary change) offer no simple way for innovators to capture the benefits, and thus there is little incentive to produce them. On the other hand, when large sums of money are available to put good ideas into practice, most of the money is not well spent. The new road primarily benefits a construction company owned by a senator's brother-in-law, the new antismoking campaign is highly visible and impresses voters but doesn't keep children from lighting up, and the new sex education program for teenagers is so dreary that they only use it to make jokes. Even if we know exactly how much to spend on public goods, it is doubtful that all the money will be well spent. Because no single individual has much of an interest, those who are able to capture a piece of the action will distort the program to benefit themselves, and the objective of meeting the needs of the public will be compromised.

14.5 MARKET FAILURE

Monopoly

For public goods, the marginal cost of additional consumption is $0. The production of some private goods has such high fixed costs and low marginal costs that the average cost per unit continually falls as output increases. Such goods (telephone networks, power and water supply) are called **natural monopolies.** Declining average cost means that the largest firm can underbid all the others, and competition will lead to a single firm that dominates the whole market. However, to break even, that firm must charge a price above marginal cost (the high fixed cost overhead means that average cost per unit is always above marginal cost). Since there is no competition, the monopoly firm may push prices up to extract extra profits from consumers, stopping only when the profits are so great that another firm is tempted to enter the market, even at an inefficiently small scale. In a rural area, ambulance transport, hospital services, even a doctor's office, may all be natural monopolies. In addition to the technologically induced natural monopoly, there are monopolies created by political action. For example, a certificate-of-need law may give a hospital an effective monopoly in its local market by barring the construction of new competitors, licensure laws may give a profession monopoly control over supply, quality regulations may give a manufacturer monopoly control over a special medical device, and requirements to hold clinical trials demonstrating safety and efficacy can give a pharmaceutical firm monopoly control over a type of drug.

The desire to maximize profits and the lack of competition leads a monopolist, unlike a firm under perfectly competitive conditions, to charge a price above the average cost per unit, thus generating excess profits known as **monopoly rents.** Monopoly pricing causes the market to be inefficient. With prices above average cost, some consumers choose not to buy even though goods could have been produced and sold for an amount less than their willingness to pay. The amount of consumer welfare foregone is traditionally estimated by the "welfare triangle," which under appropriate conditions is approximately one-half the difference between the monopoly price and the average cost per unit multiplied by the number of units not purchased due to the excessive price.

$$\text{Welfare Loss (triangle)} = (P_{monopoly} - AC) \times (Q_{optimum} - Q_{monopoly})$$

The magnitude of inefficiency due to monopoly pricing is shown by the shaded welfare triangle in Figure 14.2. Monopoly rents (shown as dots) resulting from high prices are a loss to consumers, but are a gain to the seller, and are regarded by most economists as a pure transfer that does not in itself create any loss of market efficiency. However, consumers tend to get upset about being charged extra just because a firm has a monopoly. Also, there is likely to be some fighting between firms for the right to become the monopolist that takes home the rents, and this fighting is a waste of resources that generates inefficiency.

FIGURE 14.2   Welfare Loss Due to Monopoly Pricing

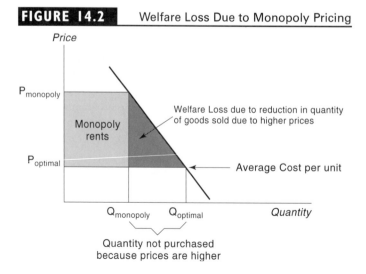

There are four ways for government to deal with the problems created by a natural monopoly:

- Take over the process and let government become the producer.
- Subsidize the fixed cost overhead and set a government-controlled price equal to the marginal cost per unit.
- Set a government-controlled price equal to the average cost, which causes some inefficiency but avoids using taxpayers' money to subsidize a monopoly firm.
- Do nothing and let the firm set a monopoly price.

Some economists claim that government production is so inefficient that the first option should always be avoided. Options 2 and 3 depend on the government's ability to accurately estimate marginal and average cost, which is always difficult and is inevitably made worse by firms' attempts to overstate costs and hide revenues to make extra profits. However, allowing firms to become monopolies often costs much more than the traditional welfare triangle loss, because firms waste millions of dollars making donations to politicians, hiring lawyers, and competing for (and competing away) the potential monopoly rents. Natural monopoly is a cornerstone of applied welfare economics, but is relatively less important in health care. Most medical monopolies arise from government intervention (licensure, regulation, reimbursement rules) designed to ameliorate market failures caused by risk and information difficulties (discussed in Chapter 6) rather than market failures caused by production conditions of declining average costs.

Paternalism

Market efficiency depends on consumers' ability to choose, to correctly balance their demands with prices and available income. Some types of consumers—notably children, the mentally ill, addicts—are considered incapable of making reasonable choices. There is a biological necessity for parents to care for and make decisions on behalf a child, forcing it to learn by doing many things it does not initially want to do (hence the term *paternalism*). Market failure due to mental incapacity is dealt with by having a parent, legal guardian, social service agency, or government bureau make decisions on behalf of those individuals rather than allowing them to do so for themselves. Addicts are prohibited by law from buying drugs they are willing to pay for. To that extent, these people are wards of the state, not fully participating citizens of the country.

Recently there has been a move to provide more freedoms and more rights to people who are mentally ill. "Deinstitutionalization" emptied state mental hospitals as patients were released into the community. In principle, inpatient hospital services were going to be replaced by community services so that former patients could operate at a higher level of functioning and be integrated into the community. The rise of a new generation of homeless people is evidence that things did not work out as planned. Economics, or rather the *failure to consider* the economics of deinstitutionalization, was a contributing factor. The public was more willing to recognize that people with mental illness had rights, and to vote for a change in the law making it difficult to keep people in mental hospitals, than to provide money for the community services needed to take care of these people. Once it cost something, voters approached the issue from a different perspective. Unlike a manager or a factory owner, voters are under no obligation to be consistent. Thus, they could vote for their principles one day and for their pocketbooks on another. Deinstitutionalization created a need for services, but not the taxes to pay for these services. Furthermore, the expected transfer of funding from hospitals to community programs did not occur. Employees at state mental hospitals fought to maintain their jobs and their budgets even though most patients were being discharged.

The initial proponents of deinstitutionalization were ordinary citizens who had worked with people with mental disorders and were convinced that most of them could function better and enjoy life more if they lived in the community. Like doctors, they were agents and even advocates for their clients. Yet they were not balancing the interests of all the parties involved. Although living in the community might be beneficial to a patient, it might not be beneficial to the community. Deinstitutionalization has had a large and unrecognized externality that we call the homeless problem.

14.6 INCOME REDISTRIBUTION AND CARE OF THE POOR

Every civilized society takes care of its poor. It is generally accepted that no one in the United States should die because he or she cannot afford a necessary operation or medications. However, the poor cannot afford to buy insurance or medical care generally available to most members of society. Not being able to buy is what being "poor" means. Countries that provide health services as a public good just as they provide water and mail delivery services, such as Sweden and the United Kingdom, automatically provide medical care to the poor. In a pluralistic system where individual income affects access to the system, a more explicit mechanism to protect those least able to pay is required. In the United States, Medicaid is the most important program to guarantee that poor people have access to medical care. Originally directed toward impoverished families with dependent children, Medicaid has been broadened to include all people who are medically indigent, and now pays for almost half of all nursing home care, even for the middle-class elderly (see Chapter 11).

Medicaid and Medicare: Dependency or Rights?

Medicaid is fraught with ambiguity and compromise because of an unresolved conflict at its core: Is it charity or a form of social insurance? Is it a program for taking care of people who can't take care of themselves and whose dependency, like that of children, addicts, and the mentally ill, makes them inherently less qualified than other citizens to make decisions? Or is Medicaid the provision of a basic necessity of life, such as safe water and national defense, that poor people can claim as a right of citizenship and, therefore, should not involve giving up any decision-making power?

Some people (liberals) believe that most or all of the benefits of economic development should belong to society as a whole, and they favor broad government activity to ensure a relatively equitable distribution of goods and services. In Sweden, for example, more than half of gross domestic product (GDP) moves through the government sector. Other people (conservatives) believe that individual initiative and luck should determine who gets to consume what and thus want to limit the role of government to referee and safety net provider. Medical care for the poor is caught between these opposing positions. Conservatives who believe in reducing taxes and the role of government are willing to make an exception for medical care, but expect the indigent (like other dependent beneficiaries) to give up some autonomy and self-respect. Liberals want a more equitable distribution of all goods and services, but are willing to settle for a few (medical care, education) rather than none.

In general, rich people will rationally favor a conservative position since any redistributive government activity is likely to cost them more in taxes than they will receive in benefits. Conversely, the self-interest of poor people rationally favors a liberal position. The motivations behind these two positions are in conflict on several levels and it is, therefore, almost impossible to design a practical program that satisfies both at the same time. This tension and its policy implications are well illustrated by comparing Medicare and Medicaid.

Medicare is a universal and popular program to pay on a national basis for the medical care of all the elderly.[6] Medicaid is a much reviled and unpopular part-federal part-state (local) program that requires each beneficiary to meet a "means test" and covers a complicated patchwork of special programs. Even conservatives are not foolish enough to attack Medicare, and even liberals are not foolish enough to support an expansion of Medicaid.[7] Why are these two programs perceived so differently? Medicare is constructed like a public good for all citizens, whereas Medicaid has the punitive elements of a qualified dependency assistance program. To qualify for Medicare, one need only be 65 or older, and it covers everyone, rich or poor, sick or healthy, black or white. Every voter expects to benefit from Medicare and views it as vital to their financial planning for old age. Medicaid is the opposite. Applicants must submit to probing questions and must sometimes misrepresent their economic positions to qualify for benefits. Most voters believe they personally will never benefit from Medicaid, and often feel shame when they help Grandma (and themselves) do so by transferring ownership of her car and her house to their own name so that she can qualify for assistance. Medicaid is not designed to provide satisfaction to its beneficiaries; it forces them to acknowledge dependence and serves as a necessary social backstop so that no one is deprived of minimal (but not comfortable) care.

The expansion of a Medicare-type program (universal access, no means testing, the same care for all) furthers liberal political goals by broadening participation in government activities viewed as helpful and high quality. Replacement with a Medicaid-type program (means tested, differential standards of care by payment class) furthers a conservative political agenda by making government programs unpopular. Thus, how a public health program is put together affects not just the services people get, but also their future voting behavior and attitude toward government. Each political party fights to get programs that make it easier to say, "I told you so," and that favor the economic interests of its supporters. Attitudes toward public health activities and the design of programs thus depend on political ideology and self-interest as much as any objective evaluation of costs and benefits or morbidity and mortality.

14.7 HOW GOVERNMENT WORKS

Government influence on various parts of the economy ranges from watchful oversight to total control (Table 14.2). Government is least intrusive when it confines its activities to creating a foundation of property rights and contract enforcement within which the market can operate freely. Government is most controlling when it takes over production and replaces private ownership completely. Through regulation and third-party financing, the health care sector has a high degree of government involvement. **Government production** is mostly limited to certain core public health functions, such as setting and monitoring standards, controlling infectious disease, and conducting medical research.[8] Direct contracting with production tailored to government specifications, which occurs in military health insurance, federally qualified neighborhood health centers, immunization programs, and so on, offers extensive, yet not complete, public control since the workers are employed by private firms. With **subsidies,** government can exert influence, but rarely control. For example, tax-exempt municipal bond financing can encourage construction of hospital facilities, but only rarely and indirectly affects the type of clinical services offered. **Entitlement financing,** such as Medicare, may leave behavior essentially unconstrained since it is designed to be the equivalent of privately purchased insurance.

TABLE 14.2	Varieties of Government Action
	Examples
Public production	Centers for disease control & prevention
	Veterans administration hospitals
Public financing	
• Contract	Neighborhood health center
• Producer subsidy	Vaccine liability insurance
• Consumer subsidy	Employee health benefits
• Entitlement	Medicare
Public regulation	
• For the market	Financial standards for insurance companies
• Superseding market	Price controls
Private production	Self-paid visit to therapist

A large part of **health regulation** is intended *to make markets more efficient* by providing standard definitions, quality assurance, uniform insurance contracts, and other measures that reduce transactions costs. Other regulations attempt to change the shape of the market *or to supersede the market entirely* and dictate prices and quantities. The regulatory apparatus can be tightened or loosened to allow government to exert more or less control, and can be made compelling without resorting to legal action by combining regulation with financing. Medicare, initially a passive entitlement financing program that provided essentially private funding for the purchase of physician services, now sets prices within a narrow range and may virtually prohibit the use of some medical technology by refusing to pay for it. Direct regulatory control is exercised by government in only a few areas where the threat to public safety is compelling: water and air quality, production and prescribing of pharmaceuticals, and performance of surgery. For the most part, medical care is "regulated" through control over finances rather than laws.

The Voluntary Sector

The public good is sometimes best served neither by a government bureaucracy nor a private firm but by independent "voluntary" organizations. Nonprofit status can free hospitals, social service agencies, professional societies, and other voluntary organizations from the dictates of profit maximization and make it easier for them to pursue the goal of maximizing health. Independence from government often makes voluntary organizations more flexible and creative than the public sector in meeting social needs.[9]

Government as the Citizen's Agent

Government exists, to paraphrase the quote from Abraham Lincoln at the opening of this chapter, to do for the people things that they cannot do for themselves. However, what guarantee is there that a government agency will act as the agent of the people rather than of special interest groups or of the bureaucrats themselves? When information problems cause market failure and thus preclude private action, governments will also have a difficult time collecting information and voters will have a difficult time evaluating the performance of an agency to make sure that it is, in fact, operating in the public interest. Economists examine the performance of government agencies from four perspectives:

- Maximizing public welfare
- "Capturing" of regulatory agencies by profit-maximizing firms
- Maximizing bureaucratic objectives
- Balancing political interest groups

Public Welfare Maximization The starting point for the economic analysis is to assume that regulation does what it says it does—maximize public welfare. The British Empire, the state of Pennsylvania, and other governments argue as much when they define themselves as a *commonwealth*. However, to define *public welfare,* assumptions about whose preferences count, and how much, must be made. Is everyone equal? Do people who harm themselves through drug use or lack of exercise deserve the same services as people who try to stay healthy? Do people with genetic defects that shorten their lives deserve more, or less, than people without genetic defects? Does a desire for lifesaving heart surgery count as much as a desire for face-saving cosmetic surgery? Even if all these issues are resolved, there still may be no way to reach a decision about which government policy is best, as demonstrated in the proof of the famous "Arrow impossibility theorem."[10] The theoretical problems of welfare maximization pale beside the practical problems of public incentives. Unlike a firm, which has an owner, no one has an interest in maximizing the benefits of government. An individual seeks to maximize his or her own welfare. Acts and votes are usually directed by self-interest, even when the cost to others far outweighs the benefits to the individual. Many government programs are characterized by *concentrated benefits* and *diffuse costs.* For example, lengthening patent restrictions would raise the price of drugs several cents per prescription thus adding millions of dollars to the profits of a few pharmaceutical firms, but would cause just a slight, almost unnoticeable, rise in the medical bills and insurance premiums of millions of consumers.

Regulatory Capture The concentrated interest of the firms most affected by a regulation makes it worthwhile for them to lobby government and try to "capture" the regulatory agency. For example, a hearing on the safety of cardiac pacemakers is sure to be attended by lawyers for the device manufacturers, but few patients will to travel to Washington to testify and will not be paid $400 an hour for doing so. Contributing to political campaigns is an obvious way of attempting to exercise control, but usually is not the most effective way. It is common for firms in regulated industries to appeal directly to bureaucrats, not with money or gifts (which are illegal), but by hiring former regulators and holding informational seminars in Hawaii. It is natural for someone who has worked for years in regulating health to take a job with a company in the same field, but such a **revolving door** is likely to compromise regulatory objectivity. How can a junior analyst in an agency remain clear when asked to make a difficult judgment call if the person on the other side of the table is the well-respected former chairman? Even a bureaucrat who wants to do a good job performing daily tasks can be influenced by the asymmetry between concentrated producer interests and diffuse consumer interests. There are many more patients than producers, yet most complaints to regulators (or complaints to politicians about regulatory decisions) come from producers, because they stand to gain so much from any change in the rules.[11]

Bureaucratic Objectives Bureaucrats, just like consumers, profit-maximizing owners, union workers, and all other individuals in the economy, prefer not to be harassed. Most people get paid to do tasks that are occasionally unpleasant in order to maximize long-term gains (e.g., impose discipline on second-graders, redo a botched repair job for free, fire an incompetent employee, hold the HMO doctors within budget). The difficulty of evaluating how well a government agency is performing can reduce the competitive pressure to take on unpleasant tasks. This can lead to an agency that is bloated and excessively risk averse. Unlike an owner, who can gain large profits from taking on risk, a bureaucrat will continue to be compensated on a civil service pay scale. Any effort to make changes or take risks could go wrong and cost them their jobs, so they tend to play it safe. If an owner believes that the additional revenues gained are less than the additional cost in wages, then an employee may be let go. A bureaucrat, on the other hand, has almost no incentive to reduce the number of workers. Instead, an increase in employment usually means a larger salary for the director (since they now run a bigger agency) and better working conditions (since the tasks are spread out among more employees, giving them more time to do the job). Unlike a profit-maximizing firm, there is no internal incentive to limit the size of a government agency; therefore, control must be imposed from the outside. Unfortunately, outsiders are, by definition, less familiar with the tasks, workload, and performance of the agency than the employees and managers inside, or the industry experts who lobby them. This does not mean that most government agencies are too large, since the fear of "waste" may lead legislators to preemptively cut regulatory budgets. What it does mean is that the difficulty of evaluating performance, which is why this task was taken out of the market and given to government in the first place, also makes it much harder to tell whether the agency is too big or too small or to manage the agency so that the use of employees and other resources is optimized.

Political Interest Group Balance   The actual behavior of government agencies is not determined by the public interest, self-interest of the industry, or of the bureaucrats, but by a complex and shifting balance of all interest groups. Transactions costs shape politics just as they shape markets, and are lower when interests are concentrated or uniform across a large group of people (e.g., all of the elderly tend to favor increased Medicare budgets). However, political deals cannot be negotiated, specified, and enforced by precisely weighing conflicting interests the way the market can so precisely and quickly weigh dollars, making outcomes less predictable. Economists and political scientists devote considerable attention to studying how the process of making decisions affects the decisions made. For example, a majority rule implies that 50 to 49 wins while 49 to 50 loses, thus providing politicians with a great incentive to seek the median (50th percentile) voter rather than maximize the average level of support. Other political structures favor different parts of the voting spectrum. In union representation, for example, seniority is important; thus, the desires of older workers for more health benefits and higher pensions tend to outweigh the desires of younger workers for fewer benefits and higher wages. Several critiques of the health care industry claim that it is dominated by an "iron triangle" of providers, insurance companies, and government agencies, all of whom benefit from higher health care spending rather than difficult, but potentially worthwhile, cost cutting.[12]

Winners and Losers

Although economists try to evaluate how a regulation changes the overall efficiency of the system, most hospital administrators, physicians, and patients are far more concerned with how it affects them personally. Even if a change in Medicare reimbursement is good for the country, a medical equipment vendor will fight it with everything he owns if that regulation would force his business into bankruptcy. Changes in the regulatory structure often have more to do with finding paths that have less resistance than the achievement of noble ends. Many issues have solutions that are nearly the same in terms of overall efficiency, but quite different in terms of who bears the costs or receives the benefits. For example, it may not make a great deal of difference in terms of economic efficiency whether an expanded Medicare drug benefit is paid for through increases in enrollee premiums or an income tax surcharge for the elderly, but the former falls mostly on the poor while the latter falls mostly on the wealthy (who pay more taxes) with predictable consequences in the political support for these alternatives by different groups. Research suggests that when a necessary change in policy involves two mutually exclusive options, the wealthy, even if less numerous and initially less powerful than the poor, may be able to hold out longer and obtain a result more favorable to their interests.[13] A disproportionate share of benefits, from Medicare reimbursement to subsidized medical education, goes to those in the highest income groups, who have the power to make their demands on government effective. Yet, without government intervention, the poor would surely be much worse off.

14.8 PROS AND CONS OF REGULATION AND COMPETITION

Even when markets are suppressed, there is always competition. Physicians try to attract patients with their reputations for quality and with evening office hours. Hospitals try to attract physicians with subsidized office rentals, access to new equipment, and helpful staff. HMOs try to attract enrollees with special benefits, picnics, or free radios. Conversely, even the most open market in health care is highly regulated, with oversight of safety, professional qualifications, and long-term side effects, even when prices are freely set. The issue is not "regulation" or "competition," but what combination and compromises to make (see Table 14.3).[14]

Many problems are created by reliance on government intervention. First, regulation itself costs money: agencies must be staffed, salaries must be paid, and information systems must be maintained. Many of these costs have to be paid for with taxes. Other costs, such as for the compilation of mandated reports and time spent in preparing for regulatory inspections, are imposed on private firms, which then pass them on to the public in the form of higher prices. When government takes over production from private firms, it has sometimes been inefficient and inept at customer service. Even if the market is superseded by direct government provision of services, some form of rationing must still take place. Since prices are not used to match demand and supply, the amount distributed often will be too large or too small, and the people served may not be the ones who value the services most highly. Both discrepancies cause deadweight losses of consumer welfare. Government suppression of the price mechanism prevents desirable trades from occurring, and will also distort related markets for inputs and substitute goods.

Government responds well, perhaps too well, to focused interest groups willing to lobby for their positions. Markets are better able to respond to diverse and diffuse consumer groups, and the prices people pay are a superior mechanism for publicly revealing the value of the services they use. Politicians are constrained by public scrutiny to "do no harm," and every dollar spent becomes a "federal case"; therefore, services that are valued by consumers and raise average health levels (e.g., mass immunizations, fluoridation, birth control) may not be available. Government is subject to so much criticism that agencies can become very risk averse. This exacerbates bureaucratic formalism. Government programs designed to deal with the public must impose universal standards and thus are less able to respond to the variation in individual preferences or to make individual exceptions. Legal constraints make bureaucracies rigid and may stifle innovation. A central failing of regulation is its reliance on precedent. There is no flexible equilibration of supply and demand through prices to create automatic adjustments as conditions change, and little

TABLE 14.3	Pros and Cons of Regulation and Competition

Limitations of Regulation

- Regulatory agencies are costly to operate.
- Government is sometimes an inefficient producer with inadequate customer service.
- Rationing must still take place, and without prices, deadweight welfare losses are larger.
- Suppression of prices distorts markets in inputs and substitute goods as well.
- Government responds to narrowly focused interest groups, not broad consumer interests.
- Regulators must "do no harm" and avoid losses (except the hidden kind).
- Bureaucracies rigidly impose uniformity, treating everyone according to the same standard.
- All regulation is based on the past as a precedent, not directed toward the future.
- No automatic adjustment is made to changes in supply or demand.
- There are no incentives to be an entrepreneur developing new technologies that anticipate demand.

Limitations of Markets

- Markets are costly to operate and must be policed.
- Entrepreneurs maximize profit, not health or social welfare (which are not paid for).
- Under competition, prices pay for services valued by individuals, not public goods (education, research).
- Health care is not very price sensitive, so it is difficult to control behavior through prices.
- Consumers are willing to pay to avoid using prices to make health care decisions.
- Somebody must still take care of the poor, the chronically ill, and the seriously injured.
- Adverse selection may cause private insurance markets to collapse unless government steps in.
- The ethics of competition do not blend well with the ethics of medicine as a *caring* profession.
- Licensure, insurance, and other erosions of the medical marketplace must do more good than harm or they would not be built into the health care system of every country.
- Even the U.S. government must be doing something right, since it has been given increased funding responsibility and control over the medical marketplace.

scope for entrepreneurs who are willing to make mistakes and go out on a limb to create the next generation of technology.

Markets have their flaws as well. They, too, are costly to operate, requiring salespeople, billing systems, and policing mechanisms. Entrepreneurs are apt to push the newest and most expensive technology because it is the most profitable rather than a more cost-effective substitute that would do more to improve health.[15] Markets reward those who provide what consumers want, not those who provide public goods such as medical research, infection control, and ethical standards of professional education. Furthermore, markets for health do not appear to be very price sensitive, perhaps because of information problems and the potential for death from even small errors; therefore, reliance on prices to motivate behavior seems ill-placed. Even when people can use prices to make decisions about medical care, they seem to want to avoid doing so. For example, the elderly, although well insured with Medicare, overwhelmingly opt to obtain supplemental insurance that reduces the marginal price to zero.

Although advocates of competition emphasize the beneficial effect of creating incentives to win, what about the losers? Who will care for people with mental retardation, an alert but alone and alienated 92-year-old, people with genetic defects, the truly unlucky accident victim? Although markets can enable socially beneficial risk pooling through insurance, adverse selection may be so severe that insurance can become unstable or fail to cover many of those most in need unless government intervenes. Medical *care* is so grounded in a concern for the health of others that any competition sufficiently vicious to really cut costs and close all the unnecessary hospital beds may entail such a fundamental violation of human caring that it is socially unacceptable. One might ask, "If the erosion of the marketplace due to licensure, insurance, and nonprofit organizations is so terrible, why are these anti-competitive features an integral part of every health care system in the civilized world?"

The approach to health care in the United States is among the most highly privatized and most responsive to individual needs. Yet even in the United States, government is the largest funding source, paying 45 percent of the bills directly, subsidizing much of the remainder through tax relief, and regulating virtually every dollar spent. It is the mixture of competition and market forces, the matching of programs to needs, that must be evaluated, not the pros and cons of one or the other alone.

SUGGESTIONS FOR FURTHER READING

Ronald Coase, "The Problem of Social Cost," *Journal of Law & Economics* 3 (1960):1–44, 1960.

Paul Feldstein, *The Politics of Health Legislation: An Economic Perspective* (Ann Arbor, Mich.: Health Administration Press, 1988).

Douglass North, *Structure and Change in Economic History* (New York: W.W. Norton, 1981).

Joseph Stiglitz, *Economics of the Public Sector* (New York: W. W. Norton, 1986).

Burton Weisbrod, *The Non-Profit Economy* (Cambridge, Mass.: Harvard University Press, 1988).

Charles Wolfe, *Markets or Governments: Choosing Between Imperfect Alternatives* (Cambridge, Mass.: MIT Press, 1994).

SUMMARY

1. **Government accounts for 45 percent of health care spending.** Most government spending pays for private medical services of special populations (the aged, the indigent, veterans). **Only one-tenth pays for core public health** activities such as infectious disease control, research, and monitoring of drugs, food, air, and water.

2. Under certain conditions, a **purely competitive market allocation** of goods and services, where marginal benefits equal marginal costs enforced by the price mechanism, is most efficient.

3. Perfect competition is rare in the real world. There are **market failures** resulting from uncertainty and information problems, transaction costs, **externalities,** and the existence of **public goods.** Government or another paternalistic agency must step in when an individual is incapable of making appropriate market choices due to immaturity, substance abuse, or severe mental illness. Civilized societies **redistribute income** to protect the poor and disabled.

4. Since most benefits of government are public goods available to all without restriction, many people would be **free riders** who avoid paying unless forced to do so through **compulsory taxation.**

5. Government is formed to act as the agent of the citizens to **maximize public welfare.** However, the ability of special interests to exert undue influence may lead to **regulatory capture,** where government favors the industry rather than the public. Also, the employees of a government agency may pursue **bureaucratic self-interest,** avoiding risks and controversy, and increasing budgets to obtain higher salaries and more employees to ease workloads. The most realistic model of government action combines all three of these perspectives and a consideration of **transaction costs** in achieving **political interest group balance.**

6. Although people say that they want to do what is best for everyone, **they tend to vote for what is good for themselves.** That is why some government programs, such as

Medicaid to care for the poor, are unpopular and grudgingly supported, while Medicare, which most voters believe will benefit them now or in the future, and which incidentally helps keep politically connected doctors and hospitals well off, is very popular.

7. To some extent, **politics is a type of market,** albeit a slow and imperfect one, with legislators trying to get elected by promising the best package of benefits and costs in return for votes. Special-interest legislation benefiting a small group at the expense of the many is most apt to occur when benefits are concentrated on a particular group, making it worthwhile for them to organize and lobby, while the costs are widely dispersed across all of society. **Prices change much faster than laws.** Public goods take longer to adjust because groups and individuals with different interests must agree before any changes can occur.

8. The **voluntary sector,** composed of **nonprofit organizations independent of government** whose objective is to foster the public good, dominates the ownership of hospitals in the United States, and the important private disease control and medical research firms.

9. **For the most part, government works with the market,** regulating and financing private activities. Government supersedes the market when it exerts control over prices and quantities and when it prohibits certain kinds of trades. Some critical functions, such as law and order (police and courts) and national defense (military), are produced directly by government employees. The important question is not whether government or markets are "better," but how to **balance and blend regulation and competition** to optimize social welfare and meet necessary constraints. To do this, a consensus about what constitutes **a just society** is needed.

PROBLEMS

1. {*flow of funds*} What fraction of total health expenditures in the United States are paid for by government? Which government programs are the largest? Were the same, or similar, programs at the top of the list for government funding in 1900?

2. {*market failure*} Which aspects of the economic organization of U.S. medical care result from market failure?

3. {*distribution*} In several marches on Washington, demonstrators have carried signs saying, "No Justice, No Peace." Explain what this slogan means, and how it relates to the level of funding for Medicaid.

4. {*incidence*} Why is more dental care paid for privately while more hospital care is paid for publicly?

5. {*welfare*} Which results in lower prices, competition or regulation?

6. {*incidence*} Why is Medicare more popular than Medicaid?

7. {*public goods*} Does the demand for public health increase or decrease as the size of a city increases?

8. {*rents*} How are rents different from other input payments? Which of the following are rents?

   a. Royalties from a biotechnology patent

   b. Lease payments for use of a laboratory

    c.   Payments to subjects who are observed while sleeping

    d.   Surgical fees

    e.   A bonus paid to a research assistant who finishes an experiment ahead of schedule

    f.   A bonus paid to a Nobel Laureate for switching to another university

9.   {*transactions costs*} What is the Coase Theorem? What does it imply about the extent of immunization among herds of cattle? What does it imply about the levels of immunization among schoolchildren in a classroom?

10.   {*regulatory capture*} Explain how the Food and Drug Administration might be subject to regulatory capture. Who would favor, and who would be opposed to, regulations that limited regulatory capture?

11.   {*regulatory capture*} Name several medical professional/trade organizations that have made large donations to political campaigns. Did they get their money's worth?

12.   {*incidence*} Who benefits and who loses from deinstitutionalization of people who are mentally ill? Which factors thwarted the original plans for transfer of funding to community treatment facilities?

13.   {*flow of funds*} Which of the following are funded as entitlements?

    a.   Medicare

    b.   Medicaid

    c.   Medical research

    d.   Public health statistics

14.   {*voting*} Who counts for more in political calculus:

    a.   The sick or the well?

    b.   The old or the young?

    c.   The rich or the poor?

15.   {*incidence*} Medical savings accounts (discussed in Chapter 5, Section 4) tend to favor which groups of people?

16.   {*dynamics*} Why does it often take longer for a government program to change in response to shifts in external conditions than it takes a private company? Is this good or bad?

17.   {*dynamics*} Which is harder to close, a public hospital or a private clinic? Why? Which is more likely to take advantage of information asymmetry to cheat patients?

ENDNOTES

1.   Oliver Williamson, *Markets and Hierarchies* (New York: Free Press, 1975).

2.   Douglass C. North, *Structure and Change in Economic History* (New York: Norton, 1981), 21.

3.   Joseph E. Stiglitz, *Economies of the Public Sector* (New York: W.W. Norton, 1986), 77.

4.   John Rawls, *A Theory of Justice* (Cambridge, Mass.: Harvard University Press, 1971).

5.   Ronald H. Coase, "The Problem of Social Cost," *Journal of Law & Economics* 3 (1960): 1–44.

6.   Marilyn Moon, *Medicare Now and In the Future* (Washington, D.C.: The Urban Institute, 1993); Mark V. Pauly and William L. Kissick, eds., *Lessons from the First Twenty Years of Medicare: Research Implications for Public and Private Sector Policy* (Philadelphia: University of Pennsylvania Press, 1988).

7.   SCHIP (the State Childrens Health Insurance Program) discussed in Chapter 5 is the sort of "exception that proves the rule." Expansion of coverage to include children is so hard to resist politically that conservatives

have pushed to limit funding to poor—lest there be another popular universal health insurance entitlement program on the books. However, for an intriguing contrary view of the relative political merits of Medicare and Medicaid, see Lawrence D. Brown and Michael S. Sparer, "Poor Program's Progress: The Unanticipated Politics of Medicaid Policy," *Health Affairs* 22, no. 1 (January 2003): 31–44.

8. A significant exception is the Department of Defense/Veterans Administration health care system. Although national defense is a pure public good, the fact that VA/DOD health is an adjunct to defense does not necessarily make it public, and indeed large parts of the VA/DOD health care are now being privatized through subcontracting.

9. Burton Weisbrod, *The Non-Profit Economy* (Cambridge, Mass.: Harvard University Press, 1988).

10. Peter J. Hammond, "Social Choice: The Science of the Impossible," in George R. Feiwel, *Arrow and the Foundations of the Theory of Economic Policy* (New York: New York University Press, 1987), 116–134.

11. "Money and Politics: AMA's Lobbying Tab Surges in Second Half of 2000," *Modern Healthcare* (November 12, 2001).

12. Lawrence R. Jacobs, "The Politics of America's Supply State: Health Reform and Technology" *Health Affairs* 14, no. 2 (Summer 1995): 143–157. See also Lawrence D. Brown, "Politics, Money and Health Care Reform," *Health Affairs* 13, no. 2II (Spring 1994): 175–184, and "Commissions, Clubs and Consensus: Reform in Florida," *Health Affairs* 12, no. 2 (Summer 1993): 7–26.

13. Alberto Alesina and Allan Drazen, "Why are Stabilizations Delayed?" *American Economic Review* 81, no. 5 (1991): 1170–k1188.

14. Charles Wolfe Jr., *Markets or Governments: Choosing Between Imperfect Alternatives* (Cambridge, Mass.: MIT Press, 1994).

15 Eleena de Lisser, "Ready or Not, Firms Rush to Sell the Public on Laser Eye Surgery," *The Wall Street Journal* CCXVI, no. 38 (August 24, 1995): A1, A8.

CHAPTER 15

PUBLIC GOODS AND PUBLIC HEALTH

QUESTIONS

1. Should treatment of syphilis be part of the public health system or private medical care? What about psoriasis? Psychosis? Scoliosis?
2. Why not charge people full price for vaccinations?
3. Why are new surgical techniques developed with public funds while pharmaceutical research and development is conducted privately by for-profit firms?
4. Who paid for Pasteur to discover bacteria?
5. Why pay for cost-benefit analysis to decide which public programs are worthwhile instead of using prices to let the market decide?
6. Do the preferences of smokers, patients who are mentally ill, or unborn children count when assessing the efficiency of the public health system?
7. Is medical care for homeless and terminally ill AIDS patients a public good or a waste of money?

15.1 CHARACTERISTICS OF PUBLIC GOODS

It is not possible to charge for some goods because no one can be excluded from using them (e.g., clean air), and there are other goods no one wants to charge for because there is no cost to accommodate additional users (e.g., a news release reporting the discovery that eating oranges cures scurvy). How easy and how desirable it is to use market pricing to ration goods or to exclude people from using a service determines whether it is part of public health or private health care. The two dimensions of "publicness," the ability to enforce exclusion with prices and the marginal cost of accommodating additional users, are illustrated in Figure 15.1. A knee brace is costly to produce and easy to charge for. Therefore, it is a pure private good. Arthroscopic surgery for knees falls between being a private good and a public good. Although the surgery has a relatively constant average cost per unit, the development of surgical techniques and instruments is more like a public good. Once knowledge is obtained, it can be used over and over again. It is relatively easy to charge for the surgery, but a bit difficult to charge for the years of developmental work. Polio vaccine is more of a public good. Once discovered, the cost of production per dose, although constant, is almost negligible. Although it would be relatively easy to charge users for vaccination, it would not be economically desirable to do so, since the benefits of freeing the population of disease are externalities that benefit everyone, not just the user. The monitoring of infectious disease by the Centers for Disease Control and Prevention (CDC) to discover epidemics is a pure public good. If the agency is successful, there are fewer epidemics, and there is no way to charge individuals for preventing a mass tragedy that does not happen. Also, once CDC's *Morbidity and Mortality Weekly Report* is printed, there is essentially no additional cost for having more physicians use CDC data to protect their patients.

Publicness can vary with local conditions. A congested suburban hospital can readily charge for services, whereas a quiet rural hospital that is three-quarters empty most of the time cannot. Most of the benefits the community derives from the rural hospital come from the hospital just being there in case of an emergency (option demand) rather than from use of services. There also are goods that are publicly provided, even though some amount could be sold privately. Motor vehicle inspections are required, and thus do not depend on owners' willingness to pay, because there is a compelling public interest in having a car's brakes and emission control system work properly to protect other people. A social calculation of costs and benefits must supersede market pricing.

Privatizing Public Goods

Prescription drugs are an interesting case of a public good being privatized. Once a discovery is made and validated through clinical trials, the actual costs of production are nearly zero. However, unlike vaccine, which benefits the public by inhibiting communicable disease, most of the benefits from a prescription drug accrue to the user. Patent law gives the firm a monopoly on the drug for seventeen years so that it can charge users for

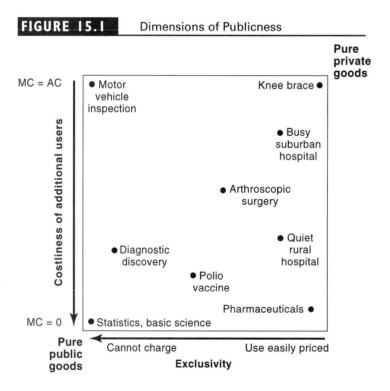

FIGURE 15.1 Dimensions of Publicness

the sunk costs of discovery and testing.[1] Geographic enclosure also privatizes public goods. Thus, residents of a resort community will pay privately for maintaining the cleanliness of a lake and have private agreements to limit noise and pollution. Externalities arise primarily because the costs and benefits are borne by different people so that one or the other is external to the market transaction. Patent laws, enclosed communities, and membership clubs are examples of internalizing effects so that government intervention is less necessary.

Social Costs Depend on the Number of People

The extent of externalities depends on the magnitude of the costs and the number of people involved. For example, very strict sterilization procedures are followed for spacecraft because of the possibility that extraterrestrial bacteria could threaten the health of the entire world. Airplane accidents are scrutinized by government safety inspectors more carefully than automobile accidents, and nuclear power plant failures are even more closely scrutinized. The larger the number of people who could be hurt, the more thorough the investigation.

Garbage disposal is an example of how the treatment of public goods changes with the number of people involved.[2] In prehistoric times, people did whatever they pleased with their garbage and no one worried about a waste disposal system. The same is true today in isolated rural areas where people toss the garbage out in the woods or bury or burn it. Keeping one's own house tidy and the neighbors happy is sufficient incentive to maintain a social optimum, and no government rules are needed. However, as people move closer together, creating a town, the divergence between private and social costs widens. Dumping trash in fields, or in the yards of strangers, rapidly creates a problem. Therefore, rules are formulated designating when and where garbage can be dumped. As the town becomes larger, public spending becomes necessary to handle all the garbage produced. Land is purchased and set aside to serve as a dump. As the town becomes a city, it is not enough just to have a dump; the city must actively collect all the trash and carry it to the dump. Taxes are imposed and trucks drive around to collect garbage at people's houses. In this way the private costs of conforming to the social optimum are minimized. Garbage collection is a public activity that requires collective financing through taxes, but the actual work can be done by a private firm, and often is.

Insurance Makes Any Good More Public

Whenever a service is financed through third-party insurance rather than directly by individual purchasers, the service becomes more of a public good. When individuals purchase a good, one person may choose high quality, another low; one wants the color to be blue while the other wants it green; and so on. Within a risk-pooling group, they all become the same. Whether the person being treated is a vice-president of marketing or an assistant janitor, the hospital gets paid the same amount. It is possible for insurance companies to provide extensive coverage for plastic surgery and 200 days of mental health coverage, but everyone in the benefit plan must get it. The differentiation between individuals by payment is eliminated. The quality of services covered by the insurance package is a public good. There is no gain to the janitor for seeking out a cheap hospital, since even if the company does obtain some savings, it won't make insurance any cheaper to the janitor personally. Thus, once medical care is financed on a group basis, any change in quality or standards of service affects everyone and requires collective action.

15.2 INFORMATION

Research on new drugs, new surgical techniques, and new methods of diagnostic imaging is popular and receives billions of dollars in public funding. However, it is the collection of statistics over many years and from millions of patients that makes it possible to determine how medical discoveries work in practice. Statistics and scientific discoveries are both forms of information and are almost pure public goods.[3] Once statistics have been tabulated or a discovery has been made, there are no additional costs incurred as more and more people use them (zero cost). Once discoveries are known, there is no way to stop anyone from using them, regardless of whether or not they have paid for them (zero charges). The discovery of bacteria by Louis Pasteur began a revolution in the treatment of disease. It also saved the wool industry from the plague of anthrax, which had been decimating sheep (Pasteur's original research project); the wine and beer industries, which were having trouble with fermentation irregularities; and the dairy industry, whose unpasteurized products caused diarrhea and many fatalities among infants.[4] Much of Pasteur's work was supported by government grants, just as medical research is today. No single person or firm could obtain enough benefits to justify spending the money required to fund such a large research and development project. It was a collective enterprise. However, there were still many free riders. Although the costs were paid mostly by France and, to a lesser extent, by some industrialists in Belgium and Germany, people in the United States, Africa, China, and the rest of the world benefited. To the extent that those who benefit do not contribute, there is underinvestment in the development of knowledge.

Information is created not only through new discoveries, but through the compilation and organization of existing data. A landmark breakthrough in the history of medicine and public health was the printing of *Observations on the Bills of Mortality,* by John Graunt, in 1662.[5] Graunt studied death records in the city of London and tabulated the number of people dying each year and their causes of death, thus creating the first modern work in the science of epidemiology. With the causes of death plainly laid out, the years of plague and the probable effects (or lack of effects) of government attempts to improve the health of citizens could be seen.

Measurement and statistics do not come into being just because it is a good thing to have them; they must serve an economic purpose. The census that recorded Mary and Joseph at the birth of Jesus of Nazareth was mandated to enable Caesar to collect taxes. Deaths historically have been recorded to establish inheritance, not to study the effects of medical treatment. The provision of universal public benefits, such as Social Security, made it possible for the United States to easily enforce the requirement that all deaths be recorded. The fact that collecting information is costly explains why there are more statistics on health care expenditures (which must be recorded on each transaction to pay employees, bill insurance companies, and so on) than on medical diagnosis or treatment effectiveness. The U.S. Centers for Medicare and Medicaid Services (CMS) (which has power because it controls the funds) is setting standards for a "uniform bill" that will be submitted electronically by all hospitals and doctors and thus provide an integrated database for comparing the costs and effects of all types of medical care. Potentially, this will not only reduce the administrative costs of running the system, it will also make it possible for researchers to tap into an online database with hundreds of millions of patient years of experience and, therefore, rapidly determine which treatments, types of hospitals, drugs, and so on are most cost-effective.

The National Institutes of Health (NIH) has overall responsibility for medical research in the United States, and the National Center for Health Statistics (NCHS) is responsible for data collection and distribution. NCHS's oldest and most important publication is its *Vital*

Statistics Reports on births and deaths. NCHS also conducts surveys on health and nutrition status, insurance coverage, and the characteristics of patients treated in doctors' offices, and compiles statistics on patients discharged from hospitals using billing records. All this information is made available in "public use data tapes" and in free publications (which can be obtained from the library or the Web for your term paper) because it is a public good produced with public money. Those running the agency want to maximize the value of this "free" good so that they can argue for more funding from Congress—and, not incidentally, benefit all of us.

Rational Consumer Ignorance

Why does the government have a better information base for making decisions than most citizens? Because the government paid for it. From safety standards for seatbelts to the efficacy of vitamin supplements, millions of dollars have been spent to determine the best possible answers. Massively wasteful duplication would result if each consumer collected such information individually. If consumers banded together to share the costs of gathering information, such banding would constitute a form of government. Consumers are rationally ignorant of many health and safety issues because it is more efficient to have the government collect information once than for each of us to do it separately. Rational consumer ignorance is sensible free riding. Even for a private good, such as a bottle of vitamins, it is cheaper to perform quality control once in a government laboratory than to do it over and over again in each individual's home.

Consumers remain rationally ignorant by delegating their decision-making powers to the government because it is more efficient for them to do so—they are being smart by staying stupid! Thus, the Food and Drug Administration (FDA) tests the safety of food and drugs, the Environmental Protection Agency (EPA) conducts studies on the effects of pollution, and the Department of Transportation (DOT) monitors the safety of highways and motor vehicles.

Milk or Bread: Which Is More Public?

Whether a particular set of health concerns should fall in the public or private arena depends on the characteristics of the goods and the way they are produced and transacted. In general, if something is produced collectively so that one person's consumption cannot easily be separated from another's, more government intervention is called for. If the relevant characteristics are readily observable by consumers at the time of purchase, more reliance on private markets is appropriate. Consider two products that are consumed by almost everyone: milk and bread. Milk was subjected to government regulations more than a hundred years ago, and public milk dispensing stations were set up in New York and other cities.[6] It is now illegal in most states to sell milk that has not been inspected and processed according to government standards. Bread, while under routine surveillance as a food, is largely unregulated. Why is there such a difference in standards for these two foods?

Bread may be mixed in batches, but each loaf is baked separately, and the baking process kills most germs. When bread gets old after sitting on the shelf too long, it becomes stale and hard, and green and white furry spots start growing on it. These signs of deterioration are readily visible to consumers. Milk from many dairies is mixed together when it is being processed for sale; thus, contamination at any one dairy potentially threatens thousands of consumers. Contamination is most likely to occur during the milking process and can best be prevented by keeping the cows clean, keeping the equipment sterilized, and sweeping the manure out of the barn. On-site inspection is the best way to cheaply enforce cleanliness and can be performed at moderate cost by government agents, but it would be prohibitively costly for consumers to visit all the dairies their milk comes from each week and check the floors. Bacteria are killed during the processing of milk, but how is a consumer to know that the "pasteurized" label on the carton is to be believed? When the crucial quality-control step can be monitored efficiently only during processing and compliance is not easily discernable at the point of sale, government oversight and labeling are called for. Most of the dangerous bacteria that people can get from milk, particularly salmonella, do not make milk curdle or smell bad; and thus are hard to detect. Milk is an ideal culture medium for many bacteria, making milk distribution, in effect, a perfect way to spread disease. Contamination from one farm cannot be determined later because milk from all the farms is mixed together. The bacteria rapidly grow to infect all the milk and are delivered invisibly, with much of the product going to the most vulnerable segment of the population, children.

Many factors make milk more suitable for government regulation, but the crucial issue is which information consumers can easily obtain at the point of sale. Bad bread is visible to consumers; bad milk is not. The information necessary to protect the safety of the public is available at low cost if regulations are enforced *during production,* a process that would be prohibitively costly for consumers to carry out on their own. The asymmetry of information costs makes milk quality a public good, while the quality of bread is largely private.

Given the benefits of good information for both science and political management, it seems that often there is too little of it around. Problems frequently have to reach the crisis stage before the necessary information is collected, and decisions regarding thousands of lives or billions of dollars are made without adequate study. The difficulty lies in the conflict between individual and collective incentives. A lot of data may be useful in solving a public problem, but it is in the interest of no particular person to collect that data unless that person can benefit from it. Even if the person can benefit, he or she will not be able to devote enough resources to the problem because their personal benefits are much less than the total benefits to society as a whole. To see more clearly why free-riding leads to persistent underproduction, it is necessary to consider the theory of pure public goods in more detail.[7]

15.3 THE THEORY OF PURE PUBLIC GOODS

Information is a public good, but it can be provided privately as well as publicly. For example, people may purchase cable television by paying for each channel or show, or they may tap into a broadcast, which is a public good paid for through taxes, donations, advertising, or other collective means. To more meaningfully address the question, "How much of a public good should society produce?" we will consider a society made up of three people, Ann, Bob, and Carl, who can either purchase TV from the cable company at $5 per channel or contribute through taxes to have the signal broadcast to everyone at a collective cost of $10 per channel. The private demand and supply for TV channels for Ann, Bob, and Carl is shown in Figure 15.2a. The total private market demand for this three-person market is obtained by adding horizontally the quantity demanded by each person at any given price, as shown in Figure 15.2b. For example, at a price of $10, Ann would purchase one channel, Bob would purchase three channels, and Carl would not purchase any channels; therefore, total market demand at $10 would be 1 + 3 + 0 = 4. Similarly, at a price of $5 per channel, market demand would be 2 + 5 + 0 = 7, and at a price of $1 per channel, it would be 3 + 7 + 4 = 14. The market equilibrium with a perfectly elastic (flat horizontal line) supply curve at a price of $5 per channel is for seven channels to be sold, two to Ann, five to Bob, and none to Carl.

The demand for a public good is different. If the government provides one public channel paid for with taxes, everyone gets to watch it. The value of that public good is the value of the service to each member of society added together. In this example, the marginal value of the first channel is $10 to Ann, $15 to Bob, and $4 to Carl, for a total social value of $29. Similarly, the second channel has a marginal value of $5 + $12.50 + $3 = $20.50, the third $0 + $10 + $2 = $12, and the sixth $0 + $2.50 + $0 = $2.50. Whereas the

---

FIGURE 15.2   Public and Private Demand Curves

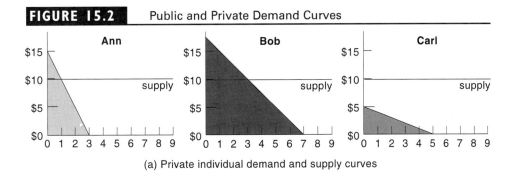

(a) Private individual demand and supply curves

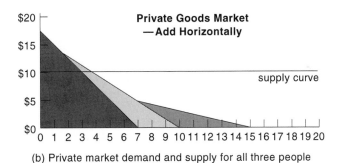

(b) Private market demand and supply for all three people

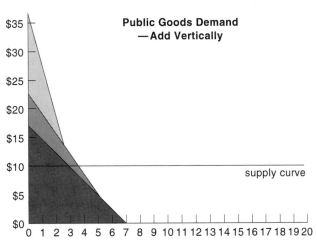

(c) Public goods quasi-demand curve and supply for all three people

quantities are added horizontally in Figure 15.2b to find total market demand at a specified price for a private consumption market, the values are added vertically at a specified quantity to find total social value for a public good, as in Figure 15.2c.[8]

PUBLIC VERSUS PRIVATE DEMAND CURVES

Social Demand Curve for Public Goods: for each quantity Q,

$$\text{Value}_{total} = V_A + V_B + V_C$$

Market Demand Curve for Private Goods: for each price P,

$$\text{Quantity}_{total} = Q_A + Q_B + Q_C$$

The cost of broadcasting a channel to everyone is $10, twice as much as the price of providing it on cable to just one person. It is beneficial for society to produce more of the public good as long as the marginal cost is less than the additional value; therefore, the social optimum is reached at the intersection of the public good marginal cost "supply" curve and the public good quasi-demand curve. In this example, three channels would be supplied at a total cost of $30, because the marginal cost of a fourth channel ($10) exceeds the value to the members of society ($0 + $7.50 + 1 = $8.50).

Public Goods Make Most People Better Off, But Few Happy

In the private market, with channels selling for $5 each, Ann paid $10 for two and Bob paid $25 for five. Who will pay the $30 to broadcast three public channels? Suppose that a tax of $10 is collected from each person. Ann is indifferent to public versus private provision. Although giving up some flexibility, by participating in society she gets one additional channel for the same amount as she was previously paying. Carl is mad and wants to start a taxpayer's revolt. He paid nothing before and now must pay $10 for stations he barely wants. The consumer's surplus ($4 + $3 + $2 = $9) he obtains from getting three TV channels "for free" is worth less to him than the new taxes he has to pay. Carl has an incentive to understate his demand to get the government to provide less. He might say, "I hate the stuff and, as you can tell, did not watch it before (although he does watch it now that it is public and 'free'). If it has to be there, don't make me pay for it." If Carl could force the government to back down from the social optimum and provide just one channel, he would be better off, although both Bob and Ann would be worse off.

Bob loves TV and gets a large consumer's surplus. The value of three stations to him ($15 + $12.50 + $10 = $37.50) far exceeds the new $10 tax. But he is not happy, either. He complains that he used to get five channels and now that the government has taken over, he only gets three! Bob wants five public TV channels. Although these two extra channels would cost $20, he would only get taxed to cover a third of the cost, or $6.67. To a certain extent, Bob would be a partial free rider. He would push for more TV channels than he would be willing to buy in a private market. Even though Bob and Ann are unhappy, they are both better off. Carl is only slightly ($1) worse off. The group as a whole is clearly better off using public provision, but each individual has a reason to complain and try to get a different deal.

For public goods, cost-benefit analysis must replace market pricing as a mechanism for resource allocation and rationing. Voting and administrative procedures are used to make public decisions. In a private market, people who value services more highly pay more to get them. Since a social optimum depends on values, why doesn't government tax people depending on how much they want the services? Besides being unfair (imagine saying to someone, "Since your broken leg forces you to stay at home, we want to double your public TV taxes"), it cannot readily be done because there is no way to tell how much someone values a public good. In a private market, the act of purchasing demonstrates people's willingness to pay and reveals how much they value the good. With public goods, however, there is no purchase. In our example, both Bob and Carl watch all three public TV stations, but Bob values them more. Suppose we sent a questionnaire asking how much each person likes TV to adjust individuals' tax rates. Why should Bob reveal how much he likes TV and then pay more? His paying more will not increase the number of stations. Conversely, Carl will say, "I don't care one bit, nothing, nada, zilch," because he wants to pay $0 and still be able to watch all three channels. This is why Figure 15.2c is only a *quasi*-demand curve. It does not show choices people make in a market, only what we estimate they should do to optimize social value.

To get the government to provide more "free" services, Bob and people like him have an incentive to overstate their demands because most of the cost will be borne by the rest of the public. Since public goods are provided at no charge, there is no way to use market behavior to gauge demand. Everyone's self-interests might lead them to lie on the questionnaire to get more services. The sensible thing for Bob and every other interest group to do is to act as a rational free rider: always tell their elected officials that they want more and the tax collector that they want less. There is no simple way to get everybody to agree on the social optimum once we consider not only the benefits and who will get them, but also the costs and who will pay them. The social value function is only a quasi-demand curve, because the voluntary actions of individuals will never allow society to reach the optimum and will only lead to name-calling, avoidance, and unstable coalitions (also known as "politics").

The provision of a public good poses two problems: how much of it to provide and how to pay for it. Neither is solvable through individual action. For example, a swimming pool is a semi-public good after it is built; it does not cost very much to allow one more person to use it, yet people can be easily excluded. The pool could be paid for collectively through taxes so that each person would pay the same amount or according to income. It is also possible to pay for the pool with user fees. This way the people who value swimming the most, and go to the pool often, will pay more. However, neither method will get to the social optimum. If we depend entirely on taxes, taxpayers will not be willing to build as many pools as the social demand curve indicates. If user fees are imposed, some swimmers (such as the poor ten-year old who wants to train for the Olympics) will be denied entrance even though the marginal cost of using the pool is $0. The actual method chosen to fund a service depends on the transaction costs particular to that case (pools, yes; clean air, no; TV used to be no and now yes, sort-of). How purely public is the good? Can users be easily charged for use? Can we tell what aggregate demand will be? Are people able and willing to acknowledge their demand up front and promise to pay or vote for the proposed program? (schools, maybe; venereal disease clinics, maybe not). Is a dedicated revenue source available? (such as recurrent proposals to put a tax on hospital bills to fund indigent care, and the near-universality of room and airport taxes to extract money from tourists). Is anyone likely to sue?

Purchasing of public goods is problematic even if the money can be raised. Since no particular person has a comprehensive interest in making sure that all the goods contracted for are delivered or that the quality is adequate, a supplier may extract some of the social benefits by providing poor service or inferior goods. Even if we all want a good army, or hospital, or national weather service, none of us individually is willing to spend our time making sure that those who are paid to provide these public goods are actually doing their jobs and doing them efficiently. The free-rider problem goes beyond payment; it makes the enforcement of public contracts more difficult.

15.4 INFECTIOUS DISEASE EXTERNALITIES

One way of looking at the publicness of a good is to ask how much one person's action affects the welfare of other people. As discussed earlier, a mistake by the bread baker will have only a limited effect on consumers, while a failure in sanitary procedures at the dairy could cause illness or even death among thousands. Economists observe that milk has more externalities than bread. Infectious disease is a classic example of externalities and the basis for many public health laws. The author's first job was as a sexually transmitted diseases (STD) investigator for the city of New York. Why were tax dollars used to pay civil servants to find out who was infected and who they had sex with, and to bring these people to the clinic for penicillin shots? Didn't people who were infected already have sufficient incentive to come in for treatment? No. Infection creates externalities. The one who is infected bears the personal costs of disease and treatment, but does not bear the cost imposed on society by increasing everyone else's risk of infection. The divergence between private and social costs means that people are not sufficiently motivated to seek treatment. Consider what would happen if you discovered that you are infected. Whether you get treated this week or next week may not make much difference to you, but may significantly affect the risk you impose on others.

Sexual transmission of diseases heightens the divergences between private and social costs of infection because stigmatization makes information harder to come by. The desire for privacy increases transaction costs. With the flu, everyone knows when you are sick. With syphilis or gonorrhea, the symptoms are usually unobservable, even by your sexual partner. Whereas coughing is a costless signal of flu infection, you must be told that you have been exposed to an STD. This is difficult for most people because it marks them as infected and involves the admission that they have been having sexual relations with others. While it is beneficial to society as a whole that all your sexual partners be notified that you are infected, it is often costly to you personally—it may cost you some friends, a marriage, or a job. The U.S. Public Health Service (PHS) developed a rule of anonymity to minimize the costs of acting in the interests of society. When sexual contacts are notified to come in for treatment, they are not told who has given their name. One client showed up with his wife and three girlfriends (yes, all at once, in the same room) and demanded to know who had been infected. While it may have been in his interest to know, violating confidentiality would make it more difficult for the PHS to get people to divulge sensitive information.

Day care centers are a useful and familiar example of infection externalities. Parents with a child who is slightly sick, or who might be coming down with a cold, face a difficult choice. If they stay home, they miss a day of work; if they send the child to day care, other children will be exposed. The first cost is borne personally, but the costs of other children getting sick is a social cost borne by the other parents. Therefore, many busy parents faced with deadlines at work make a decision that is in their own best interests and drop the slightly sick child off at day care. Day care workers hate this and have developed a rule that if a child does get sick at day care, the parents must come immediately and take the child home or they will be fined and/or barred from the facility. The day care facility is deliberately trying to increase the costs of bringing in a sick child to force parents to act in accordance with the collective good, to take account of social costs.

Epidemics

Sudden upsurges in disease have had profound effects on the course of human civilization: the black death of the Middle Ages; the Biblical plagues that afflicted the people of Egypt; tuberculosis, syphilis, a pandemic (worldwide epidemic) flu outbreak in 1918 that killed hundreds of thousands of young people; and most recently, AIDS.[9] The externality imposed by contagion was recognized long before germs were identified as a cause of disease. Quarantine was among the earliest forms of public health action. In primitive societies, those who were visibly ill were sometimes banished from the tribe. As early as 1400 A.D., ships from ports where plague had been reported were kept out in the harbor for months to see if any of the sailors would die. Only after sufficient time had passed for the authorities to convince themselves that the ship was not carrying disease was it allowed to unload. The public interest in disease reduction conflicted with the private interests of ship owners. Most of the costs of an epidemic (i.e., deaths) would fall on the population of the city, while the benefits of continuing to trade accrued to the merchants. The plot of the famous play "An Enemy of the People," by Henrik Ibsen, centers on the disastrous consequences of ignoring the long-run risks of disease to pursue short-run profits.[10]

Leprosy may have been the first communicable disease brought under control by public health measures. Now known as Hansen's disease, after the scientist who discovered the causative agent, leprosy is a slow-growing bacterium that destroys the neural sheath and hence sensation. The infection itself is often less damaging than its side effects. People with leprosy cannot feel pain in the affected area; therefore, they may scratch an itch until they gouge their flesh away, or get burned without even knowing it, and so on. The bacterium is hard to transmit from person to person; thus, infection usually requires intimate contact over an extended period of time. People with leprosy were isolated from the rest of the population to halt the spread of the disease. Although the United States still had leper colonies until 1953, effective treatment with antibiotics has now removed the threat of contagion.

Permanent quarantine in hospitals appears to have played a significant role in reducing the incidence of leprosy. In the twelfth century, there were more than 200 hospitals for the confinement of lepers in France alone. By the end of the Middle Ages, leprosy had become much less common throughout Europe. But consider the cost. Leprosy is a progressive disease. Without treatment, the person sent to a hospital was put away for life, without visitors. The church would hold a funeral for the leper, the family would mourn, and all the person's property would be passed on through inheritance, just as if that person had died. The signs and symptoms of leprosy (a scaly rash) are common to a variety of ordinary, non-serious disorders (psoriasis, scabies, skin allergy), making diagnosis difficult. Therefore many people without leprosy must also have been permanently confined in such hospitals (where they presumably caught leprosy after awhile anyway). The uncertainty of diagnosis and the severe consequences probably made people very reluctant to visit the doctor for a rash or to share information with neighbors. Claims of leprosy were more apt to be made against people who were not welcome within society (gypsies, Jews), and a disgruntled family member or impatient heir might assert that the wealthy grandfather had leprosy purely out of self-interest. Permanent quarantine probably did help protect the community, but at the cost of making a person with leprosy, or who was suspected of having leprosy, a non-person. Only when epidemics caused high rates of mortality did the interests of the community (disease prevention) outweigh the interests of the individual (property, freedom).

HIV/AIDS

HIV/AIDS also illustrates economic issues in disease control and public policy.[11] When first diagnosed, in the early 1980s, the costs of treatment were very high. The first official estimate, made in 1987, was $147,000 per patient. Subsequent estimates became lower over time. One reason for declining costs was economies of scale. As more cases were treated, unit costs went down. There was specialization of labor as dedicated AIDS units were established, and movement down the learning curve as infectious disease specialists became better at managing the opportunistic illnesses that affect immuno-compromised people. There was a growing recognition that medical care served an important humanitarian purpose. A crash program of medical research brought about major advances in an incredibly short time span—less than a decade. However, the new protease inhibitor combination treatments that successfully reduced symptoms and increased a patient's ability to function did not cure the infection, it only suppressed it. Thus the extension of life implied increasing the number of years of expensive medical therapy.

HIV/AIDS also increased insurance market failure, due to adverse selection. The association between frequency, type, and number of sexual partners and HIV/AIDS means that the individual may possess private information about risk not available to an insurance company. People who are HIV-positive know they will need considerable medical care in the near future; therefore, insurance companies offering individual policies covering HIV/AIDS would be swamped by purchasers from this 100 percent risk group. The inevitability of illness makes it almost impossible for someone who is HIV-positive to change jobs and switch insurance plans if there is any exclusion of pre-existing conditions. The appearance of a fatal disease at an early age disrupts many economic relationships. A bank might wonder why an 83-year old man wants to borrow $250,000 and be unwilling to lend without security since he no longer has a job, but be quite happy to lend this amount to an employed 33-year-old man to buy a house. However, if the young man is HIV-positive, he might actually want the money to pay his medical bills and the living expenses of his partner, and may figure that there is little the bank can do to collect on the debt when he dies. Therefore, the bank is inadvertently thrust into the role of supplying life insurance to people at high risk. Developing the social mechanisms to deal with the consequences of the AIDS epidemic on economic contracts will take awhile, and it is hoped that a cure will be available long before financial institutions have to make a full adjustment.

The Sanitary Revolution: A Moral Campaign for Public Health

The public health reforms that reduced the threat of cholera, diphtheria, typhoid, and other communicable diseases were part of the nineteenth century social revolution that imposed Victorian middle-class values on society as a whole.[12] Posters that attacked working conditions in the coal mines did not stress that workers had to eat stooped over while standing in pools of water that collected human waste, but the fact that women working underground were stripped to the waist because of the heat. Mandating that children under the age of twelve work no more than ten hours a day seemed an act of kindness, not an attempt to prevent premature disability. Above all else, Victorians hated dirt, and so the social reformers wanted cleanliness and light—which happened to be effective in reducing the spread of infectious disease, although there was no way to know that given the science of the time. A belief in what was morally right, not scientific evidence, underlay the English sanitary revolution.

Not all attempts to remove dirt and immorality proved to be healthful. Sending women to maternity hospitals instead of having a midwife attend birth at home caused the spread of puerperal (childbirth) fever and a rapid increase in maternal mortality. The replacement of breast-feeding with sterile bottles deprived middle-class infants of maternal immunities. Diseases of poverty, such as pellagra, were so consistently blamed on lack of cleanliness and insects that the mounting evidence of dietary deficiency was ignored. The sanitary revolution did much to clean up the environmental mess created as industrial urbanization brought masses of people together in cities, but science was decidedly secondary to morality and ideology. The net result was beneficial overall, but quite unbalanced. These historical lessons are worth remembering as we attempt to evaluate the hazards of environmental carcinogens and other public health issues today.

Formation of the U.S. Public Health Service

The U.S. Public Health Service had it origins in the merchant seamen's hospital founded in 1798.[13] The rationale for government involvement was threefold. First, seamen were engaged in international trade and ships frequently carried diseases between countries, so the government had an interest in making sure that the seamen were willing to report any illnesses. Second, medical care was mostly provided at home by one's family, but sailors spent years abroad on ships and rarely had families to depend on. Ordinary laborers without kin who became sick or disabled were the responsibility of local communities, but sailors were travelers who might have been born in Boston or Chicago or Kankakee or anywhere, and thus could not always rely on a town to support them in their time of need. Third, international trade was vital to the economic growth of the nation. Unless the national government was willing to take care of people who became ill or disabled, few would have been willing to leave home and become sailors.

Public health activity was much more limited in the United States than in England during the nineteenth century. American cities were not as old, or as crowded. There were fewer innovations in the United States, but European social programs and sanitary reforms were quickly adopted. Massachusetts set up the first state board of health following the Shattuck report in 1850. By 1900 the New York City health department had become an active center with special support programs for immigrants and free sterile milk distribution for mothers and children. The Pure Food and Drug Act was passed in 1906, and in 1920 the Shepard-Towner Act provided the first national government-sponsored medical care for mothers and dependent children. Other milestones in U.S. public health include the formation in 1952 of the National Institutes of Health, now by far the largest public health agency, to conduct medical research; the 1965 passage of amendments XVIII and XIX to the Social Security Act, which established Medicare and Medicaid; and the 1970 acts creating the Environmental Protection Agency (EPA) and the Occupational Safety and Health Administration (OSHA).

15.5 SEX, DRUGS, AND WAR: PUBLIC HEALTH IN ACTION

Government uses police powers to enforce health and safety regulations. It acts as the agent of all citizens to perform collectively beneficial activities more efficiently than individuals could on their own. Rules made by the people and for the people are not an intrusion on liberty, but a way of making the people more free by maintaining order. Government is not there to enforce public health standards because people are too ignorant to know what is in their own best interests. Instead, government exists so that citizens can remain rationally ignorant and devote their time to sports, making money, and art rather than checking the temperature at the pasteurization facility each hour. However, government does sometimes intercede directly against the will of the individual, overruling his or her own desires. Such paternalism is based not on ignorance, but on a determination that the individual is incompetent; thus, it is reserved for people who are assumed to be unable to make decisions on their own: children, addicts, the mentally ill and retarded.

Sexual behavior reveals some of the underlying value judgments that are at the heart of any paternalistic decision to override individual decision-making authority. For centuries, children's sexual behavior fell under the control of parents because inheritance was a major form of economic exchange. Thus, the rules regarding whom to have sex with for the aristocracy (who had inheritable land) were much different than the rules for the peasantry. Aristocrats, who were not allowed to have sex with the 17-year-old sons and daughters of neighboring lords, could have sex with their serfs because any children born from such a union had no property rights.

Sexual preferences are value laden, with active debates over homosexual marriage and the acceptability of gays and lesbians serving in the military and holding public office. The

American Psychiatric Association listed homosexuality as a disease until 1974 and, although difficult to imagine today on a college campus with prominent gay organizations, young men and women then were treated for having the illness of "abnormal" desires. The labeling of behavior as illness is not limited to homosexuality. Activities such as eating pork, piercing lips and noses, circumcision, lying down to sleep with the dead, taking hallucinogenic drugs, speaking in tongues, and mortification of the flesh are viewed as normal or exemplary in some cultures and as clear signs of illness in others. The line between using power to make someone "do something for your own good" and dictatorial thought control is not always easily drawn, and it is rarely more contentious than when it touches on the continuation of society through procreation. In one society, it may be routine for a young person to be taken to a prostitute or religious center for sexual initiation, while in another such behavior would be seen as cruel or immoral.

Advocates for people with mental illness and mental retardation are willing to push for the fullest participation in "normal" activities, but are often placed in a quandary regarding the desire of the mentally disabled to have children, especially when the disability is genetically related. Can that person understand the consequences? Is it fair to the unborn child? Even if the child has no genetic abnormalities, is it fair to the child to be raised by parents whose capacity is severely constrained, making it likely that he or she will be raised in a foster home? Externalities forcefully raise the question: Who counts, and do some count more than others?

Who Counts as a Citizen? Abortion and Other Dilemmas

Nowhere is the conflict over whose views are to count more apparent than in decisions regarding abortion. American society has been unable to achieve a clear resolution, and we will not attempt to do so here. What we can do is see how abortion poses a dilemma that affects many other problems in public health, and thus we will use it to clarify the nature of a general issue: Who is to be counted as a citizen, and do everyone's views count equally?

In the marketplace of third-century Rome, there was a law stating that no citizen could be sold a fish that was more than three days old (which, given the lack of refrigeration, seems plenty).[14] What happened to fish more than three days old? They were sold to noncitizens. Although this kind of blatantly discriminatory behavior seems inconceivable to us today, most countries follow similar policies. Pharmaceuticals that are not approved for use in the United States are routinely sold overseas, and for years many drugs whose shelf lives had expired were disposed of profitably this way. The most forceful statement regarding who is not a citizen, and what the country is willing to do to protect and enrich those who are its citizens, is war.

Even more difficult questions are posed by pregnancy. The right of a mother, as the one most proximately involved, to make decisions regarding her pregnancy seems reasonable, but it does elevate her rights over those of others. Could this position, if accepted logically, be used to claim that someone else is even more proximate (a grandparent for example, especially if the mother is incapacitated by substance abuse or illness)? This position is also directly in conflict with what pro-life activists describe as the right to life of the unborn child—*if* such an entity can be said to be a citizen. In general, societies seem to accede that mothers have special rights over their infants, and this extends with even greater force to before their birth. Yet this interest is not absolute. Similarly, it is accepted that a fetus does not have the same standing as a child. Consider how differently a court would treat a pregnant woman who took heroin because she was anxious and upset and a mother who gave the drug to her baby to keep the baby quiet. There is no social resolution to these issues other than in crafting some new set of rules and in agreeing to live, however uneasily, within them. It is possible that for many years two or more sets of rules will be in effect for different groups of people who can only agree not to talk about the issue or to fight in the courts rather than in the streets.

Ultimately the question of who counts as a citizen, and how much, is a moral one, but it is heavily conditioned by economic considerations, and transactions costs in particular. Experience has shown that it is virtually impossible to stop women who desperately want an abortion from having one. Making the practice illegal leads to many unsafe operations that cause infertility, disability, and death. Furthermore, any woman who can afford an airplane ticket to a country where abortions are legal can choose that option; thus, the practical effect may be to limit access for those who are young and poor and perhaps less able to care for a child. Indeed, the cost-benefit argument (that abortion is much cheaper than years of social services) may have sufficient appeal to some people that their moral positions are influenced by it. How strongly we support another person's right to self determination depends in part on our own self-interest.

Addiction

Addiction, which is sometimes treated as a mental illness, also reveals the tensions surrounding overrule of the individual by the state. Economists do not really understand addiction, but then, doctors don't either.[15] Many foods and substances are habit-forming, and many people have bad habits without engaging in self-destructive addictive behavior. Yet legally, a rather sharp distinction must be made between substances that are legal (e.g., candy, coffee, cigarettes, alcohol) and those that are not (e.g., steroids, marijuana, cocaine, heroin). The distinction is sometimes as much social and historical as it is biological. Heavy alcohol use is probably more likely to impair judgment and lead to injury than marijuana, and heroin taken regularly over years has fewer adverse physical effects than cigarettes. Yet alcohol has been a part of human culture for thousands of years and thus is not only well accepted, it is also subject to some social controls. Cigarettes are a relatively recent innovation. Only in the last fifty years have large numbers of people been able to afford to smoke many cigarettes daily. They are also a rather mild addiction and are cheaply available. Heroin, on the other hand, is such a powerful drug that addicts will do almost anything to get it, and illegality raises the price so high that it becomes necessary for many to steal to stay high. It is the externalities (stealing, dirty needles) rather than use that makes heroin so harmful to society. Cigarettes may be bad for your health, but they provide income to farmers, bring us sporting events, elect senators and representatives, and contribute mightily to the profits of large multinational firms. In trying to understand how morality is shaped by economics, it is useful to point out that the British Empire started a war with China to enforce its "right" to cross the border and sell opium to Chinese workers, a practice the Emperor wanted to prevent.

There is no way to fully separate the moral issues from the economic ones. Who is or is not a person, and how much their wishes are to be respected, is ultimately more than an economic decision, but is always conditioned by economic factors. Government usually acts as a collective agent to carry out the wishes of (most) people, not as an omniscient ruler dictating standards of good behavior. Borderline cases can never be solved to everyone's satisfaction, and there will always be conflict over the appropriate boundaries of action for criminal and social justice.

War and Public Health

A common wall poster during the 1960s read, "War is not healthy for children or other living things." Activity dedicated to killing seems obviously inimical to public health, and indeed, the American Public Health Association has passed several resolutions condemning war. Yet many advances in public health have been associated with war: Florence Nightingale's reform of field hospitals during the Crimean War led to modern nursing, malaria was eradicated during the Spanish-American War, and the campaign against venereal disease and the development of rapid psychotherapy occurred during World Wars I and II. The number of times that medical breakthroughs occurred during or because of a war raises the question: How (un)healthy is war?

As economic historian Douglass North points out, competition between states forces them to meet the needs of the people.[16] A government with no rivals does not need to develop new technologies. When kings or countries are vying for people's loyalty, it is in their interest to build hospitals, clean up the water supply, and perform all the other public health activities that are costly but also yield net benefits to society. North points out that we cannot understand the development of laws and political organization unless we recognize that rulers put their own interests first. War has a positive long-term effect on medical science because it heightens the interest of rulers in the health of the population—sick civilians make lousy soldiers.

In every war throughout history, at least until the twentieth century, many more soldiers died from diseases than from wounds inflicted on the battlefield. Armies of 20,000 or more would gather and camp in open fields with no toilets or running water. Contamination of food and drink were a more likely cause of death than enemy attack. Even in battle, it was often infection rather than bullets that killed, because lack of sanitation made minor wounds fatal. Conscripts were often drawn from isolated villages and so had never been exposed to common diseases. The result was uniformed disaster. Armies that spent any long period together were decimated by disease. Rulers' incentives for finding ways to keep large numbers of people living in close proximity without illness and epidemics were much greater in war than in peacetime.

When the United States entered World War I, the first thing it did was to call up an army of young, healthy men. To the chagrin of leaders at that time, one out of every four volunteers was medically unfit for service. They had tuberculosis, or syphilis, or vision so poor that they could not shoot straight. Prior to this time, it had been assumed that Americans were much healthier than their European counterparts who lived in crowded conditions with less food. The 1917 mobilization was the first time the nation collected information on the health of its citizens on a large scale, and the results were appalling. After the war, campaigns for the control of disease and malnutrition were promoted based on the data collected at induction centers.

The war also radically changed the practice of medicine. What had been a local trade practiced without a license was transformed in the military. Standards to determine how diseases should be treated and which doctors should be in charge were established. Physicians who had never seen modern medicine were educated by three years of practice in an organized setting, with antiseptic surgery under anesthesia saving thousands of lives. New occupations were developed to assist the harried field surgeons, and the organization of medicine was decisively changed from solo individual practice to cooperative expertise centered in the hospital. Although most people were skeptical of medical science at the turn of the century, the stories and living examples of what medicine could do were spread as the injured soldiers returned home throughout America.

War changes the calculus of individual costs and benefits. As the collective interest looms larger, massive investments in new knowledge and infrastructure are made. The attempt to place as many men as possible on the front lines leads to the rapid acquisition of knowledge on nutrition, surgery, psychology, and infectious disease. Without ignoring the shameful horror of death and destruction that wars impose on humankind, the fact that they have been a powerful force in advancing public health must be recognized.

SUGGESTIONS FOR FURTHER READING

American Journal of Public Health and *Public Health Reports*, published monthly.

U.S. Centers for Disease Control and Prevention (www.cdc.gov).

Institute of Medicine, *Public Health in Crisis* (Washington, D.C.: National Academy Press, 1990).

Senator William R. Frist, M.D., Public Health And National Security: The Critical Role of Increased Federal Support," *Health Affairs* 21, no. 6 (November 2002): 117–130.

John R. Lumpkin and Margaret S. Richards, "Transforming the Public Health Information Infrastructure," *Health Affairs* 21, no. 6 (November 2002): 45–56.

George Rosen, *A History of Public Health* (New York: MD Publications, 1958).

Paul Samuelson, "A Diagrammatic Exposition of a Theory of Public Expenditure," *Review of Economics and Statistics* (November 1955).

SUMMARY

1. A **pure public good** is something that is **consumed collectively** by all. It is indivisible so that **no one can be excluded** (zero charges), and one person's consumption has no effect on another's **(zero marginal costs)**. Examples are clean air, statistics, and the discovery of penicillin.

2. Many goods are both public and private. The degree of **publicness** of a good increases with **the number of people,** the use of **insurance,** and the **transactions, information, and measurement costs.**

3. Although decisions about private goods can be made through the market, the **indivisibility** of public goods **means that governments must make these decisions through voting,** political compromises, or cost-benefit analysis. Invariably, this means that there is a **moral or social justice** dimension, as well as an economic one.

4. **Externalities** are said to exist when the actions of one person affect another (e.g., smoking, disposing of garbage). Infectious disease externalities have shaped public health, from the foundation of the U.S. Public Health Service as the homeless seaman's hospital to the pasteurization of milk. The increased risk of infecting others is a cost the individual does not bear, and government intervention is required to achieve (or get closer to) an optimum level of prevention.

5. To improve public health, it is necessary to determine exactly **who the public is;** whether some people or **some preferences count more than others.** Conflict over who is and is not worthwhile and able to make decisions lies at the heart of some of the most contentious public health issues: abortion, substance abuse, and care of people with mental illness.

6. People's **attitudes toward a particular public good** are always affected by their **private interests.** Universal access to high-quality medical care and redistribution of income *may* be an important public good. Whether you think so depends a lot on whether you are poor or identify with those who are.

7. **Competition** between governments over the provision of public goods may be just as important as competition between people or firms in creating economic efficiency, particularly in **forcing beneficial change over time.**

PROBLEMS

1. {*property rights, public goods*} Why is most drug research paid for by companies, while most medical research is paid for by the government?

2. {*public goods*} Explain which item in the following pairs is more "public" and why:

   a. AIDS or lung cancer

   b. Milk or bread

   c. Saturday morning cartoons or a Sunday night late show

   d. Stroke or lung cancer

3. {*externalities*} Why not charge people full price for vaccinations?

4. {*welfare*} Which type of good is apt to have a larger consumers' surplus, a public good or a private good? Why?

5. {*property rights, scale*} Why have wars often given rise to improvements in medical technology?

6. {*property rights*} Caring for the poor costs money, much more than they are able to pay directly or in taxes. Why would different government jurisdictions compete to provide medical care for the poor?

7. {*incidence, voting*} Many goods are desired by some people and not by others. Since diversity of tastes is universal, why does it create more problems for public goods than for private goods?

8. {*aggregation*} Draw the demand and supply curves for (a) a public good and (b) a private good for two people, Adam and Barbara, and (c) the market demand for a two-person (Adam + Barbara) market.

9. {*exclusivity, marginal cost*} Some forms of health care are public because the marginal cost of serving additional people is zero. Other types of health care are public, even though marginal costs are positive, because it is impossible to exclude beneficiaries who do not pay. Some forms of care meet both criteria—zero marginal costs and a lack of exclusivity. Give examples of all three categories (recognizing that no real goods or services are perfectly public or fall entirely in one category or another).

10. {*welfare*} Why pay economists to conduct a cost-benefit analysis if the market will show the value of a new medical technology to consumers?

11. {*public goods*} Which has more externalities, cigars or chewing tobacco? Guns or knives? Laptop computers or portable telephones?

12. {*externalities*} What are the externalities of heroin addiction?

ENDNOTES

1. After seventeen years, other firms can manufacture the drug in generic form if they meet certain standards and obtain approval from the FDA. See chapter 12 and also Sam Peltzman, *The Regulation of Pharmaceutical Innovation: the 1962 Amendments* (Washington, D.C.: American Enterprise Institute, 1974).

2. Elizabeth Fee and Steven Corey, *Garbage: The History and Politics of Trash in New York* (New York: New York Public Library, 1994).

3. Donald A. Dunn and Aristides C. Fronistas, "Economic Models of Information Services Markets," in Robert Goldberg and Harold Lorin, eds., *The Economics of Information Processes* (New York: Wiley, 1982), Vol. 1:141–162; Michael R. Rubin, *Information Economics and Policy in the United States* (Littleton, Colo.: Libraries Unlimited, 1983).

4. Bruno Latour, *The Pasteurization of France* (Cambridge, Mass: Harvard University Press, 1988).

5. John Graunt, *Natural and Political Observations on the Bills of Mortality,* London (1662), see Charles Creighton, *A History of Epidemics in Britain*, 2nd ed. (New York: Barnes & Noble, 1965), 532.

6. George Rosen, *A History of Public Health* (New York: MD Publications, 1958), 354–360.

7. The classic paper setting out these results is Paul A. Samuelson, "A Diagrammatic Exposition of a Theory of Public Expenditure," *Review of Economics and Statistics,* November 1955.

8. Note how difficult pricing is in the real world of broadcasting. The network stations are in effect "priced" by making the consumer watch advertisements, while the "PBS public broadcasting" uses a mixture of taxes and voluntary donations. Such pricing problems, and the blandness of much government programming, may also explain why cable and satellite TV are doing so well in newly developing countries.

9. David Rosner, ed., *Hives of Sickness: Public Health and Epidemics in New York City* (New Brunswick, NJ: Rutgers University Press, 1995).

10. Henrik Ibsen, "An Enemy of the People" (1882) in *Henrik Ibsen, The Complete Major Prose Plays,* translated by Rolf Fjelde (New York: Farrar, Strauss, Giroux, 1978), 277–388.

11. Paul Farnham, "The Economic Cost of HIV/AIDS," in J.M. Pogodzinski, ed., *Readings in Public Policy* (Cambridge, Mass.: Blackwell, 1995). Treatment using protease inhibitors is effective against the HIV virus, but only under such strict treatment regimens and at such great cost that a new set of economic issues is raised.

12. George Rosen, *A History of Public Health* (New York: MD Publications, 1958).

13. Fitzhugh Mullan, *Plagues and Politics: The Story of the United States Public Health Service* (Basic Books: New York, 1989). Odin Anderson, *Health Services as a Growth Enterprise in the U.S. Since 1875* (Ann Arbor, Mich.: Health Administration Press, 1990).

14. George Rosen, *A History of Public Health* (New York: MD Publications, 1958).

15. The attempt to explain why people do things to their bodies that are clearly not in their own best interests and hence seem to contradict the assumption of rationality has led to a spate of research by economists on "rational addiction." While these models have been well received within economics, they have had limited effect on the substance abuse and psychiatric community. See Donald S. Kenkel, Robert R. Reed III, and Ping Wang, "Rational Addiction, Peer Externalities and Long Run Effects of Public Policy," NBER working paper w9249 (October 2002); or Jonathan Gruber and Botond Koszegi, "Is Addiction 'Rational?' Theory and Evidence," NBER working paper w7507 (January 2000), (www.nber.org).

16. Douglass North, *Structure and Change in Economic History* (New York: Norton, 1981).

CHAPTER 16

ECONOMIC HISTORY, POPULATION GROWTH, AND MEDICAL CARE

QUESTIONS

1. Does economic growth cause population growth?
2. Is medical care the main reason life expectancy is increasing?
3. Must a society be wealthy to invest in medical care?
4. Do economic failures cause plagues and other mortality?
5. Was Malthus right? Will populations continue to expand until food supplies are exhausted?
6. Why do families have fewer children today?
7. Does medical technology create economic growth or does economic growth create new medical technology?

16.1 ECONOMIC GROWTH HAS DETERMINED THE SHAPE OF HEALTH CARE

In order for a modern health care system to develop and be supported economically, four conditions must exist:

- Effective medical technology
- A sufficiently low risk of death that improving health is worthwhile
- Ample wealth to pay for advanced medical treatment
- Financial organization through insurance and government programs to pool funds from many people

While medical care has been provided for as long as human society has existed, these four conditions have been met only within the past hundred years, and only in developed countries. Most of Africa and parts of Asia and Latin America are still characterized by high mortality, subsistence farming, and a lack of social and financial organization so that the risks of dying are high and heavily influenced by the amount of income available.[1] Economic development creates the foundation for modern medicine. As large numbers of people live longer and have more wealth, they become more willing to pay for medical care. They pool funds to finance care through insurance (Chapters 4 and 5) and to support medical research so that collectively they can obtain the technological wonders that none of them could afford individually (Chapters 14 and 15).

Food was the primary limitation on the number of people in a population and their health until perhaps two hundred years ago. Only after the Industrial Revolution did medical technology become important. Yet close study indicates that changes in economic organization, from simple tribes to complex multinational corporations and global markets, have done more to increase human health and welfare than the technological discoveries themselves.[2]

16.2 BIRTH RATES, DEATH RATES, AND POPULATION GROWTH

Population growth is determined by the number of births minus the number of deaths (ignoring immigration, which just transfers people between different parts of the world). Stated in percentage terms:

Natural Rate of Population Increase = Birth Rate – Death Rate

If the birth rate is 4.2 percent and the death rate is 3.9 percent, the rate of increase is 4.2 percent – 3.9 percent = 0.3 percent per year. As a first order of approximation, the death rate ≈ 1/(life expectancy), thus a life expectancy of twenty-five years implies that 1/25, or 4 percent, of the population will die each year.[3] Birth and death rates fluctuated wildly through most of history, but were forced on average quite close to each other because of the uneasy equilibrium between population and food supply. If births were high for a while, there would be too many mouths to feed in the winter and starvation became more likely. If food was scarce for many years, people delayed marriage, thus reducing the birth rate. On the other hand, years of bumper crops meant people were more likely to survive and reproduce.

It is important to recognize the numerical effects of **compounding**: how small differences in rates turn into large differences in size over time. If births and deaths are both 4 percent per year, the population is stable, neither growing nor shrinking. If there is a slight increase in births, to 4.1 percent a year, the natural rate of increase becomes 0.1 percent and population will double in seven hundred years, as it did through much of the Agricultural Age. If births rise further to 4.2 percent (i.e., 0.2 percent net increase), the population will be four times larger in seven hundred years. A growth rate of 1.0 percent a year means the population will double every seventy years, a total population growth of 106,000 percent in a seven-hundred-year time span.[4]

16.3 THE STONE AGE

Time span: 5 million to 10,000 B.C.	**Economy:** Subsistence hunter-gatherer
Total population: Beginning to 4 million	**Distribution of income:** Roughly equal
Growth rate (doubles): .0007% *(100,000 years)*	**Medical care:** Shaman/witch doctor
Life expectancy: 28 years	**Medical $:** Not applicable

The **Stone Age** began with the emergence of the first hominids in Africa about 5 million years ago. People lived in small bands as hunter-gatherers, with a simple family/tribal social structure and little physical or intellectual capital to improve productivity. Population was limited by the amount of food in the immediate area. Life expectancy was less than thirty years, and more than half the children did not live long enough to start families, although some elders lived into their forties or fifties.[5] For millennia upon millennia, the rate of population growth was so slow as to be almost unnoticeable. It took about 100,000 years for global population to double, an annual growth rate of 0.0007 percent. At the end of the prehistoric Stone Age around 10,000 B.C. there were about 4 million people in the world, mostly in Asia, Africa, and the Near East, with only a few in the Americas. For stone age hunter-gatherers, everyone lived pretty much equally at a subsistence level. Violent death and starvation in the winter were constant threats, but during the good times, life was relatively easy. Studies of remaining hunter-gatherer tribes that rely on Stone Age "technology" in the Amazon, Philippine jungles, and Africa indicate that only two to four hours per day is required to obtain food and repair simple shelters and tools, with much of the rest of the time taken up by pursuits such as socializing, singing, and art. Exchange between groups was rare, so there were no organized trading systems.

Population growth during the Stone Age occurred primarily by expansion into new territory. As a tribe got too large for the local area, some family groups split off and occupied new land. Evolution and new technology (i.e., bows and arrows, flint knives) meant better exploitation of the existing food supply, not increased productivity. *Homo sapiens* displaced *homo erectus* because the former was more efficient at hunting and killing, gathering and storing food, and building shelter. This increased efficiency did not increase the productivity of the land, and in some cases even reduced it as large game species (mammoths, sloths) were exterminated. Each additional person required more land, and the ultimate size of the population was limited by the area under settlement. By the end of the Stone Age, those limits had already been reached in some fully populated areas. The rising population pressure in long-settled lands overfilled with people may have contributed to the development of animal husbandry and plant cultivation to feed the excess population, initiating the Agricultural Age.

16.4 THE AGRICULTURAL AGE

Time span: 10,000 B.C. to 1800 A.D.	**Economy:** Farming and harvesting
Total population: 4 million to 400 million	**Distribution of income:** Top-heavy, unequal
Growth rate (doubles): .046% (1,500 years)	**Medical care:** Empirical
Life expectancy: 24 years	**Medical $:** Perhaps 1%

Population growth accelerated with the development of agriculture, but only slowly at first. Agriculture appears to have originated around 10,000 B.C.–7,000 B.C. in the river valleys of the Tigris, the Euphrates, and the Nile, and subsequently developed independently in China and the Peruvian highlands. People began to settle permanently in one place. Irrigation canals were dug and roads were built. The same acreage could support more permanent farmers than roaming hunter-gatherers. The productivity increases that made agriculture a stable way of life depended on countless and often incremental innovations occurring at different times and places. Furthermore, the geographic diffusion of ideas was slow, only about one kilometer a year. As late as 4000 B.C., global population was still growing at a rate of only about 0.01 percent a year (doubling in 7,000 years). Agriculture meant greater reliance on just one or a few crops so there was less diversity in foodstuffs and nutrients, reducing health. Cultivation of a single food also exposed the population of a village to catastrophic declines as drought or infestation caused crop failure. Thus, although the population grew larger, life expectancy declined.

Investment and Trade

Farming takes investment. Seed must be saved, fields plowed, and animal pens erected. A hunter might have worked at making a sharper spear or better root gatherer, but the increase in output was small compared with the gains obtained from farm improvements (building an irrigation ditch, selection of superior seed, the invention of the harrow or plow). In the **Agricultural Age,** many farm investments, such as building a road or a large corral, were collective, benefiting the entire village. The returns on investment became larger when more people were involved. There is a synergy in bringing people together. While each person could know something about farming, a hundred could compare experiences and draw on the best ideas. Each person could make tools, but collectively, in a village of a hundred, the few people who were best at it could spend more time making tools for others, and get food in return. Specialization, trade, and division of labor arose. Towns and cities were built. Trade between regions became a regular part of economic activity.

For trade and investment to occur, societies must develop property rights. To have farms, people needed to be able to stay on their land and improve it from year to year. They had to own a portion of the extra grain that was stored for times of famine or traded for tools, salt, and other necessary items. Stored grain had to be defended against the marauding bandits who showed up at harvest time. Once an agricultural society formed an army, it quickly discovered that force was useful for things other than defense. Neighboring tribes were displaced from their more productive lands or conquered and made into slaves. Leaders who successfully rallied the troops in battle gained power and, through a hierarchy of princes and priests, effectively controlled most of the wealth of society. Yet the development of governance was more than a military necessity. To grow, agricultural societies needed rulers who could accumulate and manage the excess output necessary for collective investments in irrigation, laws, and war making.

Civilization, War, and Government

With the advent of the first great civilization—the Sumerians—population began to increase rapidly. Population growth rates increased to 0.07 percent per year (doubling in 1,000 years), about a hundred times the hunter-gatherer growth rate. Although the Sumerian empire soon fell, the Pharoic theocracy established along the banks of the Nile in Egypt endured for centuries. Between 1,000 B.C. and 1 A.D., many other large and vigorous civilizations developed. The classical Greeks rose to unprecedented heights, and Alexander conquered the world before being displaced by the Romans. In China, the Han dynasty unified 50 million people, and in the Americas the great Inca and Olmec/Maya/Aztec civilizations began. By 1 A.D., empires spanned continents and trade routes stretched for thousands of miles. World population exceeded 200 million and was growing about 0.12 percent per year (doubling every 600 years).

As cities grew, the population split into two classes: peasants who worked the land and continued to live at subsistence level and rulers who controlled all the wealth. While hunter-gatherers were all at the same level, working two to four hours a day to obtain subsistence plus a little extra, farmers had to work much harder, eight to twelve hours a day, to obtain the same amount of food. Why, then, did anyone become a farmer? People became farmers probably out of necessity rather than choice. When a climatic change caused a succession of bad years, or a stronger band of tribes pushed people out of favored territory, they were forced to try to get more out of what was at hand: husbanding animals rather than just hunting them, planting roots and grain rather than just picking them wild, and so on. Many peasants were "recruited" as they were captured and placed under the domination of a warlord. Once the shift from hunting to farming occurred, farming acquired a momentum of its own and the trend became irreversible. There were too many people in the valley to go back to the old ways and the kings did not want to give up the wealth they obtained by ruling others. Even if doubling the population of the city did not make the average person better off, it made the king and the court twice as well off.

Prosperity depended on the willingness of people to support (or at least tacitly cooperate with) the existing system and to work toward improving it. While the king might coerce peasants into paying taxes, he had to deliver order and a stable standard of living in return or face rebellion. The taxes collected had to be directed toward appropriate public works and services to maintain progress. The rapid growth in population could only be sustained by new forms of social organization, by creating the cultural, political, and economic institutions that make up civilization. Having enough wealth left over to indulge idle priests and philosophers as they researched mathematics, astronomy, chemistry, physics, and medicine also fostered the conditions for technological advance. This process of economic development was mutually reinforcing, because growth required more government and investment, and made it possible to free up resources to support them.

The Decline of Civilizations Leads to Population Declines

The amazing growth of classical civilizations was followed by almost equally sensational declines when social order decayed. There were more people in ancient Greece at its apex in 440 B.C. than at any time during the next 2,000 years, and it was not until 1850 A.D. that the population again exceeded 3 million. As the Roman Empire shrank, the total population of Europe fell from 44 million in 200 A.D. to 22 million in 600 A.D. By 1000 A.D., European population had only partly recovered, to 30 million. Similar though less severe declines occurred in China and Africa. A recent example is found in the traumatic transition of the Soviet Union as communism disintegrated in 1990. The sharp drop in economic output, widespread moral and social disorder, and precipitous decline in life expectancy has been dubbed Katastroika (catastrophic construction) by some commentators.

IMPLOSION OF THE SOVIET ECONOMY CAUSES DRAMATIC DECLINES IN LIFE EXPECTANCY

Life expectancy in Russia in 1990 was 63.8 years for males and 74.3 years for females, slightly higher than it had been thirty years previously.[6] The reconstruction (perestroika) of the Union of Soviet Socialist Republics (USSR) under Mikhail Gorbachev brought hope, and then disaster. The Soviet economy crumbled, the USSR fragmented, and quality of life declined. For some people on fixed incomes, hyperinflation took food prices beyond their reach, causing malnutrition. More important, the loss of jobs and hope meant despair. In such a grim situation, deaths from alcohol poisoning and accidents soared. By 1993, life expectancy had fallen four years for males (to fifty-nine years) and three years for females (to seventy-one and a half years), a decline that is virtually unprecedented in modern industrial countries. Fertility dropped below replacement level and total population declined. In 1992, births exceeded deaths by 184,000. By 1993, there were 800,000 more deaths than births.[7] For every live birth, there were 2.2 abortions. Only now are the true dimensions of this contemporary social and demographic catastrophe being measured.

The Plague

As European populations began to recover robustly toward the end of the Middle Ages (500–1500 A.D.), they were hit by a new and rampantly destructive force, the plague. Bubonic plague, or black death, swept through Europe in 1347-1352 and repeatedly thereafter, wiping out a quarter of the population.[8] Half the citizens of Genoa and Naples died as a result of the plague of 1656.[9] Although bouts of plague continued to appear until 1700, changes in immunity, social structure, the plague bacillus itself, or a combination of these, reduced the impact over time, and population growth resumed after 1500 A.D. The peoples of the New World were not as fortunate. After contact with the Spanish conquistadors, plagues of measles and smallpox spread rapidly, with devastating effects. The native population of Aztecs dropped from 17 million in 1532 to 2 million in 1580, and fell to just 1 million by 1608. It was not just disease, but the collapse of social order that caused the permanent decline in numbers. Much of the repopulation of the Americas after 1600 came from the growth of immigrant populations from Europe and Africa.

Food Supply Determines Population

From 1500–1750 the European and world populations grew at an average annual rate of 0.25 percent (doubling in 300 years). Food supply was the fundamental constraint on growth since the great majority of people lived at a subsistence level. A study of the Italian district of Siena from 1550–1715 shows that increases in prices for grain were associated with malnutrition and death.[10] Each time the cost of food rose, the meager salaries of the residents were stretched thinner and mortality climbed. The cycle is self-correcting and self-reinforcing. As people die, there are fewer mouths to feed; therefore, demand falls and prices fall. When food is abundant and prices are low, peasants are more able to marry and have children, the number of mouths to feed rises, demand increases, prices jump, and the cycle starts over again.

As the Agricultural Age drew to a close and the transition to an urbanized industrial society began, scarcity of food continued to be a major issue. Salaried workers were little better off than peasants, because it took 80 percent their salaries to get enough to eat. For example, in 1790, France was a highly developed country, with perhaps the greatest cultural and political influence in the Western world, yet most of its citizens were impoverished and undernourished. The average thirty-year-old Frenchman of 1790 had to live on 2,250 calories per day, was just 5 feet, 3 inches tall, and weighed only 110 pounds.[11] The bottom 10 percent of society had so little food that they were usually ill, and most people below the twentieth percentile did not get enough food to meet the caloric energy demands of regular work. Even relatively well-off people at the eightieth percentile were sufficiently stunted and wasted (height and weight below current U.S. standards) that they were at substantially higher risk of chronic health conditions and premature mortality.

The Rise of Economics

The intellectual ferment of the Renaissance (1350–1650 A.D.) and Enlightenment (1650–1800 A.D.) brought advances in government, science, and commerce (although major changes in medicine did not occur until 1900). In 1662, John Graunt published his *Natural and Political Observations on the Bills of Mortality* in London, a work now recognized as the beginning of the science of epidemiology. In 1671, Sir William Petty made the first estimate of national wealth (gross domestic product [GDP]) in his essay *Political Arithmetik* (economic statistics). As people moved from rural estates, where they had been cared for (and/or owned) by a feudal lord, into cities where they worked at jobs for wages, the economic organization of society evolved from one based on tradition to one based on money. Only after exchange became standardized through the use of money could regularities be observed and statistical analysis be performed.

The development of accounting and statistics marked the emergence of a new "information technology" that revolutionized trade. Financial markets in London and other cities traded government bonds and shares in joint stock companies, shifting tons of gold with the stroke of a pen. Factories were built and thousands of people changed occupations and even nationalities to better their standard of living. Capital investment and labor mobility of this magnitude had been impossible during the Middle Ages because the necessary economic structure was not available or was too rudimentary. Corporations, rental contracts, taxes, ownership, and other property rights had to be refined before trade between individuals, firms, and governments could be conducted on a large scale. *The Wealth of Nations*, Adam Smith's insightful analysis published in 1776, is recognized as the start of modern economics.[12] Yet Thomas Malthus's *Essay on the Principle of Population* (1798) often has been more influential, clearly presenting the consensus of thinkers at the end of the agricultural age and responsible for labeling economics "the dismal science."

The Malthusian Hypothesis

Malthus's hypothesis was that any increase in productivity could provide only a temporary boost to the standard of living.[13] Over time, increases in the number of people to be fed would use up all the productivity increase; therefore, on average, people would be no better off than before—still living at a subsistence level. The **Malthusian hypothesis** is based on two key assumptions: that (1) *food supply* is a primary constraint on population growth and (2) any increase in the number of people would inevitably lead to more crowding or to farming of less desirable land so that the *declining marginal productivity* of labor (and hence, wages) would bring down the standard of living.

Ireland became a natural experiment for testing the Malthusian hypothesis. The importation of a new crop, potatoes, led to a tremendous increase in yields per acre. Using the new crop, the acreage that could support only one family in 1700 could be split up and support three families by 1800. Potato farming was so much more efficient than other types of agriculture that the peasants ate little else, consuming up to ten pounds per day. The population of this small and already fully settled island grew 50 percent in the half century before Malthus wrote, and by another 50 percent over the next thirty years. Farms were divided into smaller and smaller parcels, and the Irish people, with a diet consisting almost entirely of potatoes, lived no better than before—there were just more of them. Then came the fungus blight that damaged the potato harvest of 1845 and destroyed the crop of 1846 entirely: 1.5 million people died and another 1.5 million people emigrated, mostly to America. Those who were left tightened their belts and stopped having children (the women born before the blight who remained in Ireland were four times as likely to remain unmarried as those who emigrated to America).[14] Out of a population of 8 million in 1840, there were only 4.5 million left by 1900, and by 1950, only 2.8 million.

The assumptions in the Malthusian hypothesis had been valid through the thousands of years that spanned the agricultural age, and continued to apply in countries that remained essentially rural, such as Ireland. The law of diminishing returns, as elaborated by Malthus, was a major intellectual contribution to economics. However, it applies only if the technology of production stays essentially the same. In England, Germany, France, and the United States, the same intellectual revolution that stirred Malthus to write his treatise led others to create a technological and commercial revolution so profound that productivity increases were continuous, and output grew much more rapidly than any natural increase in the number of people.[15] A continuous excess of food and other goods became available for all to enjoy.

16.5 THE INDUSTRIAL AGE

Time span: 1800 to 1950 A.D.	**Economy:** Manufacturing
Total population: 0.4 billion to 1.6 billion	**Distribution of income:** Mixed
Growth rate (doubles): .65% (108 years)	**Medical care:** Empirical
Life expectancy: 35 years	**Medical $:** 2% to 4%

Life was difficult at the start of the Industrial Revolution and often got worse for those who moved into cities to work in factories. Crowded slums and harsh working conditions caused disease. Whereas diets on a farm could be supplemented by gardens and occasional hunting, in the cities food was monotonous and lacking in vitamins. As the countryside became enclosed (put under ownership of a lord rather than held in common) and people moved into cities, illness increased. Life expectancy in England, about thirty-eight years in 1600 A.D., declined throughout the next hundred years and did not regain earlier levels until about 1850.[16] Yet as the Industrial Revolution took hold, productivity increases caused the average person's standard of living to improve. There was a sharp rise in the rate of population growth to 0.43 percent from 1750–1800, almost twice the rate of the preceding three centuries, rising to 0.53 percent in 1800–1900, 0.88 percent per year in 1900–1950, and surging to 1.8 percent since 1950. World population quadrupled from about 750 million to 2.5 billion. Overall life expectancy rose by more in these two hundred years than it had in the previous two thousand, going from twenty-seven to thirty-five years. The rise was even more remarkable in the most developed countries, such as Sweden, where life expectancy rose from thirty-seven years in 1750 to 71.3 years in 1950.

Why Malthus Was Wrong

There are two reasons Malthus' gloomy predictions were wrong. First, technological advance, rather than being a one-shot improvement, became a continuous process. Output expanded at an exponential rate as one invention led to another. In the Agricultural Age, the primary productive inputs were land and labor. The total supply of land is fixed, and any increase in the supply of labor meant more mouths to feed. In the **Industrial Age,** capital equipment, skilled labor, and knowledge became more important than land and unskilled agricultural labor. By 1950, a single farmer, sitting in an air-conditioned cab operating a combine, harvesting genetically engineered wheat, could feed more people per 100 acres than a dozen farmers could in 1750. Although the rate of productivity increase during the Agricultural Age averaged about 1 percent a year, in the Industrial Age it rapidly tripled and sometimes exceeded 5 percent a year. A second reason that Malthus's immiserating population growth failed to occur was that as death rates declined, birth rates also declined. With fewer children dying, parents chose to have fewer babies, and invested more in the education, medical care, and nutrition of each one. Parents acted in what they saw as the best interests of their families as they made decisions regarding how many children to have and how to care for them. Cumulatively, these individual decisions brought about a social revolution. It also changed the character of labor and accelerated technological advance, leading to higher wages and a rising standard of living.

Why did Ireland suffer a Malthusian catastrophe and lose two-thirds of its population while most other European nations experienced surging growth during the Industrial Revolution? Ireland was not a self-governing nation, but a colony exploited by absentee landlords from England. Profits from Irish estates were not invested in Ireland, but used to build factories in England or sent overseas through joint stock companies. Irish farmers did not own their land, but were tenants working the fields for the benefit of the landlord. As crop yields went up, rents were raised, keeping workers in subsistence conditions typical of the Agricultural Age. With no claim on the profits, the tenant farmer had no incentive to raise crop yields and had little ability to save and improve the lot of the family in the next generation. The only way for Irish farmers to capture any of the economic surplus created by increased agricultural productivity was to have more children, and so they did. Irish citizens wishing to leave the farm and build a better life in the city had to leave their country and go to New York. The lack of property rights for citizens and restrictive colonial economic organization were significant factors in keeping Ireland from joining the ranks of industrialized countries during the nineteenth century.

Malthus's predictions were never as dismal or as wrong as his critics claimed. He hoped that by clearly laying out the logical conclusions of agricultural demographics, he would encourage people to delay marriage and have fewer children. Birthrates did, in fact, decline, but for other reasons. Women gained more opportunities and spent less time on child rearing. More children survived; thus, fewer births were needed to make sure that one or two children in a family lived to maturity. Dependence on children in old age was replaced by reliance on savings. Perhaps most important, children went from being a form of supplemental income (as productive family farmworkers) to a form of consumption (bringing joy but costing money). All these changes either raised the price of or reduced the demand for children. Average total fertility per mature female in England fell from 5.3 births in 1750, to 4.6 in 1850, to 1.96 in 1900 (below the replacement rate of 2.0; therefore, national population would actually have decreased over time if not for foreign immigration).

Demographic Transition

The process of economic development is linked to a dramatic change in national population known as "demographic transition." When societies are in the agricultural stage, many children die before reaching adulthood. High rates of mortality (4 to 5 percent) are matched by high rates of fertility (also 4 to 5 percent), so the total number of people is stable or just slowly increasing. This equilibrium between births and deaths is radically changed during the process of economic development. With greater material well-being, mortality rates decline toward 1 to 2 percent. Since birth rates are still high, the rate of population growth (births–deaths) is very rapid, 2 to 4 percent a year, enough to double the population in each generation (every fifteen to forty years). Such explosive growth does not continue indefinitely. Although constantly increasing economic output should not necessarily cause birth rates to fall, it is observed that birth rates do in fact fall in virtually every developed country. As children cease to be productive farm assets and become a costly form of family consumption, families decide to concentrate more care and investment on fewer children.[17] This decline in fertility does not require the use of modern birth control techniques. Delayed marriage, extended breast feeding, infanticide, and other methods have been used to restrict population to desired levels in many countries without recourse to contraceptives. As economic development continues, low mortality (1-2 percent) is eventually matched by low fertility (1–2 percent) so that the total population is again stable or slowly growing, and the process of demographic transition is complete (see Figure 16.1).

FIGURE 16.1   Demographic Transition

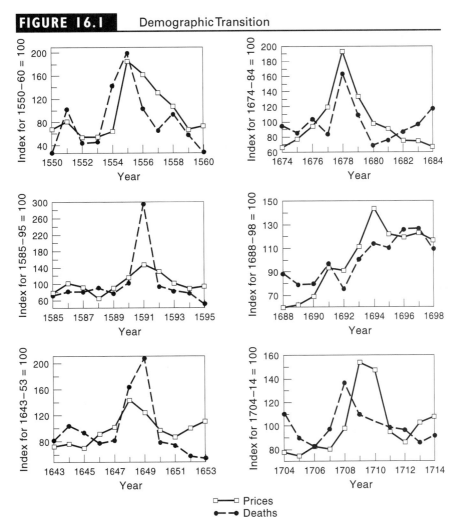

Source: Massimo Livi-Bacci, *A Concise History of World Population,* Cambridge, Mass.: Blackwell, 1992, p. 80; G. Parenti, *Prezzi e mercato a Siena,* 1546–1765, Florence: 1942, pp. 27–28.

Population growth spurts during the agricultural age occurred when settlement of new territories caused an increase in births, whereas population growth during demographic transition is caused by a decline in deaths. These two demographic patterns have different long-run consequences on the average level of individual wealth. When new territories are settled, the pioneers have much more land per person than in the country they came from and thus initially enjoy a much greater marginal productivity of labor and greater wealth. This advantage is eroded over time as more and more people are born in the new territories. Eventually, the new territories are just as crowded as the old country, the marginal productivity of labor reverts to the subsistence level, and the total population, although larger, is not much better off. In contrast, the economic advances that mark demographic transition, rather than fading over time, are reinforced with each succeeding generation. Healthier adults can work longer and harder and thus accumulate more surplus for investment, while a smaller number of children means that each one receives more in the way of education, nutrition, and inheritance. These gains lead to even lower mortality, even fewer children, and so on. Each generation is better off, and material advantage is concentrated among an ever smaller number of offspring until transition is complete. By then, the amount of family income required to buy food has fallen from 80 percent to 20 percent. Getting enough to eat is no longer a significant factor in demographic change or labor productivity.

Demographic Change, Income Distribution, and the Rise of the Middle Classes

In a hunter-gatherer society, there are no wealthy people. The tribe as a whole is living at the subsistence level with only a little accumulated wealth in the form of weapons or religious objects. One or two bad years can spell disaster. An agricultural society, in contrast, is hierarchical and often has considerable wealth, almost all of it concentrated at the top. Most of the agricultural population consists of rural peasants. As agricultural civilizations develop, the number of traders, soldiers, craftspeople, merchants, and other members of the bourgeois who live as free "citizens" in (mostly small) cities increases, but they are always a minority. The king's authority is absolute, and almost all of the wealth stays under his control.

To industrialize, the bulk of the population has to move into cities. People who leave the land are no longer under the control of the lord, and they enter into wage labor contracts with factories. As businesses and bureaucracies replace the feudal manor as a means of organizing production, the fruits of economic development are spread more widely. Although the wages of industrial workers are near the subsistence level at first, real earnings rise rapidly for two reasons. First, the decline in the number of births during demographic transition means fewer new workers entering the market; thus, the supply of labor grows less rapidly than demand, putting upward pressure on wages. Second, the labor market becomes specialized. Initially the threat of starvation drove unskilled workers off the farm to take subsistence wages in the city. However, the later movement of skilled mechanics, clerks, and managers to the city was driven by the premium wages required to attract these workers. These well-paid workers and shopkeepers could afford some luxuries. They could also save for retirement, and in so doing, contribute to the pool of capital funds for investment and entrepreneurial ventures.

Although feudal blacksmiths took pride in their art, most of the benefits went to the lord. Master mechanics in the industrial era had a much greater incentive to improve their skills, because they were paid more for the increases in quality and productivity. Furthermore, they were apt to take the risk of innovating and starting new businesses, because they might become rich. Even if their ventures failed, they would only lose some money, not their lives. They could still get other jobs and keep their families from starving.[18]

In the city-states and empires of the agricultural age, lords and kings exercised centralized bureaucratic power to raise taxes, build roads, and support armies. Building factories and inventing new technologies in the industrial era required decentralized entrepreneurs who acted as managers on their own behalf rather than on behalf of the king. Working independently or in small groups, entrepreneurs convinced investors to put up capital and attracted skilled labor with high wages. By the end of the industrial age, even people of modest means could go to school, start a business, and save for retirement. A startling change in the distribution of income and wealth had occurred—the bulk of the money was held by the large and growing middle class of laborers, tradespeople, and small-business owners. In 1750 the market for art, education, travel, housing, and almost everything except food was concentrated in the upper 2 percent of families who were truly wealthy. By 1950, the market for such goods in the United States, England, Germany, and other developed countries was dominated by the middle class. The wealthy bought luxury in a few shops, while the millions shopped in department stores (see Figure 16.2).[19]

The hierarchies that dominated the Agricultural Age were broken up by tremendous increases in economic mobility and a general improvement in wages. The crowd at the bottom was replaced by a bulging middle class of people who actively participated in a monetary economy. This shift in social and economic structure, rather than the discovery of new technology per se, was the driving force that powered the growth of the Industrial Revolution. Many countries today remain poor and rural, struggling to make the demographic and economic transition to development. It is not because they lack technology (which can be found in many textbooks, ordered from catalogs, or shared in commercial joint ventures), but because they lack the property rights, social order, and administrative structure to create a context in which technology can be applied productively.[20] The deficit that allows starvation to remain a threat to people's health is not a lack of knowledge, machinery, or money for investment, but a lack of economic organization.

16.6 THE INFORMATION AGE

Time span: 1950 to future	**Economy:** Services
Total population: 1.6 billion to 20 billion?	**Distribution of income:** Not yet clear
Growth rate (doubles): 1.88% (40 years) but slowing	**Medical care:** Scientific
Life expectancy: Up to 80 years	**Medical $:** 6% to 15%

The advent of a post-industrial **Information Age** is marked by the ubiquitous appearance of the television and the computer. The labor force is concentrated in services rather than agriculture or manufacturing. Information specialists, the dominant workers, spend their entire childhood and many years of adulthood in school investing in the skills required for active participation in a global economy linked by communications networks where massive amounts of capital flow between countries with a few keystrokes. Such training can be prevalent only in a population with long life expectancies and few children per family. In this era, most people are healthy and wealthy enough that personal income affects longevity and fertility primarily through lifestyle choices, rather than lack of food or shelter. What was rare throughout history, the ability to retire with independent means and sufficient fitness to travel the world after age sixty-five, has become not just attainable, but an ordinary reality for most people in post-industrial economies.

U.S. life expectancy was about thirty-five years in 1750, forty-nine years in 1900, rose to sixty-eight years by 1950 and seventy-seven years in 2002. Although people will continue to live longer, incremental years of life expectancy are added at a slower rate as infectious diseases and childhood maladies are removed as major causes of death. More important from a demographic point of view is that almost all the gains in longevity after 1950 occurred for mature adults who had already completed their families. Each generation may live longer, but will not have more babies. Additional increases in life expectancy

FIGURE 16.2	Distribution of Income at Different Stages of Development		
Upper classes	$$$$$	$$	$$$$$$$$
Middle class	$	$$	$$$$$$$	$$$$$$$$$$
Lower classes	$$$$$	$	$$$	$$$$$$$
	Hunter-Gatherer	Agricultural	Industrial	Informational

will not increase the number of children and thus will have no long-run effect on the total size of the population.

During the demographic transition of the industrial age and its final phase, the 1950s baby boom, rapid population increase created expansive economic growth as more houses, roads, and factories were built. However, the rapid expansion due to demographic transition is a one-time occurrence. After transition, population returns to a steady state of slow or zero growth, typically a small natural decrease offset by immigration of people from less-developed countries seeking higher wages. It is important to recognize that the "normal" conditions of industrializing countries from 1770 to 1970 were actually abnormal periods of spectacular but transitory growth. In comparison, the recent era's 1 to 2 percent growth rates can seem inadequate, particularly since most of the added value comes in the less visible form of service improvement and information content, rather than in the number of count-able goods (cars, houses, tons of corn) that are more readily measured in GDP accounts.

Much of the world is still undeveloped, caught somewhere between an agricultural society and the modern information era. A world map shaded to show which nations today still have economies dominated by agriculture is almost identical to a world map showing which nations have the most premature mortality under age thirty.[21] Such nations have the potential for fantastic growth as they industrialize (e.g., Korea, Singapore, Indonesia), but also for tragic population explosions without economic advancement, leading to starvation and social ruin (e.g., Somalia, Rwanda). In a developing country, such as Mexico, the average age of the population is about seventeen, longevity is less than sev-enty years, many people still work on farms, and a sizable fraction still live at the subsis-tence level. Such countries have a tremendous "population momentum." Even if every family immediately limited fertility to the replacement level of 2.2 births, the total popu-lation would still double in size because so many young women have already been born. In the United States, as in most developed countries, the natural population growth is already zero to negative; thus, the increase in population is due to immigration from less developed countries. If current trends continue, almost every country in the world will be developed within a hundred years (by 2100) and have a steady or shrinking population.[22] Total world population will stabilize somewhere between 10 to 20 billion, Mexico City will be much larger than Los Angeles, and food supply will be a trivial health problem com-pared to pollution and congestion (see Figure 16.3).

16.7 INCOME AND HEALTH

The connection between poverty and poor health was noted long ago. The connection is described in ancient Greek and Chinese commentaries, and detailed empirical studies were conducted in London and Paris in the nineteenth century.[23] As economic historians care-fully review the data, it becomes clear that although economic growth may have been the major contributor in lengthening life expectancy, its effects were neither uniform across groups nor steady over time. Average health appears to have declined significantly in the United States during the early decades of the nineteenth century despite rising per capita incomes; therefore, life expectancy was probably not much greater in 1900 than it was in 1800.[24] Most commentators assume that extreme poverty has the most deleterious effects and that the relationship between income and health is nonlinear, with gains in life expectancy becoming smaller as one moves up the income scale (see Figure 17.4). However, the famous "Black Report" on civil service employees in the United Kingdom

FIGURE 16.3   Timeline: Economic History, Population Growth, and Medical Care

	Stone Age	Agricultural Age				Industrial Age			Information Age	
	5 million–10,000 BC	**4000 BC**	**1 AD**	**1200 AD**	**1800 AD**	**1900**	**1950**	**1975**	**2000**	**????**
World population	beginnings to 4 million	8	250	400 million	950	1.6 billion	2.5 billion	4 billion	6 billion	stops @ 20 billion
Rate of growth	*.0007%*	*.01%*	*.09%*	*.04%*	*.14%*	*.52%*	*.88%*	*1.88%*		
(years to double)	*(100,000)*	*(7,000)*	*(800)*	*varies*	*(500)*	*(130)*	*(80)*	*(40)*		
Life expectancy	28 years		24 years			35 years			80 years	
Organization	family/tribe		fief/city/empire			national states			global village?	
Information	oral		written			statistics			electronic	
Economy	hunter-gatherer		farming & harvesting			manufacturing			services	
Incomes	subsistence		rich rulers/subsistence serfs			wages			wages & entitlements	
Equivalent $ per cap	$200		$300			$300 rising to $5,000			$25,000 (developed countries)	
% Spent on food	all		almost all—90%			80% falling to 30%			12%	
Income distribution	roughly equal		highly unequal			mixed			not yet clear	
Type of medicine	witch doctor/shaman		healer priest			empiricist			scientifically trained physicians	
Medical spending	—		? maybe 1%			2% rising to 4%		6%	10%	?

established that, even among high-income people, mortality was lower for those at the very top. In addition, the report established that although the absolute effect got smaller over time as general life expectancy increased, the relative importance of rank did not disappear and perhaps even widened between 1930 and 1981 (Table 16.1).[25] This finding is often viewed as indicating that health insurance cannot reverse the effects of poverty, because this period includes the formation of the National Health Service in the United Kingdom, which provides essentially free medical care for all citizens. Studies of U.S. populations show a similar gradient, with smaller but still significant income effects even at very high income levels.[26]

The relationship between income and health is strong, but the nature of that relationship is far from clear. The Social Security "notch" (some people receive higher retirement incomes because they are born a week earlier than others) provided a natural experiment—which showed that giving people bigger checks did not make them live longer.[27] It is not income per se that makes people healthy, but all the things associated with higher income: more education, better nutrition, social connections, family stability, and so on. Research to determine how greater income is related to better health is just beginning.

Income and the Value of Medical Care

Given the strong relationship between mortality and income, questions have arisen regarding the importance of medical care in increasing life expectancy. Although perhaps hard to believe, it is difficult to demonstrate conclusively that medical care has an independent effect on average life expectancy. One complication is that more and better medical care is usually associated with higher incomes, making the independent effect of medicine harder to disentangle. However, just as the Black Report showed that the formation of the National Health Service did not significantly reduce the differential mortality advantage of high-income persons in the United Kingdom, several studies have shown that the introduction of Medicare in the United States, while bringing the poor nearly equal to the rich in their use of medical services, did not eliminate, or even substantially reduce, the large differential in mortality. Empirically, there is no discernable effect of Medicare on the generally declining trend of mortality in the United States between 1900 and 2000.[28]

Many researchers agree that medical care has had some, but not a large, effect on life expectancy—perhaps attributing 10 percent of the gain from forty-seven years to seventy-seven years during the 20th century to the increased use and effectiveness of medical care. Of course, the gains from medical *science* are much larger, because the advance of medical knowledge is responsible for demonstrating the importance of hand washing, sanitation, smoking cessation, food sterilization, a balanced diet, and a host of other lifestyle factors that contribute to health. It is sometimes difficult to believe that as recently as the 1920s,

TABLE 16.1	Mortality Rates by Social Class, 1931–1981				
Class	**1931**	**1951**	**1961**	**1971**	**1981**
I Professionals	90	86	76	77	66
II Managerial	94	92	81	81	76
III Skilled manual	97	101	100	104	103
IV Semi-skilled	102	104	103	114	116
V Unskilled	111	118	143	137	166

Source: The Black Report (note 25). Standardized Mortality Ratios, Men 15–64, England and Wales, age adjusted: 100 = average mortality rate for that year.

vitamin deficiency disease (pellagra), parasites (hookworm, malaria), and such infections as typhoid, diphtheria, and smallpox were major drains on the vitality of the nation. The importance of science is demonstrated in the mortality trends in Africa during the 1970s and 1980s. There, despite disastrous decades in which dysfunctional governments and economies led to declining per capita income, there were still continued increases in life expectancy and worker productivity due to advances in health science.

16.8 REDUCING UNCERTAINTY: THE VALUE OF LIFE AND ECONOMIC SECURITY

Economic development not only meant that most people had more; it also meant that the risks of losing it all were vastly reduced. For the first time, it was possible and reasonable for ordinary people to plan for the future—to decide how many children to have, whether or not to go to school or start a business, and to save for retirement. The improvements in health and income brought about by economic development had a powerful and paradoxical effect: the more secure the future became, the more afraid workers became of losing that security.

The Value of Risk Reduction

Even if medical care is responsible for only a small incremental improvement in health, the value of that increment is increasing. Consider how the value of reducing the risk of dying in the next ten years by 1 percent changes as workers become more well-off. If the average person has a 50-50 chance of dying in ten years, it is not worth changing the probability to 51-49. Yet if a healthy person has only a 1 percent chance of dying, eliminating this risk, or just cutting it in half, is worth a lot.[29] The value of risk reduction also depends on the level of income. In a subsistence economy where workers get paid only enough to buy food and rudimentary housing, they cannot afford to give up much of what they earn to buy medical care, even if such care would help them avoid future illness and death. On the other hand, a skilled industrial worker earning $40,000 a year can probably afford to pay $300 a month for health insurance and another $100 for vitamin supplements and a health-club membership. A rock star or corporate CEO earning $5 million a year can afford to spend hundreds of thousands of dollars just to keep looking young.

By reviewing a number of studies conducted during the twentieth century, Dora Costa and Matthew Kahn constructed a consistent set of estimates of the value of life (reducing mortality risk) for workers. Valuation increased by thirty-fold, from $427,000 to $12,000,000 in inflation adjusted dollars, during the last one hundred years (Table 16.2).[30] The value of life tends to increase more than proportionately as income rises, since life itself is necessary to enjoy the benefits of having goods. Costa and Kahn estimated that the income elasticity of the value of life is about 1.6 (i.e., a 160 percent increase in value for every 100 percent increase in income), indicating that life itself is a "luxury good" in economists' terms (see Chapter 18, Section 2).

Social Security and Health Insurance

Even though the poor agricultural masses may have been happy to get a chance to stay alive and perhaps get ahead, the industrial middle-class expected progress. If their lives did not constantly improve, or if something went wrong, they expected their employers or the government to do something to correct the problem. Originally, coal miners went underground

TABLE 16.2   Changes in the Value of Life, 1900–2000

Year	Estimated Value of Life (2002 dollars)
1900	$ 427,000
1920	895,000
1940	1,377,000
1950	2,426,000
1960	2,884,000
1970	5,176,000
1980	7,393,000
2000	12,053,000

Source: Dora L. Costa and Matthew E. Kahn (Endnote 29).

to work to get higher wages. They began to demand safe working conditions, compensation for accidents and disability, and retirement plans. As early as 1700, a few English industrialists offered health insurance to their workers. Such employee benefits made the workers loyal to these firms and willing to work harder. The risks of disability and sickness were no longer borne by the workers individually, but by the firm. This sharing of risk reduced the uncertainty and variability of wages to workers (Chapters 4 and 5).

Industrialization and the change to wage labor shifted the distribution of political power. Workers' revolts spread across Europe during the nineteenth century, stretching from Paris in 1798 to Russia in 1917. Economic, legal, and health security were fundamental demands of what became known as "socialism." In 1883, to forestall further labor unrest, Chancellor Bismarck created the first national social security system in Germany, providing pensions to workers over age 65, sick leave, and health insurance.[31] In the United States, private insurance provided by employers became the dominant mode of health care financing in the 1950s. These plans have been supplemented by the government Medicaid program for the poor and Medicare for the elderly. Today 77 percent of all health care spending, and 95 percent of hospital costs, are paid for through third-party financing mechanisms. In 1850, medical care was still largely a personal transaction. Workers paid, or did not pay, for what they thought they could afford, rather like they bought clothes, food or heating oil. Although in less-developed countries, medicine must still rely primarily on personal purchases for financing, pooled financing through government and private insurers has dominated the economic organization of medical care in developed countries since 1960. Now the shape of the health care system is determined by negotiations over benefit packages and government appropriations, not consumers' personal purchasing decisions.

Preconditions for Changing Medical Organization

This chapter began with a list of four preconditions for the development of modern medical care: effective technology, sufficient wealth, low risk of death, and insurance financing. These factors are not independent of each other, but mutually reinforcing. Increasing wealth meant more food, which reduced the risk of dying. Increased longevity also meant greater productivity and hence even more wealth. As trade developed, financial markets increased in complexity and insurance contracts were needed to better manage capital. Broad participation in pooled financing could only occur when most workers were relatively healthy and well-off.

The development of medical technology was the result of an interactive process, requiring advances in biology, chemistry, physics, statistics, and data management. Gaining knowledge and reducing the uncertainty caused by illness takes both science and economics. It is now quite possible that the most commonly used medical instrument is the computer.

16.9 THE RISE OF MEDICAL TECHNOLOGY

Medicine is as old as humankind. One of the earliest-known written documents, the "Code of Hammurabi," contains references to medical price controls and malpractice in the laws of this Assyrian kingdom circa 2200 B.C. The Hippocratic oath, written about 1 B.C. and still quoted in medical writings today, put forth the principle that physicians should "first, do no harm." Good advice, because for thousands of years physicians could do little to cure illness or reduce the risk of death. Despite the vast amount written about medicine, and the great store of practical knowledge transmitted orally in many cultures, this knowledge was largely unsystematic and did not create therapies that made a significant impact on the health of most people.[32] Medical theory, such as it was, usually consisted of a strange mixture of mysticism; serious looks and kind words; some sound advice about eating, sleeping, and getting fresh air; and a few favorite remedies, some of which might sometimes be useful. Hospitals were places where sick or disabled people were housed, and little was expected in the way of treatment. Physicians were counselors who could make someone feel better and preside over the deaths they prognosticated, but could do little to change the course of illness. Many were also priests, and the distinction between morality and medicine was often unclear. Plagues were more likely to be blamed on infidelity or blasphemy than on unseen organisms in the blood.

The change from mysticism and fear to scientific investigation was the defining characteristic of the Enlightenment. Some milestones include the demonstration of proteins in urine by Paracelsus in 1500, the discovery of the microscope and "little worms" (bacteria and protozoans) by Athanasius Kircher in 1569, William Harvey's discovery of the circulation of blood in 1619, and Anton von Leewenhoek's microscopic description of red blood cells in 1668. The growing accumulation of knowledge presaged a form of medical practice that eventually would be able to provide effective treatment against disease. The crucial link, however, was organizational rather than technical; more a matter of changing the way knowledge was collected, used, and transmitted than any particular scientific breakthrough or discovery. The formation of "clinics" in the great hospitals of Paris around 1750 is particularly noteworthy.[33] These clinics were organized by what would now be called specialties: one for the eye, another the hand, another mental illness, and so on. Instead of trying to create a holistic theory that covered all aspects of health, the clinics broke medical problems into component parts. A single doctor would become an expert in diseases of the hand, or the eye, and so on, and then train others. The clinic provided the working classes with access to trained physicians whom they otherwise could not afford. The physician was provided with a large group of compliant patients all suffering similar illness so that he could experiment with new therapies, teach students, and perfect his techniques. Practicing on the masses of poor workers allowed him to charge higher fees to wealthy patients and to collect tuition from students eager to learn the latest advances. The creation of clinics was a success because they provided a social exchange mechanism that yielded gains to both parties.

Organizational innovation was complemented by an intellectual innovation, statistics. Clinic doctors began to count how many people were treated and how many got well. Numerical comparisons of outcomes began to replace doctors' personal assessments.

Determining which treatment was best previously depended mostly on the reputation and experience of the physicians who vouched for it, but now experiments and statistical observation were used. The impact of this new approach to medical science is well illustrated by Edward Jenner's discovery of vaccination for smallpox in 1798. The act of making a healthy person sick (inoculating them with cowpox) to prevent possible future illness is a form of therapy that can only be defended statistically. No single patient feels better or gets cured because of what the doctor does.

Scientific advances accumulated rapidly throughout the latter part of the nineteenth century; Pasteur, Semmelweiss, and Koch determined that bacteria cause anthrax, childbirth fever, tuberculosis, and other infectious diseases; Eijkman discovered vitamins; and Roentgen discovered X-rays. Whereas France was preeminent in the eighteenth century, Germany was arguably the world leader in medical technology by the end of the nineteenth century when Chancellor Bismarck provided the landmark social insurance legislation. American physicians tried to improve the quality of practice in the United States with the Flexner Report of 1910, promoting the "Johns Hopkins model" (actually the German model, but Americans needed a local champion to make it more acceptable). By the end of the 1930s, a license and modern scientific education were required to enter the practice of medicine, and most doctors treated their difficult cases in the hospital using a range of technical devices and nursing support (Chapter 7).

Information systems and access to capital gave hospitals economies of scale and made them necessary adjuncts to medical practice. As modern surgical techniques using anesthesia and antiseptics turned what were formerly warehouses for the sick into technologically sophisticated treatment facilities, written medical records became the locus for storage and communication of test results, diagnostic information, and treatment documentation that linked all the trained medical practitioners together. Florence Nightingale, through her work in military hospitals during the Crimean War and subsequent books, is most often credited with developing the hospital as an organization. Her patients may have seen nurses as "angels of mercy," but she saw them as soldiers gathering intelligence and carrying out orders as part of a grand campaign against disease. As technology became more advanced and specialized, it cost more—too much for individual physicians to purchase on their own. In 1816, Laennec invented the stethoscope to investigate the body, and every doctor bought one. In 1885, Roentgen's X-ray machines peered inside the body, but the equipment was so large and so expensive that most doctors had to join the staff of a hospital to use one. The computed axial tomography (CAT) scan developed in 1973 costs millions of dollars, depends on software that few radiologists understand, and can transmit images through the Internet to be digitally enhanced and read by a specialist thousands of miles away in another country.

Although medicine has been actively practiced since ancient times, only fragmentary technological advances were made until the end of the industrial era. In the eighteenth and nineteenth centuries, scientific discoveries came more and more rapidly, yet there was still little improvement in treatment outcomes. Only after 1900 did effective medicine start to become available, 150 years after the productive expansion that marked the beginning of the industrial age. Between 1900 and 1950, a virtual revolution took place, and medicine became one of society's most valued occupations.

Medical progress resulted more from planned effort and massive public investment than serendipitous discovery or any preordained march of ideas: Florence Nightingale's scientific hospital was supported by kings who wished to cut the cost of putting soldiers into battle; Pasteur's discovery of bacteria was made under contract to the French wine and beer industry; and Walter Reed worked to conquer yellow fever so that construction of the Panama Canal could be completed in tropical jungles. Rising incomes, falling mortality, and commercial organization were more than just contributing factors; they were the central forces driving the demand that created medical technology.

Although all four conditions needed for the development of modern medicine (technology, wealth, low mortality, organized financing) operate concurrently and reinforce each other, medical technology is more a result of the process than a cause. Society's accumulation of the necessary prerequisites for modern medicine began with the rise in wealth brought about by trade and technology, which quickly led to a decline in mortality, and subsequently to a decline in the birth rate. The application of science and industrial technology to medicine not only took time, it took money and an independent profession dedicated to continuous improvement. Both organized medicine, with its schools and professional associations, and organized financing, with insurance risk pooling and government funding, were necessary to carry out that research and pay for years of trial and error as treatments were perfected. The development of integrated health care systems and decentralized contracting will bring medicine to the final stages of the Industrial Revolution's productivity enhancements, and will evolve in new directions to meet the challenges of the information age.[34]

SUGGESTIONS FOR FURTHER READING

Angus Deaton, "Health, Inequality and Economic Development," working paper, Center for Health and Wellbeing, Princeton University, May 2001, (www.wws.princeton.edu/~chw/).

Robert G. Evans, Morris Barer, and Theodore Marmor, *Why Are Some People Healthy and Others Not? The Determinants of Health of Populations* (New York: Aldine De Gruyter, 1994).

Robert W. Fogel, "Economic Growth, Population Theory and Physiology: The Bearing of Long-Term Processes on the Marking of Economic Policy," *American Economic Review* 84, no. 3 (1994): 369–395.

Massimo Livi-Bacci, *A Concise History of World Population* (Cambridge, Mass.: Blackwell, 1992).

Angus Maddison, *The World Economy: A Millennial Perspective* (Paris and Washington D.C.: Organization for Economic Co-operation and Development (OECD), 2001).

Douglass C. North, *Structure and Change in Economic History* (New York: Norton, 1981).

Roy Porter, *The Greatest Benefit of Mankind* (New York: Harper-Collins, 1998).

Mancur Olson Jr., "Big Bills Left on the Sidewalk: Why Some Nations are Rich, and Others Poor," *Journal of Economic Perspectives* 10, no. 2 (1996): 3–24.

James P. Smith, "Healthy Bodies and Thick Wallets: The Dual Relation Between Health and Economic Status," *Journal of Economic Perspectives* 13, no. 2 (Spring 1999): 145–166.

SUMMARY

1. Four conditions must be met for modern medicine to develop:

   a. The risk of dying must be low enough (i.e., **life expectancy** long enough) that spending money to improve health is worthwhile.

   b. People must have **sufficient income** to pay for medical care.

   c. There must be a way to pool funds and **organize financing** for large numbers of people through insurance or government programs.

   d. **Medical technology** must be effective enough at improving health to be worth paying for.

2. **Life expectancy** averaged about twenty-eight years from 10,000 B.C. to 1 A.D., and populations grew slowly, taking 100,000 years to double. From 1 A.D. to 1750, life expectancy averaged twenty-two to twenty-eight years, and population doubled every 1,000 years. From 1750 to 1900, life expectancy averaged thirty to forty-five years, and population doubled every 200 years. Today, life expectancy in the United States is more than seventy years, and the number of births is almost identical to the

number of deaths, making the total population stable. In less-developed countries, life expectancy is still less than fifty years, and population growth is still very rapid, doubling every thirty years.

3. **Demographic transition** involves the movement of the population into cities, a rise in output per capita, a decline in mortality rates followed by a decline in birth rates, concluding with the stable and well-off populations characteristic of a developed country.

4. **Growth in population and increase in life expectancy have been influenced more by economic development than improvements in medical care.**

5. Development has always had some adverse effects (crowding, pollution); however, improvements in nutrition, security, and technology make the overall effect of economic development positive.

6. The dismal hypothesis of Thomas **Malthus** was that any increase in productivity would bring an uncontrolled increase in population, eventually making people worse off as the number of mouths to feed expanded faster than the food supply. While Malthus's analysis provided insight into forces that had previously governed population growth, he did not foresee the rapid and continuous rise in productivity due to the Industrial Revolution, nor did he understand how the newly emerging middle-class families would choose to have fewer children so that they could invest more in their care and education.

7. In the hunter-gatherer economy of the pre-historic Stone Age, no one had much more than basic necessities. In the Agricultural Age, most people lived at a subsistence level, but the rulers controlled vast wealth and made major investments. In the Industrial Age, workers' wages rose rapidly above the subsistence level, economic organization became more complex, and most income was held by a large **middle class.**

8. A 1 percent reduction in mortality is worth more to people with a seventy-year life expectancy than to people with a life expectancy of only twenty-five years. With good salaries and savings, people can afford to pay more to protect their health than could their grandparents, who barely earned enough to eat.

9. The **reduction in uncertainty** brought about by lower mortality and better jobs made it possible for ordinary people to plan for the future. Having a taste of freedom from fear and loss, they wanted more. In time, the demand for insurance and social security became universal.

10. The development of **medical technology** came after the Industrial Revolution was already well advanced. Improvements in the productivity of medicine (ability to actually heal and extend life expectancy) began about 150 years after technological change had begun to raise industrial productivity. While scientific advances are to some extent accidental, **the rate of technological change in medicine is largely determined by the economic resources** devoted to making new discoveries and applying them in practice.

11. The **economic organization** of medical care is rapidly evolving. From pre-historic times until 1900, most care was given by doctors practicing alone as independent practitioners. By 1950, the hospital and an organized medical staff funded through third-party payment were common. By 2020, most care probably will be provided by integrated health care systems with thousands of employees. **The most important medical advances are being brought about by improvements in information technology,** not pills and scalpels.

PROBLEMS

1. *{life expectancy}* What is the current average life expectancy? What was life expectancy one hundred years ago? One thousand years ago? Ten thousand years ago? Is life expectancy likely to increase more rapidly or less rapidly during the next 100 years?

2. *{population growth}* How rapidly is the population growing in the United States? Is population growing more rapidly or less rapidly elsewhere in the world? Was it growing more rapidly or less rapidly one hundred years ago? One thousand years ago?

3. *{population growth, dynamics}* What were the causes of the baby boom? How long did it last? How long will it affect the U.S. economy? Which part of the health care system was (is, will be) most affected?

4. *{population growth}* If the birth rate is 5 percent and the death rate is 3.5 percent, what is the rate of population increase? What life expectancy is consistent with this death rate? The death rate is consistent with a life expectancy of approximately how many years? The birth rate is consistent with approximately what family size? *(hint, family size = number of children per year times number of fertile female years)*

5. *{population growth}* If population is growing 1 percent a year, how long will it take it to double? If it is growing 0.1 percent a year?

6. *{distribution}* Is the distribution of income per capita more equal or less equal now than in the past? Is the distribution of life expectancy more equal or less equal now than in the past?

7. *{life expectancy}* Which has been more influential in raising life expectancy, economic growth or the development of medical technology? What evidence would support your answer? What evidence would contradict your answer? What evidence would support either answer?

8. *{population growth}* What is the Malthusian hypothesis? How did Malthus link population growth to declining marginal productivity?

9. *{population growth}* What are the most common reasons for population declines in the world today? Give examples.

10. *{family dynamics}* Will a family with higher income have more or fewer children? Which other economic factors affect choice of family size?

11. *{demographic transition}* Why do birth rates fall during demographic transition? How can population growth be accelerating if birth rates are declining?

12. *{demographic transition}* Why might death rates rise at the end of demographic transition? Can you give an example of a country where death rates might be rising now for this reason? Would such a situation imply more or less growth in per capita income? Why?

13. *{flow of funds}* Why is the development of a middle class a precondition for the development of medical insurance? Why is insurance necessary for the development of a modern, high-technology medical care system?

14. *{risk}* Does an increase in uncertainty, especially life-threatening uncertainties such as famine and plague, make medical care more or less valuable?

15. {*dynamics*} Did the productivity of medical technology start to increase before or after improvements in the productivity of industrial technology? Why? What determines the rate of technological change in medicine?

16. {*productivity*} Assume that you are writing a science-fiction book that takes place in the year 2050. Which would be more devastating to the health of the world, loss of the drugs that cure HIV/AIDS or loss of computers?

17. {*productivity*} Which has grown more rapidly, the productivity of farmers or the productivity of doctors?

18. {*statistics, productivity*} The application of statistics was necessary to improve productivity in which field: industry, agriculture, or medical care?

19. {*health production*} If the cities were the growing centers of economic opportunity, why did many of the families that moved to the city during the Industrial Revolution experience shorter average life spans than those who remained in the country?

20. {*industrial organization, dynamics*} Was it economic organization, social organization, political organization, medical organization, or technology that lead to the creation of a national medical insurance plan in Germany in 1883?

21. {*distribution*} Does health insurance make income distribution more equal or less equal? Who is favored by such income redistribution? Would a national health plan such as that proposed by President Clinton in 1994 be more redistributive or less redistributive than the current mixed public/private health insurance system in the United States? Which groups were most likely to benefit from the Clinton plan? Which groups were most likely to lose? Who is likely to gain or lose from President Bush's proposals to privatize Medicare?

22. {*distribution*} What is the difference between income and wealth? Which has grown more rapidly in the United States?

23. {*social insurance*} What is the difference between "social security" and "insurance"?

24. {*pricing, productivity, risk*} To whom will a drug that provides a 1 percent increase in ten-year survival be most valuable? List factors that will increase or be ambiguous with regard to the effect of that factor on the market value of such a drug.

ENDNOTES

1. *Mortality* is the death rate, the number of deaths per 100 (or 1,000 or 100,000) persons alive at the beginning of the period. *Morbidity* is the incidence of illness or ill health, the number of cases per 100 (or 1,000 or 100,000) persons. While clearly related to mortality, morbidity should also be clearly distinguished from mortality rates. While it is possible to obtain mortality rates from a variety of sources throughout history and so to create a reliable record, morbidity rates are available only under special circumstances (i.e., epidemics, aboard ships or in school or prison populations) until the advent of routine health surveys in the twentieth century, and are still lacking in many low-income countries with less comprehensive government statistical capabilities.

2. Douglass C. North, *Structure and Change in Economic History* (New York: Norton, 1981).

3. Note that this relationship, death rate = 1/(life expectancy), is a stock/flow equation analogous to the relationship between interest rates and the value of an annuity, interest = coupon/(price of bond), presented in finance texts, and is also rather similar to the stock/flow relationship between medical graduates and physician supply discussed in Chapter 7, Section 3.

4. A rule of thumb for compounding is known as the *"rule of seventy-two."* If you divide seventy-two by the interest rate, it gives the approximate length of time required to double your money. For very small rates of increase, such as those discussed here, a better approximation is to use seventy rather than seventy-two. Thus 70 ÷ 2 = 35 years to double at 2 percent per year, 70 ÷ 0.35 = 200 years to double at 0.35 percent, and

70 ÷ 0.1 = 700 years to double at 0.1 percent rate of growth. This rule is quite accurate for rates less than 5 percent, and can be computed by hand or with a simple calculator until you have time to check the result with a spreadsheet.

5. For a large empirical study of conditions in the Americas, see Richard H. Steckel and Jerome C. Rose, eds., *The BackBone of History: Health And Nutrition in the Western Hemisphere* (Cambridge, UK: Cambridge University Press, 2002). An earlier assessment is found in Mark Nathan Cohen and George J. Amelagos, eds., *Paleopathology at the Origins of Agriculture* (New York: Academic Press, 1984), and a general overview in Mark Nathan Cohen, *Health and the Rise of Civilization* (New Haven: Yale University Press, 1989). It must be recognized that "life expectancy" varied widely (plus or minus ten years or more, even for groups living within a few miles of each other during the same time periods). Hence any comparisons of relative health are only rough indicators subject to many caveats and assumptions. The demographic data in this chapter is drawn largely from the books and articles by Deaton, Fogel, and Livi-Bacci listed among the Suggestions for Further Reading, as well as Wrigley and Schofield (note 16) McKeown (note 32) and McEvedy and Jones (note 9).

6. Theodore Tulchinsky and Elena Varavikova, "Addressing the Epidemiologic Transition in the Former Soviet Union," *American Journal of Public Health* 86, no. 3 (1996): 313–320.

7. Barrie Cassileth, Vasily Vlassov, and Christopher Chapman, "Health Care, Medical Practice, and Medical Ethics in Russia Today," *Journal of the American Medical Association* 273, no. 20)1995): 1569–1573.

8. Johannes Nohl, "The Black Death: A Chronicle of the Plague, Compiled From Contemporary Sources" (London: Unwin Books, 1971); Philip Ziegler, *The Black Death* (New York: John Day Company, 1969).

9. Massimo Livi-Bacci, *A Concise History of World Population* (Cambridge Mass.: Blackwell, 1992), 47, 106; Colin McEvedy and Richard Jones, *Atlas of World Population History* (Middlesex: Penguin, 1978), 25.

10. Massimo Livi-Bacci, *Population and Nutrition* (Cambridge: Cambridge University Press, 1991).

11. Robert Fogel, "Economic Growth, Population Theory and Physiology: The Bearing of Long-term Processes on the Marking of Economic Policy," *American Economic Review* 84, no. 3 (1994): 369–395.

12. Maurice Brown, *Adam Smith's Economics: Its Place in the Development of Economic Thought* (London: Croon Helm, 1988); E. G. West, *Adam Smith and Modern Economics: From Market Behavior to Social Choice, Aldershot, Hants* (England: Edward Elgar Publishing, 1990).

13. Thomas Robert Malthus, *An Essay on the Principle of Population*, 1803, new edition by Patricia James for the Royal Economic Society (Cambridge: Cambridge University Press, 1992).

14. Livi-Bacci (1992), p. 65.

15. Gary D. Hansen and Edward C. Prescott, "Malthus to Solow," *American Economic Review* 92, no. 4 (September 2002): 1205–1217.

16. E. A. Wrigley and R. S. Schofield, *The Population History of England, 1541–1871: A Reconstruction* (Cambridge, Mass.: Harvard University Press, 1981).

17. Gary Becker, *A Treatise on the Family* (Cambridge, Mass.: Harvard University Press, 1981).

18. A surprisingly large number of successful entrepreneurs and inventors go bankrupt several times before and after they strike it rich. Such risk taking is not feasible if two bad years in a row means starvation.

19. Note that the rise of the middle class economy applies only within the small subset of developed countries. For most of the world's population, sharp divisions between rich and poor continued to be the rule. Francois Bourguignon and Christian Morrisson, "Inequality Among World Citizens: 1820-1992," *American Economic Review* 92, no. 4 (September 2002): 727–744.

20. Mancur Olson, Jr. "Big Bills Left on the Sidewalk: Why Some Nations are Rich, and Others Poor," *Journal of Economic Perspectives* 10, no. 2 (1996): 3–24.

21. The World Bank, *World Development Report 1993: Investing in Health* (Oxford: Oxford University Press for the World Bank, 1993), 237.

22. United Nations, *World Population Prospects*, New York (1989); The World Bank, *World Development Report 1986* (Oxford: Oxford University Press, 1986); Livi-Bacci, 199–208.

23. Angus Deaton, "Policy Implications of the Health & Wealth Gradient." *Health Affairs* 21, no. 2 (March 2002): 13–30.

24. Clayne L. Pope, "The Changing View of the Standard-of-Living Question in the United States." *American Economic Review* 83, no. 2 (May 1993): 331–336.

25. "The Black Report," reprinted in *Class and Health*, Richard G. Wilkinson (London: Tavistock, 1986). See also, G.D. Smith, Mel Bartley, and David Blane, "The Black Report on Socioeconomic Inequalities in Health 10 Years On." *British Medical Journal* 301 (August 18, 1990): 373–377.

26. E. Rogot et al., *A Mortality Study of 1.3 Million Persons by Demographic, Social and Economic Factors: 1979-1985 Follow-Up* (Bethesda, Md.: National Institutes of Health, 1992); P. McDonough et al., "Income Dynamics and Adult Mortality in the United States, 1972 through 1989," *American Journal of Public Health* 87, no. 9 (September 1997): 1476–1483; Angus Deaton, "Health, Inequality and Economic Development," *Journal of Economic Literature* XLI (March 2003): 113–158.

27. Stephen E. Snyder and Wiliam N. Evans, "The Impact of Income on Mortality: Evidence from the Social Security Notch," NBER working paper 9197 (September 2002),(www.nber.org).

28 Angus Deaton and Christina Paxson, "Mortality, Income and Income Inequality over time in Britain and the United States," Working paper, Center for Health and Wellbeing, Princeton University (August 2001), (www.wws.princeton.edu/~chw/); William H. Dow, "Introduction of Medicare: Effects on Elderly Health," presented at American Economic Association Annual Meetings, Washington, D.C., January 4, 2003.

29. The value of risk reduction is also high at the other extreme, where a person faces near certain death. If you knew that otherwise you would die, you might well be willing to give up half of your money for just a 1 percent chance of continuing to live.

30. Dora L Costa and Matthew E. Kahn, "Changes in the Value of Life, 1940–1980," NBER working paper 9396 (December 2002), (www.nber.org); and "The Rising Price of Non-Market Goods," paper presented at the American Economic Association Annual Meetings, Washington, D.C., January 4, 2003.

31. Isidore S. Falk, *Security Against Sickness* (New York: Doubleday, 1936); Jesse George Crownheart, *Sickness Insurance in Europe* (Madison, Wisc: Democrat Printing Company, 1938).

32. Thomas McKeown, *The Modern Rise of Population* (London: Edward Arnold, 1976).

33. Michel Foucault, *The Birth of the Clinic* (New York: Pantheon Books, 1973).

34. Institute of Medicine, *Crossing the Quality Chasm* (Washington, D.C.: National Academy Press: , July 2001), (www.nap.edu/books/0309072808html).

CHAPTER 17

INTERNATIONAL COMPARISONS OF HEALTH AND HEALTH EXPENDITURES

QUESTIONS

1. In which aspect of the health care system is there more trade between countries: goods, services, people, or ideas?

2. Is health care trade more or less international than other goods and services?

3. Which country has the largest health care market?

4. Are the differences among countries larger in terms of doctor supply, hospital technology, or per capita spending?

5. Is it high income or high medical expenditures that makes wealthy countries more healthy?

6. Does the distribution of income within a country determine the distribution of health?

17.1 WIDE DIFFERENCES AMONG NATIONS

There were more than 6 billion people in the world in 2002, distributed across some 200 countries. Health care expenditures for these 6 billion people totaled $3.5 trillion that year.[1] The 285 million people living in the United States represented 5 percent of the worldwide total, but U.S. health care expenditures, $1.5 trillion, accounted for more than 40 percent of total spending. Although China was the world's largest country, with 1.3 billion people, it accounted for less than $0.3 trillion in health care spending. Health expenditures per person in the United States were 10 times the worldwide average in 2002, twice as much as the $2,009 per person spent in Japan, and 20 times the per person average of $45 (approximately $205 in international purchasing power parity [PPP] exchange rates) in China (see Table 17.1).[2] The extra $1,200 billion purchased a lot more hospitals, physicians, drugs, and technologically sophisticated equipment for U.S. citizens. But how many additional years of life, how much reduction in morbidity and mortality, did all these extra medical inputs yield? Could the United States have done as well, or become even more

TABLE 17.1 Comparison of Health and Expenditures Across Nations, 2002

	Population (millions)	Growth % Rate	Life Expectancy	% Age 60+	Mortality Under 5	Mortality (15–59)	GNP (per capita)	GNP (ppp)	% Urban	% Agr.	Health % of GNP	Expenditures (international $)	% Govt.	Private	Out-of-Pocket	Prepaid Plans
World	6,122	1.6	65.1	9.8	.064	.247	$ 4,890	$ 6,490	46	4	5.7	$ 573	.62	.38	.32	.08
Sudan	32	2.3	55.9	5.5			330	1,298	??	??	4.7	51	.21	.79	.79	.00
Kenya	31	2.5	48.9	4.2	.114	.537	360	975	32	27	8.3	115	.22	.78	.56	.05
Pakistan	145	2.6	61.3	5.8	.110	.216	470	1,757	36	26	4.1	76	.23	.77	.77	.00
India	1,025	1.8	60.8	7.7	.094	.257	450	2,149	28	28	4.9	71	.18	.82	.82	.00
China	1,292	0.9	71.2	10.0	.037	.132	780	3,291	32	17	5.3	205	.37	.63	.60	.00
Turkey	68	1.7	69.0	8.5	.043	.162	2,900	6,126	74	18	5.0	323	.71	.29	.29	.00
Mexico	100	1.7	74.2	7.1	.030	.140	4,400	7,719	74	5	5.4	483	.46	.54	.50	.04
Poland	39	0.1	74.0	16.6	.009	.150	3,960	7,894	65	4	6.0	578	.70	.30	.26	.00
U.K.	60	0.3	77.5	20.7	.007	.089	22,640	20,883	89	1	7.3	1,774	.81	.19	.11	.17
Canada	31	1.0	79.3	16.9	.006	.079	19,320	23,725	77	2	9.1	2,534	.72	.28	.16	.71
Japan	127	0.3	81.4	23.8	.005	.072	32,230	24,041	79	2	7.8	2,009	.77	.23	.19	.01
Germany	82	0.3	78.2	23.7	.005	.091	25,350	22,404	87	1	10.6	2,754	.75	.25	.11	.50
U.S.A.	285	1.1	77.0	16.2	.008	.114	30,600	30,600	77	2	13.0	4,499	.44	.56	.15	.63

Source: World Health Report 2002, World Bank Development Report 2000.

healthy, while spending less? Many factors other than hospitals and doctors are responsible for differences in health among China, the United States, and other countries, but $1,200 billion is a significant amount to spend on health care.

Any assessment of health economy across the world must take into account the tremendous diversity in population, economic growth, and health status. Mozambique, Tanzania, and Ethiopia are among the world's poorest countries. These predominantly rural countries depend on subsistence agriculture and have limited government, little accumulation of savings or investment, per capita incomes of less than $500, and rapidly expanding populations facing repeated threats from starvation. One out of ten children die before age five, and life expectancy is less than sixty years. At the other extreme are Sweden and Switzerland, whose urbane citizens enjoy incomes of more than $30,000, where most deaths occur after age seventy-five, and where average life expectancy exceeds 78 years. Development economists categorize countries as low, middle, or high income. More than half the world's population still lives in low-income, rural agricultural countries. Most countries in Africa are toward the bottom of the distribution. The two undeveloped giants, China and India, have 1.292 and 1.025 billion people, respectively. China's recent rapid development could, if maintained, transform the economy within twenty years. Middle-income countries ($1,500 to $7,500 per capita income), in which 1.5 billion people live, include many Latin American countries; most of the formerly socialist countries of the former Soviet Union and Eastern Europe; South Africa, Saudi Arabia, and other oil-rich states of the Middle East; and Asian countries with emerging economies such as Korea. High-income countries ($10,000 per capita income), in which 850 million people live, include Western European countries and the United States, Canada, Japan, Australia, and New Zealand

A nation's health resources generally increase with income, while the extent of illness and need for medical care is reduced. The high-income countries had 2.5 doctors and 8.3 hospital beds per 1,000 people in 1990 (1990 statistics used to enable greater range of international comparisons).[3] The average life expectancy was seventy-eight years, with more than half of all deaths occurring after that age. The perinatal mortality rate was nine per 1,000 births, and the rate of tuberculosis (TB) infection was 0.2 per 1,000. In contrast, the low-income countries of sub-Saharan Africa could afford to spend only $12 per person on health care and had just 0.1 doctors and 1.4 hospital beds per 1,000 people. Life expectancy averaged fifty-two years, the perinatal mortality rate was sixty-eight per 1,000 births, half of all deaths occurred in children under age six, and the TB infection rate was 2.20 per 1,000.

Size of the Market

From the perspective of the marketing department of a profit-maximizing health care firm, the importance of a country is determined not by the number of people, illnesses treated, or unmet needs, but by the number of dollars spent there. In these terms, the United States is by far the largest market in the world, with a 42 percent share. In contrast, the world's most populous country, China, has only a 7 percent share, and the second most populous, India, has only a 2 percent share. In dollar terms, China's market is roughly the same size as the state of Ohio. All of the very-low-income countries together, 2.5 billion people, account for less than 2 percent of the world's health care spending (about one-third as much as the state of California) (see Figure 17.1).

The disparity in health resources is not as great as the disparity in health spending because wages are lower in low-income countries; therefore, 75 percent less health care spending usually translates into a somewhat less severe reduction in the number of doctors

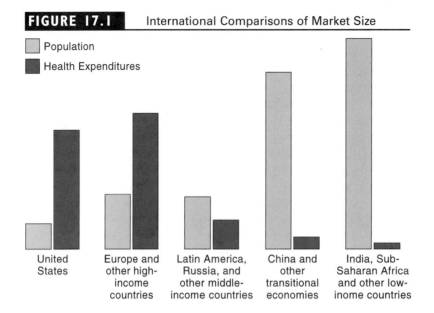

FIGURE 17.1 International Comparisons of Market Size

or nurses.[4] Still, the gap between high-income and low-income countries is substantial (see Table 17.1). Some goods, such as pharmaceuticals, are traded internationally, and their prices are somewhat consistent across countries; thus, any decline in spending causes an equivalent decline in usage. Such internationally traded items take a much larger portion of health care budgets in low-income countries (25 to 50 percent) than in high-income countries (5 to 15 percent). There are vast disparities between rich and poor. Haves and have-nots face such different choices that they almost seem like inhabitants of different planets or different centuries. What is common and readily accessible to most citizens of high-income countries are the favored privileges of a few government officials, industrialists, and celebrities in low-income countries. Medical care as practiced in the developed world is but a dream, as distant as Hollywood for most of the world's population.

17.2 MICRO VERSUS MACRO ALLOCATION: HEALTH AS A NATIONAL LUXURY GOOD

Economists call entertainment, travel, and other expenditures "luxury goods," not as a judgment regarding the necessity or importance of such items, but because they observe that the percentage of income spent on these goods increases as income increases. Items for which a 10 percent increase in income leads to a greater than 10 percent increase in spending (i.e., income elasticity > 1.0) are labeled luxury goods, regardless of their use. Differences in relative wages between countries may complicate dollar comparisons, but a country that spends 12 percent of its gross domestic product (GDP) on health care is using more of its resources for medical care than a country spending 8 percent.[5]

Nations spend more money on health care because they have more money to spend, not because they have greater medical needs. This conclusion is not very surprising when considering whether Bangladesh (GDP $400 per capita) will spend more or less than Belgium (GDP $24,000 per capita) on health (see Figure 17.2). Yet the finding that health care

FIGURE 17.2   Health Expenditures Related to Income

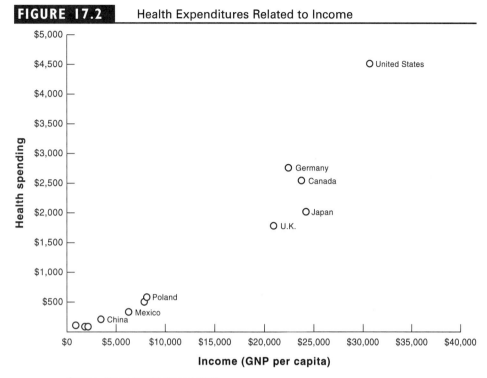

Source: World Health Report 2002.

spending is unrelated or inverse to medical needs contradicts most personal experience—individuals spend more on health care if they become sick. Decisions on how much will be spent by or for a particular individual (micro) are significantly different from, and based on different factors than, national decisions made collectively through the political process about how much of the budget or GDP should be spent on health (macro). Health expenditures come mostly from pooled funds raised through taxes and employee benefit plans. Given that pooled set of funds, decisions will be made about how to spend these funds on a covered individual based on personal medical need. Insurance and government financing are ways to make sure that a person's ability to pay does not limit the care they receive when they need it. Yet collectively, the ability of all to pay, their aggregate prior contributions in taxes and insurance premiums, puts an absolute limit on how much can be spent in total on all the individuals treated. As the focus shifts from micro to macro allocation, the significant determinant of spending shifts from "medical need" to "available income" (see Figure 17.3). For example, most countries spend two to five times as much on elderly people as they do on young and middle-aged people. However, this does not mean that if a country's population is older it will spend more on health care (take it to the limit and suppose everyone were old and retired—who, then, would be working to pay for the extra nursing homes, hip replacements, and heart medications?).[6] As shown in Table 17.1, England has an older population than the United States and health statistics that are roughly equivalent on many measures (life expectancy 77.5 years versus 77.0 years, infant mortality 7 percent versus 8 percent), but England spends significantly less on health care on average ($1,774 versus $4,499), largely because per capita income is lower ($22,640 versus $30,600).[7]

FIGURE 17.3 Micro and Macro Determinants of Health Spending

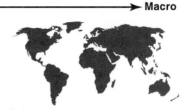

Micro ◄──────────────────────────────► Macro

Health status

Individual differences
in medical spending
are determined mostly
by differences in health
status, i.e., whether or
not the person is sick

GDP per capita

National differences
in spending per person
are largely determined
by differences in income.

17.3 CAUSALITY: DOES MORE SPENDING IMPROVE HEALTH?

Wealthier countries are healthier, and they spend more on medical care. Can one then conclude that more spending buys better health? Not necessarily. Many factors associated with higher incomes, such as education, nutrition, and sanitation, are also known to improve health (see Chapter 16). Furthermore, life expectancy has increased greatly in many poor countries over the past twenty years, even when the availability of doctors and GDP per capita declined. A full assessment of all the influences on health status and relative contribution of each factor is not possible, but a rough appraisal of the relative importance of *economic growth,* advances in *public health and medical research,* and the *use of medical care services* can be made. However, it must be recognized that all these influences interact with and modify one another. With no knowledge of what to do, money is worthless, and medical knowledge alone is useless in the face of extreme poverty, which leads to death from starvation. Any specific estimate of how much each factor contributes to health is to some extent artificial and is also limited to what can readily be observed (i.e., differences noticeable within the range covered by statistics, such as those presented in Table 17.1). Perusal of data from many countries indicates that only large differences, increases of ten-fold or hundred-fold, consistently affect health outcomes. Income differences on the order of 50 percent or 100 percent are not reliably associated with increases or decreases in life expectancy and appear to be within a range of indifference, minor variation, or measurement error. Hence, they should either be treated with caution or ignored. It is the big picture that matters in this appraisal of relative importance.

Figure 17.4 illustrates that there is a relationship between per capita income and average life expectancy, and that the relationship has changed over time. A plausible interpretation is that movements along the curve reflect the combined effects of more income and more medical care, while the shifting of the curve reflects the universal effect of increased knowledge, which is a public good. Between 1960 and 1990, life expectancy in Africa increased by about ten years, from 43 to 52, despite the lack of improvement in living standards or incomes. Another piece of evidence for the effect of knowledge on health is provided by studies of childhood mortality in the United States around 1900.[8] In that era, children of well-to-do physicians were just as likely to die before age five as children of poor laborers living in tenements, since both the wealthy and the poor used the same ineffectual health practices. As the importance of infection and nutrition were revealed, physicians'

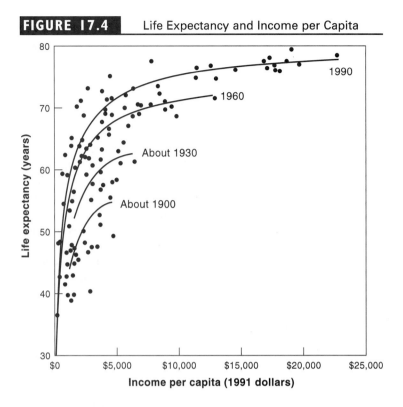

FIGURE 17.4   Life Expectancy and Income per Capita

families were able to take advantage of their better education and resources so that child mortality declined much more rapidly in this group than among low-income laborers. In poor countries today, sanitation, basic nutrition supplements for infants, and control of preventable disease are still of primary importance. In these situations, studies have indicated that maternal education and literacy is often more important than income in preventing childhood disease and death.

Separate assessment of the effects of living standards and utilization of medical care is difficult because both generally rise or fall together. Japan, for example, has achieved a phenomenal twenty-five-year increase in life expectancy since World War II, but there is no easy way to determine how much is due to the rapid economic growth and how much is due to the deployment of modern medical care. The achievement of relatively high life expectancies in some low- or middle-income countries with relatively low use of sophisticated medical treatments (72 years in Malaysia, 75 years in the Czech Republic, 76 years in Costa Rica) suggests that the incremental effect of medical care alone is probably modest. Analysis across many countries reveals that the absolute level of income may not be as important in many cases as **income distribution.**[9] It is not surprising that where there is greater equality of income, the average level of health is higher. The relationship between income and health is nonlinear. A 20 percent drop means much less at the middle or top of the distribution than it does toward the bottom. High rates of illness are a function not of poverty, but of extreme deprivation. The greater the degree of inequality, the more likely it is that some families will be so lacking in food and amenities that deaths from infantile diarrhea, tuberculosis, and other preventable or treatable illnesses occur.

17.4 LOW-INCOME COUNTRIES

Low-income countries face very different health care problems from wealthy, industrialized countries. Their populations are rural, with many children, and a heavy burden of infectious disease and stunting (abnormally low height and/or small body size) due to occasional malnutrition. However, government officials living in the capital have incomes, tastes, and health care needs much more like those of developed countries. This can lead to a major misallocation of resources, such as building a modern research hospital in the capital providing excellent **tertiary care,** while much of the country lacks access to a doctor or a nurse and children remain unvaccinated so that preventable disease epidemics remain common. It is not unusual for as much as half the entire health budget of a low-income country to be spent in the capital city, with a large part going to equip and staff the leading hospital (in contrast, the Johns Hopkins University Hospital takes about 0.6 percent of the U.S. health care budget). Convincing local medical leaders to change the allocation of resources to a more appropriate emphasis on low-technology primary care is difficult, since they do not wish to give up their expensive research hospital, which might bring the doctors and government officials prestige and international fame. The world may admire a European doctor trained at a leading university who spends years alone treating cases in an isolated river village, but a local physician who spends his days treating diarrhea and wound infections without any chance to practice in a modern surgical facility is simply considered to have minimal skills of little importance to outsiders. Incentives are not aligned with the health needs of the majority of citizens. Both ruling politicians and leaders of the medical profession will naturally tend to favor maintaining a state-of-the-art facility with modern technology and capability for research, even when doing so drains funds from the village clinics and nursing care that can do more to reduce infant mortality and raise life expectancy. Even in very-low-income countries, medical schools train many specialists who want to perform technologically advanced procedures rather than primary care generalists able to treat most common illnesses.

Studies by the World Bank have found that the status of women is a major determinant of health in low-income countries. Access to knowledge is one factor. In countries where most women are illiterate and uneducated, there is no way for them to know about sterilization of water, proper nutrition, or care of childhood infections. Women are also more likely than men to make family health a priority. In subsistence economies where women have some control over spending (because of tradition or because they have a job with wages), a larger fraction of the household budget gets spent on food and less on alcohol and tobacco.

Starvation remains a problem in many of the lowest-income countries. In Nigeria, 43 percent of children aged two to six are stunted (low height for age), 32 percent in Kenya and 65 percent in India, compared with 22 percent in Mexico, 4 percent in Japan, and 2 percent in the United Kingdom and United States.[10] This situation occurs not because food supply is insufficient, but because the supply is maldistributed. Organizational disarray, lack of transport, disruptions due to war and political upheaval, and poorly functioning markets mean that food does not get to where it is needed most. No simple solution presents itself, since the defects in economic organization that cause mismanagement of food are the same as those responsible for a lack of economic development in the first place. National governments that maintain order, handle their budgets and money supply prudently, and support market-oriented policies are able to grow out of the low-income category.

Sudan

Sudan* is a low-income, highly indebted poor country on the northeastern coast of sub-Saharan Africa. Sudan's population of 32 million people is spread out over 2.5 million square kilometers and is growing rapidly at a rate of 2.9 percent a year despite desperate poverty. Per capita income is estimated at $330 for 2001. As has been the case in most African countries, the public health system was the main provider of health care services, employing physicians, nurses, pharmacists, and paramedical and other support staff on a salary scale comparable to the public service salary scale. Physicians and facilities were over-concentrated in urban areas, although indicators point to the rural areas as being the most in need. Taxation was historically the primary source of funding, with all premises and equipment owned and maintained by the government.

Although historically services were offered free of charge at the time of use, economic retrenchments and severe natural and man-made disasters, including floods, droughts, and armed conflict in the southern part of the country, have caused serious dislocations in the national health system. The promise of free health services for all citizens became increasingly hollow as inadequate budgets left buildings, equipment, and professional time of salaried health personnel seriously underutilized. Economic waste was further aggravated by purchases of capital equipment, building materials, and medical staff training using scarce foreign exchange. Spending on social services in general and on health in particular was low and declined during the 1980s and 1990s. In times of financial stringency, the obligations to pay salaries and rent, and to pay for maintenance and replenishment of assets frequently used by physicians (e.g., cars, stethoscopes), are given priority, making the impact of reduced spending on services even more severe than the financial figures alone indicate.

The adverse economic situation since the 1980s has had a great impact on health services, health status, and funding. The private sector in medical care witnessed a qualitative and quantitative expansion. Traditionally the private sector was restricted to after-hours consultations by government-employed doctors during their free time in the evening. But more doctors have converted to full private practice, and private inpatient hospitals are being built. A World Health Organization (WHO) consultant estimated that the central government spent $2.50 per person on health care in 2002, about 0.065 percent of GDP.[11] Most total health spending, 62 percent, comes from fees paid by private households, 17 percent from the compulsory National Health Insurance Scheme, 19 percent from ministry of health and other central government ministries, and 2 percent from international organizations (mainly WHO and United Nations Children's Fund [UNICEF]). Other sources of financing for health services include small company-based health insurance schemes, humanitarian national and international nongovernmental organizations, and private expenditures on traditional healers. Because most of the public and private health facilities and personnel are concentrated in urban areas, the actual coverage by health services is expected to be very low. By law the health insurance scheme is supposed to cover all employees of public and private enterprises that employ at least 10 people, but currently this plan covers only 6 percent of the population.

People who can afford to use the current fee-based health services system more tend to benefit most. Reliance on private funds has increased inequity. With less public funding, many individuals wait until their illness reaches a serious stage before contacting the health services system. There is less spending on routine care and prevention and more on

---

*This section on Sudan was contributed by Muneef Abdelbagi Babiker, Assistant Professor, Department of Economics, University of Khartoum.

catastrophic events. The trend toward privatization has even encroached on public health services. In Khartoum, the upkeep of a number of previously unattended, filthy, and deserted public lavatories attached to mosques, market areas, bus stops, and other public areas have been contracted to private individuals or institutions. The average annual rents for a lavatory unit are 615,000 Sudanese dinars (approximately $2,460). The contractors can charge a small fee ranging between 10-20 dinars (4-8 cents) for every episode of use. Although no formal study has been conducted to evaluate this privatization experiment, a limited survey revealed that contractors and users were satisfied. This, along with the fact that these arrangements have been functioning since 1995 and that more units are being constructed, indicates success.

Health Care in Kenya

The economy of Kenya is dominated by agriculture. Its most significant exports are coffee, tea, cotton, and minerals. Kenya's 24 million people had a per capita income of about $340 in 1990. Income is much more difficult to measure or define in a traditional agricultural economy; therefore, any figure should be considered approximate. The population is growing very rapidly (3.8 percent per year), with almost half under the age of 15. Enrollment of children in primary school is 88 percent, and more than half of all adults are literate. About a quarter of the population lives in cities. The single-party KANU government, in power since 1963, is relatively stable for such a poor country. Life expectancy, 59 years, is among the highest in sub-Saharan Africa. However, half of all deaths occur in children under the age of 15, and adults are about three times as likely to die in any given year as they are in the United States.

The health system is split almost equally between the public and private sector (see Table 17.2). The Ministry of Health runs 80 hospitals, 41 district health centers in the provinces, 178 rural health centers, and about 1,200 sub-centers and dispensaries. District medical officers are physicians, usually assisted by one or more nurses and a hospital secretary (administrator).[12] Below the district level, most facilities are operated by paraprofessionals, and at the dispensary level, by community workers or untrained auxiliaries. Despite a stated emphasis on primary care and rural development, more than 35 percent of the entire national budget is spent on the showcase Kenya National Hospital in Nairobi. Some government agencies, such as the Ministry of Transport and the Coffee Board, run health services for their workers, as do the dozen or so corporations with more than 500 employees.

Religious missions are a very important part of the health care system, running 40 hospitals, 84 health centers, and 173 clinics. Although the origins and management of these facilities are religious, 60 percent of their funding comes from patient fees, about 25 percent from government subsidy, and only 15 percent from donations. Thus, they are considered part of the private sector. Overall, about 22 percent of Kenyan health expenditures are derived from foreign aid.

The government actively encourages private sector health care. Private hospitals, supported entirely by fees, are viewed as being of higher quality and are growing rapidly. The government runs a National Hospital Insurance Fund for high-income workers through a mandatory 2-percent wage tax (there is no employer contribution) designed to reimburse people for stays in private and religious hospitals or private rooms of public hospitals. However, this plan covers only 12 percent of the population. The effectiveness of the plan may be further limited by its low payout rate: only 60 percent of the hospital insurance premiums collected were used to pay claims or administrative expenses, allowing 40 percent to be held by the central government.

TABLE 17.2	Health Expenditures in Kenya, 1990	
	$ Millions	**Percentage**
Government		
Ministry of health	204	42%
Municipalities	27	6%
Other government	6	1%
Private Sources		
Voluntary agencies	6	1%
Religious missions	28	6%
Corporate clinics	2	*
Household spending		
Hospitals	45	9%
Physicians & healers	36	7%
Drugs	114	24%
Other	16	3%
Total	484	approximately $20 per person

Source: The World Bank Development Report 1993, and Bloom et al., 1986.

Most physicians (70 percent) work full time in private practice. The 30 percent who work for the government or missions also engage in private practice after clinic hours. There are, perhaps, 2,000 physicians actively in practice in Kenya, almost half of them in Nairobi (although it has only 7 percent of the nation's population). In contrast, there are about 19,000 traditional healers and herbalists practicing in Kenya, most of them in the countryside. A physician earns roughly thirty times as much as a traditional healer. A small fraction of the population, the 2 or 3 percent who belong to upper-income families living in the major cities, accounts for more than half of all private expenditures for medical care. About one-third comes from the 10 percent who are middle-income city dwellers. The poor who have flocked to the cities account for less than 2 percent of private spending, and the bulk of the population still living in rural areas (about 75 percent) accounts for just 17 percent of private expenditures. The flow of medical resources clearly follows the flow of funds. The disparity between members of the elite who live in the capital and the vast rural population that subsists by farming is clearly visible in morbidity and mortality statistics, and remains the largest problem facing health care in Kenya.

17.5 MIDDLE-INCOME COUNTRIES

Turkey, Mexico, Thailand, and South Korea are examples of countries that are in the process of industrialization. Subsistence agriculture and poverty is still the norm in the remote rural regions, but the bulk of the population has moved into cities and works for wages. The shift from rural agricultural labor to urban wage labor presents a major organizational problem: how to develop a comprehensive health insurance system able to fund a higher level of health care. Rapid economic growth allows some countries to expand government services; thus, a predominantly public system is created. In other countries, such as Korea, a strong tradition of industrial paternalism leads to private insurance based on employment benefits. Some countries began with a public system and switched to reliance on the private sector, while others are moving in the opposite direction. In almost every middle-income developing country the health insurance system is in transition. Even when coverage is universal by law, the reality is that access to medical care is very uneven. The urban ghettos and impoverished rural villages frequently lack sanitation. Restrictions and incompleteness in the health insurance system may prevent poor citizens from using medical facilities even when these facilities are accessible geographically. Thus, the disadvantaged populations are disproportionately represented in morbidity and mortality statistics. At the same time, expanding incomes have brought the lifestyle illnesses of the wealthy countries, such as heart disease and lung cancer, to prominence. The growth markets for cigarettes in the twenty-first century are China, India, and Asia, not Europe and North America. Finally, the middle-income countries are still likely to misallocate resources, emulating the advanced health care systems of high-income nations: large research hospitals in the cities matched by a lack of village clinics in the countryside and the training of too many specialists and not enough primary care physicians or public health experts.

The Health Care System of Mexico

With a 2001 per capita GDP of $6,200, an average life expectancy of seventy-three years for males and seventy-eight years for females, and a young population (34 percent under age fifteen) of 101 million that is growing rapidly (1.4 percent per year), Mexico is similar to many other countries with transitional economies.* The bulk of the people have moved off the farms into cities to find industrial and service jobs, but agriculture and export of raw commodities still make up a substantial part of the economy, and illiteracy is still a problem in rural areas. The government is politically stable, with a new party coming to power in 2000, shifting away from eighty years of single-party rule to a more open, multiparty democracy.

The government enacted a comprehensive social security system (IMSS, in 1943) relatively early for a transitional economy, but it only covered industrial workers and their dependents.[13] A nationwide network of IMSS health centers, polyclinics, and hospitals was built. The Ministry of Health and IMSS-Solidaridad provide services for around 40 million uninsured Mexicans, mainly the rural and urban poor. In 1960, a plan for government employees, ISSSTE, was established, and a modern and technologically sophisticated network of hospitals and clinics was built with generous funding to accommodate this favored group of employees. ISSSTE, IMSS, and the medical services for the armed forces and employees of the national oil company (PEMEX) provided the top tier of health insurance, and covered about half the population (see Table 17.3).

The organization of services is rigidly segregated, and quality is considerably heterogeneous. The Ministry of Health, IMSS, and ISSSTE provide primary, secondary, and tertiary services, with specialty services concentrated in the three largest cities; Mexico City, Guadalajara and Monterrey. The private market provides services both at the bottom of the income distribution (where SSA is inadequate) and at the top (where wealthier people can buy state-of-the-art medical care), with the middle occupied by three separate tiers of public care. The private sector consists of providers working in hospitals, clinics, offices, and folk medicine units on a for-profit basis. In theory, this component should provide services for around 10 percent of the population. However, according to recent surveys, around 25 per cent of the people enrolled in social security agencies report a private provider as their usual source of ambulatory care. In the same

---

* This section was revised by Julio Frenk, M.D., Ph.D., Minister of Health, and Octavio Gomez, M.D.

TABLE 17.3	Health Insurance Coverage in Mexico	
Mexican Institute of Social Security (IMSS)		39%
Institute for Governmental Workers (ISSSTE)		8%
Other federal agency health plans		2%
Secretariat of Health & Welfare (SSA)		21%
Marginal families program		13%
Private medical care		5%
Unprotected population		12%

Source: Milton Roemer, *National Health Systems of the World*, 1991.

vein, around 40 per cent of the uninsured population report a private practitioner as their usual source of primary care.

Most physicians in Mexico work in salaried positions for ISSSTE, IMSS, or SSA and also have a private practice as well. Yet even though Mexico has considerably fewer physicians per 100,000 population than in the United States (about one-fourth as many), there is a large pool of unemployed or under-employed physicians (more than 30 percent of all physicians) who cannot find a government job or attract enough private patients to make a living from medicine.

The present administration has identified three main challenges for the Mexican health system: equity, quality, and financial protection. To meet them, three basic initiatives have been implemented: (1) programs to confront the backlog of common infections and reproductive health problems that mostly affect the poor, (2) a major initiative to improve the quality of care both in the public and private sectors, and (3) an ambitious effort to provide universal health insurance. The universal health insurance program will provide regular access to quality care and financial protection to almost 40 million Mexicans who are presently uninsured. Relative to that in other transitional economies, the health care system in Mexico seems to work reasonably well. Yet glaring deficiencies in finance (the per capita expenditure in Mexico is below the Latin American average) and in organization (lack of coordination and production efficiency) remain.

Poland

Poland* has 39 million people, with an average per capita income of $8,200 and a life expectancy of sixty-nine years for males and seventy-eight years for females. There are about twenty-two doctors, forty-nine nurses, and fifty hospital beds per 10,000 people. Total expenses for health care in Poland were about $540 per capita (6.6 percent of GDP) in 2002.[14] The main sources of financing are public sickness funds (Kasy Chorych), but private resources have recently grown to contribute almost 40 percent. Since 1999, social insurance funds have accounted for 80 percent of public resources. Insurance is mandatory for all workers. The amount of the premium (7.5 percent of wages) is established by Parliament as a part of personal income tax. Employers do not finance the premiums, but withhold the amount from wages and submit them for collection by a nationwide public agency. The government pays premiums for about 35 percent of the citizens (farmers, the unemployed, people collecting social security payments). Administrative information systems have many weak points; thus, these estimates must be used with caution. Payments

* This section was contributed by Katarzyna Tymowska, Director of Postgraduate Study in Health Economics, Warsaw University.

between sickness funds are equalized to account for differences in participants' income and ages. The sickness funds practice cost control by establishing rates and limiting the number of services. However, administrative inefficiencies and the difficulty of enforcing agreements mean that budget limits are frequently broken. Hospital services accounted for approximately 50 percent of the total expenditures of public funds in 2002. Cost shifting also takes place. Teaching hospitals receive financial resources for research from a special quasi-budget fund and from pharmaceutical company grants. Part of these resources covers expenses for patients' treatment. Thanks to the extra funding, quality of care rises, which attracts good physicians and more patients. Due to the lack of standards, these specialized hospitals also admit patients with minor health problems.

Pharmaceuticals account for one-third of total health expenditures. The percentage is high not only because drug consumption is high, but also due to the relatively low cost of medical staff. Half of households' private expenditures for health are for buying pharmaceuticals. Drug expenses, both public and private, have increased considerably during recent years. Among the causes are the elimination of the state monopoly in the drug market, intensive marketing by pharmaceutical companies, and the strong belief of many Poles in the efficacy of expensive drugs produced by foreign companies. Hospital managers have responded to the squeeze caused by rising drug expenditures and limited budgets by introducing standardized pharmacological procedures and prescription books and requiring approvals by the head of a hospital unit to order expensive drugs.

In Poland, co-payment for services is unimportant. Because patients incur few charges, services are overused (moral hazard). However, there exists a culturally conditioned custom of giving gifts to facilitate access to services or obtain greater kindness from hospital employees. Such informal gratuities constituted 36 percent of private out-of-pocket health spending in a recent study.

Private resources are of increasing importance in Poland. Earnings are going up, educational levels are rising, and social expectations regarding easy access to health care (and to higher-quality care) are escalating. Medical services have become consumption goods, which has encouraged development of private medical companies. Unlike the times of communist rule, one no longer needs administrative permits to establish a firm. These companies, often operating with foreign capital, react quickly to a growing demand for medical services. Some have signed contracts with public payers, while others are planning to take part in the competition offering medical services to the insured. Dissatisfaction with the low quality of public sector medical services has been a major cause of increasing demand for the private companies. Large employers are able to buy services in advance, especially ambulatory care, using prepayments (called "subscriptions"). This is not the same as the workers' health plans, but has similar benefits: tax advantages for employers and employees and "golden cuffs" to keep valued workers. Another factor favoring this development is the partial transfer of treatment costs so that the private sector does not bear full financial responsibility. High-risk patients are directed to specialized diagnostic centers and hospitals financed with public money. In Poland, private facilities act as a kind of "gate" through which patients can get into a facility maintained by public resources more easily.

The present system of contracts creates a special inducement for cost shifting through the use of capitation payments to primary care physicians. Primary physicians receive a fixed amount of funds to pay for their work, for the work of nurses and record-keepers, and for basic diagnostics (physicians are not allowed to own pharmacies, but can own diagnostic centers). In some regions, capitation fees also cover specialized health care and diagnostic services. A primary care physician, especially one with an individual practice, prefers to send a patient to a specialist. The primary care physician keeps the capitation payment, the specialist takes over the patient's treatment, and public insurance pays a fee-for-service amount to the specialist.

Both primary and specialist physicians have reason to transfer diagnostic expenses to hospitals, especially when ambulatory diagnostics are underdeveloped or require a long waiting list. Patients, who eagerly accept hospital referrals, contribute to this situation. Despite attempts to limit the number of admissions, the number of hospitalized patients has increased greatly, as has the amount of hospital diagnostic testing. The contracts signed by ambulatory care physicians as well as those signed by hospitals create hidden incentives for cost shifting.

These comprehensive capitated payment plans, resembling managed care in the United States, have caused many conflicts between primary and specialist physicians. Primary care physicians created their own network of service providers, paying for the specialists' work and supervising them. This supervision, a type of utilization review, has brought many complaints from specialists. Very soon all capitation fees will cover primary medical care and an extended range of diagnostics. Some primary care physicians, having funds for a wide range of services, have been motivated to limit the number of referrals. These restrictions are seen as threats to the quality of care, particularly given the lack of standards and of treatment monitoring. Strong protests and lobbying by specialists have resulted in a number of changes, but it is unlikely that the problems of cost shifting and quality deterioration will go away soon.

17.6 HIGH-INCOME COUNTRIES

Among high-income countries, there is considerable variation in the use of medical care inputs (doctors per 1,000 population ranging from 1.4 to 4.3; hospital beds per 1,000 ranging from 3.9 to 16.1), organization of services, reliance on taxpayer financing, and total cost (from $450 to $4,500 per capita), but remarkably little variation in health outcomes. Life expectancy in the twenty-two high-income countries is between seventy-six and eighty-one years and infant mortality is between four and eight per 1,000 births. More variation in health statistics exists between regions within any one of these countries than across all twenty-two of them. Given the small differences in average health outcomes, it is difficult to say that one country's system is better or worse than another. What is clear is that many health problems are concentrated in specific, underserved populations, usually ethnic minorities or areas of extreme poverty.[15] Although tremendous resources are available for advanced experimental treatment, electronic scanning for diagnosis, and long-term rehabilitation, there is still a lack of primary care resources ensuring that every child is immunized, that all pregnant women receive adequate prenatal care and nutrition, and that every person has a primary physician to contact when in need of advice or care. In many ways, high-income countries face the same problems of maldistribution and misallocation in the delivery of medical care as low-income countries, but at a different level (see Figure 17.5).

Costs and Cost Control

Rapidly rising health care costs created fiscal difficulties in all high-income countries during the 1970s and again in 2002. Although the attempts at cost control varied widely, there has been a degree of convergence across nations so that most spend between 6 percent and 10 percent of GDP on health care, with the notable exception of the United States, which spent 15 percent in 2002. The United States spends by far the most on health care, yet ranks twenty-second out

FIGURE 17.5 Health Expenditures and Life Expectancy Across Countries

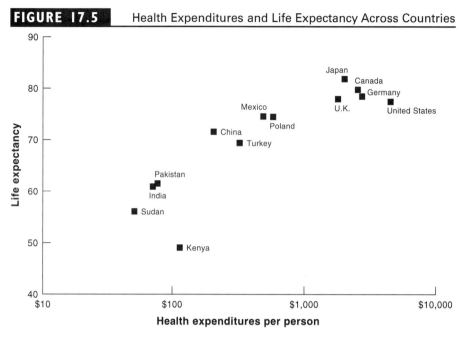

Source: World Health Report 2002.

of twenty-three countries in number of patient bed days per 1,000 population (only Greece is lower), ninth out of fourteen in number of physician visits per person, and twelfth out of eighteen in number of prescriptions.[16] There is no consistent correlation between costs per capita and the number of services provided, hospital beds, physicians employed, or extent of public or private insurance. Reducing the number of visits, drug prices, hospital days, and other micro level variables have not been successful in controlling macro system costs. Changes in the method of payment and administration do not seem to hold much promise, either. A comprehensive examination concluded "There appears to be no relationship between success in containing costs and ways of organizing services."[17]

How were Japan and Europe able to keep health care costs so much lower than the United States while maintaining equal or better health outcomes and patient satisfaction? Many attempts to control costs in the United States have been motivated at the individual level, using deductibles and co-payments to moderate demand, yet the use of pooled financing that protects patients from risks also insulates them from costs. Consumer choice does not lead to lower expenditures when consumers are spending someone else's money. European countries have operated largely on the supply side, constraining the provider system rather than individual demand. The number of health care workers and their wages has been limited and is often subject to nationwide bargaining and controls. Purchasing of expensive new diagnostic and therapeutic technology has been restricted (see Table 17.4).[18] Open-ended entitlements that reimburse patients for all bills have been avoided in favor of contracts for large groups of patients on a per capita or fixed-budget basis. In analyzing the evolution of payment systems, it has been argued that the flaws of bureaucratic governmental control (lack of innovation and consumer responsiveness) and the flaws of insurance markets (lack of cost control and gaps in coverage) are leading toward a convergence of public and private in a blended contractual model—what is known in the United States as managed care (Chapter 10).[19] Government will be responsible for setting the rules and the overall limits on the amount to be spent and ensuring that everyone receives coverage, while market competition will be used to maintain the quality and amenity of services and provide local control.[20]

TABLE 17.4	Medical Technology per Person in Three Countries, 1992-1993					
	Canada		**Germany**		**United States**	
	Number	**Per Million Persons**	Number	**Per Million Persons**	Number	**Per Million Persons**
Open-heart surgery	36	1.3	61	0.8	945	3.7
Cardiac catheterization	78	2.8	277	3.4	1,631	6.4
Organ transplant	34	1.2	39	0.5	612	2.4
Radiation therapy	132	4.8	373	4.6	2,637	10.3
Lithotripsy	13	0.5	117	1.4	480	1.9
MRI	30	1.1	296	3.7	2,900	11.2

Source: Dale A. Rublee, "Medical Technology in Canada, Germany, and the United States: An Update," *Health Affairs,* 13, vol. 4 (1994): 113–117.

Japan

Life expectancy in Japan* is the highest in the world: seventy-eight years for men and eighty-five years for women. However, the level of health care spending is only half that of the United States, about $2,000 per person, 7.4 percent of GDP. This figure is perceived in Japan as a sharp rise in comparison with 5.5 percent of GDP in 1990, the peak of the boom years. Health care spending has risen by 40 percent while the economic system has suffered from the after-effects of the asset "bubble," with essentially no growth in income for the past 10 years.

While the technology used in the Japanese health care system is similar to that used in the United States, the organization and flow of funds and, hence, the quantity and intensity of use, is considerably different.[21] In Japan, all citizens are covered by some form of insurance and are able to choose any physician or hospital they wish, with no bills other than modest co-payments per visit or per day. Japan's universal health insurance system functions as more than just a financing mechanism, it also functions as the means of health policy implementation. By using the uniform fee schedule, the government is able to macro-manage provider behavior as well as national health care spending.

Physicians are clearly split into two groups. Generalist physicians are private solo practitioners providing primary and secondary care as small businesses, earning a substantial portion of their income from mark-ups on pharmaceuticals and laboratory tests. Specialist physicians work in hospitals on salary and generally earn much less. Unlike in the United States, a patient undergoing surgery at a hospital in Japan receives a single bill that includes both room and board and the surgery fee. Surgeons are employees of hospitals and are not allowed to charge patients independently. Some argue that this combined bill may be one reason that giving gifts to the doctor is a customary practice in Japan. Private practitioners cannot attend to hospitalized patients, and hospital physicians are not allowed to have a private practice on the side. A government survey showed that the average private practice had revenues of 146 million yen and expenses of 122 million yen in 2001, making the average family doctors' income about 24 million yen ($200,000). This is three times the average annual income of salaried workers and much higher than the annual salary of $100,000 to $150,000 earned by hospital specialist doctors.

Hospitals are also split into two groups. Large public and university hospitals contain medical schools and research facilities, but may also have large outpatient departments providing primary care. Small facilities owned by private practitioners provide less sophisticated treatments and simple therapeutics. For-profit, investor-owned hospitals

* This section was contributed by Ato Z. Okamoto, M.D., M.P.H., National Institute of Public Health, Saitama, Japan.

are prohibited in Japan. Controls over utilization are not stringent. There is no preauthorization for surgery, no requirement for a second opinion, and no statistical profiling or concurrent review as under managed care in the United States. With no limits imposed, length of stay tends to be very long, 30.4 days for general acute hospitals and 377 days for psychiatric hospitals.

Universal health insurance coverage is obtained through myriad funding bodies, all regulated by the Ministry of Health, Labor, and Welfare (MHLW) (see Figure 17.6). Society managed health insurance (SMHI) covers the employees of the large corporations. Corporations with a minimum of 700 employees may opt to establish their own health insurance societies as distinct legal entities whose assets are shielded from liabilities of the parent corporation. Approximately 1,800 such SMHI societies exist, and virtually all corporations known worldwide, such as Sony and Toyota, have them. SMHI premiums are 6 to 9 percent of salary, split equally between the employer and the employee. Large-company employees tend to have the best salaries, with young workers (typical retirement age is 60) in good health, making these societies financially viable without subsidy. Small- and medium-sized corporations are covered by government-managed health insurance (GMHI). The premium for GMHI, 8.5 percent of salary, is not

FIGURE 17.6 Flow of Funds in the Japanese Health Care System

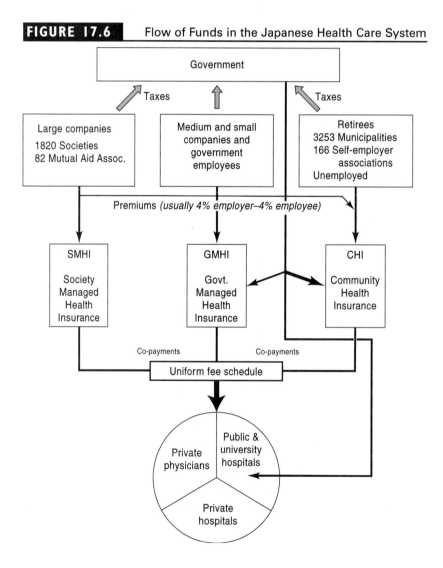

sufficient to cover costs, and subsidies are provided through the MHLW, amounting to about 14 percent of funding. The self-employed, the unemployed, retirees, and all others are covered by local community health insurance (CHI) plans administered by the 3,200 municipal governments (cities, towns, and villages ranging in size from a few hundred to several million people). Premiums for CHI are levied on household income but vary widely by municipality and are subject to a cap of $4,300 per household. Although enrollment in municipal CHI and payment of premiums is compulsory for all people not covered by SMHI or GMHI, about 10 percent of families default on payment, and penalties are rarely enforced because most defaulters have few assets. Most CHI spending is for health care of the elderly, whose incomes are small. Substantial subsidy (almost 50 percent) is required from the central government to maintain solvency of the CHI plans. Hence, although the Japanese health care finance system superficially resembles a large number of independent insurance pools, the extent of transfers and cross-subsidies means that these plans are linked through the MHLW into what is, in effect, a form of social insurance that equalizes medical purchasing power across all people.

In contrast to the fragmentation among insurance plans, reimbursement to providers is standardized, with little concern for differences in the type of facility, severity of illness, or geographic variance. The fee schedule and drug prices are set by the government every two years after negotiation with the Japan Medical Association and insurance plans (see Table 17.5). These fees are administratively negotiated provider payments, not "prices," and are adjusted in response to political agreements, not changes in demand. The fee schedule implemented in 2002 introduced a 30 percent cut for hospitals whose surgical cases do not reach specified minimum numbers in each category, giving an obvious incentive to concentrate surgery into a smaller number of hospitals.

Since all reimbursement is regulated by the uniform fee schedule, it is possible for the government to exert rather rigid control over total expenditures, even in the absence of a

TABLE 17.5	Japanese Medical Fees—Examples

1) Acute Nasopharyngitis: visit outpatient clinics twice, direct dispensing

Initial consultation fee	2,700
Follow-up visit	740
Medication	1,580
Total	5,020
(patient co-payment)	1,510

2) Acute Appendicitis: emergency surgery and hospital stay 7 days

Initial consultation fee	2,500
Hospital charge (7 days)	116,270
Laboratory	31,690
X-ray	18,760
Medication	1,510
IV	14,950
Bandage, etc.	3,520
Surgery (appendectomy)	64,200
Anesthesia	10,680
Total	264,080
(patient co-payment)	63,600

MHLW fee schedule revision, March 2002.

Charges for typical cases, in Yen (125 Yen = $1)

global budget. The financial incentives regarding specialization and high technology are almost exactly the opposite of those in the United States, where doctors doing high-tech procedures garner the most prestige and the most income. In Japan, a doctor who chooses to become a specialist gets prestige, but must give up the lucrative office-based primary care practice. The administrative operation of the fee schedule system can reverse the dynamics of a market (where the services most in demand have higher prices, which in turn, brings forth a larger supply). In Japan, if a procedure becomes popular, its fees are often cut to discourage provision. A notable effect of this shift in remuneration is that there are two-thirds fewer surgical operations in Japan than in the United States.

The structural flaw in Japan's universal health insurance system is that all employees will eventually retire and migrate to the under-funded CHI. A 1983 reform established the Elderly Health System (EHS) to redistribute financing among insurance plans. A second reform, Long-Term Care Insurance (LTCI) was introduced in 2000. Unification of Japan's fragmented insurance plans (with the attendant rise in premiums to cover the costs of the elderly) is a potential solution that has been repeatedly debated, but political divisions have prevented action. Japan's complex and bureaucratic health care system has remained viable because of strong price regulation, constant economic growth, and a relatively young population. The Japanese system is a way of reaching equilibrium through consensus, which is vastly different from the sprawling mixture of regulated and competitive markets in the United States.[22] However, many of the conditions that previously favored Japan are now being reversed: the economy is stagnant and weakened by a long slump, the population is rapidly aging, and calls for deregulation are increasingly popular. How Japan copes with these daunting challenges will be one of the great social experiments in health economics.

The German Health System

The German* health system has its roots in legislation initiated by Chancellor Bismarck in 1883 that made enrollment in pay-as-you-go sickness funds mandatory for certain groups of workers nationwide. This system of statutory social insurance, financed by payroll taxes, has since been greatly expanded to include more and more groups of workers and now covers more than 90 percent of Germany's population. The remaining 9 percent have chosen private insurance. The objectives of the social insurance system are equality in access to medical care and a progressive distribution of the financial burden. Yet since the reunification of East Germany and West Germany in 1990, the share of GDP devoted to health has risen to more than 10 percent and challenges the economic future of the country.

Social insurance contributions are made through sickness funds (Krankenkassen) and set at a specified percentage (usually around 15 percent) of gross wages, half of which is deducted in the form of a payroll tax and half of which is paid by the insured to the sickness funds of her choice. The list of legally mandated medical services leaves little scope for product differentiation, and prices of medical services are determined in centralized negotiations with provider organizations, not by individual sickness funds. The opportunity to make special deals with preferred providers is generally nonexistent. Thus, sickness funds are limited in their ability to lower costs and compete on price. Lower rates are achieved primarily through reduced administrative spending and risk selection. The evidence suggests that cream skimming, by providing inconvenient service for the chronically ill and by offering attractive extra services for the young and healthy, has been a successful strategy. Free aerobics classes and health food cooking courses have proved particularly popular.

---

* This section was contributed by Dr. Michael Stolpe, Institute of World Economics, University of Kiel.

Private health insurance is confined to the self-employed, civil servants, and the relatively small number of workers making more than 40,000 euros per year who may, therefore, opt out of the statutory system. Premiums are based on the age, sex, and individual health risks of an applicant, who usually must answer a long health-related questionnaire and often undergo a medical examination. After a contract has been signed, an insurer cannot unilaterally change its terms in response to changing health risks of the individual; the insurance promise is for the rest of the insured's life, and premiums are allowed to rise only by the same percentage as the general rise in medical care prices. In a similar vein, people opting for private insurance cannot revert to the statutory social insurance plan, but must remain with private insurance for the rest of their lives.

The reimbursable fee for an individual service can be three times higher under private insurance than the official prices listed in the Federal Health Minister's list; therefore, doctors prefer to treat patients with private insurance. To lure them, waiting times in the physician's office tend to be shorter and treatment is sometimes more generous than for the socially insured. Many private health insurance plans provide strong financial incentives to refrain from seeing a doctor for small, self-limiting health problems. If an insured makes no claims during a given year, the insured can often get a refund of up to half his or her annual premium payments. Because income is positively correlated with health status, the privately insured tend to be healthier and utilize medical services less frequently than the enrollees of statutory sickness funds. To foster consumer choice and competition, insurers are allowed to offer, in addition to regular full-coverage plans, a type of supplemental insurance, mainly used to upgrade the level of hospital amenities, to enrollees of any sickness fund.

There is a **strict separation of ambulatory care from hospital care in Germany,** with too little cooperation and too much competition between the two sectors. Only one-third of doctors in the ambulatory sector are general practitioners, while two-thirds are specialists with their own private practices. Independent specialists often invest heavily in diagnostic and surgical technology, sometimes setting up their own clinics to rival the services offered by small hospitals. This high degree of medical specialization in ambulatory care has long been encouraged by Germany's system of fee-for-service payments. New technology creates more and more billable events, and patients are free to take themselves to any office-based physician, but not to a hospital.

Fee-for-service remuneration for the individual physician is combined with global budgeting for the ambulatory sector as a whole. Budgets are periodically negotiated between the collective of sickness funds and regional physician associations, called "Kassenärztliche Vereinigungen," which operate like a cartel. The associations negotiate the contracts for delivery of care and administer overall budgets for various categories of care. They allocate funds to individual practitioners according to a uniform relative value scale for all services delivered to patients with statutory insurance. In addition, office-based physicians have the opportunity to generate income from private patients.

German **hospitals** employ their own salaried physicians, and physicians in private practice do not have admitting privileges. However, chief physicians of German hospital departments have strong incentives to increase the amount and quality of care since they are allowed to treat private patients, and thereby supplement their personal income in proportion to the number of beds filled with patients with statutory insurance. Hospital reimbursement has been on a per diem basis. Rates vary considerably depending on the type, size, and location of a hospital. The sickness funds must reimburse the charges of any hospital to which patients were referred by their general practitioners. Hence, the use of resources was often inefficient and the provision of care per case excessive. There is a significant oversupply of hospital beds per capita despite regulatory threats of capacity cuts if a hospital's utilization falls below 85 per cent. This has not only encouraged longer and more frequent inpatient treatment of domestic patients, but also the export of stationary care to foreign patients (mainly from Scandinavia and the United Kingdom, where rationing of hospital services has created long waiting lists for certain procedures).

In the **pharmaceutical sector** a reference price (set by the government) system limits drug spending. Sickness funds are required to reimburse retailers for part of the cost of any drug they dispense, using fixed reference prices for drugs with similar properties. In practice it is often difficult to delineate therapeutically comparable drugs. Moreover, the net effect on prices is unclear because generic drug competition almost collapsed as generic prices were brought into line with reference prices. Political lobbying by doctors and the pharmaceutical industry has averted a long proposed "positive list" of reimbursable pharmaceuticals based on effectiveness.

Reforms in the 1990s aimed at cost control by introducing competition among sickness funds and a prospective payment (diagnostically related group [DRG]) system now implemented in the hospital sector. However, restrictions on sickness funds' ability to become efficient buyers (by negotiating prices differentially with individual providers and bundling medical services in novel ways) have been left in place. Changing this would destroy the corporatist cartel of ambulatory physicians and meet fierce resistance from this well-organized and powerful political lobby. The ambulatory sector has been targeted by introducing co-payments, global budget limits for pharmaceuticals, restrictions on the adoption of costly new technology, and limits on the number of ambulatory physicians allowed in any given geographic region. However, these efforts did not prevent sickness funds' contribution rates as a percentage of gross wages from rising sharply after Germany's reunification, when mass unemployment eroded the tax base and East German per capita health spending rapidly caught up with the levels in West Germany, while GDP per capita remained much lower in the East. Moreover, global budgets in pharmaceuticals apparently led to cost shifting through an increased number of referrals from general practitioners to specialists and hospitals not subject to the budget limits.

In retrospect, the structure of the German health system survived the Second World War and accommodated the country's reunification almost unmodified, but is no longer well suited for the rapid changes that are occurring in demographics and technology. Within the statutory insurance system, any increase in spending is seen as a threat to social stability because increased payroll taxation automatically increases non-wage labor costs and further aggravates Germany's structural unemployment problem and decreases its international competitiveness.

17.7 INTERNATIONAL TRADE IN HEALTH CARE

Health care is among the world's largest industries, accounting for 10 percent of gross world product, but only a tiny fraction of world trade. Products (drugs, equipment) are much more likely to be bought and sold across national boundaries than services. Although in principle there is no reason why an X-ray performed in Seoul cannot be read in San Francisco, licensure and other regulations currently make such international service flows difficult or impossible. Trade in services is usually limited to a small amount of border crossing; for example, when a Canadian citizen disgruntled with a long wait for elective surgery crosses into the United States or an uninsured Hispanic worker from Texas crosses to Mexico for cheaper hospital and physician care. The part of the health care system most subject to international movement—trade in people and skills—does not appear in the world economic accounts.

Pharmaceuticals

The pharmaceutical trade is one of the world's truly global businesses (see Chapter 12). Drugs made in England or France cross pharmacy counters in the United States as readily as drugs made in Chicago, and research is as likely to be conducted in Genoa or Geneva as it is in Georgia. Companies such as Rhone-Poulenc Rorer and Astra-Merck cross international boundaries and link major markets. Protectionist legislation still gives local firms an advantage, but it is common for more than 25 percent of a large pharmaceutical company's sales to occur outside the country where it is headquartered, and some, such as Ciba-Geigy, are mostly international. There are three major markets: Japan, the United States, and the European Union. The ability of Japanese doctors to profit from prescribing gave them the highest rate of prescription drug use in the world. Thus with only half as many consumers, the Japanese market was larger than the U.S. market in 1990 ($51 billion versus $48 billion). However, the decade-long recession in Japan has caused a relative decline even though the percentage of health expenditures spent on drugs there still exceeds that in the United States (16.8 percent versus 10.4 percent). The European Union accounted for about $40 billion, and all of the developing low- and middle-income countries accounted for $44 billion.[23] Only the major market countries have the research infrastructure and a protected domestic market of sufficient size to cover the massive fixed costs of discovering and testing new drugs. Canada presents an interesting case. Because the nation lacked significant pharmaceutical development capacity, it decided to free ride on the technology produced by the rest of the world. Canada refused to recognize the property rights created by patents and mandated that foreign companies license their drugs for manufacture or use in Canada in return for set royalty payments. This way the Canadians could obtain the benefits of research, but not pay the cost. Vigorous protests eventually led to this system being overturned, and now Canada recognizes international patent protection, as do other industrialized countries. However, free riding is still the rule for many developing countries, either through mandatory licensing or simple failure to enforce patents, which allows local companies to make copycat versions of brand name drugs. Clinical tests constitute a sizable portion of drug companies' costs and provide an interesting opportunity for international trade. By carrying out trials in a foreign country, a firm may be able to significantly reduce the cost per patient of developing a drug and may face lower liability from adverse reactions the experimental drug might produce.

Equipment

Medical equipment is less amenable to international trade because it cannot simply be packed in a box and shipped. Skilled technicians are required to maintain and use these sophisticated devices, and the ongoing labor costs are much larger than the manufacturing cost. Once a new technology is developed, it will usually be produced and supported by a local firm or the local branch of a global firm within a few years.

Services

Health care is sharply demarcated at national boundaries. The U.S. Medicare program does not pay for operations in Mexico, nor will it cover Canadians who come to the United States. Therefore, the border-crossing trade in services that does occur is usually paid for privately. Private investment in the small fee-for-service or insured hospitals and clinics that exist alongside national health facilities in the United Kingdom, Sweden, and elsewhere is often international. The largest hospital in Singapore used to be owned by an

American firm, National Medical Enterprises. Yet the true test of international trade in medical care looms in the proposals for full integration of service markets within the European Union. A Belgian patient might prefer heart surgery in one of the major Parisian hospitals, or a Swiss factory worker might decide to seek psychiatric care in Germany. Conversely, a German hospital would find it cheaper to obtain nurses or doctors from Greece and pay travel expenses rather than hire them locally. To date, every country has jealously guarded its health care system, and such freedom of choice is available only to a few employees of international companies.

People and Ideas

In stark contrast to the lack of international trade in medical services is the substantial movement of medical personnel and ideas across national boundaries. Most specialists in developing countries receive some of their training in Europe or the United States, bringing home skills of immense value. The extraordinary increase in life expectancy that has swept over the world is perhaps one of the greatest benefits of international trade, made no less significant by the fact that, as public goods, information and scientific discoveries cannot be owned or charged for by a particular firm or country. What is somewhat surprising is the extent of trade in the reverse direction—doctors and nurses who come to work in the United States from low-income countries. At its peak, in 1978, more than half of all medical residents who were in training (and providing care) in urban teaching hospitals were foreign medical graduates. In the less remunerative and attractive specialties, such as psychiatry, this is still the case today. More than 12 percent of all U.S. physicians are immigrant doctors. Similarly, a large number of licensed nurses were educated overseas. There are more Filipino nurses practicing in the United States and Canada than in the Philippines. This anomalous flow of highly trained labor from less-developed to more-developed countries has much to do with the economics of restrictions on labor supply and with the incentive structure created by the size of the market. Limits on the numbers of physicians and nurses imposed through the U.S. educational system mean that there is room for those who have received training overseas and are willing to work for less. Also, truly outstanding neurosurgeons are able to earn more in the United States than in Mexico, and may be tempted to go where their skills command the highest reward—just as Latin baseball players and movie stars do. There is also a niche at the bottom of the market that attracts foreign labor. Caring for the elderly in nursing homes is so demanding and underpaid that it is difficult to find competent staff willing to work for the minimum wage. These positions are attractive to immigrants who are able to obtain steady employment and benefits in jobs that require a lot in the way of patience, endurance, and strength, but not in language or education. The lack of dollar-denominated trade obscures the extent to which medicine and health care became globalized in the twentieth century.

SUGGESTIONS FOR FURTHER READING

World Health Organization, *World Health Report 2002* (http://www.who.int/whr/2002/en).

Bruce J. Fried and Laura M. Gaydos, eds., *World Health Systems* Chicago: AUPHA Press, , 2002).

The World Bank, *World Development Report 1993: Investing in Health* (New York: Oxford University Press for the World Bank, 1993).

Rupa Chandra, "Trade in Health Services," *Bulletin of the World Health Organization* 80, no. 2 (2002): 158–163, (www.who.org).

David M. Cutler, "Equality, Efficiency and Market Fundamentals: The Dynamics of International Medical Care Reform," *Journal of Economic Literature* 40 (September 2002): 881–906.

"The Danish Health System," special issue of *Health Policy* 59, no. 2 (January 2002).

Naoki Ikegami and John Campbell, (Medical Care in Japan,) *New England Journal of Medicine* 333, no. 19 (1995): 1295–1299.

Philip Musgrove, Riadh Zeramdini, and Guy Carrin, "Basic Patterns in National Health Expenditure," *Bulletin of the World Health Organization* 80, no. 2 (2002): 134–1146, (www.who.org).

SUMMARY

1. There is **a tremendous disparity in health** between rich and poor nations. The poor countries of sub-Saharan Africa have very little health care and low life expectancies. Many people there die before the age of 5. The wealthier countries of Europe, North America and Japan have more health resources to be applied to much less need. People in these countries have a longer life expectancy, with most deaths occurring after age 70.

2. Average **spending** on health care **is determined primarily by national income** per capita, not the health needs of individuals. Increased per capita income is also a major factor explaining increased life expectancy.

3. More health expenditures usually mean more health professionals and more use of technology, not more visits to physicians or days in the hospital. It is the **intensity of service, rather than quantity,** that increases as spending is increased.

4. **The United States is the world's largest health care market,** accounting for 40 percent of all health expenditures, even though it has only 5 percent of the world's population. U.S. health expenditures per person are 10 times the worldwide average and 100 times the average per person in India. With more than 15 percent of the world's population, India accounts for less than 1 percent of the global health care market.

5. Significantly **higher medical expenditures do not** appear to have made U.S. citizens significantly healthier. U.S. life expectancy ranks about in the middle of developed high-income countries.

6. The curve depicting the relationship between national income per capita and life expectancy has shifted upward over time. This illustrates the productive impact of **new knowledge** as well as the **transmission of that knowledge across national boundaries.**

7. The **distribution of income** across people and social groups, as well as the average, is important in explaining differences in health and life expectancy.

8. **Lack of organization, maldistribution, and political instability** are perhaps even more important than low income in causing poor health among many low-income countries. Even in mid- and high-income countries, many of the worst health problems result from the uneven distribution of health care and an inability to effectively target care to those most in need.

9. Most countries assert that their health care systems emphasize **primary care,** but their **funding favors specialty training and tertiary hospital care.**

10. **Cost control** in Europe, constraining supply and putting limits on the system as a whole, appears to have been more effective than in the United States. Japan's inexpensive health care system is much less technology-intensive than that of the United States, using only a third as much surgery, but more drugs.

11. There is very little **international trade** in health care services. Global trade in health care is dominated by pharmaceuticals. However, the invisible trade in knowledge and health professionals has the largest effect on national health care systems.

PROBLEMS

1. {*flow of funds*} How many people are there in the world today? What fraction of them live in high-income developed economies? What fraction of total health expenditures is accounted for by high-income countries?

2. {*flow of funds*} How much is spent per person on health care in China? How much is spent per person on health care in the United States? In the United Kingdom? What are the primary factors accounting for these differences?

3. {*market size*} What is the largest global health care market?

4. {*correlation v. causality*} Is more spending on health care associated with more health?

5. {*incidence*} As an officer of the World Health Organization with a budgetary allocation of $100 million, which programs would you fund if you wished to make the greatest impact on health, measured as the increase in life expectancy multiplied by the number of people affected?

6. {*nominal v. real*} Mexico spends less than a tenth as much per person on health care as the United States. Does it have more than or less than a tenth as many hospital beds? Physicians? Is the real amount of health care provided overestimated or underestimated by dollar comparisons? Why?

7. {*international trade*} Which types of health care labor are most likely to be traded between countries? Why?

8. {*international trade*} Which types of health care goods are most likely to be traded between countries? Are there more or fewer barriers to trade in health care than in other sectors?

9. {*trade*} Which aspects of medical care are most international? Which are the most parochial?

ENDNOTES

1. World Health Organization, *World Health Report 2002*, (http://www.who.int/whr/2002/en).
2. In converting local expenditures and income into U.S. dollars, two methods are used. The value in local currency can be converted using the foreign exchange rate (the rate at which dollars are traded for local currency in the market) or it can be converted in terms of "purchasing power parity" (PPP), the amount required to purchase an equivalent amount of goods and services. In India, GNP per capita was $450 measured in terms of foreign exchange, but $2,149 in terms of the value of goods. This is largely because the cost of food, transportation etc. is much lower than the price of such goods in the U.S., converted at the currency market exchange rate (i.e., whereas 100 rupees = $2.08 U.S. dollars, that amount cannot buy a good meal in the U.S., but would be sufficient to purchase more than three good meals in India).
3. The World Bank, *World Development Report 1993: Investing in Health* (New York: Oxford University Press for the World Bank, 1993). This report provides comparative data on a number of health issues not available elsewhere, and thus is used here despite the age of the data (mostly 1990). Making comparisons requires not only that the data exist, but also that the data be made comparable in terms of definitions, time periods, etc., a tremendous task for 191 countries.
4. Victor Fuchs, "The Health Sector's Share of the Gross National Product," *Science*, 2 February 1990, 534–38.
5. Mark Pauly, "When Does Curbing Health Costs Really Help the Economy?" *Health Affairs*, 14, no. 2 (1995): 68–82.
6. Thomas Getzen, "Population Aging and the Growth of Health Expenditures," *Journal of Gerontology*, 47, no. 3 (1992): S98–104.
7. Thomas E. Getzen, "An Income-Weighted International Average for Comparative Analysis of Health Expenditures," *International Journal of Health Planning and Management* 6 (1991): 3–22.

8. Samuel H. Preston, *Fatal Years: Child Mortality in Late Nineteenth-Century America* (Princeton, NJ: Princeton University Press, 1991).

9. G. B. Rodgers, "Income and Inequality as Determinants of Mortality: An International Cross-Section Analysis," *Population Studies,* 33, no. 2 (1979): 343–351; also The World Bank, *Population Change and Economic Development* (New York: Oxford University Press, 1985).

10. The World Bank, *World Development Report 1993: Investing in Health* (New York: Oxford University Press for the World Bank, 1993).

11. Eladreesi Zainuelabdeen, *Summary Report of the Establishment of the Sudan Health Economics Unit,* planning section, Sudan Federal Ministry of Health, November 7, 2002.

12. Milton I. Roemer, *National Health Systems of the World* (New York: Oxford University Press, 1991), which includes information reproduced from G. M. Bloom, M. Segal, and C. Thube, *Expenditure and Financing of the Health Sector in Kenya* (Nairobi: Ministry of Health, 1986). The World Bank Statistics, used for most of the tables in this chapter, estimate national health spending in Kenya at $375 million for 1990, of which 63 percent came from the public sector. Roemer argues that private sector spending is much less visible and usually under-reported since no regular statistics are kept. Bloom et al., through extensive surveys and several alternate methods, estimate that private sector spending actually slightly exceeded public sector spending, 51 percent to 49 percent, in 1986. Table 17.2 takes the World Bank estimate of public spending of $237 million, derived from government budget reports, as correct. Private sector spending is then estimated to be 51 percent of the total, or $247 million, following Bloom et al. The percentages of total spending within each category in Bloom et al. for the year 1986 are then applied to the $484 million total to create breakdowns by category. The net effect of the adjustment for under-reported private expenditures is to raise the estimate of per capita health expenditures in Kenya from $16 per person to $20 per person.

13. Milton Roemer, *National Health Systems of the World* (New York: Oxford University Press, 1991), 345–51.

14. Katarzyna Tymowska, "Health Care Transformation in Poland," *Health Policy* 56 (2001): 85–98.

15. WHO Regional Office, *European Health Report 2002,* (http://www.euro.who.int/document/e76907.pdf).

16. *OECD Health Systems: Facts and Trends 1960-1991* (Paris: OECD, 1993).

17. Brian Abel-Smith, *The Reform of Health Care Systems: A Review of Seventeen OECD Countries* (Paris: OECD, 1994), 49.

18. Dale A. Rublee, "Medical Technology in Canada, Germany and the United States: An Update," *Health Affairs,* 13, no. 4 (1994): 113–117.

19. Jeremy Hurst, *The Reform of Health Care: A Comparative Analysis of Seven OECD Countries* (Paris: OECD, 1992), 140–151. See also, Alan Maynard and Karen Bloor, "Introducing a Market to the United Kingdom's National Health Service," *New England Journal of Medicine* 334 (1996): 604–608.

20. The fact that so many health policy experts in so many countries all agree on the essential elements of what the future of health care organization and financing will and should be is probably reassuring, although such a consensus has not always guaranteed either insight or good results in the past.

21. Some of the information presented here came from conversations with Naoki Ikegami, M.D., Professor of Health Administration at Keio University, and is well presented in Naoki Ikegami and John Campbell, "Medical Care in Japan," *New England Journal of Medicine,* 333, no. 19 (1995): 1295–1299. See also Margaret Powell and Masahira Anesaki, *Health Care in Japan* (New York: Routledge, 1990); and Kyoichi Sonoda, *Health and Illness in Changing Japanese Society* (Tokyo: University of Tokyo Press, 1988).

22. Can you imagine a group of U.S. executives or lawyers suspecting heart failure being willing to wait patiently for hours in a public clinic to be served alongside the unemployed, or accepting a situation in which two out of three who currently would be receiving a bypass graft or new pacemaker are sent home with pills instead? Then, when adversity strikes, can you further imagine that they would not sue? The sources of such a disparity go beyond language, currency, and government. Although cultural studies lie a bit beyond the scope of this book, it is clear that culture profoundly affects the health systems of the two countries just by looking at the differences in physician salaries, relative differences in the uses of drugs versus invasive therapy, and ownership of facilities and equipment.

23. The World Bank, *World Development Report 1993: Investing in Health* (New York: Oxford University Press for the World Bank, 1993), 145; *OECD Health Data 2002,* Paris: OECD, (www.oecd.org).

CHAPTER 18

DYNAMICS OF NATIONAL HEALTH SPENDING

QUESTIONS

1. What determines wage levels in the health care industry?

2. How does a nation decide the right amount to spend on health care?

3. How does a person decide what is the right amount to spend on food, housing, clothes, and everything else each year?

4. Why do general tax revenues pay for so much personal health care? Who will pay if (when?) the Medicare trust fund runs out of money?

5. Which is more important in determining how much to spend on health care: how sick people are or how much money is available?

6. Does inflation affect health care spending? If so, does it affect health care spending permanently or temporarily?

7. Do professional licensure, third-party reimbursement, and nonprofit organization make it easier or harder to adjust health care spending to changes in prices?

8. Is it easier to adjust to growth or to a recession?

9. Do price controls work? If not, why might people think that they do?

18.1 MICRO AND MACRO PERSPECTIVES ON SPENDING

Looking at health care spending from an individual perspective and from a community perspective reveals why micro and macro analyses can arrive at different conclusions. Consider hospital expenses. From the point of view of an individual, there are no hospital expenses unless one is admitted for treatment. From the point of view of the community, however, the hospital must be maintained, the laundry washed, staff paid, and magnetic resonance imaging (MRI) devices calibrated regardless of the number of patients receiving treatment on a particular day. From the community perspective, the hospital is a system resource. Only a small fraction of the total cost of hospital care (drugs and supplies, food, nursing overtime) varies with the number of patients. Most costs are relatively fixed.

An individual assumes that if he or she becomes sicker, additional care will be provided. However, if all hospital beds are full, the next patient cannot be admitted, and the hospital must displace someone whose need for the bed is less pressing. A capacity constraint limits total resource use: the total amount of resources available. If everyone in the United States got twice as sick next winter, the nation could not suddenly double the number of doctors. To some extent, each doctor would work harder and see more patients, but the capacity constraint means that for the most part this surge in demand would be met by doctors giving each patient fewer minutes of attention, keeping some patients who are mildly ill from making return visits, and other adjustments.[1] Insurance shows the same disparity between individual and group perspectives. To an individual, medical expenses resulting from an accident are something the insurance plan has to pay—their personal insurance premiums are fixed and paid in advance. Yet from the point of view of the group, all expenses must be paid out of premiums. If more accidents than anticipated occur, a premium increase for all group members is required, or the insurance plan becomes insolvent.[2]

In Chapter 17, comparisons were made regarding medical spending among different countries. The main reason Sweden spends more on health care than Sudan, because they have more money, was so obvious it hardly needed to be explained. Yet among the employees of General Motors, the janitors and clerks with low wages get the same kind of health care, and spend just as much, as the engineers and executives. Why should income matter so much in one case (comparisons between nations) and barely matter at all in another (comparisons between employees)?

The funding of a health care system is a macro system characteristic. For most countries, including the United States, funding is national in scope. Thus, we do not expect to see major differences in health care as we cross the border from Texas into Arizona, or in Mexico as we cross the border from Sonora into Chihuahua. Yet crossing the national border from Arizona into Sonora, or Texas into Chihuahua, reveals a vast disparity in the use of medical resources, costs, and prices.

Disparities in health care of this sort were once found within a single country. At the end of the nineteenth century, New Yorkers living on Park Avenue and those living in the tenements of lower Manhattan occupied different social and medical worlds. To some extent, disparities still exist within a country today—between the suburbs and the inner city, between the mainstream medicine provided to most Americans and the care available to residents of isolated Indian reservations in the United States or the remote Inuit villages in Canada. In Australia, studies have demonstrated that the health and health care of aboriginal populations is much worse than that of the majority white population.[3] In South Africa, studies showed large differences in health spending per capita for blacks and whites under apartheid, which has been greatly reduced, but not entirely removed, under the new political system. The crucial determinant of the health care available to a group of people is the amount of resources available to that group, often measured by average income per capita. The essential question then becomes, what is a group? Why are Mexican-Americans living in San Diego getting more medical care than their relatives and friends across the border in Tijuana? Why are some Indian tribes not sharing in the wealth of the average American? Why are the aboriginals of the outback not sharing in the wealth of the average Australian? Defining who is and who is not part of the group determines who does and who does not have access to health care.

18.2 THE CONSUMPTION FUNCTION

The relationship between income and spending is known as the **consumption function.** Some people spend less than they earn so that they can save. Some people spend more than they earn, dissaving or going into debt. What is always true is that *consumption + savings = income*.[4] This is an accounting identity, a definition that cannot be changed by obfuscation or by wishing it were not so. A corresponding accounting identity holds across people and nations: for each person who borrows, there must be someone who saves and can lend the borrower money. Unless there are people with savings to lend, people (or nations) that want to spend more than they earn cannot do so. This accounting identity is easily obfuscated when dealing in money; therefore, it is better to think in terms of food. If country A wants to consume 80 tons of lettuce, but produces only 60, it has to borrow 20 tons from country B. Country B can do so only if it produces more lettuce than it consumes. Country A will usually pay off the debt with oil or wheat or money instead of lettuce, but the mechanics of transfer are clear—total consumption of all people (nations) globally = total production (+ amount saved for next year or – amount taken from storage). For services and perishables that cannot be stored, the relationship simplifies to *total production = consumption + investment*.

A 10 percent increase in income must result in a 10 percent increase in spending if all possible uses of income, including savings, are counted. By construction, the average income elasticity for all goods (with each good weighted by its share of the total budget) must equal 1.0, unit elasticity (see Chapter 2). Economists are interested in why one good, such as food, or entertainment, or medical care, increases more or less than proportionately as income increases. For many years, economists were perplexed by the following observation: rich individuals tended to save a larger percentage of their incomes than the poor, making the income elasticity of individual savings greater than 1.0 (thus "saving" was categorized as a superior or luxury good).[5] In contrast, rich countries and poor countries both save about the same percentage of national income. Furthermore, when gross domestic product (GDP) rises over time, there is no tendency for a larger percentage of national income to be saved. The disparity between individual and national income elasticities of consumption and savings posed a major puzzle, one that forced economists to scrutinize and reconsider the relationship between individual and national spending.

The Permanent Income Hypothesis

A major conceptual advance coming from the micro and macro economic analysis of consumption is that of **permanent income**—the hypothesis that the amount consumed is determined by expected average earnings over the long term rather than current earnings today. Thus, a medical student entering a surgical residency buys a new Volvo and a house for a growing family because she is confident that although her current earnings are near $0, they will jump to $40,000 next year and to several hundred thousand dollars per year as soon as her residency is completed. Conversely, a trial lawyer who has just earned $15 million from a case will not spend it all this year. He is aware that such big paydays are rare, and that the next major settlement, *if* it occurs, may take five, ten, or twenty years. Thus, while earnings and consumption are matched in the long run, they can deviate widely in any given period. Nobel Laureate Milton Friedman began his economics career as an assistant in the construction of the first national income and product accounts used to measure GDP, GNP, current account surplus and deficit, and so on.[6] His task was to measure the incomes of doctors, lawyers, and engineers. These people were problematic because their spending did not seem to match their incomes. Employees with steady wages seemed to consume about the same amount each year—but so did these professionals, whose incomes fluctuated widely from year to year. Friedman hypothesized that the spending of doctors, lawyers, fishermen, farmers, and other groups with highly variable earnings was based not on their actual income, but on their expected long-run income.[7] Franco Modigliani (Nobel Laureate in 1985) examined how people's income and spending varied over their lifetimes, showing that they typically began with a period of borrowing at the start (to buy a home, automobile, furniture and other goods), followed a period of saving in their 50s and 60s, and then dissaving in retirement.[8] Like Friedman, Modigliani found that spending is related to average long-run income rather than the size of the current paycheck. Together, the ideas of Friedman and Modigliani have become known as the life-cycle permanent income hypothesis.

The permanent income hypothesis resolved the empirical inconsistency between micro and macro studies of consumption and savings. It recognized that a disproportionate number of high-income individuals are people who only temporarily earn so much money (such as the malpractice lawyer who just received $15 million, or the 59-year-old house carpenter saving for retirement) and hence would naturally hold some for later periods, while a disproportionate number of low-income individuals (such as the surgical resident, the carpenter in winter, and most undergraduate economics and finance students) are only temporarily poor and hence rationally spend more than they currently earn. For countries, however, the budget constraint is binding. Total national consumption is limited by what the country produces each year (except for the limited flexibility allowed by international borrowing and investment) and thus automatically adjusts to match national income.

Income Elasticity and Shared Income

What is your income? If you are not working and your parents are sending you to school, the more relevant question is: What is your family's income? For the child of the young surgical resident, it is the parents' earnings, not the child's, that matter. The surgeon may also eventually have to support her aged parents. Families tend to share income; therefore, it is usually the resources available to all family members on average, not the amount earned by an individual family member that determine personal consumption. How extensive is such sharing? Who counts as a member of your family? Do you owe anything to your brother, who moved to Alaska twelve years ago and only contacts you once a year when he sends a Christmas card? Do you owe him more if he loses his leg and his job due to an accident and moves back home? Do you owe anything to a neighbor who lost his job, or a homeless person sleeping on the street? The surgeon may or may not feel that she owes a lot to a neighbor or a homeless person, but will pay taxes that are used to help both of them.

Just as the permanent income hypothesis suggests that long-run expected earnings rather than current measured earnings determine current spending, a similar **shared income hypothesis** suggests that the average income of a group of people who share determines their consumption, rather than the earnings of each person individually. Most consumption is shared within the family, and some public goods are shared within the community (schools, roads, fire and police protection). Clothes, food, entertainment, and most other private goods are shared within a family, and perhaps within a circle of friends, but not within a larger community. What about medical care? Although care of an individual may seem like a private good, the infrastructure (hospitals, medical education, pharmaceutical companies), clinical standards and funding of care are arranged collectively. Shared group spending is not just the 45 percent paid by taxes, or the 5 percent paid by charity and community programs. The 35 percent paid by private insurance is regulated by the Employee Retirement Income Security Act of 1974 (ERISA) and state insurance commissioners to meet public policy objectives. Even the remaining 15 percent paid out of pocket by individuals is subject to special treatment in the tax code and thus is affected by collective political decisions. A physician office practice and a for-profit hospital may be private enterprises, but both are subject to regulation and social expectations much greater than those faced by other firms.

Studies of individuals show that utilization of medical resources is only slightly related to income (elasticities of 0.0 – 0.4), but studies of nations show that rich nations spend more on health than poor nations (with income elasticities > 1.0). The reason for this disparity is that individuals' ability to consume medical care is based not on their own personal income, but on the average income level of all the people in their family, in their community, in their insurance plan, and in the nation as a whole.

Consider two people employed by a company that provides insurance benefits. Both employees, who are covered by the same insurance plan, a file clerk and the chief financial officer, have the same illness. They do not live in the same type of house, drive the same type of car, or take the same vacations, but they will receive similar hospital care. Even if the clerk does not make much money, most of the hospital bill is already taken care of. It would be foolish for him not to take advantage of his employee benefits when he is sick just to save a few dollars on co-payments. Now consider the chief financial officer. There is little more medical care that she can buy, no matter how much she is willing to spend. If she wants to have the new gene therapy or positron scans she has read about, the decision is up to the medical staff, not her. Indeed, every effort is made to keep such medical decisions from being influenced by payment considerations. This is not to say that there are no differences in the treatment of the rich and the poor, but the differences are deliberately kept small by professional ethics within the system. Government provision of care for the poor and tax subsidies to pay for health insurance are parts of that system. The consequences, relatively similar sorts of care for all people with the same illness, are not an accident; they are some of the reasons that these collective policies receive wide public support. Insurance converts personal medical care into a public good, and as a society we have collectively decided that all citizens should have reasonable access to quality medical care.

For public goods, such as clean air, national defense and control of communicable diseases, society's willingness to pay determines how much will be provided (see Figure 15.2). Since everyone is able to consume the same amount of a public good, individual income is irrelevant except for its contribution to the total tax base. For a public good, or within a group insurance plan, the individual's income is not a binding budget constraint. It is possible to spend more curing one sick child than the child could earn in three lifetimes, and the amount of money spent to clean up the air in Los Angeles is hundreds of times greater than the money earned by a Hollywood movie star. It is the resources available to the group as a whole that determines the average level of spending.

The shared income hypothesis implies that income becomes more important in determining spending as the unit of observation gets larger and becomes similar to the budgetary unit.[9] For individuals, income is relatively unimportant, and income elasticities are near 0. For small areas, such as a census tract, average per capita income is somewhat more important, with income elasticities rising to perhaps 0.4. For counties or states, their budgets are a constraint, but it is still possible for them to obtain money from the federal government. Per capita income is significantly more important as a determinant of health care spending than health status, and elasticities are about 0.9. For the nation as a whole, the budget constraint is binding. No other country is going to reimburse us for our medical bills. Every dollar paid to doctors, nurses, and drug companies must be collected in taxes, insurance premiums, or direct fees. Income thus becomes the dominant determinant of spending at the national level, with elasticities greater than one, usually about 1.3 (see Figure 17.2).

18.3 DYNAMICS

If per capita income falls, health care spending must also fall. Yet it is impossible to make this economic adjustment all at once. Usually the country goes into debt during the transitional period. Even for an individual, adjustments to changes in income are not instantaneous. If you were to lose your job today, you would not immediately move into a smaller apartment, drive an older car, or wear less fashionable clothes. In fact, if you lose your job today, you will probably go out and spend a little extra money to keep up your spirits. Next week you will cut back, but not too much, because you probably expect to find another job soon. If you are still out of work six months later, you will find that your clothes and your house and your car start getting shabby and you think about downsizing your lifestyle. Once you do get a new job, it will take years to build your savings back up.

When college students graduate and begin to earn good wages, they find it easy to live and save part of their salary because their lifestyles are still somewhat geared to being a student. Consumption for the newly employed does not usually rise as fast as their incomes rise. During this "I can't figure out how to spend it all" period, savings accumulate. Later on, with a fancy lifestyle suitable for a young stockbroker or lawyer, they find it difficult to see how one could have lived on so little money as a student, or even on what they earned three years ago. Consumption is geared to expected income, whether $15,000 or $150,000. The amount of income saved depends not so much on how high the income is, but on transitional (permanent income/life-cycle) factors and the extent to which a person is willing to give up current pleasures for retirement or future consumption.[10] If a young lawyer who has just bought a new Mercedes loses his job, he will discover one of the underlying asymmetric truths of human behavior: it is a lot easier and more fun to adjust spending upward rather than downward.

The dynamics of adjustment for individuals (micro) and for nations (macro) are similar, except that it usually takes longer for macro adjustment, because the system as a whole must change. People who still have their jobs must be convinced that it is necessary to cut back, to reduce the provision of public goods, or to change the tax code. Achieving a consensus to alter organizations and revise institutional structures is extremely time-consuming. The health care system, based on professional ethics, institutional obligations, and shared public values, is even more reliant on a complex set of public and private financing mechanisms, is even more difficult to change than most other sectors of the economy. In the stock market, expectations of the future are traded every day, and prices change by the minute. Commodity sectors, such as farming and metals, are forced to respond quickly due to market discipline. Although the number of houses cannot change rapidly, housing sales are sensitive to macroeconomic conditions. The decision to buy a house is based on an individual's assessment of job prospects. The effective price of a house, the monthly mortgage payment, depends on interest rates, which are volatile and forward-looking. For both these reasons, housing tends to be one of the sectors that leads the economy into or out of a recession. Health care is slow to change, and lags behind other sectors in adjusting to macroeconomic conditions.

How long does it take for health care to adjust? From one to five years on average, but some parts take even longer. Even if everyone in Congress decided today that we need more health care or less health care, this decision could not be carried out for months, and its full effects would take years to work their way through the system. If a medical school decides to accept more students, it takes at least a year to enroll them, and to build new medical schools takes much longer. Medical students take four years to graduate, and another three or four years to complete a residency and enter practice. Thus, eight years after a decision to expand a medical school has been made, there are still no extra doctors in practice. Something might be done to reduce the rate of retirement, but effectively the quantity of doctors in practice who graduated in a particular year in the past was fixed once they leave school. It took until 1985, twenty years after the Health Professions Educational Assistance Act of 1963, before the expansion in physician supply was a real force in the market—and by then Congress had changed its mind. It takes forty years, until all graduating physicians have retired, before the full effects of such decisions work through the system (see Chapter 7).

Not everything in health care takes as long to adjust as physician supply. The supply of nurses is much more flexible because typically there are many licensed nurses who are temporarily not working or working part-time; therefore, an increase or decrease in demand is quickly translated into a change in the numbers employed. Clerical, maintenance, and other less-specialized labor adjusts even more smoothly and rapidly because people can move between health services and other sectors of the economy in response to changing conditions. Although we do not have data to look at each segment of the health care sector separately, the National Health Expenditure (NHE) Accounts, the analogue to the National Income and Product Accounts established by the U.S. Department of Commerce to track GDP and the economy as a whole, do categorize health care spending by type (hospitals, physicians, dental care, drugs, nursing homes) and enable us to examine the patterns of adjustment separately for each component.

Hospitals, the largest component of health care expenditure, are quite rigidly institutionalized and dependent upon public or third-party financing. As one would expect, they took a bit longer to adjust, 3.0 years, than the average for all medical spending, 2.7 years.[11] Physician services are somewhat more flexible and adjust a bit more quickly, with a lag of 2.5 years. Spending on drugs, much of which depends on direct consumer decisions and is paid for out-of-pocket with current income, takes only 1.3 years. Long-term care, a mixture of flexible personal spending and rather inflexible Medicaid spending, adjusts in 2.5 years on average. The component that takes the longest to adjust is construction, at 3.5 years. Capital must be accumulated in advance to fund new construction, and the decision to build depends on long-run future economic considerations, not just revenues and expenses today.

It is difficult to pinpoint the timing of adjustment in a complex area with many segments and subsegments. Consider hospital expenditures again. Because of the way NHE Accounts are kept, construction is listed as a separate component, making it possible to see that construction took longer to adjust than labor. However, some construction (clinics, equipment installation) probably takes less time than others (new buildings), but we cannot tell because they are categorized together. If supplies were listed separately, they would probably be seen to adjust more quickly than labor. The "average lag" is just that, an average. Some parts are moving faster, and some slower. It is also an average over time—in some periods the organization may respond more quickly than in others. In particular, it appears that managers are quicker to step up purchasing when the economy expands than they are to cut back when the economy contracts. Everyone hopes that a slowdown is just temporary, and delays firing people or closing clinics. The time required to adjust also depends on the magnitude of the change. The statistical techniques used here can only detect changes in the one-to-ten-year range, but a truly massive revision of the system, such as that which occurred in 1965, may take several decades to complete. Some argue that one reason health spending is so high in the United States is because it is still stuck with a health care system constructed on the lines of the Great Society envisioned during the 1960s, when economic growth was steady and strong. This system is not appropriate to the more constrained conditions and budget deficits prevailing in 2003.

Permanent Income and Adjustment of Health Spending to GDP

Government is based on stable rules that change slowly and only with the consent of citizens. For example, any amendment to Medicare must be approved through the courts, the legislature, and public opinion. What are the consequences of slow adjustment in the health care sector? Importantly, it buffers the economy. During a downturn, Medicare and Medicaid spending usually continue; therefore, health care workers are less likely to lose their jobs than workers in the farming, housing, or financial services sectors.[12] Conversely, an increase in employment during an economic recovery is delayed.

The delay in adjustment can have adverse budgetary consequences. Because spending continues to rise in a recession even though government tax revenues fall, a deficit builds up. In theory, such periods of excess spending average out over time with under-spending during periods of rapid growth. However, it is easier to obtain agreement to pour money into the health care sector and save jobs during a recession than it is to hold back and save money during good times. In a recession, people hope that normal growth will soon return, and they may bend their spending rules to temporarily soften the impact of macroeconomic disorder. An economic boom feels so good that people may not realize that such high growth rates are abnormal, that another recession is bound to come eventually. People may claim that this time around will be different and that we never have to worry about going hungry again, thus we do not need to save money for bad times or give up much to pay off old debts. As a consequence, it is much easier to accumulate deficits than build up surpluses.

Politicians want to get elected. They need results that will affect the economy and the voters in the near term. Extra government spending during a recession meets these needs; extra saving when the economy starts to grow again usually does not. The benefits of a balanced budget—low inflation, steady or falling interest rates, strengthening the dollar in foreign exchange, stability for businesses to invest in productivity improvements, and a modest but sustainable path of optimal growth—are long term. But none of these benefits can be realized quickly enough to help the politician worried today about the next election. In a pinch, a politician (or a professor) will sacrifice the long-term good that helps others in favor of near-term benefits they can capture for themselves. It is difficult to get politicians to behave in a way that benefits the long-term public interest, because it is difficult to get voters to behave that way. One consequence of this is well known—a U.S. deficit of a trillion dollars. Eventually, just like the out-of-work lawyer running up his charge cards, we will have to bring spending back into line and balance the budget. But that is in the long term, and the elections keep coming up fast.

Adjustment to Inflation

The slow adjustment of the health care sector to inflation means that during a period of rising prices, spending is less than expected.[13] To see why, trace the process of adjusting spending to changing price levels, as illustrated in Table 18.1. Suppose that a hospital spent $100,000 in 2000 and wanted to spend the same amount in real terms (e.g., full-time equivalents [FTEs] in labor, gallons of fuel, square feet of office space) in each succeeding year. If the expected rate of inflation is 5 percent, 105 percent of 2000 spending will be budgeted for 2001; that is, $105,000. If actual inflation equals the expected 5 percent, the same quantity of all inputs bought in 2000 can be bought with the 2001 budget. If inflation is again expected to be 5 percent in 2002, $110,250 is budgeted for that year. However, suppose that inflation actually turns out to be 12 percent in 2002. The budget does not buy $100,000 worth of goods in constant inflation-adjusted dollars, but only $110,250 ÷ (1.05 + 0.12) = $94,000. With a 12 percent rise in prices, the budgeted 5 percent wage increase leaves employees worse off, with less purchasing power. The budgeted

5 percent increase in the supply budget is not enough; thus, equipment purchases will have to be cut back. In 2003, inflation is expected to be, and actually is, 5 percent. However, the hospital has to make up for the lost purchasing power resulting from underestimating inflation the previous year. Therefore, the budget for 2003 will be up 12 percent to $123,480. Having caught up, spending will once again be $100,000 in real (year 2000) terms (see last line of Table 18.1).

National health care spending shows this type of lagging adjustment to unexpected changes in the price level for several reasons. First, the government and nonprofit organizations such as hospitals usually set a budget at least a year in advance, which limits their flexibility. Second, most wage contracts run for at least one, and usually several, years. A set of inflation adjustments is already built into raises, and any difference between what negotiators expected to happen to prices and what actually happens falls on the workers. If inflation is less than expected, workers are lucky and can buy more. If inflation is worse, they have to tighten their belts. Estimates calculated from Bureau of Labor Statistics (BLS) data indicate that for any 1 percent change in the rate of inflation, only about 0.5 percent shows up in the wages of health workers in the first year, and another 0.3 percent in the following year. It takes three years for wages to fully adjust to a change in inflation. In the long run, all wages do adjust, making inflation neutral, neither raising nor lowering real health care spending. The government can only temporarily trick workers and firms into accepting a dollar that is only worth $0.90. Any government that tries to "save" money by printing lots of currency ends up with chronic inflation, as Brazil and Russia have had. Therefore, most governments aim for price stability and a sound currency. Yet the year-to-year fluctuations caused by temporary inflation adjustment problems may be larger than any real changes in health care spending due to GDP growth or changes in health care policy.

The distorting effects of a surge in inflation are shown in Table 18.2, which traces prices and employment in Canada during the oil price shock of 1973. Inflation, which had previously been averaging 3 to 5 percent, suddenly leapt to 9 percent in 1973, peaked at 14 percent in 1974, and remained high at 10 percent in 1975. However, by this time, the health sector had begun to build in expectations of high inflation. It looks as if spending, measured by the fraction of GDP devoted to health care, fell during 1973 and 1974. However, real resources, as measured by the number of nurses working in the Canadian health system, continued to rise throughout this period.[14] Indeed, employment for nursing rose not only in absolute numbers, but also as a fraction of total employment. In terms of real labor,

TABLE 18.1	Adjustment to Inflation			
	2000	**2001**	**2002**	**2003**
Nominal spending	$100	$105	$110	$123
Price index	100	105	117	123
Real spending	$100	$100	$ 94	$100

Note: Hypothetical example of adjustment to inflation. The hospital tries to spend exactly the same amount ($100 in year 2000 dollars) in each year. In the first year, inflation is 5% and spending increases 5%, so there is no change in real deflated expenditures. In the second year, spending increases by 5% again, but inflation is 12%, so the real spending power declines. In the third year, inflation is 5%, and the hospital catches up by increasing spending 12% (7% to catch up and 5% for current inflation).

TABLE 18.2		How Inflation Distorts Reported Health Expenditures			
		Employment			
Canada	**Inflation**	**Nurses**	**Total**	**Ratio**	**Health Share of GNP**
1972	5.6%	152,005	8,447,000	.0180	7.3
1973	8.9%	159,274	8,860,000	.0180	7.0
1974	14.4%	168,530	9,220,000	.0183	6.9
1975	9.8%	177,182	9,364,000	.0189	7.4

Note: Inflation rates, nurses and total employment, and health spending as a share of GNP show how sudden price increases distort budgetary measurement of the relative size of the health sector.

Source: OECD 1990.

spending was rising. It only appeared to decline because the nurses were temporarily underpaid, getting raises smaller than the rate of inflation. Their wages had gone up somewhat during 1973 and 1974, but not as rapidly as the prices of the things they bought with those wages. Thus, the nurses' real purchasing power fell, which is why the fraction of GDP spent on health declined. This "decline" was entirely transitory, because the nurses were not willing to make less than everyone else and were able to get their wages revised upward to take into account the increase in inflation during the next contract period. In the long run, whatever was taken away by a delay in adjustment had to be given back. When this was done, in 1975, there appeared to be a jump in the share of GDP spent on health care. Actually, this rapid rise is accounted for by the removal of the earlier distortion—eventually the health care sector had to catch up with the rest of the economy.

Although expected inflation is built into contracts, a surge in overall prices is not immediately matched in the health care sector. Because wages are slow to adjust, workers bear the burden by being made worse off temporarily. Because budgets are slow to adjust, health care organizations must make do with fewer supplies, drugs, buildings, and so forth, or temporarily go into debt. However, in the long run, inflation has no effect on real health care spending. After about three years, health care wages and other contracts have fully taken account of earlier shifts.[15]

A Dynamic Model of U.S. Health Expenditures

Using the permanent income hypothesis and the lagging inflation adjustment hypothesis allows us to create an econometric model of U.S. national health expenditures. Analysis of the correlation between actual spending, fluctuations in prices, and per capita income indicates that health expenditures are a function of the average percentage rate of growth in real per capita GDP during each of the preceding five years (but not the current year), and over the preceding 25 years. This analysis also indicates that health care expenditures lag by 40 percent of the change in inflation for the current year and 20 percent of the change in inflation for the previous year. This model can be used to project future national health care spending, and is shown in Figure 18.1.[16] This forecast, made in January 2003, used actual GDP growth to forecast 2003 national health expenditures (because only prior years' GDP up to 2002 were required), but had to use the consensus estimates of professional economic forecaster's for 2003 and 2004 inflation. For 2005 and beyond, more assumptions about macroeconomic trends are required, and the forecast becomes increasingly less reliable the further into the future projections must be made.[17]

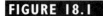

FIGURE 18.1 Annual Percent Change in U.S. Health Expenditures—Econometric Forecast

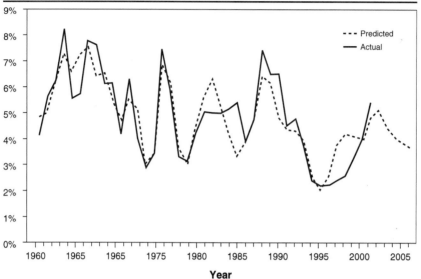

18.4 GOVERNMENT COST CONTROLS: SPENDING GAPS AND THE PUSH TO REGULATE

Analysts have questioned why a cost-control policy that seems so successful in one instance, or so successful among individuals or physicians or hospitals alone, fails to reduce total costs. It is because the consequences of income for spending are established only at the level where the budget constraint is fixed. For some types of health care, this is the individual household, for others, the hospital, region, or the insurance plan, but for much of medicine it is the national budget constraint that is most relevant.

The lagging response of the health care sector to macroeconomic changes makes management easier in one respect—budget forecasts are usually accurate because the system is inertial and slow to change, and much of the movement over the next few years will reflect what has already occurred in the broader economic indicators such as the consumer price index (CPI) and GDP. However, this same inertia also makes it difficult to balance the budget. In a recession, expenditures continue to climb even as revenues fall. The budgetary gaps created by delays in the adjustment of spending to changing macroeconomic conditions may force governments to put cost controls on health care. Almost every inflationary spike or sharp recession is followed by a new attempt to regulate hospital rates, ration health care, establish price controls, cap revenues, or use another method to stem rising costs. For example, Figure 18.2 shows the progress of a recession in the state of Washington and the legislative implementation of a hospital cost control commission. In 1965, Washington was a robustly growing state with above average per capita income, 108 percent of the U.S. average. Growth continued in 1966 and 1967 with per capita income rising above 110 percent of the U.S. average and state population growing 3 percent a year as people migrated to the state to look for good jobs, particularly in the aerospace industry. Growth slowed in 1968 and again in 1969, before the recession caused real per capita incomes to fall in 1970 and 1971. Boeing, which accounted for one in four jobs in metropolitan Seattle, eventually laid off half its work force. Local businesses were devastated and many retail stores closed. In 1972, state population declined and per capita income fell to the U.S. average. The state suffered a fiscal crisis

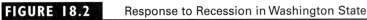

FIGURE 18.2   Response to Recession in Washington State

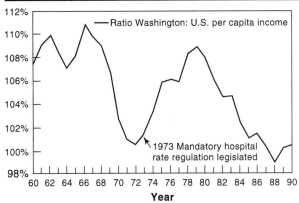

as tax revenues fell. In 1973, the legislature passed an act creating a mandatory Hospital Rate Review Commission that was among the toughest in the nation. In 1974, hospital expenditures per capita declined 2.8 percent in real inflation-adjusted terms.

Hospital expenditures would have declined anyway because of the recession, even if the legislature had failed to pass any acts. A dynamic model that incorporates lagging income and inflation effects shows that the decline resulted from a delayed response to the severe state recession, not regulation. Eventually, the state legislature came to the same conclusion, and the hospital rate commission was disbanded. If the researchers responsible for the initial analysis of the cost commission had been able to wait ten years for more information, then they would have concluded that the controls did not have much effect, since the level of per capita hospital expenditures in Washington state was essentially unchanged relative to projected levels or the U.S. average in 1990 compared with 1973.

ARE RECESSIONS GOOD FOR YOUR HEALTH?

Just as spending may respond differently to permanent and transitory income, it is possible that the effect of income on health may differ in the long run and the short run. The evidence reviewed in Chapters 16 and 17 made it clear that long-term trends in health are strongly and positively related to growth in GDP per capita. Since that is well known to be the case, many economists assumed that disruptions in economic growth, recession and the unemployment that accompanies it, would temporarily cause health to worsen. Christopher Ruhm, in a series of careful empirical articles, has shown that exactly the opposite occurs.[18] For every 1 percent increase in unemployment, there was a 0.5 percent *decrease* in mortality rates. The primary reason recessions appear to be good for health is that peoples' lifestyles improve; they exercise more, eat better, lose weight and smoke less. Motor vehicle fatalities show a large drop, in part because unemployment means less work and less money, so people drive less. Back injuries decline, perhaps because people no longer have to do so much heavy lifting. Diseases that are less affected by lifestyle, such as cancer, do not show much correlation. Contrary to the general trend, suicides increase during recessions, as do some forms of mental illness. This is consistent with the common perception that the fact or threat of unemployment increases stress. What is fascinating about these studies is how clearly they illustrate the fallacy of composition. The short-run effects of macroeconomic fluctuations in this case are, for most conditions, exactly the opposite of the long run effects.

The ineffectiveness of rate controls in Washington state does not mean that no state regulatory program can reduce costs. The Maryland cost-containment legislation, passed without the pressure of a severe fiscal crisis, did reduce costs.[19] Prior to implementation, Maryland costs were 111 percent of the U.S. average, and by 1990 costs had fallen to just 95 percent of the U.S. average. Other state mandatory cost-control programs in New York, Massachusetts, and Connecticut may have had some impact, but the evidence is less clear. The national cost controls contained in the Balanced Budget Act of 1997 had a large impact on Medicare expenditures, but that was offset to some extent by the shifting of costs to the private sector.

Substantial ability to control costs is built into existing government administrative mechanisms. Consider the state of California, which has never proposed or enacted hospital rate regulation. The combination of strict limits on taxation imposed by Proposition 13 and a massive recession caused what was once one of the most generous of health care systems to tighten down so much that by 1998, hospital expenditures per capita were 9.8 percent below the U.S. average.

Legislatures don't get together to pass cost-control measures for health care because the economy is doing well. Macroeconomic crises bring about a call for legislatures to do something, but these crises eventually push spending down, regardless of whether legislatures act. The ability of politicians to dictate spending independent of the rest of the economy is limited, particularly during the next one to four years, which are usually all that remain before the next election. The process of adjustment is shown in Figure 18.3. Incomplete adjustment to inflation and recession is apt to simultaneously exert pressure on legislatures to do something about excessive health care costs and force future spending downward, thus often creating a spurious correlation between the enactment of regulation and the temporary moderation in costs.

Price Controls: The "ESP" Program

Economic growth slowed toward the end of the 1960s, and a recession occurred in 1970. Unlike previous recessions, however, there was no moderation in prices. This combination of slow or negative GDP growth with high inflation, called stagflation, rudely ended the dream of permanent stability and prosperity. President Nixon stepped in to impose shock therapy in the form of wage and price controls with the Economic Stabilization Program (ESP) on August 15, 1971. All prices were frozen for ninety days in Stage I, which was followed by rules and procedures for Stages II, III, and IV. In retrospect, the U.S. experience from 1971 to 1975 served mostly to confirm the lessons learned from wage and price controls imposed by other governments around the world over the last two millennia. The underlying pressures created by excess monetary growth and the fiscal imprudence of waging a war without raising taxes could not be contained, controls were routinely evaded, and prices shot up as soon as controls ended in April 1974. Paul Ginsburg, an economist who worked with the Price Commission, which was responsible for implementing the ESP, wrote an article that provided a detailed look at the practical difficulties of writing and enforcing regulations.[20] The problems of ambiguity in the definition of "price" (per item, per day, or per admission), crudeness in the construction of adjustment indexes, use of a

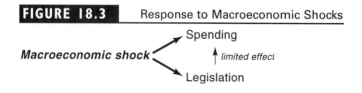

FIGURE 18.3   Response to Macroeconomic Shocks

"fudge factor" for technological change, arbitrariness in implementation, and the inability to provide a consistent and fair mechanism for determining exceptions, became cumulatively worse as time went on. Price control rules were frequently changed, became administratively complex, and lost credibility. Ginsburg also pointed out that cost-based reimbursement insulated many hospitals from the effects of controls over charges and that hospital price inflation had already begun to decline even before controls were imposed.

Yet at the time, the public, government officials, and even many economists thought that price controls on health care had been successful. They thought so because there was a clear moderation during 1971 in both nominal and real health care costs from the 1966–1970 trends; falling from 11.1 percent to 9.3 percent and from 6.1 percent to 3.5 percent, respectively. The dip was even more pronounced for the narrower measure, hospital costs, which grew 8.3 percent in 1970 but only 3.4 percent in 1971. Comparing trends before and after ESP makes it appear that the controls were effective in reducing spending, yet most of the decline would have occurred anyway due to the slowdown in GDP growth and lagging adjustment to a rapid increase in inflation. To get a true picture of the incremental effect of ESP price controls, it is necessary to compare the actual rate of increase in health care costs with the predicted value from a dynamic macroeconomic forecasting model such as the one shown in Figure 18.4. Spending was indeed 1.5 percent below expectations in 1971, and ESP could have been responsible for this decline, but ESP was in effect only for the last three months of the year. In 1972, spending was slightly above expected, 1973 spending was below, and 1974 and 1975 spending was slightly above again, but none of these differences are significantly different from the residual variation in the series. Econometric estimates of the ESP effect show that ESP may have reduced costs, but the evidence is inconclusive. At most, the reduction was perhaps 1 percent during the four years that price controls were in effect—far less than the 10 percent and greater reductions that were claimed at the time.

The Voluntary Effort

After the expiration of ESP, health care costs were freed from external economywide controls, although they continued to be regulated by cost reimbursement rules (see Chapters 5 and 8). Medicare, in particular, attempted to constrain costs, but without notable success.

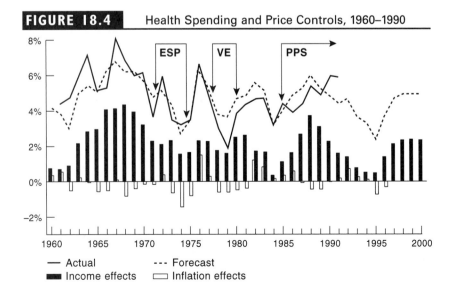

FIGURE 18.4 Health Spending and Price Controls, 1960–1990

— Actual   --- Forecast
■ Income effects   □ Inflation effects

The genesis of the voluntary effort (VE) lay in President Carter's April 1977 legislative proposal to regulate hospital revenues. The hospital industry was strongly opposed to the measure and formed the VE coalition of providers and payers in December 1977. Flyers and buttons were printed to promote voluntary efforts to reduce the rate of cost increases. The VE coalition promulgated a national target for holding cost increases to 2 percent less than the previous rate or to 3 percent above the rate of inflation (the 1978 target was 13.6 percent). More flyers and buttons were printed as industry representatives lobbied Congress. After several modifications, the House of Representatives voted on a new version of the Carter bill in November 1979, which was soundly defeated, removing the potential threat of federal regulations that had sustained the VE coalition.

This tale of voluntary regulation would normally have been forgotten and relegated to footnotes, yet the story lingered on because claims of effectiveness were uncritically accepted. Three reasons for the persistence of the impression that VE worked are that (1) hospital price increases did moderate in 1978 and 1979, (2) claims of VE's effectiveness were loudly voiced, and (3) Congress cited these claims in debate before Carter's legislation was defeated. It is difficult to understand how flyers and buttons could accomplish what the force of law could not, but the claims appear plausible until the data is examined more closely. Hospital costs had already begun falling in 1977 before VE. They declined further in 1978 and were below the target (12.8 percent versus a target of 13.6 percent). Even VE believers referred to the American Hospital Association's luck, because the VE coalition did not even convene a meeting until December 1977 and, therefore, had no time to directly affect hospital behavior. The financial reports on which the 1978 NHE figures were based came mostly from hospitals whose fiscal years ran from July 1, 1977, to June 30, 1978. For these hospitals, fiscal year 1978 was half over before the VE coalition met.

Luck, however, was only one factor in the fortuitous "success" of VE. The main reason that nominal health care expenses were lower than expected was that hospital wages and supply prices, because they lag the CPI, had not yet caught up with the surge of inflation that began in 1977. There was no decline in hospitals' use of real inputs (labor FTEs, supply items), only a delay in price adjustment that made nurses and technicians temporarily cheap relative to the CPI (as in the Canadian example in Table 18.2). In 1979, however, there was a real decline in health care spending. Nominal expenditures per capita rose by only 10.8 percent, 0.5 percent less than the year before. This drop placed spending almost 2 percent below the predicted value. Is this a real VE effect? Probably not. VE was a program promoted by the hospital industry to control *hospital* expenditures. Therefore, the effect of VE should have been greatest in the hospital sector, resulting in a lower rate of increase in hospital spending than nonhospital spending, which was not under the purview of VE. In fact, the opposite was the case: nonhospital expenditures rose more slowly in 1979, less than half the rate of hospital expenditures.

Prospective Payment System with Diagnosis-Related Groups

In October 1983, Medicare radically changed its method of paying hospitals from cost reimbursement to a new prospective payment system (PPS) based on the expected cost of each admission, categorized into diagnosis-related groups (DRGs). This new cost control plan did work, in some ways. There was a significant reduction in the rate of increase in Medicare Part A (inpatient) expenses and in hospital expenses generally. However, this was accomplished primarily by hospitals shifting services to outpatient and day surgery categories covered under Medicare Part B. Total health care expenditures per capita continued to rise at historically high rates (see Figure 18.4). In 1985, 16.9 percent of the $407.2 billion spent on health care was paid for by the federal government, and by 1990, the fraction actually increased to 17.7 percent of the $643.4 billion spent that year, even though reduction in the federal deficit was an explicit objective of the Medicare legislation. PPS clearly had a large effect on the health care system. Administrators and doctors panicked, employment was (temporarily) held below trends, and the average length of stay for patients fell sharply. However, there were no long-run reductions in the total costs of health care.[21]

Why Do People Believe Cost Controls Work?

The idea that ESP, VE, and PPS regulations were "effective" in reducing expenditures lingers because a superficial before-and-after comparison in each case showed a decline in spending that the public and legislators could understand, which was quickly reported in the newspapers. People did not recognize that these declines were delayed effects of the adverse macroeconomic conditions that had caused the regulations to be proposed in the first place. Also, the declines in spending in one reimbursement category (Part A) due to regulations look like effective cost controls, until it is realized that these costs were just shifted to another area (Part B). A more human reason for the persistence of this belief is that many analysts and politicians worked thousands of hours to draft and implement these regulations, becoming so personally committed that it was hard for them to accept that so much well-intentioned effort had so little effect over the long run.[22] It is possible to objectively assess the actual effects, or lack of effects, of regulation only by examining the aggregate total of all health expenditures in the context of a dynamic model showing how spending adjusts over time to macroeconomic changes.

Health care expenditures are never too high or too low in an absolute sense; rather, they are out of line with the spending that can be afforded under current economic conditions. A theory of health care cost regulation must start with the realization that shared costs, and governmental expenditures in particular, are always regulated even when no external regulatory agency is in operation. Furthermore, costs can be ratcheted up or down within the existing framework by making administrative procedures tighter or looser, even if no legislation is passed. Regulation is always an integral component of health care system management in a modern nation. It is part of the process, not an external shock. What an economist can evaluate is a *change* in the regulatory regime. To do so, one must first ask why the change took place at a particular time.

18.5 "SPENDING" IS MOSTLY LABOR

What does it mean to control costs? Because health services are mostly labor, costs are primarily a function of the number of people employed in the health sector and the wages (or professional incomes) that they are paid. Cost control must be employment control. Yet it is easier for politicians to say that they will control costs than to say that they will have people laid off or cut wages, which is one reason that there is so much more rhetoric than action in health care cost control.

The most significant government interventions in the health care labor markets have been (1) cooperating with the medical profession in the formulation of effective licensure laws and making medical schools the restrictive gateway for entry into the profession during 1910–1930, (2) extending the medical licensure model to other health professions throughout the remainder of the twentieth century, and (3) enacting the Health Professions Education Act of 1963 to expand health care labor (see Chapter 7).

Every occupation within the health services field has its supply and demand most strongly influenced by the particulars of licensure statutes and relations with the dominant medical profession. Yet what is true of each of the parts is not true of the whole. Most of the growth in health employment comes from adding new occupational categories rather than by expanding numbers within an existing occupation. Therefore, to study how health care labor is related to the economy as a whole, it is necessary to look at aggregate employment in the health sector rather than a single occupational category.

Employment

There are two separate sources of data on U.S. health care employment. The decennial census began recording information on the occupation of respondents in 1850 and thus can be used to create a long series of health-related occupations with fifteen observations over the past 150 years (see Table 18.3). The Bureau of Labor Statistics (BLS) records employment within industries by Standard Industrial Classification (SIC) codes and has identified health care services (SIC 808) as a category since 1958 (SIC 80806 is the subcategory "hospital employment."), providing 45 annual (or 540 monthly) observations from 1958 to 2002 (see Table 18.4). The definition of the two series is quite different. The census data is based on *occupation of the individual;* therefore, a secretary, chemist, or accountant employed at a hospital would not be counted as a health care employee. The BLS data is based on the *SIC code of the employer;* therefore, a nurse, medical technician, or doctor employed at a manufacturing firm would not be counted as a health care employee, but a hospital secretary would.

Employment in health care has grown more than twice as rapidly as total U.S. employment over the past hundred years, 3.4 percent versus 1.5 percent for the period 1900–2000. Consequently, the share of total employment accounted for by health care has increased from 1.2 percent at the turn of the century to 7.7 percent (1 out of every 13 workers) now. Yet the 0.6 percent percentage of total employment accounted for by physicians in 2002 was up only slightly from 0.5 percent in 1900. The health care sector (SIC 808) has enjoyed positive employment growth every year for the past three decades. The average annual growth rate of this sector between 1958 and 2002 was 4.8 percent—more than double the annual average growth of total U.S. employment. During this period, health care sector employment never contracted (see Figure 18.5), in contrast to total employment, which experienced four major contractionary episodes. Total U.S. employment contracted in the 1960s, after the oil price shocks of the 1970s, and again at the start of the 1980s and 1990s. Although health sector employment grew more slowly during the mid-1970s and early 1980s, annualized year-on-year growth never fell below 2 percent. Health care employment shows less fluctuation because it adjusts more slowly and gradually to macroeconomic shocks. When total employment is shifted upward or downward 1 percent from trend, health care employment moves by only 0.2 percent after one year, 0.17 percent after two years, and so on (see Figure 18.6).[23] The cumulative rise or fall in health care is proportionately larger, about 1.2 percent for each 1 percent shift in total employment, but spread out over the entire decade that follows, so that on average shifts in health employment lag by 2.6 years.

The slow rate of adjustment to government intervention is shown in Figure 18.7, which presents the estimated impact on health care employment resulting from the enactment of Medicare and Medicaid in 1965. Although this legislation created a fundamental change in reimbursement and flow of money into the system, and was ultimately responsible for a rise of more than 10 percent in the number of health care jobs, it had no visible effect on health employment during 1965 or 1966. Not until 1967 did employment begin

TABLE 18.3   U.S. Health Employment 1850–2000

	1850	1860	1870	1880	1890	1900	1910	1920	1930	1940	1950	1960	1970	1980	1990	2000
Population	23,192	31,443	39,818	50,156	62,948	75,995	91,972	105,711	122,775	131,669	150,697	180,671	205,052	227,726	249,973	275,372
Employed civilians	5,372		12,925	17,392	23,318	29,073	37,371	42,434	48,830	51,742	59,230	67,990	79,802	104,058	123,473	131,720
All health occupations	46	61	103	114	170	346	486	634	900	1,020	1,450	2,064	3,277	5,403	7,580	10,103
Fraction	0.8%		0.8%	0.7%	0.7%	1.2%	1.3%	1.5%	1.8%	2.0%	2.4%	3.0%	4.1%	5.2%	6.1%	7.7%
H/pop	1.97	1.93	2.58	2.26	2.70	4.55	5.29	6.00	7.33	7.75	9.62	11.42	15.98	23.73	30.32	36.7
MD/pop	1.76	1.75	1.62	1.71	1.66	1.73	1.66	1.43	1.33	1.33	1.31	1.29	1.45	1.90	2.35	2.8
Aid/MD			0.2	0.2	0.5	1.0	1.4	2.1	3.2	3.7	5.1	6.7	8.7	10.1	10.6	10.9
Physicians	41	55	64	86	105	131	152	151	163	175	198	234	297	433	587	772
Dentists	3	6	8	12	17	30	40	56	71	71	76	83	95	125	156	168
Diagnosticians, NEC	2						8	22	38	40	53	68	40	54	132	94
Pharmacists			18			46	54	64	84	83	89	93	116	146	182	208
Nurse (practical)				15	47	120	166	212	236	200	224	276	267	435	429	679
RN-nurses			13	1	1	12	51	104	214	284	406	592	762	1,285	1,885	2,290
Att-hosp/nurse aides, orderlies									41	102	212	409	951	1,378	1,860	1,834
Att-phy/health aid							4	7	14	35	42	73	134	292	249	490
Dent asst							2	7	14				100	158	216	251
Dent hygienist													17	46	72	148
Opticians, lens grinders						6	9	11	13	12	20	21	31	47	38	67
Therapists (licensed)									14	18	25	37	78	224	332	296
Psychologists											5	12	30	93	192	***
Dieticians											23	27	43	67	90	97
Med technicians											78	141	260	508	927	1,057
Managers, medicine & health													58	111	234	***

U.S. Health Labor: Annual % Rates of Growth

	1850	1860	1870	1880	1890	1900	1910	1920	1930	1940	1950	1960	1970	1980	1990	2000
Population		3.1%	2.4%	2.3%	2.3%	1.9%	1.9%	1.4%	1.5%	0.7%	1.4%	1.8%	1.3%	1.1%	0.9%	1.0%
Employed civilians		4%	4.5%	3.0%	3.0%	2.2%	2.5%	1.3%	1.4%	0.6%	1.4%	1.4%	1.6%	2.7%	1.7%	1.9%
All health occupations		2.9%	5.4%	1.0%	4.1%	7.4%	3.5%	2.7%	3.6%	1.3%	3.6%	3.6%	4.7%	5.1%	3.4%	2.6%
Physicians		3.1%	1.6%	2.9%	2.0%	2.3%	1.5%	-0.1%	0.7%	0.7%	1.3%	1.7%	2.4%	3.8%	3.1%	3.1%
Dentists		6.7%	3.6%	4.4%	3.6%	5.4%	3.0%	3.5%	2.4%	0.0%	0.6%	1.0%	1.4%	2.8%	2.2%	1.3%
Nurse (practical)					11.9%	10.0%	3.3%	2.5%	1.1%	-1.6%	1.1%	2.1%	-0.3%	5.0%	-0.1%	
RN-nurses					7.2%	28.0%	15.6%	7.5%	7.5%	2.9%	3.6%	3.9%	2.6%	5.4%	3.9%	2.7%
Att-hosp/nurse aides, orderlies										9.6%	7.6%	6.8%	8.8%	3.8%	3.0%	
Att-phy/health aid								5.5%	7.1%	9.7%	1.7%	5.6%	6.3%	8.1%	-1.6%	
Therapists (licensed)										2.5%	3.3%	4.0%	7.7%	11.2%	4.0%	
Psychologists												9.4%	9.3%	12.1%	7.5%	
Dieticians												1.5%	4.9%	4.5%	3.0%	3.8%
Med technicians												6.0%	6.3%	6.9%	6.2%	
Managers, medicine & health														6.7%	7.8%	

Source: U.S. Census and Bureau of Labor Statistics, various publications.

TABLE 18.4		Trends in Employment in the Health Care Sector		
Year	Total U.S. (000s)	SIC 808 Health Services	SIC 80806 Hospitals	SIC 808 % of Total	SIC 80806 % of 808
1960	54,189	1,548	1,030	2.9%	67%
1970	70,880	3,053	1,863	4.3%	61%
1980	90,406	5,278	2,750	5.8%	52%
1990	109,403	7,814	3,549	7.1%	45%
1991	108,249	8,183	3,655	7.6%	45%
1992	108,601	8,490	3,750	7.8%	44%
1993	110,713	8,756	3,779	7.9%	43%
1994	114,163	8,992	3,763	7.9%	42%
1995	117,191	9,230	3,772	7.9%	41%
1996	119,608	9,478	3,812	7.9%	40%
1997	122,690	9,703	3,860	7.9%	40%
1998	125,865	9,853	3,930	7.8%	40%
1999	128,916	9,977	3,974	7.7%	40%
2000	131,720	10,103	3,989	7.7%	39%
2001	131,922	10,381	4,096	7.9%	39%
2002	130,793	10,673	4,225	8.2%	40%

Source: Bureau of Labor Statistics, *Employment and Earnings.*

FIGURE 18.5   Annual Percentage Change in Employment

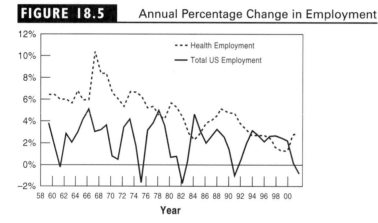

to soar, leaping 3.7 percent above trend in that year, 2.4 percent in 1968, 1.2 percent in 1969, 0.6 percent in 1970, and 0.4 percent in 1971 (see Figure 18.7). The average lag between the enactment of Medicare and the creation of an additional job was 3.5 years.

Wages

Health care wage data for the United States are available from the BLS for hospitals from 1968 on, and for all health employment from 1972 on. There were rapid increases in real inflation-adjusted wages of more than 5 percent per year in the late 1960s post-Medicare period. During the 1970s, health care wages were essentially flat, just keeping pace with wages in other industries and with inflation, and growing less than 0.5 percent per year. From 1980 to 2002, while real wages in the rest of the economy were essentially flat (rising by less than 2 percent), average health care wages rose by 26 percent, and the increases for

FIGURE 18.6   Health Employment Adjusts Slowly

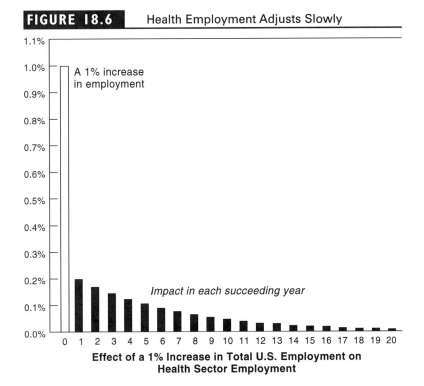

A 1% increase
in employment

Impact in each succeeding year

**Effect of a 1% Increase in Total U.S. Employment on
Health Sector Employment**

FIGURE 18.7   Effect of Medicare on Health Employment in Subsequent Years

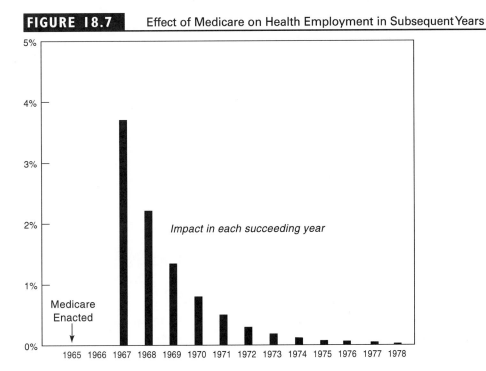

Impact in each succeeding year

Medicare
Enacted

hospital employees and self-employed physicians were even greater. There does not appear to be any consistent correlation between economic growth (GDP) and health care wages, but the thirty years of data available is not enough to be certain of this. Other than the apparent surge due to Medicare (which occurred before health care wage data was collected) no government policy appears to have significantly altered the health care wage trend. The adjustment of health care wages to changes in the rate of inflation is slow. More than 60 percent of the rise (or fall) in inflation from one year to the next was not incorporated in health care wages until the following year, and 11 percent was still missing after two years, indicating substantial contractual rigidity in health care wages.

Real health expenditures per capita in the United States grew 5 percent a year from 1960 to 2002, outpacing the 2 percent rate of growth in per capita incomes and thus consuming an ever-larger share of GDP. The labor portion of this 5 percent annual increase can be decomposed into a 4 percent increase in employment and a 1 percent annual increase in real wages; therefore increased intensity of medical services, more nurses and perfusionists and occupational therapists per patient day, is by far the more important cause of increased spending over this time span. However, since 1980 excessive compensation growth in the health care sector relative to the rest of the economy has accounted for a significant proportion of spending increases. With both wages and employment increasing faster than in other occupations, it may well be that health care professionals are getting more than a fair share of the nation's economic growth, a concern that health economist Uwe Reinhardt of Princeton University has humorously identified as "feasting on healthcare, or the allocation of lifestyles to providers."

Although the power of licensed health professions to control entry and wages is a major cause of delayed adjustment, it is not the only one. The dominance of nonprofit firms and third-party financing is also an important factor in creating labor market rigidity. Health services in the United States are currently undergoing significant institutional changes. The pattern of slow and delayed adjustment over the last forty years indicates that the ultimate outcome of these changes will not be revealed for a considerable period of time.

SUGGESTIONS FOR FURTHER READING

Cynthia Engel, "Health Services Industry: Still a Job Machine?" *Monthly Labor Review* (March 1999): 3–14 (www.bls.gov).

Milton Friedman, *A Theory of the Consumption Function* (Princeton, N.J.: Princeton University Press, 1957) and with Simon Kuznets, *Income from Independent Professional Practice* (New York: National Bureau of Economic Research, 1945).

Thomas E. Getzen "Forecasting Health Expenditures: Short, Medium and Long (Long) Term," *Journal of Health Care Finance* 26, no. 3 (Spring 2000): 56–72; and "Health Care Is An Individual Necessity and a National Luxury: Applying Multilevel Decision Models to the Analysis of Health Care Expenditures," *Journal of Health Economics* 19 (2000): 259–270.

Marian Osterweis et al, eds., *The U.S. Health Workforce: Power, Politics, and Policy* (Washington, D.C.: Association of Academic Health Centers, 1996).

Shiela Smith et al., "The Next Ten Years of Health Spending: What Does the Future Hold?" *Health Affairs* 17, no. 5 (September 1998): 128–141.

SUMMARY

1. Consumption and savings decisions are not based on current income, but on expected **permanent income** over the entire life cycle.

2. Shared financing through government and insurance makes health care into a **quasi-public good,** so that group or national income is the relevant budget constraint, not individual income.

3. The major determinants of total health spending are macroeconomic (inflation, population, and GDP).

4. Professional licensure, nonprofit organization, third-party reimbursement, and other institutional features **make the health care sector slow in adjusting to changes** in macroeconomic conditions.

5. These delays in response create **pressures for regulatory change.**

6. Many of the effects associated with the passage of health care cost control regulations are actually **delayed effects** of inflation and recession.

7. Real **increases in health care spending** are largely **increases in labor.** Much of the growth shows up in the form of new occupations, and some shows up as higher wages and professional incomes.

PROBLEMS

1. {*dynamics, productivity*} How many nonphysicians are currently employed in the health care sector for each M.D.? Is this ratio more than or less than it was fifty years ago? Does the change in the ratio of physician to nonphysician labor imply that productivity has increased or decreased? Which adjusts more rapidly to changes in demand, ancillary employment or physician supply?

2. {*flow of funds*} Which factor has accounted for more of the increase in the cost of hospital care per patient: increases in the number of physicians, the number of days of care, physician incomes, wages of nonphysician employees, or number of nonphysician employees?

3. {*dynamics*} Do delays in adjustment cause deficits, surpluses, or both?

4. {*elasticity*} If the income elasticity of NHE spending is 1.4 and per capita income increases from $12,000 to $15,000, how much will health care spending increase? If income elasticity is 0.9?

5. {*elasticity, aggregation*} Since the amount of income spent on health care for a group is just the sum of the amounts spent on each member, why would the income elasticity be different if the economist measured one person, or groups of ten, or one hundred, or 1 million? Is individual income elasticity for health care spending larger or smaller than national income elasticity for health care spending? If so, why?

6. {*fallacy of composition*} What determines how much is spent on your health care: how sick you are or how much money you earn? What determines how much is spent on average in the United States: how sick people are or how much money they earn?

7. {*price controls*} Suppose that you read Sunday's newspaper and learn that price controls have been put in place to limit the cost of health insurance to $2,500 per employee, which is significantly below the current average. What effects would you predict to occur?

8. {*inflation*} **a.** Assume that inflation is 4 percent for the years 2000 to 2004, jumps to 14 percent for the years 2005 and 2006, and then falls to 3 percent for 2007 to 2009. Calculate the price index using 2000 as the base year. What is the price in each year of a good whose price changes matched the overall level of inflation and cost $27.42 in 2002?

    b.   Suppose that service "L's" price adjusts with a lag, causing a third of the change in the rate of inflation to show up in L's price in each succeeding year. Calculate the annual percentage rates of price increase for L.

    c.   Suppose that good "A" anticipates future price increases, causing half the change in next year's inflation rate to show up in its price in advance. Calculate the annual rate of price increase for good A.

    d.   Which prices in the health care system might show delayed adjustment, lagging behind changes in the general rate of inflation? Which prices might show anticipatory response, changing in advance of the general rate of inflation? (*hint*: who sets premiums in advance?) What problems would this pattern of delay/advance present to administrators trying to work within a budget?

9.   {*inflation*} Will changes in the rate of inflation affect health care spending? In your answer, distinguish between real and nominal expenditures and between short- and long-run effects.

10.   {*dynamics*} Are decisions regarding health care budgets and medical school enrollments based on the past or the future?

11.   {*consumption*} What is the permanent income hypothesis? For which type of person would the permanent income hypothesis lead one to expect the greatest error from using tax returns to predict consumption?

    a.   Assistant manager at Macy's

    b.   Management intern at Macy's

    c.   Chief executive officer at Macy's

    d.   Retired vice president of Macy's

    e.   College student

    f.   Medical student

    g.   High school teacher

12.   {*dynamics*} Why might it take longer to adjust health care expenditures downward than upward? Frame your answer in terms of the economic incentives facing those who make the decisions.

13.   {*equilibrium, segregation*} What determines the level of wages among health care occupations?

14.   {*public good*} Why does insurance turn private medical care into a public good?

15.   {*price controls, dynamics*} Did health care costs rise less rapidly after President Nixon introduced price controls in 1971? Why or why not?

16.   {*dynamics, price controls*} Which forces cause the public to want price controls?

17.   {*price controls*} What was the effect of Medicare PPS, which paid a fixed price per DRG after 1983, on the length of hospital stay? Outpatient surgery? Nursing home admissions? Total Medicare hospital expenditures? Total Medicare expenditures for all types of care?

18.   {*voting*} If price controls and crazy tax proposals are the economic equivalent of voodoo, why do such proposals continue to gain support? For that matter, why has voodoo continued to be profitable?

19.   {*dynamics*} How long is the "long run"? How much difference can the length of the period used for measurement make on the estimates of price and income elasticity?

20. {*productivity*} Is it be possible to raise both employment and wages while still controlling total costs through the development of new technology that increases the productivity of medical care? Why or why not?

ENDNOTES

1. Understanding how capacity constraints interact with service delivery requires a shift in perspective that is sometimes difficult to grasp. The disconnect between individual and group perspective is, however, easily seen by considering what happens when people try to win a gold medal at the Olympics. While additional training and effort can increase the probability that any individual can win the gold, for the group as a whole the number of medals is fixed, there is only one gold. If everyone tries harder or trains more, there is no corresponding increase in medals. Similarly, studying harder may increase my chances of getting into Harvard medical school, but whether all applicants study harder, or watch more reality TV shows, does not affect the number of medical students at Harvard next year. Many resources have capacity constraints, and hence the determinants of individual and group consumption are not connected. If there are ten hearts available for transplant, then only ten people can get a heart transplant. Being young, a better match with donor tissue, having better insurance or political connections can all help an individual increase their personal chance of getting a transplant, but for the group as whole the number of transplants is fixed.

2. Thomas E. Getzen, "Health Care is an Individual Necessity and a National Luxury: Applying Multilevel Decision Models to the Analysis of Health Care Expenditures," *Journal of Health Economics* 19 (2000): 259–270.

3. David Mayston, "Disadvantaged Populations, Equity, and the Determinants of Health: Lessons from Down Under," in *Health, Health Care and Health Economics: Perspectives on Distribution*, Morris L. Barer, Thomas E. Getzen and Greg L. Stoddart, eds. (Chichester, U.K.: John Wiley & Sons, 1998).

4. Note that savings may temporarily be negative, as they are for many students who go into debt to support a lifestyle. Yet in the long run savings aggregated across all people must be positive (or at least zero). It is not possible for everyone everywhere to have more by going into debt. Note also that economists consider savings very different from food, clothing and other consumer goods because savings determine investment, interest rates, growth, the price level, and many other macroeconomic variables.

5. The economic definitions of "necessity" or "inferior good" and of "superior" or "luxury goods" depend solely on consumer buying behavior, whether income elasticity is less than or greater than 1.0, and not on any judgments regarding the usefulness or importance of the items, or how most people think of them. Thus bottled water, new cars and organic baby food all qualify as luxuries, while hot dogs, cheap costume jewelry and bus tickets are all termed necessities.

6. Milton Friedman and Simon Kuznets, *Income from Independent Professional Practice* (New York: National Bureau of Economic Research, 1945).

7. Milton Friedman, *A Theory of the Consumption Function* (Princeton, N.J.: Princeton University Press, 1957).

8. Franco Modigliani, *The Collected Papers of Franco Modigliani: Vol. 2: The Life-Cycle Hypothesis of Saving* (Cambridge, Mass.: MIT Press, 1980).

9. Getzen, op. cit., 2000.

10. Take-home advice: if you want to become rich, get in the habit of saving *now*, while you are still in school.

11. Thomas E. Getzen, "Macro Forecasting of National Health Expenditures," *Advances in Health Economics and Health Services Research* 11 (1990): 27–48.

12. William C. Goodman, "Employment in Services Industries Affected by Recessions and Expansions," *Monthly Labor Review* (October 2002): 1–15 (www.bls.gov).

13. Angus Deaton, "Involuntary Savings Through Inflation," *American Economic Review* 67 (1977): 899–910.

14. The data for all health workers are, unfortunately, not readily comparable across these years.

15. Shiela Smith et al., "The Next Ten Years of Health Spending: What Does the Future Hold?" *Health Affairs* 17, no. 5 (September 1998): 128–141.

16. Thomas E. Getzen, "Macro Forecasting of National Health Expenditures," *Advances in Health Economics and Health Services Research* 11 (1990): 27–48.

17. Thomas E. Getzen, "Forecasting Health Expenditures: Short, Medium and Long (Long) Term," *Journal of Health Care Finance* 26, no. 3 (Spring 2000): 56–72.

18. Christopher J. Ruhm, "Are Recessions Good For Your Health?" *The Quarterly Journal of Economics* CXV (May 2000): 617–650; "Good Times Make You Sick," December 2002, and "Healthy Living in Hard Times," January 2003, working papers for University of North Carolina Greensboro and NBER.

19. David Dranove and Kenneth Cone, "Do State Rate Regulations Really Lower Hospital Expenses?" *Journal of Health Economics* 4, no. 2 (1985: 159–165; C. Eby and D. Cohodes, "What Do We Know About Rate

Setting?" *Journal of Health Politics, Policy & Law* 10 (1985): 299–327; Michael Morrisey, Douglas Conrad, Steven Shortell, and Karen Cook, "Hospital Rate Review: A Theory and Empirical Review," *Journal of Health Economics* 3, no. 1 (1984): 24–47.

20. Paul Ginsburg, "Impact of the Hospital Stabilization Program on Hospitals," in M. Zubkoff, I. E. Raskin, and R. S. Hanft, eds., *Hospital Cost Containment: Selected Notes for Future Policy* (New York: PRODIST for Milbank Memorial Fund, 1978), 293–323.

21. Congressional Budget Office, *Rising Health Care Costs: Causes, Implications and Strategies* (Washington, D.C.: U.S. Government Printing Office, 1991).

22. Karen Davis, Gerard Anderson, Diane Rowland, and Earl Steinberg, *Health Care Cost Containment* (Baltimore, Md.: Johns Hopkins University Press, 1990).

23. Michael Kendix and Thomas Getzen, "U.S. Health Services Employment: A Time Series Analysis," *Health Economics* 3, no. 3 (1994): 169–181.

CHAPTER **19**

VALUE FOR MONEY IN THE FUTURE OF HEALTH CARE

QUESTIONS

1. What, how, and for whom is medical care produced?
2. Is Medicare likely to go broke, or continue to grow?
3. Will investors put more money into biotechnology or nursing homes?
4. How will economists affect the allocation of health care? Of health care incomes?
5. Are people willing to spend more and get less health?
6. Why is it so hard to reach a consensus if everyone knows what the problem is?

19.1 FORCING THE QUESTION: WHO GETS HEALTHY AND WHO GETS PAID?

The most important contribution economists can make to the operation of the health care system is to be relentless in pointing out that every choice involves a trade-off—that certain difficult questions regarding who gets what, and who must give up what, are inevitable and must be faced even when politicians, the public, and patients would rather avoid them. In the words of Paul Samuelson, "Every economy must answer a triad of questions: *what, how,* and *for whom.*"[1] In the case of cancer, for example, one could ask what symptoms or diagnoses are to be treated, whether inpatient or outpatient, by generalists or specialists, and who is to receive first priority for treatment (those who plan ahead and show up first, those who are most ill, most likely to recover, or best insured). Although these questions can be asked independently, the answer to one influences all the others: "for whom" affects "what" and "how," and vice versa. Any answer also determines who pays, who gets paid, and how much; that is, it determines the distribution of income as well as the distribution of health care.

It is the job of health economists to give economic advice, not patient care. They estimate, evaluate, and elucidate the decisions to be made; they do not make the decisions or carry them out. The analysis of decision making can be divided into three levels:

- What are the questions?
- Who is going to decide?
- What are the answers?

For most economists, it is necessary to work backward, starting with the data collection required to make comparisons among different treatments (i.e., cost-benefit analysis), then considering how different systems for making medical care decisions can affect efficiency (e.g., indemnity insurance versus managed care, network providers versus solo providers), and only then approaching the top level—framing the questions. Tracing the flow of money over the last eighteen chapters reveals that while data can be used for clarification, the questions are fundamentally *economic;* they are about choices and thus have to do with values as well as numbers. Are some lives worth more than others? What does it mean to be human? How much should a surgeon be paid for a one-hour operation if it saves a life? Which product of the health care system is more important, social justice or cancer mortality?

The pragmatic and detailed collection of data for comparing the costs and outcomes of different drugs, different surgical procedures, and different treatment settings has grown rapidly over the last decade. Doing such work requires a tremendous amount of clinical knowledge and an understanding of basic economic principles: equilibrium at the margin, production functions, comparative advantage, opportunity cost, and so on. Increasingly, such work is being carried out by clinicians who have training in economic concepts, while economists concentrate on developing theory and new measurement techniques.

Upon this mass of detailed data collection and analysis rests the second layer of issues regarding how to design a better health care system. At this level, the question is not whether radiation is better than chemotherapy, but whether capitation or fee-for-service leads to better decisions, or whether group practice is more efficient than solo practice. The focus shifts from the particular decision being made to the issue of who is making the decision—physicians, patients, or payers.

As economists trace how the flow of money follows the path of decision making, the assumptions embedded in the current medical care system become more evident. Analysis at the third level becomes reflective. What does "better" mean? According to which value system? Better for whom? Analysis transcends the current system as it is by asking: What are the questions? Reaching beyond the veil of money and grasping the concept that every dollar spent on health care is a dollar earned by a health care provider makes it clear how the distribution of income and health are connected, and suggests some fruitful directions for assessing the health implications of changes in economic organization.

19.2 SPENDING MONEY OR PRODUCING HEALTH?

The distribution of health is unequal and has a profound impact on economic well-being. Some people work productively for years and die contentedly with wealth and happiness in old age, while others struggle for a few months or decades in agony as they are relentlessly drawn down into premature mortality. The question is not whether the distribution of health is fair, or whether it determines or is determined by income, but whether it is amenable to change. More precisely, the questions are: How, and how much, change can be brought about by spending more on medical care? What is that change worth? The marginal productivity of medical care spending declines as more is spent. Increasing spending from $4,000 to $5,000 per person increases average life expectancy, but not by as much as increasing spending from $2,000 to $3,000, which, in turn, does not have as large an effect as going from $0 to $1,000. As more and more money is spent, fewer and fewer gains are achieved in life expectancy as the "flat of the curve" is reached, where marginal productivity, although still positive, is barely above zero.

Reaching a consensus on how much to spend becomes more complicated when there are two or more types of people who are to receive care. Suppose one group is relatively healthy and would maintain a high level of health even if no money were spent on them, while another group begins at a disadvantage and, even with maximal effort, would still remain less healthy. If the same amount is spent per person on each group, the total and marginal impact of medical care will be very low in the healthy group, which seems wasteful, while the sicker group would still be forced to do without a lot of potentially beneficial care. To jointly maximize the average healthiness of all people for a given health care budget, it would be necessary to equalize the marginal productivity of medical care (increase in health per additional dollar spent) across both groups, spending much more per person on the sicker people. Such an allocation of medical care resources might seem both fair and efficient, but it also might not. Suppose the healthy group consisted of employed people who paid insurance premiums while the sicker group were heroin and cocaine users. Most voters would not be willing to cut funding for those who take care of themselves and go to work every day in order to provide more funding to people who stick needles in their arms. Further complications are posed by groups such as infants born with genetic defects who are likely to die young even with the best medical care. Should they be denied treatment on the grounds that it would not do them much good anyway?

Although stating that the goal of medical care is to maximize health seems superficially accurate and appropriate, a little reflection (or reading the last eighteen chapters) shows how inaccurate and irrelevant such a measure often is. If taken literally, maximizing health would mean that most hospitals in the United States would close so that more food, clothes, books, and medicine could be provided to China, India, Mozambique, and other less developed countries. It would also force most surgeons to give up their operating rooms in favor of sewage treatment plants, and force psychiatrists to give up the provision of therapy and the prescription of psychoactive drugs in favor of immunization campaigns and early childhood education. Stating that the goal of medical care is to maximize health for all is not only inaccurate, but profoundly misleading. It confuses a measure of social welfare with the incentives of the groups that make up society to maximize their own welfare. Doctors, nurses, hospital supply company executives, National Basketball Association players, healthy industrial workers, college students, and other definable groups have multiple objectives, including the health of their families and their own incomes, many of which are more important to them than the advancement of global health averages.

It is relatively easy to understand why most Americans do not want all of their hospitals to close, and why most of the doctors who work in them are not eager to practice in Mozambique, even if they are certain that the number of additional life years produced would be higher. It is less obvious why Americans keep spending more and more on medical care if technological advances are making medicine more productive and efficient. Given that the baseline life expectancy at birth, even in the absence of medical care, is much higher now than it was a century ago, each year of life expectancy added becomes more difficult and more expensive to obtain; therefore, marginal productivity (gain in life expectancy per additional dollar spent) is much lower today than it was 50 or 100 years ago. If society optimized by choosing the point at which the value of health matched the price of health, and the value of health were the same, then less money would be spent as technology improved.[2] Instead, we now spend more per person, implying that the incremental increase in health per additional dollar is even smaller. Extrapolating from the comparisons with Japan, Germany, and England in Chapter 17, it appears that it would be possible to cut spending by a third or more, with only a minor decrease in health, leaving average life expectancy in the United States almost unchanged at 77 years.

The declining marginal productivity of health care is offset, to some extent, by the increasing aggregate wealth of society, which raises the dollar value of each additional year of health gained (see Table 16.2). The increased medical buying power of specific groups of people who are likely to be high utilizers of care (the elderly, children with disabilities) is perhaps more important as a factor in augmenting demand. Yet even so, the vastness of the increase in medical spending cannot be explained purely in terms of productivity and relative prices. It must be recognized that medical care has become largely a consumption good. Economists do not seek to explain increased spending on clothes in terms of warmth or durability, or gourmet takeout food in terms of calories and vitamins, and they should not try to explain all of the increase in medical expenditures in terms of health or life expectancy. Although it may seem inappropriate to compare arthroscopic surgery to the cut of a jacket, or organ transplants to organic vegetarian sushi, it is impossible to avoid the conclusion that medical care has a significant consumption component that is not well explained by production theory. Medicine is beginning to more and more resemble the service industries studied by marketing researchers.

If surgery is sold like automobiles, and mental health like entertainment,[3] what role is there for the dismal science of economics with its insistent "on the other hand"? Perhaps economists relate to the public and politicians in a manner similar to the way personal trainers relate to their affluent and often overweight clients: as someone whose expertise is required to in order to establish authority and make compliance with an unpleasant regime easier, even though all of the exercises and advice are pretty simple and mostly well known in advance. It may be that economists, like politicians, are being paid to talk about the old-fashioned values of thrift and efficiency that everyone is eager to hear about, if not always to follow.

19.3 ALLOCATION, ALLOCATION, ALLOCATION

When asked which three factors are most important in determining value, real estate appraisers reply, "location, location, and location." In a similar vein, health economists asked to determine the value of the money spent on health care must focus primarily on allocation: the distribution of resources, the distribution of health, the distribution of medical care, and the distribution of provider incomes. Although a high value is often placed on the quality of nursing care, the skill of the physician, or the use of new medical technology, none of these matters much if the care is provided to the wrong person or at the wrong time. The health economist is asked to assess economic efficiency, how well the health care system has used the resources available to achieve its stated (and unstated) goals. The following short list contains a few of the questions that must be answered in this regard:

- Which diseases should be treated?
- Which people should be treated?
- How much care should be given?
- Who will pay?
- If the money is to come from taxes, who should be taxed most—those who benefit most or those who can most afford to pay?
- Should more money be spent on prevention or cure?
- How much should healers be paid?

- Should treatment be given by specialists or primary care providers?
- How should the power to make decisions be allocated?

Allocation is the subject of economics. Why, then, haven't economists been more successful in reforming health care? First, it must be recognized that the study of health economics has indeed improved efficiency to some degree. It has made the system better, although it is still far from perfect. Cost-benefit analysis has led to a reduction in the over-investment in hospitals, to the support and improvement of immunization programs, and to the more rapid and objective evaluation of new drugs. Assessment of incentives and risk bearing has led to the creation of new types of insurance and to the refinement of managed care contracting. The application of microeconomics to decisions regarding individual allocation has only limited potential, however, because the most crucial issues in health are likely to involve public goods, macro allocation, and the contentious questions of how the costs and benefits are to be distributed between different groups of producers and consumers.

It is quite possible to spend less on health care and simultaneously improve the average level of health by changing the allocation of resources. Yet just as U.S. citizens are unlikely to vote for a program that cuts Medicare in half and sends 80 percent of the remaining funds overseas to clinics in poor countries to raise average global life expectancy, almost any reallocation that improves efficiency makes some concerned group with decision-making power worse off, and is, therefore, likely to be opposed even if it clearly improves overall efficiency. The difficulty for health economists is that the question of "how to improve efficiency" is less relevant to reform of health care than the question of how to make a deal so that the various interests can agree to make a change that, at the cost of harming some identifiable groups, yields an increase in average benefits.

19.4 DYNAMIC EFFICIENCY

Deals are difficult to make, even when clearly beneficial overall, because groups that will be harmed find it hard to be sure that their concerns are adequately weighed and that the harm done to them is somehow offset by benefits gained from other programs and policies. Assurances of fair treatment are harder to believe the more distant in time and uncertain the compensating benefits are. Thus, while a group of elderly people may possibly be willing to accept less technologically advanced treatment for a reduction in their premiums and out-of-pocket costs, they might not be willing to make such a sacrifice in order to fund research that will only bring results twenty or thirty years from now. Although this reluctance may be short-sighted, it is perfectly reasonable.

The problems of allocation are often formalized by economists in terms of technical productivity (maximizing the output from any given set of resource inputs), cost minimization (choosing the least expensive set of inputs), and current economic efficiency (balancing marginal costs and marginal benefits). More sophisticated analyses may also consider how systems are structured to deal with transactions costs and public goods. In medicine, the most important allocation may be that between current consumption and future productivity. The difference between adequate and outstanding current practice is far smaller than the gap between what was possible twenty years ago and what is expected within the next decade (gene therapy, real-time imaging, robotic laser surgery, in vitro diagnoses). The challenge is to structure a health care system for *dynamic efficiency,* creating technological and organizational change to improve health and productivity. Some current allocative efficiency must be sacrificed for scientists to spend time tinkering to make new discoveries and to give managers the slack to come up

THE VALUE OF MEDICAL PROGRESS

Is the development of new medical technology worth the cost? Should we have spent so much money trying to improve health? William Nordhaus concluded that the growth in longevity in the United States during the twentieth century was approximately equal in value to the growth in all nonhealth goods and services in the economy.[4] However, a substantial portion of that increase in longevity was due to better housing, nutrition, education, heating, transportation, and other nonmedical factors. David Cutler and Mark McClellan examined technological advances in five conditions: heart attack, low birth weight, breast cancer, depression, and cataracts. Table 19.1 summarizes their findings. For heart attacks, the cost of treatment increased from $12,083 in 1984 to $21,714 in 1998 (inflation adjusted), a real increase of $9,631 per case.[5] Life expectancy increased from just under five years to a bit over six, a gain of more than a year. If society values an extra year of life at $10,000 or more, it appears that the gains in health are worth more than the cost. (Usual assumptions for the value of a year of life are in the range of $750,000 to $375,000 per additional year.) Conversely, treatment of breast and most other cancers has become substantially more expensive but has not provided sizable increases in life expectancy. Overall assessment depends on the mix of treatments and individuals considered, but it does appear clear that on net, the investment in medical technology in the twentieth century has been economically beneficial.

TABLE 19.1 Costs and Gains of Medical Technology

Condition	Period	Incremental Cost	Gains from Treatment
Heart attack	1984–1998	$9,631	One more year of life
Low birthweight	1950–1990	$40,000	Twelve years of life
Depression	1991–1996	(decreased)	Better quality of life
Cataracts	1969–1998	($0 or decrease)	Better quality of life
Breast cancer	1985–1996	$20,000	Two months of life

Source: Cutler and McClellan (2001).

with ideas for new products and service delivery systems. A purely cost-minimizing organization is not creative enough to be economically efficient in the long run.

19.5 THE FUTURE

What can be said about the future of health and medical care over the next fifty years? Table 19.2 lists expected trends. It is relatively certain that there will be continued increases in longevity, greater technological capability to treat disease, and continuous increases in expenditure. While there will be more spending overall, the sources and uses of funding will change rather markedly, and it is probable that at some point the annual rate of increase will moderate. An older and healthier population implies more long-term care, with greater emphasis on caring and rehabilitation. Thus, the fraction of medical spending accounted for by acute illnesses of the employed tax-paying population will fall. The tension between public and private financing is likely to remain unresolved, with payers operating under a mixture of market incentives and regulatory structures to provide a

TABLE 19.2	Future Trends

- Greater longevity, better health.
- More long-term and chronic care, less acute illness
- More spending overall, but a smaller fraction spent on the working population
- Less ability to shift costs by overcharging for treatment
- A middle ground between public and private control
- More assessment of cost and outcomes
- Declining trust in medicine as an organized profession
- Physicians lead teams within organizations, less autonomy and independence
- Successful organizations based on information (e.g., biotechnology) and caring (e.g., hospice)
- Special characteristics previously found mostly in medical care become more typical of many service organizations in a post-industrial economy.

middle ground. Treatment and production will become less and less important relative to the provision of caring and information. The best prototypes for studying health economics in the twenty-first century are probably biotechnology and hospice. Physicians will become technical team leaders operating within a corporate organization, rather than independent medical practitioners. Cost-shifting in the form of marked-up prices and open-ended reimbursement will continue to wither and be replaced by new forms, such as mandated benefits pools. The use of economic information and cost accounting for comparative decision making will continue to increase. Greater knowledge about actual costs and the actual effectiveness of clinical practice will provide greater clarity in the questions raised about the trade-off between dollars and health. Some fields (dietary modification, parts of mental health and disability care) are being spun off and are less likely to be counted as an integral part of medicine. Others, such as information systems and genetic engineering, are becoming more integrated and will blur the traditional boundaries between what is medicine and what is information or environmental modification.

The special institutional features that set medicine and health apart from the rest of the economy may become less so over the coming years. In part, this is because medicine is becoming more organized and more corporate, more subject to a bottom-line assessment of cost and benefits. Yet the extent to which medicine is becoming like the rest of the economy is probably of far less importance than the extent to which the rest of the economy is becoming like medicine, where information, service, and public goods matter more than manufactured commodities. Previously, health economists have taken models from the study of industrial production and applied them to health and medical care. Ideas may increasingly flow in the other direction as the issues of special interest to health economists—uncertainty, agency, trust, service delivery, and quality—become central to the economy as a whole in a post-industrial era. Models developed for the study of medical care may in the future be applied to banking, entertainment, automation, fashion, and other industries.

SUGGESTIONS FOR FURTHER READING

Victor Fuchs, "Economics, Values and Health Care Reform," *American Economic Review* 86, no. 1 (1996): 1–24.

Ian Morrison, *Health Care in the New Millennium* (San Francisco: Jossey-Bass, 2000

Institute of Medicine, *Crossing the Quality Chasm* (www.nap.edu/books/0309072808html), July 2001.

David M. Cutler and Mark McClellan, "Is Technological Change in Medicine Worth It?" *Health Affairs* (September 2001), 11–29.

SUMMARY

1. A primary role of health economists is to **force the public and politicians to consider the trade-offs** implicit in every health and medical care decision. Who gets helped? Who gets hurt? Who makes money?

2. Health economics can be viewed as answering questions in levels of ascending generality. At the base are the questions, **Which treatments are better?** and **How much do they cost?** At an intermediate level, **Who is going to have the power to make decisions?** Finally, **Which questions should be asked** to shape and judge the health care system?

3. The purpose of the health care system is to **satisfy the interests of the groups that participate** in it. Maximizing health is but one of many objectives. The average health of the population often may matter much less than *who*, in particular, gets healthy.

4. The increase in health and life expectancy that can be obtained from any given set of medical resources depends largely on the **allocation** of treatment to those most likely to benefit. Often, this is not the group that is most able or willing to pay.

5. Major **difficulties in economic appraisal** of health care policies arise because the most important issues frequently involve **public goods** and the **distribution of benefits and incomes** to different groups, as well as technical issues regarding productive efficiency.

6. Differences in the quality of care at a particular point in time are usually dwarfed by changes in the effectiveness of care over time. Hence, a health care system must provide resources and slack to make room for experiments, fostering the technological and organizational change that bring about **dynamic efficiency.**

7. **Values** ultimately mean more in health economics than the efficacy of medical technology or the estimation of costs. Analysis will increasingly focus on **the economics of caring and information,** not production.

PROBLEMS

1. {*allocation*} Will health care be more efficient or less efficient in 2020? Will people spend more money or less money on health care?

2. {*budget*} Will Medicare go broke by 2012 as some analysts predict? Why or why not? What historical evidence could you give to support your answer?

3. {*distribution*} Which matters more, how healthy we are on average or *who* gets healthy?

4. {*values*} Economists debate the future of Medicare by arguing about which set of numbers best represents reality. Do these numbers represent objective or subjective values?

5. {*economic organization, distribution*} Who will make the decisions regarding medical care in the year 2020? Which of these groups will have more or less power in 2020?

   a. Physicians
   b. Nurses
   c. Pharmaceutical companies
   d. Biotechnology investors

    e.   U.S. senators

    f.   AARP (formerly the American Association of Retired Persons)

    g.   Disability advocates

    h.   Children

    i.   Economists

6.   {*productivity*} As medical technology continues to develop, will the marginal productivity per dollar spent increase or decrease?

7.   {*economic organization, distribution*} Are health care funds spent to maximize health or to maximize the welfare of those who make the decisions?

ENDNOTES

1.   Paul Samuelson and William Nordhaus, *Economics,* 14th ed. (New York: McGraw-Hill, 1992), 19.

2.   It is possible to construct a production function that moves up and yet is steeper, with greater average productivity and yet lower marginal productivity for a given set of inputs, but it requires some contortion to do so, and such quirks are unlikely to explain the large and persistent rise in health care spending that has accompanied the twentieth-century advance of health care technology. Some other explanation must be found if the attempt is to remain plausible.

3.   In the words of Dr. John R. Ball, president of the nation's oldest hospital, "Health care used to be something perceived as mystical. Now it's something closer to marketing a product or a service," as quoted in Eric Hollreiser, "Nation's Oldest Hospital Coping With New Age," *Philadelphia Business Journal,* March 22, 1996, p. 25.

4.   William D. Nordhaus, "The Health of Nations: The Contribution of Improved Health to Living Standards. NBER working paper 8818, January 2002, NBER: Cambridge, Mass. (www.nber.org).

5.   David M. Cutler and Mark McClellan, "Is Technological Change in Medicine Worth It?" *Health Affairs,* September 2001, pp. 11–29.

GLOSSARY

Activities of Daily Living (ADLs) A checklist measure of the extent of disability and functional status.

Actuarially Fair Premium A premium equal to the expected value of the loss, although in practice all premiums must be set higher in order to cover overhead costs.

Actuary Accredited insurance mathematician who calculates premium rates and company reserve requirements using statistical studies.

Administered Prices Prices which are specified by an administrative agency, rather than being set in the market.

Administered Service Only (ASO) A self-insured health plan in which the employer bears all the risk of losses, but hires an administrator to process claims.

Administratively Necessary Days (ANDs) Payment for days when a patient's medical status is such that they should have been discharged from the hospital but were not because no nursing home beds were available.

Adverse Selection A disproportionate share of bad risks. When given a choice, the people who choose to purchase insurance are likely to be a group with higher than average losses.

Agency The process of having one party (the agent) make decisions on behalf of another (the principal).

Aggregation The process of clumping together; the creation of summary measures for a population as a whole; study at the system or group level.

Allocative Efficiency Allowing those who value a good more to consume more. Total consumption value is maximized by allowing the process to continue toward an equilibrium where for each individual, marginal benefit = marginal cost. Also, targeting medical care to those most in need so as to maximize average life expectancy.

American Medical Association (AMA) The professional organization which represents the interest of MD physicians in the United States and lobbies government agencies on their behalf.

Anti-trust Legal restrictions relating to collusion between firms and market domination.

Arbitrage The process by which the prices of a good selling to different persons or in different markets are brought together by trade. Also, the act of buying and selling in anticipation of price movements—which makes the price adjust more rapidly to information.

Assignment An agreement by a physician to take payment directly from Medicare, and to accept the amount as payment in full (i.e., with no balance billing).

Average Cost The total cost divided by the number of units.

Balance Billing Making the patient pay for the balance of any charges in excess of the amount allowed by the insurance company.

Balanced Budget Act of 1997 An act passed by the U.S. Congress in 1997 that significantly expands the role of managed care in the Medicare Program.

Branded Drugs Drugs whose production and sale are protected by a patent. Also, the brand-name drug produced by the initial firm even after its patent expires and other firms begin to sell competing generic versions.

Cap A limit on the amount that an insurance company will pay. The cap may be an overall maximum, such as a lifetime maximum of $250,000, or may apply to specific services, such as a $500 per year cap on outpatient mental health counselling.

Capitation Paying a fixed amount per enrolled person per month for a defined set of services which does not vary with **utilization**.

Case-Mix Reimbursement Adjustment of reimbursement to account for differences in patient diagnoses, and sometimes for the severity of illness as well.

Certificate of Need (CON) A legal requirement that approval from a state agency to

411

certify need (CON) must be obtained before a health care facility is built or remodeled.

Ceteris Paribus All other factors being held constant.

Charges The amount appearing on the patient's bill.

Chiropractic An alternative form of medical practice which emphasizes spinal manipulation in the treatment of disease, often to the exclusion of drugs and surgery. Although chiropractors are found in most communities, they are often not accepted by the organized medical profession.

Circular Flow of Funds The circulation of money facilitates exchange; it is not used up or consumed. Each dollar spent by a consumer goes to a producer, who in turn gives it to an owner, worker or supplier, who as consumers send those dollars on to another producer, and so on in an unending circular flow.

Clinical Pathways A protocol, or defined standard set of tests and procedures to be used in diagnosing or treating a particular symptom or disease.

Clinical Trials Testing of new drugs or medical technology on humans.

Coase Theorem The assertion that the type of economic organization (profit or non-profit, one firm or many, capitalist or socialist) and which party holds ownership rights (e.g., chemical firms or fishermen, homeowners or airport operators) would not matter if there were no transaction costs.

Coinsurance The amount of the bill not paid by insurance, but by the patient. A plan with 15% coinsurance means that the insurance company pays 85% and the person pays 15%.

Community Rating Setting the same premium rate for every person in the community regardless of age, sex or previous illness.

Comparative Statics The study of a system by comparing how the state of equilibrium differs when some set of parameters (incomes, prices, fertility) differs; in contrast to **dynamics** in which the process of change is the focus of study.

Compounding Adding to; the accumulation of growth over time; how a small percentage increase eventually leads, with interest on the interest, to doubling, quadrupling and manyfold increasing.

Concurrent Review Daily checks by an HMO on the status of a patient to monitor, and if

necessary, modify or terminate, the provision of services.

Consumer Price Index (CPI) A measure of the average change in price over time in a fixed "market basket" of goods and service purchased either by urban wage earners and clerical workers or by all urban consumers.

Consumer Surplus The difference between what consumers are willing to pay for a product and the market clearing price. As such, consumer surplus is represented by the area under the demand curve but above market price.

Consumption Function The relationship between consumption and income as income changes; the fraction of total income saved as the level or composition of aggregate income changes.

Continuing Care Retirement Communities (CCRCs) Living quarters for elderly persons with provisions for meals, transportation, therapy and other assistance, usually constructed with an adjacent nursing home. Financial risks to the individual are often reduced through prepayment. Also known as lifecare communities.

Copayment A copayment is a specified amount that the patient must pay with each service received, such as the $2 for each prescription that many drug plans make the pharmacist collect, $10 for each day in the hospital under Medicare, $5 for each visit to the doctor under some HMO plans, etc. One of the purposes of copayments is to discourage overutilization. Thus while deductibles and coinsurance may sometimes be covered under a spouse's plan or other insurance, the insured must usually pay the copayment out of pocket.

Cost Reimbursement Retrospective payment for services based upon audited cost reports, often including complex limits and rules for allocation.

Cost Shifting The process of using excess revenues from one set of services or patients to subsidize other services or patient groups.

Cost-Benefit Analysis (CBA) A set of techniques for assisting in the making of decisions, which translates all relevant concerns into market (dollar) terms.

Cost-Effectiveness Analysis (CEA) Comparison of the costs of different ways of achieving an objective (cases prevented, years of life saved). Similar to CBA, except that CEA does not require benefits to be expressed in dollar terms.

Cream Skimming Choosing to provide only the most profitable services, or to insure only the healthiest patients, so as to avoid subsidizing public goods (education, research, indigent care) and thus obtaining extra profits.

Cross-Sectional Analysis Statistics constructed using observations across different individuals or groups at one point in time, as opposed to **longitudinal** or **time-series** analysis.

Deductible An amount that must be paid by the individual before the insurance company begins to pay. For example, many policies have a $100 per year deductible. This means that if total insured medical bills were $730, the insurance would apply only after the person had paid the first $100, that is, to $630.

Demand A schedule of the amount that will be consumed in the market at varying prices.

Demographic Transition The period of rapidly increasing population which usually occurs during economic development as a poor society with high mortality and high birth rates transitions to a wealthy society with low mortality and low birth rates.

Demographics Age, sex, and other characteristics of populations.

Derived Demand The demand for an input due to the demand for output; demand for a good due to its use, rather than in itself (e.g., the demand for x-ray film is derived from the demand for medical diagnoses, which in turn are derived from a consumer's demand for health).

Detailing Marketing of pharmaceuticals to physicians by drug company representatives (detailers); offers of free samples and advice in order to increase the number of times a drug is prescribed.

Diagnostically Related Grouping (DRG) A system of reimbursement which compensates by the case (rather than per day or per charged item) based on the diagnosis of the patient.

Diminishing Marginal Returns As additional inputs of a variable input are put into the production process, holding constant all other variables, the addition to total output will eventually decline.

Discounted FFS Contracts with providers to pay a specified percentage of usual charges.

Discounting Adjustment of valuation for the passage of time, reflecting the fact that the present value of a future good is smaller. Also, adjustments to reflect risk, reductions in the quality of life, and other factors.

Diseconomies of Scale The average cost per unit rises as the quantity produced increases.

Dynamic Efficiency Use of inputs so as to maximize long-run value over time, taking account of the need for tinkering to bring about technological and organizational advances.

Dynamic Shortage A temporary deficit in supply caused by a sudden increase in demand, or sudden drop in supply.

Dynamics The process of change; the study of how change occurs over time, including the order, timing and strength of interacting forces.

Economies of Scale The average cost per unit decreases as output increases.

Efficacy The ability to actually cure a disease; how well a treatment works in practice.

Elasticity The percentage change in one variable when another variable changes by one percent.

Enrollee A person covered by a health benefits plan.

Entitlements Social insurance payments to which beneficiaries are entitled by law with little regard to actual contributions or premiums, or income qualifications (e.g., Medicare, Social Security).

Entrepreneur The person who undertakes the effort to create an organization and the network of contracts necessary for its success.

ERISA The "Employee Retirement And Income Security Act of 1974" and subsequent amendments which govern most health insurance contracts, and in particular, exempt self-insured plans from most state regulation.

Expected Value The value of an outcome multiplied by its probability of occurring. Also, the probability-weighted average of all possible outcomes.

Experience Rating Setting a group premium based on the actual losses experienced by that group during the prior year or years.

Externalities The effects of a transaction between parties on outsiders; the uncompensated effects of an action (e.g., pollution); side-effects.

Fallacy of Composition The logical error of assuming that what holds true for the individuals within a group must also hold true for the group collectively, or vice-versa.

Fee Schedule A list of approved fees for each service promulgated by an insurance company, government agency, or professional society.

Fee-For-Service (FFS) Payment for health care based on the charges for each service or item used.

Firm An organization that is responsible for coordinating the transformation of inputs, such as land, labour, capital, and entrepreneurship, into some final output or outputs.

Flexible Budget A budget that is adjusted for changes in the volume of service.

Flexner Report The critique written in 1910 which led to the reform of medical education and established the MD degree as a qualification for licensure.

Flow The amount over a period of time (i.e., income, annual mortality rate).

Food and Drug Administration (FDA) The federal agency with jurisdiction over labelling, manufacture, and sale of food and drugs for human consumption.

Formulary A list of approved drugs for reimbursement with all non-approved drugs paid at a lesser rate or not at all.

Free Rider A person who allows others to produce a public good, and then uses it without paying. For example, most poor country prevention programs are free-riders, dependent upon the research of rich countries to do the research and produce the vaccines needed to control infectious diseases.

Full Time Equivalents (FTE) A measure of the quantity of labor used.

Fundamental Theorem of Exchange Any voluntary exchange between persons must make both of them better off since they willingly agreed to trade.

Gatekeeper A primary physician who manages and approves all services for the patient who enrolls in his practice.

Generic Drugs Drugs which are identical in chemical composition to a brand name pharmaceutical preparation, but produced by competitors after the firm's patent expires.

Global Budget A fixed total budget for all health services.

Grandfathering Approving those who are already in practice to continue even if they do not meet the new standards.

Gross Domestic Product (GDP) The total market value of all production in a nation.

Group Insurance Contract for insurance made with an employer or other entity, called the policyholder, that covers a group of persons as a single unit.

Health Maintenance Organization (HMO) An organization that contracts to provide comprehensive medical services (not reimbursement) for a specified fee each month. The term health maintenance organization arose because doctors under this arrangement have a financial incentive to keep their patients healthy, since they are not paid more for providing more services.

Health Insurance Portability and Accountability Act of 1996 (HIPAA) A legislated set of rules to increase efficiency by standardizing billing and making health care transactions paperless. HIPAA also specified rules governing access to records, privacy, confidentiality, combat fraud, develop medical savings accounts, and other maters.

Homeopathy An alternative form of health practice emphasizing natural remedies used in extremely dilute solutions.

Hospital Privileges The rights of those doctors who have been voted acceptance on the hospital's medical staff to admit patients and perform surgery.

Human Capital Analysis of investments of time, effort, and money in education or health that improve productivity as analogous to investments of financial capital.

Income Distribution The fraction of all income earned by the top 10 percent of the population, the second 10 percent, and so on; the degree of disparity in incomes between the rich and the poor.

Income Elasticity The percentage change in expenditures due to a one percent change in income. Income elasticities below 1.0 mean that although spending on a good rises with income, it rises less than proportionately so that the fraction of total income spent on that good is reduced. With income elasticities greater than 1.0 (luxury goods), spending rises more than proportionately so that the share of total income spent on the good increases as income increases.

Indemnity Benefit A specified dollar amount reimbursed for a particular injury or type of care, such as $15 for each x-ray or $475 for gall bladder removal, is an indemnity benefit. Life insurance, which provides a specified dollar amount in case of death, has an indemnity benefit.

Independent Practice Association (IPA-HMO) An HMO formed by non-exclusive contracts with many providers who operate independently, as opposed to closed group staff HMO where physicians work exclusively for the HMO and are often on salary.

Inflation A measure of the reduction in the real purchasing power of currency over time.

Information Asymmetry The disparity in information between a buyer and a seller in a transaction.

Inpatient Services or goods provided within a hospital or nursing home.

Intensity (of services) The amount of inputs used to provide each unit of service. For example, an urban university hospital will typically provide complex services of high intensity, while a primary care doctor on an emergency call in an isolated rural area will use far fewer resources to treat the same injury.

Investigational New Drug (IND) A designation of FDA approval to begin the testing of a drug.

Kickbacks Surreptitious payments made in order to obtain business.

Licensure The establishment of legal restrictions specifying which individuals or firms have the rights to provide services or goods.

Life-Cycle Hypothesis Assertion that individual spending at any point in time is based on their long-run expected income over the life-cycle rather than just current income at that point in time; a common form of the **permanent income** hypothesis.

Loading Factor (or Load) The percentage of total premiums used for administrative costs, profits, and all items other than medical benefits.

Long-Term Care (LTC) Nursing homes, visiting nurses, home I.V. and other services provided to chronically ill or disabled persons.

Longitudinal Analysis Study of a set of individuals or groups tracking how they change over time.

Macroeconomics (from the Greek 'macro' meaning large) The branch of economics that studies how the economy as a whole operates, covering such topics as total output, employment and price levels. See also **Microeconomics**.

Major Medical In order to compete with the Blue Cross service benefits, commercial insurance companies came up with plans with deductibles and coinsurance that could be sold for much less. Often today, major medical is used as a supplement, while some basic services, such as hospital and doctor visits, are covered in full.

Malpractice The legal framework for failure to meet professional standards.

Malthusian Hypothesis The expectation that any increase in food supply would eventually lead to a matching increase in the number of people living at a subsistence level, so that on average, living conditions would be no better off than before.

Managed Behavioral Health Mental health and substance abuse services managed by an MCO.

Managed Care The use of a manager to control utilization of medical services and control costs. Often associated with HMOs, other forms of managed care include peer review panels, pre-approval procedures for surgery, case management for the chronically ill, formularies limiting pharmacy reimbursement to an approved list, and other contractual provisions.

Managed Care Organization (MCO) An HMO, PPO, or other organization that accepts financial risk and manages care.

Managed Competition A policy of increased reliance on competing HMO's and a fixed limit to tax subsidies so that employees would bear the full marginal cost of their health benefit plans.

Mandated Benefits Specific services (e.g., pregnancy, alcoholism detoxification) for which a state requires all health plans to provide coverage.

Marginal Incremental; a one unit increase.

Marginal Propensity to Consume The fraction of an additional dollar that would be spent on consumption, and thus not invested as savings.

Marginal Productivity The incremental output obtained with one more unit of input.

Marginal Cost The increase in total costs caused by the production of one more unit of output.

Market Failure The inability of the market to arrive at a reasonably efficient equilibrium under certain conditions, notably the existence of public goods and externalities, lack of clear property rights, inability of some consumers to act in their own best interest, natural monopoly due to constantly declining average costs of production, and excessive transaction costs or information asymmetry.

Means Testing Setting a standard of low income in order to qualify for a government benefit, e.g., Medicaid.

Medicaid Combined state/federal program to insure people whose incomes are insufficient to pay for health care; primarily those on welfare or older people in nursing homes.

Medical Savings Account (MSA) A proposal to replace regular health insurance and HMOs by allowing people to place money in a tax-free savings account to be used for medical expenses, in conjunction with the purchase of a catastrophic stop-loss health insurance plan covering expenses in excess of $3,000.

Medicare A Federal government insurance program that provides hospital benefits (part A) and medical benefits (part B) to persons over age 65 and some qualified widows and disabled.

Medigap A policy designed to pay coinsurance, deductibles, drugs, and other expenses not fully covered by Medicare.

Microeconomics (from the Greek 'micro' meaning small) A field of economics that uses economic theory to study how individual consumers and firms make economic decisions.

Monopoly A market in which there is a single provider(seller).

Monopoly Rents Profits in excess of competitive market returns due to a monopolist's ability to unilaterally increase prices.

Monopsony A market characterised by a single buyer that has the ability to influence market price.

Moral Hazard Any change in individual behavior due to insurance which increases expected losses, such as the higher utilization of covered services.

Morbidity Illness or disability, especially when expressed as a rate (e.g.; sick days per year per 1,000 employees).

Mortality Death, usually expressed as a rate per one hundred, thousand, or hundred-thousand.

Need A professional determination of the quantity that should be supplied (as distinct from market demand).

Normative Shortage When too little is supplied according to professional opinion, although not necessarily according to market behavior (e.g., there is a shortage of raw vegetables in the diet of teenagers).

Occupancy Rate The percentage of a hospital's beds filled at a specific time.

Off-Label The use of prescription drugs for diseases other than those for which it has been approved by the FDA.

Opportunity Cost What must be given up in order to do or obtain something; the highest-valued alternative which must be foregone. For example, the opportunity cost of taking the final exam may be missing out on a trip to Bermuda.

Option Demand Willingness to pay for access to a good which may or may not be used, e.g., emergency services.

Osteopathy An alternative form of medical practice which emphasizes spinal adjustment as well as surgery and drugs in the treatment of disease. Originally quite distinct from mainstream allopathic medicine, osteopathy is now almost identical so that MDs and DOs usually practice together, although DOs are more likely to be generalists focusing on primary care.

Out-of-Pocket Payments made by individuals or their family, rather than an insurance company, HMO, government, or other third party, for medical care.

Outpatient Services provided in a physicians' office, clinic, or other ambulatory setting.

Over-the-Counter A drug that consumers can purchase without a prescription from a physician.

Patents A legal monopoly for a specified period of years given to a firm which makes a discovery.

Per Diem Per day payment for services.

Per Member Per Month (PMPM) The standard form of HMO payment, also known as **capitation.**

Permanent Income Expected long-run average income, as opposed to the transitory income which a person (or group) may have during the current month or year.

Pharmacoeconomics Cost-benefit analysis of drugs; assessment of the market for a drug.

Point of Service Plan (POS) An HMO which offers partial reimbursement for services which a patient chooses to obtain outside of the HMO network.

Population Medicine Analysis and assessment of health care on the basis of the community or group rather than the individual; design of a system with services targeted to those of greatest need; making trade-offs to optimize average health, rather than doing the best possible for one specific individual under treatment.

Practice Variation Differences in the number of medical services provided not explainable by any differences in the population served. Also known as small area variation.

Pre-authorization A requirement that the doctor or the patient obtain approval from the HMO before the service is provided.

Pre-existing Condition An insurance contract may specify that it will not pay for medical problems already diagnosed or under treatment before the policy is purchased, known as pre-existing conditions. A person with AIDS who bought a policy with such a clause would find that it paid for his broken leg, and maybe even to have his tooth drilled, but not for anything related to AIDS. Often the pre-existing condition exclusion will only apply to the first 6 months or year of coverage. This, and other exclusionary clauses, are a major way of reducing adverse selection when medical insurance is marketed to individuals.

Preferred Provider Organization (PPO) A health insurance plan which offers enrollees a discount for using hospitals and physicians within an approved network of contracted providers.

Premiums Payments made in advance to provide medical services or reimbursement in the future.

Price Discrimination Charging different people different prices for the same good.

Price Index A measure of the purchasing power of money, usually set arbitrarily equal to 100 at one specific point in time (or space). The average change in prices weighted by the expenditure on each item.

Primary Care The basic medical attention provided by a physician to a patient seeking care, as distinct from referral services obtained from specialists, or tertiary care provided in technologically sophisticated hospitals.

Property Rights The right to use, sell, or to derive income from a good.

Prospective Payment Payments set in advance, especially in contrast to retrospective **cost reimbursement.**

Provider Network The set of physicians, hospitals and others with which an MCO has signed a contract to provide care for enrollees.

Public Goods Goods that are consumed or financed collectively (e.g., clean air, national defense, discovery of penicillin) either because it is impossible to include/exclude any consumer who does not pay (see **free rider**), or because once produced, there is no additional cost for additional consumers.

QALYs (Quality Adjusted Life-Years) A way of measuring the value of a medical intervention by the increase in life expectancy, adjusted for difference in disability and timing.

Rationality The notion that consumers will never purposely make themselves worse off and have the ability to rank preferences and allocate income in a fashion that derives the maximum level of utility.

RBRVS The "resource-based relative value system" developed for Medicare to reimburse ambulatory services based on the estimated time, effort, skill, equipment, and other resources needed to provide each service.

RCCAC The "ratio of costs-to-charges applied to charges" methodology used to apportion cost reimbursements.

Redistribution Policies that have the effect of changing the pattern of consumption by different income classes; allowing the poor to consume a larger share of GDP.

Regulatory Balloon The observation that any regulation pushing costs down on one side is apt to exert pressure pushing costs up in some other direction.

Regulatory Capture The subtle takeover of a regulatory agency by the industry it was meant to regulate, so that it tends to represent the interests of the industry, rather than the public.

Reimbursement The process of paying for the costs incurred, especially through a third party.

Reinsurance Acceptance by a second insurer (the reinsurer) of all or part of the risk undertaken by the first insurer; usually used to cover very large losses and protect against bankruptcy. For example, a reinsurer may agree that if total losses exceed the $5 million in expected claims by more than $1 million, they will, for a price, pick up 90% of the extra losses.

Relative Value Scales A list of point scores for each service to be used in setting reimbursement.

Rents Profits in excess of those necessary in order to call forth the requisite supply of inputs in the market. Compensation above competitive amounts obtained by professionals who are able to control supply.

Retention Ratio Agreement A contract specifying an allowed ratio of premiums to medical expenses with some fraction of any excess underwriting gains to be returned to the firm or used to reduce premiums in the following year.

Retrospective Review Monitoring records after discharge and disallowing (refusing to pay for) any services that do not meet specified standards of medical necessity and timeliness.

Revolving Door Term used to describe staff that leave a regulatory agency to work within the industry which is supposed to be regulated, and vice-versa. Such changes in employment may compromise the agency's objectivity.

Risk The chance or probability that an event will occur.

Risk Adjustment The process of setting the capitation rate for an insurance policy based on the health status and expected medical costs of an individual or group purchasing the plan.

Risk Aversion The extent to which an individual is willing to pay to reduce variation in losses or income due to random events.

Risk Pooling Forming a group so that individual risks can be shared among many people.

Risk Selection Enrollment of healthier-than-average persons into an insured group.

Sanitary Revolution The 19th-century campaign to clean up the environment and change personal behavior to conform to Victorian notions: "cleanliness is next to godliness."

Scarcity Scarcity exists when the quantity of a good or service available is insufficient to satisfy demand at a zero price. An economic good is thus any good or service which is scarce relative to our wants for it.

Selection Bias A disproportionate share of above- or below-average persons in the group.

Self-Insurance A health plan funded and controlled by the firm itself, so that no risk is transferred to an insurance company, although benefits may be administered by an outside party. Self-insurance often enables a firm to avoid regulations governing purchased health insurance.

Service Benefits If the insurance company contracts directly with the doctor or hospital to provide the service rather than setting up some form of financial reimbursement, this is a service benefit. Blue Cross provides service benefits through its contracts with hospitals. An advantage of a service benefit to the insurance company is that they usually get a discount off the price that the patient would have to pay directly for the services rendered.

Shared-Income Hypothesis Income becomes more and more important as a determinant of health-care spending as the unit of observation increases in size from the individual to the nation.

Social Insurance Pooling funded through taxes for protection against risks provided by the government for all (or almost all) of the citizens in a society. Social Security in the United States and the National Health Service in England are examples of social insurance plans.

Spend-Down The process of spending or giving away assets by elderly persons so as to qualify for Medicaid reimbursement of long-term care expenses.

Stock The amount at a point in time (i.e., total assets, population).

Stop-Loss A limit on the maximum amount a person would ever have to pay is known as a stop-loss. If a family has a $1,000 stop-loss, then the insurance company will pay everything after the family's out-of-pocket expenses reach $1,000.

Sub-capitation Carving out a specialized service (physical therapy, mental health) and paying the specialized provider on a per-member per-month basis.

Subsistence Having barely enough food and other resources to sustain life.

Tertiary Care Medical care delivered in technologically sophisticated and university hospitals.

Third-Party Administrator An organization that processes claims for a self-insured firm, but bears no financial risk for losses.

Third-Party Transaction An exchange which is indirect and often pools the funds of many individuals with money collected and disbursed by a third party such as an insurance company, voluntary non-profit organization, or government agency.

Time-Series Analysis Statistics using multiple observations of an individual or group over time; statistical analysis of the dynamics of change.

Trade-off The idea that every individual will voluntarily sacrifice some of one good or service in change for a sufficient increase in the amount of some other.

Transaction Costs All costs, monetary and non-monetary, whether counted or not, of carrying on trade.

Triple-Option A complete array of plans consisting of an HMO, a PPO, and an indemnity plan, offered by an insurer as a package. The package as a whole is experience rated, so that any one option may be significantly over- or under-priced to create cross-subsidies between plans.

Two-Party Transaction An exchange between a buyer and seller, usually trading money for goods or services.

Underwriting Gains (Losses) The amount by which premiums received exceed (fall short of) benefits paid out.

Universal Health Insurance A national plan providing health insurance or services to all citizens, or to all residents.

Usual, Customary, and Reasonable (UCR) A method for setting the maximum allowed fee for each service based on usual charges by other physicians in the area, the customary charge by this particular doctor over the preceding year, and "reasonable" adjustments for severity or special conditions.

Utilization The number of services used, often expressed per 1,000 persons per month or year.

Utilization Review (UR) Monitoring of medical records to determine if services are appropriate and should be paid for.

Variability The extent of random changes over time or between persons.

Voluntary Organization A nonprofit organization, such as a hospital or social service agency, governed by a board of concerned citizens rather than owners or elected officials.

Welfare Loss The decline in social welfare (total value of consumption/production) due to monopoly supply restrictions, price controls, rationing, taxes, or other interventions that cause misallocation of resources. Also known as deadweight losses.

Welfare Triangle The reduction in consumer's surplus caused by a reduction in quantity sold due to monopoly supply restrictions, price controls, or other distortion.

Willingness to Pay (WTP) How much a person is willing to give up in order to obtain some specified improvement in quality of life.

Withhold A pool of money for providers which is held back and distributed by the HMO only if total expenses for the year end up being at or below acceptable levels.

Workers Compensation A mandatory insurance program covering the costs of medical treatment and disability due to work-related accidents and illness.

Wrap-Around An insurance policy designed to create a more comprehensive set of coverages sold with an underlying base policy.

INDEX